Comprehensive Care of Schizophrenia

We dedicate this book to our patients whose courageous ways of coping with their illness have taught us so much. We hope that it may help to ensure that more people suffering a psychotic experience receive the good care that they deserve.

Comprehensive Care of Schizophrenia

A Textbook of Clinical Management

Edited by

Jeffrey A Lieberman MD
Thad and Alice Eure Distinguished Professor of Psychiatry,
Pharmacology and Radiology
University of North Carolina School of Medicine
Chapel Hill, North Carolina
USA

Robin M Murray FRCPsych
Professor of Psychiatry
Institute of Psychiatry
London
UK

MARTIN DUNITZ

© Martin Dunitz Ltd 2001, a member of the Taylor & Francis group.

First published in the United Kingdom in 2001.
Paperback edition published in the UK in 2002 by
Martin Dunitz Ltd
The Livery House
7–9 Pratt Street
London NW1 0AE

Reprinted 2004

Tel: +44-(0)20-7482-2202
Fax: +44-(0)20-7267-0159
E-mail: info@dunitz.co.uk
Website: http://www.dunitz.co.uk

A CIP catalogue record for this book is available from the British Library

ISBN 1-84184-150-1

Distributed in the USA by
Fulfilment Center
Taylor & Francis
7625 Empire Drive
Florence, KY 41042, USA
Toll Free Tel: 1-800-634-7064
Email cserve@routledge_nv.com

Distributed in Canada by
Taylor & Francis
74 Rolark Drive
Scarborough
Ontario M1R 4G2, Canada
Toll Free Tel: 1-877-226-2237
Email: tal_fran@istar.ca

Distributed in the rest of the world by
ITPS Limited
Cheriton House
North Way, Andover
Hampshire SP10 5BE, UK
Tel: +44 (0)1264 332424
Email: reception@itps.co.uk

Composition by Wearset, Boldon, Tyne and Wear.
Printed and bound in Italy by Printer Trento.

Contents

Contributors

Katherine J Aitchison MA MRCPsych
Honorary Lecturer
Section of Clinical Pharmacology
Institute of Psychiatry
London
UK

Alan S Bellack PhD ABPP
Director, VA Capitol Network MIRECC and
Professor of Psychiatry
University of Maryland School of Medicine
Baltimore, Maryland
USA

Anthony S David FRCP FRCPsych MD
Professor of Cognitive Neuropsychiatry
GKT School of Medicine and
The Institute of Psychiatry
London
UK

Ruth A Dickson MD FRCPC
Associate Professor
Department of Psychiatry
University of Calgary
Calgary, Alberta
Canada

Lisa Dixon MD MPH
Associate Professor and
Director of Education
Department of Psychiatry
University of Maryland School of Medicine
Baltimore, Maryland
USA

Robert E Drake MD PhD
Professor of Psychiatry
Dartmouth Medical School
Hanover, New Hampshire
USA

Ceri L Evans MBChB MA MRCPsych
Lecturer and Honorary Specialist Registrar in
Forensic Psychiatry
St George's Hospital Medical School
University of London
London
UK

David Fowler BSc MSc
Senior Lecturer in Clinical Psychology
University of East Anglia
Norwich
UK

Wolfgang Fleischhacker MD
Department of Biological Psychiatry
University of Innsbruck
Innsbruck
Austria

Philippa Garety MA MPhil PhD
Professor of Clinical Psychology
Guy's, King's and St Thomas' School of Medicine
London
UK

William M Glazer MD
Associate Clinical Professor of Psychiatry
Massachusetts General Hospital
Harvard Medical School
Menemsha, Massachusetts
USA

John K Hsaio MD
Chief, Special Projects Program
Adult and Geriatrics and Preventive Intervention
Research Branch
Division of Services and Interventions Research
National Institute of Mental Health
Bethesda, Maryland
USA

Janet Kazmer MSW
Department of Psychiatry
University of North Carolina School of Medicine
Chapel Hill, North Carolina
USA

Jane Kelly MRCPsych
Clinical Researcher
Department of Psychiatry
Institute of Psychiatry
London
UK

Roisin A Kemp FRANZCP MD
Senior Lecturer
Department of Psychiatry and Behavioural
Sciences
Royal Free Hospital and
University College Medical School
Royal Free Campus
London
UK

A Elif Kostakoglu
Department of Psychiatry
Vanderbilt University School of Medicine
Nashville, Tennesse
USA

Elizabeth Kuipers BSc MSc PhD
Professor of Clinical Psychology
Institute of Psychiatry
London
UK

Julian Leff BSc MD FRCPsych MRCP MFPHM
Professor of Social and Cultural Psychiatry
Institute of Psychiatry
London
UK

Marge Lenane LCSW-C
Senior Research Social Worker
National Institute of Mental Health
National Institutes of Health
Bethesda, Maryland
USA

Douglas Leslie PhD
Economist
VA Northeast Program Evaluation Center and
Assistant Professor of Psychiatry
Yale Medical School
West Haven, Connecticut
USA

Jeffrey A Lieberman MD
Thad and Alice Eure Distinguished
Professor of Psychiatry, Pharmacology and
Radiology
University of North Carolina School of Medicine
Chapel Hill, North Carolina
USA

Patrick D McGorry MB BS PhD MRCP(UK) FRANZCP
Professor and Director
Department of Psychiatry
Youth Program MH SKY
Parkville, Victoria
Australia

Peter J McKenna
Consultant Psychiatrist
Fulbourn Hospital
Addenbrooke's NHS Trust
Cambridge
UK

Herbert Y Meltzer MD
Professor of Psychiatry and Pharmacology
Department of Psychiatry
Vanderbilt University School of Medicine
Nashville, Tennesse
USA

Maria M Morgan MRCPsych
Stanley Foundation Research Fellow
Stanley Foundation Research Unit
St Davnet's Hospital
Monaghan
Ireland

Joseph P Morrissey PhD
Professor of Social Medicine and Psychiatry
Cecil G Sheps Center for Health Services
Research
University of North Carolina
Chapel Hill, North Carolina
USA

Kim T Mueser PhD
Professor of Psychiatry
Dartmouth Medical School
Hanover, New Hampshire
USA

Povl Munk-Jørgensen MD DrMedsc
Associate Professor
Research Director
Aarhus University Hospital
Aarhus
Denmark

Robin M Murray FRCPsych
Professor of Psychiatry
Institute of Psychiatry
London
UK

Jennifer Nieri MSW
Department of Psychiatry
University of North Carolina Medical School
Chapel Hill, North Carolina
USA

Jim van Os MRCPsych
Associate Professor
University of Maastricht
Maastricht
The Netherlands

Diana O Perkins MD MPH
Associate Professor of Psychiatry
University of North Carolina School of Medicine
Chapel Hill, North Carolina
USA

Lyn S Pilowsky MRCPsych PhD
Reader in Neurochemical Imaging
Honorary Consultant Psychiatrist
South London and Maudsley NHS Trust
London
UK

Judith L Rapoport MD
Branch Chief
National Institute of Mental Health
National Institutes of Health
Bethesda, Maryland
USA

Robert Rosenheck MD
Director, VA Northeast Program Evaluation
Center and
Professor of Psychiatry and Public Health
Yale School of Medicine
West Haven, Connecticut
USA

Chiara Samele PhD
Division of Psychological Medicine
Institute of Psychiatry
London
UK

Sukhwinder S Shergill BSc MBBS MRCPsych
Welcome Clinical Fellow/Lecturer
Division of Psychological Medicine
Institute of Psychiatry
London
UK

Susan L Siegfried MD
Department of Psychiatry
University of North Carolina School of Medicine
Chapel Hill, North Carolina
USA

T Scott Stroup MD MPH
Assistant Professor
Department of Psychiatry
University of North Carolina School of Medicine
Chapel Hill, North Carolina
USA

Donald Thompson MD
Assistant Professor and
Director of Medical Student Education
University of Maryland School of Medicine
Baltimore, Maryland
USA

Jan Volavka MD PhD
Professor of Psychiatry
New York University
Chief, Clinical Research Division
Nathan Kline Institute for Psychiatric Research
Orangeburg, New York
USA

John L Waddington PhD DSc
Professor of Neuroscience
Department of Clinical Pharmacology
Royal College of Surgeons in Ireland
Dublin
Republic of Ireland

Karen Wohlheiter MS
Senior Research Assistant
Center for Mental Health Services Research
Department of Psychiatry
University of Maryland School of Medicine
Baltimore, Maryland
USA

Marianne Wudarsky MD PhD
Senior Research Fellow
National Institute of Mental Health
National Institutes of Health
Bethesda, Maryland
USA

Richard Jed Wyatt MD
Chief, Neuropsychiatry Branch
National Institute of Mental Health
National Institutes of Health
Bethesda, Maryland
USA

Foreword

Despite its low incidence schizophrenia remains a problem of major public health importance because of its long duration and the severe consequences that it has for the individuals concerned, for their families and for their communities. Nearly half of the beds in mental hospitals in Europe are occupied by people whose primary diagnosis is schizophrenia and a large proportion of people disabled because of mental illness have the diagnosis. The World Health Organization's studies predict that schizophrenia will remain among the ten main causes of disability well into the twenty-first century. Suicide in people with schizophrenia is frequent and the stigma attached to the disease and everything related to it – for example, the hospitals in which people with schizophrenia are treated, the patients' families across generations, the medicaments used for the treatment of the condition – is overwhelming. Schizophrenia does not seem to know boundaries – the syndrome that characterizes it has been seen and well described in vastly varying settings and cultures. Until recently treatments used to deal with schizophrenia were barely satisfactory – their effectiveness was relatively low and the side-effects of treatment could be profoundly disturbing.

It is therefore a pleasure to welcome an excellent contribution to the literature about schizophrenia and its treatment. The editors, themselves highly respected and distinguished scholars and leaders in this and other fields of psychiatry, managed to mobilize a pleiad of experts each with a magisterial grasp of the issues arising in making the diagnosis, treating the disorder and living with it. The comprehensiveness of the volume is only one of its many assets: among others is the inclusion – into a textbook of psychiatry – of a chapter providing first person accounts of the disease, a review of the systems of care for people with schizophrenia in different countries and of the influence of culture on schizophrenia, all this solidly supported by a systematic review of most of the currently used treatment methods for the condition.

The material assembled in this volume is not only a textbook for those learning or teaching about schizophrenia: it is also a highly interesting account of the current knowledge about schizophrenia and can therefore be very useful for researchers in any of the related fields who sometimes find it difficult to keep up with the developments of science in fields related to but distant from their own area of preoccupation.

Norman Sartorius
Geneva, Switzerland

Foreword

It is a pleasure to contribute a foreword to this fine book. Jeffrey Lieberman and Robin Murray are among the best-known experts on schizophrenia in the United States and England, respectively. Their approach to treatment is truly comprehensive, beginning with pharmacological approaches and proceedings to psychological (cognitive behavioral) approaches and rehabilitation. Special treatment problems receive individual attention, including patients who are suicidal, violent, substance abusers, or treatment-resistant. Patient compliance with treatment, a critical but oft-neglected subject in such books, is also allotted a chapter of its own, and the importance of listening to the patients and their families is emphasized in the chapter 'Clinician interactions with patients and families'.

At the same time as books such as this outline what 'comprehensive care' should be for individuals with schizophrenia, they simultaneously highlight the gulf between what should be and what actually is. Through the work of Lieberman, Murray, and many other contributors to this volume, we know what constitutes good care for schizophrenia. However, the National Institute for Mental Health Epidemiologic Catchment Area (ECA) survey reported that 40% of all individuals with schizophrenia receive no care whatsoever in any given year. Indeed, a community survey in inner-city Baltimore found the schizophrenia nontreatment rate to be 50%. Comprehensive care for many, therefore, is an illusory concept. *Any* care at all would be an improvement.

Individuals with schizophrenia who are not receiving care are one of the great tragedies of modern medicine and social services. They constitute approximately one-third of the homeless population both in the United States and in Europe. They also constitute an increasing percentage of individuals in jails and prisons. Many are defenceless because of their illness and are victimized – robbed, raped, even murdered – with increasing frequency. Because of their delusions, thinking disorder, and other symptoms of their illness, a small percentage of these untreated individuals may act violently toward others; in the United States, it is estimated that they are responsible for approximately 1000 homicides each year.

There is probably no other disease in the Western world where the gulf between good care and what actually happens is as great as it is in schizophrenia. On human grounds alone, it is incomprehensible that we fail to treat these sick individuals who so badly need it. And on economic grounds, our failure to treat is also costly in terms of unnecessary rehospitalizations, social services costs, incarceration costs, etc. Thus, our failure to treat is not only inhumane and incomprehensible, it is also simply foolish.

The good news is that schizophrenia is a disease whose time has come. Patients, their families, and the general public are reaching the point where they will no longer tolerate the failures of the psychiatric care system. They will demand, and eventually receive, not merely care for this disease, but comprehensive care. Jeffrey Lieberman, Robin Murray, and their colleagues are pointing the way toward the future.

E Fuller Torrey
Bethesda, Maryland, USA

Preface

Bridging the gap between the optimum treatment for schizophrenia and the treatment most patients receive

People with schizophrenia should have the same right to high standards of treatment, and as good a quality of life, as people with other chronic recurrent illnesses like asthma, hypertension or diabetes. Sadly, they do not often receive the former or achieve the latter. Historically, schizophrenia has had a low priority in most health care systems around the world; consequently, the treatment facilities are often inadequate, the staff sometimes poorly trained, and the care offered far from the best. We have seen far too many people whose life has been blighted for such reasons to be contented with our profession and its practice.

This is all the more unfortunate since the potential for comprehensive and effective care of people with psychosis has improved greatly within our professional lifetimes. In particular, a wide range of evidence-based pharmacological and psychosocial treatments are now available which can be tailored to the exact needs of patients rather than prescribed or withheld on the basis of the belief system of the treating clinician. When we trained in psychiatry the prospects for such scientifically derived clinical care were limited indeed. In the United States in the 1970s treatment for most psychiatric disorders including psychosis was dominated by psychoanalytic theories. On the other hand, at the Maudsley Hospital in London, there was considerable scepticism about the effects of antipsychotic drugs and lithium was considered of little value. Thus, one of us was trained in a therapy for which there was very little evidence while the second learned more about the inadequacies of drugs rather than how best to prescribe them.

These old ideologies were slow to give way to modern methods, but now more time has elapsed since we started psychiatry than we care to remember, and much progress has been made. The remarkable advances in neuroscience, pharmacology, genetics and medical imaging have provided a solid basis on which to understand schizophrenia, and epidemiology and social science have taught us much about the factors which contribute to the onset of schizophrenia and to its clinical course. Most importantly, new treatments have become available. Now, there exists a host of antipsychotic and other psychotropic medications, each with their own advantages and side effects. In addition, more effective psychological treatments have been introduced, and the development of health services research has meant that innovative systems of care delivery can be tested as thoroughly as new drugs.

Despite this, there remains a yawning gap between the treatments that are optimum for the care of people with psychosis and the treatments which most patients receive. Far too often the prevailing dynamic in the care of the severely mentally ill is 'to leave well enough alone' rather than try to find the best treatments and continually seek further improvement in patients' conditions. Clinicians, carers, and consumers have settled for too little and the standards of care have been set too low. This is reflected in academic psychiatry by the fact that there are many more and better books describing research into the neurobiological basis of schizophrenia than its treatment. Although there are many books on schizophrenia, we could find none that provided, in a single volume, all that one would need to know in order to treat people with schizophrenia

at all stages of the illness and all clinical circumstances.

Therefore, it is our hope that this book will help to bridge the gap between the potential and actual quality of care that patients receive. To do this we have brought together a distinguished and varied group of contributors. These authorities, who come from both sides of the Atlantic, and occasionally elsewhere, are those who we believe are those most qualified to describe best practices as they are researchers, practitioners and consumers of mental health care for schizophrenia. It is our fervent wish that our collective efforts will serve the best interests and well being of those persons with schizophrenia and their caregivers.

Jeffrey A Lieberman MD
Chapel Hill, North Carolina, USA

Robin M Murray MD
London, UK

1

Diagnosing Schizophrenia

Richard Jed Wyatt

Contents • Definitions • Historical perspective • Patient evaluation • Conclusion • Acknowledgement

. . . it is irrational to attempt a discussion of schizophrenic illnesses if the meaning of the term schizophrenia is not at all explicit.

HS Sullivan, 1928[1]

After suffering for many years with a chronic psychiatric disorder, many patients display an unfortunate trait in common: deterioration. But the 'burnt-out' patient, once seen so frequently, is becoming rare. Surely the treatment advances that have occurred over the last 45 years are responsible for this improvement. And, as those treatments have become more specific, the value of precise diagnosis has become increasingly important. For example, correctly diagnosing an affective disorder determines whether it is more prudent to treat the patient with an antidepressant or a mood stabilizer, and neither class of medications is primary to the treatment of schizophrenia. In this chapter, we explore the history of schizophrenia as it has been shaped by concepts of diagnosis, and then look at the criteria currently used to diagnose schizophrenia. Before doing so, we examine a number of terms widely employed in medicine and psychiatry when discussing diagnosis. These terms are sometimes used interchangeably and with considerable confusion: symptoms, signs, syndrome, illness, disorder, disease, and diagnosis.

Definitions

Symptoms are experienced by the patient. *Signs* are what is observed, either during an examination or from laboratory tests. When a patient cannot describe his or her symptoms, they often can be inferred through signs (for example, a red, warm, swollen knee strongly suggests that the individual is experiencing the symptom of pain). Schizophrenia often presents a special problem in the assessment of symptoms and signs, because patients may not be able to describe their symptoms, and subtle signs may have to be interpreted indirectly. For example, we might infer that a patient is hallucinating because he quickly loses the focus of conversations, stares into space, or acts as if he were under the influence of a hallucination. Similarly, if a patient does not directly discuss her delusions, we must try to infer that she is having them from her behaviour.

A *syndrome* is an identifiable pattern of signs and symptoms. A syndrome can be made up of several disorders (discussed below). However, because a syndrome is a cross-sectional pattern, it does not necessarily have implications for course. The term 'syndrome' has often been used when referring to schizophrenia. For example, Leopold Bellak entitled his 10-year update reviews of schizophrenia *Schizophrenia: A Review of the Syndrome*

(1948), *The Schizophrenia Syndrome* (1968), and *Disorders of the Schizophrenia Syndrome* (1979).[2–4] By doing so, Bellak emphasized his view that schizophrenia is potentially made up of multiple disorders, a point also emphasized by Eugen Bleuler when he entitled his text *Dementia Praecox or the Group of Schizophrenias* (1950).[5]

The terms *illness* and *disorder* are often used synonymously, but illness is reserved to indicate the clinical manifestations, or what a patient experiences (symptoms). Illness does not include subclinical aspects of a disorder, which, when observed by others, are considered signs. For example, subtle motor abnormalities that appear to occur transiently years before individuals develop symptoms of schizophrenia would not be considered part of the illness, because the individual is usually not aware of them. They would, however, be considered part of the disorder or disease of schizophrenia.

The term *disorder* does imply something about course, but usually not about cause. Just as a syndrome (defined above) can be made up of several disorders, a disorder may be made up of several syndromes. Schizophrenia, for example, is thought to be made up of at least several syndromes or types (for example, paranoid and catatonic). *The Diagnostic and Statistical Manual of Mental Disorders*, fourth edition (DSM-IV)[6] and before that DSM-III and DSM-IIIR[7,8] defined a mental disorder as 'a clinically significant behavioral or psychological syndrome or pattern that occurs in an individual and that is associated with present distress (e.g., a painful symptom) or disability (i.e., impairment in one or more important areas of functioning) or with a significantly increased risk of suffering death, pain, disability or an important loss of freedom' (p. xxi). By using the term 'disorder' in the title of the manual, in addition to appending it to most diagnoses (e.g., schizophrenia disorder, bipolar disorder), DSM emphasizes that psychiatry deals with disorders. Similarly, the *Manual of the International Statistics Classification of Diseases, Injuries and Causes of Death* (ICD-10)[9] is quite explicit in

stating that schizophrenia is a disorder, not a disease. ICD-10 makes this point despite the fact that the term 'disease' is part of the title of that manual. Historically, the reason for this anomaly may be that the ICD system was originally a classification of causes of death. Nevertheless, the term disorder is less specific than disease.

A *disease* implies that there is something that can be observed physically; that there is something structurally, biochemically, or physiologically abnormal about the body or a part of the body. A disease is a distinct entity with a specific etiology, even though that etiology may be unknown. Over the last 150 years, the concept of disease has been greatly influenced by postmortem, biopsy, laboratory, and radiographic studies, as well as the finding of specific biochemical and genetic defects. How distinct an entity must be, however, to be considered a disease is rarely articulated. For example, does phenylketonuria qualify as a disease when several genetic defects are known to produce pathological elevations of phenylalanine? In practice, an exquisite level of specificity does not appear to be required. For instance, the term 'heart disease' points to that organ as a source of dysfunction, but does not tell us what is wrong with the heart. Another aspect to the term 'disease' is that, at times, it implies a progression (see discussions in Spitzer and Endicott 1978; Klein 1978; and McHugh and Slavney 1986).[10–12]

The terms described above are integral to the study of medicine. In particular, the terms *disease* and *disorder* focus attention on conditions that are neither simply extremes of normality, nor part of a normal life process. A person 7 feet tall, for example, does not have a disease, although his height is an extreme extension of normality. In contrast, if his height is caused by a pituitary tumor, height would be considered part of the syndrome, and through the identification of other signs and symptoms, a disorder or disease could be diagnosed.

One aspect of disease that is missing in modern psychiatry is consideration of the brain's reaction to insult, a noteworthy contribution of nineteenth century medicine. It is, after all, the body's reaction (defense) against many microorganisms that produces the symptoms of infectious diseases. But considering a biological reaction to whatever insult produces schizophrenia was traditionally absent in most thinking about schizophrenia. As discussed below, however, it may be the brain's reaction to insult that could account for what Bleuler termed 'accessory symptoms', and for what is being discussed when we consider positive and negative symptoms.

The idea that schizophrenia and other psychiatric problems are deviations from normality rather than diseases or disorders has at times been very popular in psychology and psychiatry. Espousing the idea that 'everyone is a little mad' suggests that being really crazy is merely an extension of normality; thus, there is no stigma attached to it. Thinking of schizophrenia as a disease, however, asks that we acknowledge a qualitative difference between being a little mad and being psychotic. Because we do not know what the 'pathobiologic' abnormality is in schizophrenia, the organizers of DSM-IV and ICD-10 may have been wise to use the term 'disorder' rather than 'disease' when referring to it. On the other hand, there is probably sufficient evidence of an abnormality within the brains of individuals with schizophrenia to suggest that the organizers may have been overcautious. Furthermore, although this caution may be scientifically wise, it has also been costly. If schizophrenia is not called or considered a disease, it is not given parity with other diseases in terms of access to treatment.

Finally, a *diagnosis* is a construct with important implications for communication, classification, prognosis, and treatment. It places an individual case in a specific class through careful consideration of a patient's and the patient's family's history, findings from physical examinations, and the results of laboratory and other diagnostic tests. Schizophrenia is somewhat of an oddity, phenomenologically, because it is largely a diagnosis of exclusion. Although laboratory studies can help differentiate other disorders, there are not, as yet, supportive laboratory tests for the diagnosis of schizophrenia. Furthermore, because the tools of a psychiatrist are more limited than in other medicinal specialities, longitudinal information that satisfies criteria is usually required to make a diagnosis.

Reliability and *validity* are two terms used in conjunction with diagnosis. Reliability is how closely correlated one diagnosis of a patient is with another diagnosis of that patient under the same circumstances and when the state of the patient remains constrained. Beginning with DSM-III in 1980, most psychiatric disorders achieved a high degree of reliability through the use of well-defined criteria for psychiatric diagnostic categories and the employment of teaching techniques such as videotaped interviews of subjects, and as a result of dropping etiological speculation.

The validity of a diagnosis refers to how closely associated the diagnosis is with the disorder. There cannot be validity in a diagnosis without reliability, but reliability does not ensure validity (for example, if six people identify tulips as roses, the reliability will be high, but the tulips will not have become roses). Although we still do not know the cause of schizophrenia (other than being able to say that some part of it is genetic and that the brain is affected), and we thus cannot tie our diagnosis of schizophrenia to a pathophysiologic expression of the disease, we have been able to achieve predictive or criterion validity. This means that when we diagnose schizophrenia, it tells us what the individual's response to treatment is likely to be and what course the illness is likely to take.

Historical perspective

Although a number of conditions resembling modern conceptions of schizophrenia exist throughout recorded history, schizophrenia does not appear to have been widely discussed in Western medical literature until the beginning of the nineteenth century. A number of clinicians in the nineteenth and early twentieth centuries – Philippe Pinel, Emil Kraepelin, and Eugen Bleuler among them – carefully studied this disease and influenced the way modern medicine thinks about and diagnoses schizophrenia. In 1801, Pinel emphasized 'the rapid ... uninterrupted alternation of isolated ideas and of trifling and unsuitable emotions, disordered movements, and continued and extravagant acts'. He went on to discuss the 'obliteration of judgement, and a kind of automatic existence' (p. 222).[13] But of the nineteenth century writers, John Haslam presented the clearest picture of schizophrenia. According to Haslam, what we now call schizophrenia had an onset at puberty with a progressive deterioration: 'The attack is almost imperceptible; some months usually elapse, before it becomes the subject of particular notice; and fond relatives are frequently deceived by the hope that it is only an abatement of excessive vivacity, conducing to a prudent reserve, and steadiness of character.' Haslam noted that patients neglect those things that had previously held their attention, their affect becomes blunted and if they read, they cannot account for what they read. As their apathy increases, they neglect their attire and personal cleanliness. Thus in the interval between puberty and manhood, he wrote, '[there] is this hopeless and degrading change' (pp. 222–3).[13]

In 1896, in the sixth and in subsequent editions of his textbook of psychiatry, Emil Kraepelin described in great detail the symptoms and course of the disease he called dementia praecox, literally, dementia of early life.[14] This term had previously been used to describe similar symptoms, but Kraepelin did much to consolidate a number of previously diverse symptom complexes or syndromes (notably hebephrenia, catatonia, and paranoia) into dementia praecox. He noted that early in the illness, external impressions were usually correctly perceived. Patients were able to recognize their environment and generally remained oriented to time, place, and person. Of

course, during times of excitement such as the acute state, a certain amount of disorientation occurred. Hallucinations and delusions further affected how the patient perceived his environment. In time, the hallucinations, or at least the fear that they sometimes generate, diminished. Kraepelin observed that even though certain patients might have varied symptoms on admission, if the onset was in early adult life, many of the patients progressed to a deteriorated state. It was also Kraepelin who used outcome (generally poor and unremitting) to differentiate dementia praecox from manic-depressive disorder.

In 1911, Eugen Bleuler introduced the term 'schizophrenia', believing that it more accurately reflected the syndrome than Kraepelin's term, dementia praecox. With its emphasis on splitting (schizo) of the mind (phrenia), it is a term that has often been misunderstood. Bleuler intended to emphasize that 'definite splitting ... in the sense that various personality fragments exist side by side in a state of clear orientation as to environment' is only found in schizophrenia (pp. 298–9). Ideas might be partially worked out with fragments of ideas connected in illogical ways to constitute new ideas. In essence the individual with schizophrenia lacked the whole of the healthy individual. Schizophrenia is not, however, a split personality, a concept that implies two or more relatively *whole* selves within one individual.

Bleuler described schizophrenia as a group of disorders characterized by hallucinations, delusions, and thought disorganization in individuals who were young, and previously and otherwise healthy.[5] Bleuler wrote that: 'By the term dementia praecox or schizophrenia we designate a group of psychoses whose course is at times chronic, at times marked by intermittent attacks, and which can stop or retrograde at any stage, but does not permit a full *restituto ad integrum*' (pp. 9, 255). Bleuler did not accept the term 'dementia', because – like Kraepelin – he noted that many patients did not go on to complete deterioration. And, in some cases, when deterioration did take place, it did not do so precociously, but only later in life. For this reason, Bleuler de-emphasized outcome.

Bleuler also introduced the concept of four primary symptoms of schizophrenia (known as Bleuler's four As). These were: *Association* disturbance; *Ambivalence* (contradictory ideas, wishes, and impulses); *Affective* disturbance (flat or incongruous affect); and *Autism* (living in fantasy and withdrawal from reality). These distortions of normal processes could be seen at any point during the illness. He felt that, because they were present intermittently, the accessory symptoms – hallucinations, delusions, disorder of person, disorders of speech and writing, somatic symptoms, and catatonic symptoms – developed out of the primary symptoms.

Furthermore, Bleuler added a fourth subtype of schizophrenia to the three previously described by Kraepelin: simple schizophrenia. Simple schizophrenia was not associated with delusions and hallucinations or thought disorder, and these symptoms were not necessary to diagnose it. Bleuler quotes Clouston: 'The patients simply become affectively and intellectually weaker; the will seems to lose its power; the capacity for work, for caring for themselves diminishes. They appear stupid and finally show the picture of severe dementia' (p. 235).

Like Bleuler, Kurt Schneider, working in the middle part of the twentieth century, stressed the importance of specific symptoms, which he called first-rank symptoms, and which he considered characteristic and diagnostic, but not basic to the disorder.[15] There are eleven first-rank symptoms, including voices speaking one's thoughts aloud, thought insertion, and feelings and actions being imposed by an external force. A number of subsequent studies,[16] however, have demonstrated that Schneider's first-rank symptoms occur with other psychotic disorders and their presence is thus not diagnostic of schizophrenia.

As the twentieth century progressed, a number of new ideas about schizophrenia emerged. Many of these are covered elsewhere in this book, but a few are crucial to how we diagnose this illness,

including the formalizing of related diagnoses such as schizophreniform, schizoaffective, and the concept of schizophrenia spectrum disorders. For instance, the term *schizophreniform disorder* was introduced by Gabriel Langfeldt in 1939 to differentiate patients having a schizophrenia-like psychosis, but generally good outcome.[17] Patients with schizophreniform psychosis did not have emotional blunting, a chronic course, or an insidious onset. Because the vast majority of patients who at one time meet the criteria for schizophreniform disorder will, with time, go on to meet the criteria for schizophrenia, schizoaffective disorder, or another psychotic disorder,[18] schizophreniform disorder is a temporary diagnosis for many patients. Nevertheless, there is a small group of patients who will not go on to develop a more chronic psychotic disorder, and for whom schizophreniform disorder is accurately descriptive.

In 1933, *schizoaffective disorder* was formalized as a term for a psychosis having the mixed features of schizophrenia and affective disorders.[19] The definition of schizoaffective disorder has changed from time to time since its introduction, but generally encompasses the concept of symptoms of a mood disorder coexisting with symptoms of schizophrenia. As noted below, it is defined slightly differently by the two major diagnostic classification systems (DSM-IV and ICD-10).

In addition, adoption studies[20] have suggested that there is a genetically based spectrum for schizophrenia – or certain psychiatric conditions that may be genetically related to schizophrenia – referred to as *schizophrenia spectrum disorders (SSD)*. The spectrum, which reaches from the psychotic to nonpsychotic disorders, includes schizophrenia, schizotypal personality disorder, schizoaffective disorder schizophrenic type, and paranoid personality disorder.

Although much of Europe held close to the Kraepelinian notion of schizophrenia, in the United States the ideas of Bleuler became predominant. By the early 1970s, it had become obvious that in the United States and some other parts of the world, little reliability existed in the diagnosis of schizophrenia. Concerns about the absence of criteria for diagnosing schizophrenia led to a series of influential studies. In the United States–United Kingdom Study,[21] the relative rates of schizophrenia and mood disorders were found to be vastly different in New York and London. But a few years later, when standardized criteria were used,[22] the relative rates of mood disorders and schizophrenia across the Atlantic were found to be almost identical. Meanwhile, the operationalized Washington University Criteria[23] were developed and gradually incorporated into the DSM by the American Psychiatric Association. Specifically, these criteria required that symptoms of schizophrenia had to be present for at least 6 months in order for a diagnosis to be made. By excluding patients who had not been symptomatic for 6 months, the criteria helped redefine schizophrenia as a chronic disorder, with relatively few individuals having full recoveries.

In the United States, the first two editions of DSM did not provide specific criteria for diagnosing schizophrenia. But, since 1980, when the third edition was published, using diagnostic criteria has become part of psychiatric practice. DSM-III and its progression to DSM-IV (1994), and the parallel ICD-10 system, have largely been adopted worldwide (even if not fully accepted). According to these texts, schizophrenia does not exist without the patient at some point having delusions or hallucinations or a thought disorder (in contrast to the simple form of schizophrenia defined by Bleuler). Also, from DSM-III on, no inferences have been made about the etiology of schizophrenia except by exclusion (what schizophrenia is not). In the United States, this was a substantial departure from the prevailing themes of postwar dynamic psychiatry, which had usually attempted to describe, name, and group disorders or advance a hypothesis (usually stated as theories) to explain and/or heal them. Furthermore, use of the multiaxial system in DSM attempts to accommodate the diverse aspects of a patient's life, including aspects such as a patient's ability to function.

As we became able safely to study the living brain with imaging techniques, it became possible to make correlations between abnormalities in brain structure and *categories* and *dimensions* of symptoms. Categories divide patients into mutually exclusive groups. This is found in Crow's (1980) distinction between types I and II schizophrenia, where type I schizophrenia was characterized by positive symptoms and an increased number of dopamine type 2 receptors, and type II schizophrenia was characterized by negative symptoms, enlarged ventricles, and a diminished cerebral cortex.[24] Positive symptoms include hallucinations and delusions, and negative symptoms include affective flattening, poverty of speech, avolition, and anergia. In some studies, a third set of symptoms – disorganized – has been posited, although these are sometimes considered to be a subtype of positive symptoms. These include disorganized speech (derailment, incoherence, and blocking) and bizarre behavior.

On the other hand, dimensions are based on statistical procedures such as factor analysis, and are not mutually exclusive; one type of disease might have a stronger correlation to a dimension than another.[25] For example, a patient with paranoid schizophrenia might have some thought disorder, but it would not be a prominent feature of that patient's illness. Thus, studying these issues through imaging techniques[26] brought about a renewed interest in positive and negative symptoms, and this interest has had an indirect impact on diagnosis; for instance, the recognition of negative symptoms has been incorporated into DSM-IV. Despite beginning to recognize the importance of negative symptoms and related syndromes such as schizophrenia spectrum disorders, today the diagnosis of schizophrenia is made on the basis of there being or having been positive symptoms.

In terms of recent diagnostic changes for schizophrenia, the major difference between DSM-IV and DSM-III is the current grouping of schizoaffective disorder with the schizophrenic disorders. In 1933, Bleuler noted that schizophrenic symptoms were of pathognomonic importance, but affective symptoms were not. Thus, according to Bleuler, affective symptoms were not considered important for diagnosis despite their common presence in patients. In a sense, the inclusion of schizoaffective disorder with the schizophrenic disorders is a return to the notions of Bleuler.

Patient evaluation

The initial evaluation
The first few times a patient is seen are probably the most important. During these early contacts, the contributions of substance abuse, as well as other psychiatric and medical conditions that may mimic schizophrenia, are evaluated and, when present, treated. Table 1.1 is a nonexclusive list of some of the medical and psychiatric disorders to consider in the differential diagnosis of schizophrenia. The initial evaluation is also a time when treatment plans are made and when patients and family members begin to learn what to expect in the future. Because there is some evidence that early treatment may improve the long-term outcome of schizophrenia, decisions here are crucial.[27]

Table 1.2 highlights some of the key components in the diagnostic process. To exclude other medical conditions, as well as determine the general health of the patient, a medical history is taken and a physical examination that includes a neurological examination is performed. If the patient is agitated or resists, it may be impossible to complete all the tasks involved during a single examination; however, the term 'deferred' should not be used in an open-ended manner. Instead 'deferred' written after a task should list a specific time when the task will again be attempted. Unfortunately, there are often logistic and financial obstacles that prevent such tasks from being completed. When such situations occur, the clinician probably should note the fact that, on more than one occasion, he or she attempted to complete these tasks and the obstacles that were encountered. At a time when the patient and/or

the family are able to understand their importance, one should remind them of their value, and urge them to undertake their completion.

All patients should undergo a mental status examination, although how detailed the mental status examination will be will depend on the patient's condition. Standard laboratory tests include a CBC (complete blood count), blood electrolytes, blood glucose, and liver, renal, and thyroid function tests. HIV and syphilis status should be ascertained when indicated and permissible. Local conditions may suggest other tests (for example, in Latin America where cysticercosis is common, one might include a CT (computed tomography) or MRI (magnetic resonance imaging) scan and/or serological tests of the sera and CSF (cerebrospinal fluid)). When substance abuse is suspected, blood can be taken for an evaluation of current alcohol use, and urine can be screened for drug abuse. In women who could potentially be pregnant, one might want to do a pregnancy test.

Most current guidelines[28,29] indicate that unless the history and neurological examination raise a level of suspicion, an EEG (electroencephalogram), CT or MRI are not indicated to exclude potentially treatable brain pathology. Although pathological anomalies are often found in patients with schizophrenia when brain imaging is used (for example, evidence of decreased brain volume), clinically meaningful anomalies are unusual when they are not suggested by a historical or neurological examination. It should be noted, however, that minor neurological signs are found in a high proportion of patients with schizophrenia. These include stereotypies, tics, dystonic movements, poor coordination, and frontal cortex release signs. Although published guidelines do not recommend a CT or MRI scan, where affordable and feasible it is probably prudent to perform one as early in the illness as possible. This would exclude the rare cases of schizophrenia caused by a neurological lesion, which would not otherwise be found.

Neuropsychological tests often help decide

Table 1.1 Disorders to consider in the differential diagnosis of schizophrenia.

Psychiatric disorders

Psychotic disorders

Bipolar 1 disorder	Bipolar 1 disorder (also known as manic-depressive illness) is characterized by one or more manic or mixed episodes, usually alternating with euthymic and depressive episodes. A patient's history may be vague early in the course of the disorder, making it difficult to distinguish between bipolar disorder and schizophrenia. Though not diagnostic, a family history of manic-depressive illness suggests bipolar disorder. Manic-like symptoms occur in the acute phases of schizophrenia, but rarely have the same infectious quality seen early in a manic episode; however, the mixed state of an individual with manic-depressive illness may be very difficult to differentiate from the many dysphoric states that patients with schizophrenia experience. The patient who describes an electrical or charge-like buildup of energy is more likely to be experiencing a mixed state of bipolar illness.
Brief psychotic disorder	Brief psychotic disorder is characterized by the same positive symptoms as the acute form of schizophrenia. Symptoms have a sudden onset and last from 1 day to 1 month, followed by a full return to the premorbid level of functioning.
Major depressive disorders with psychosis	During a psychotic episode, it can be difficult to differentiate the psychotic form of major depressive disorder from schizophrenia, but generally an individual having a major depressive disorder with psychosis spends very little time having psychotic symptoms in the absence of depressive symptoms. If psychotic symptoms last longer than 2 weeks and depression is absent, the patient is more likely to have schizophrenia or a schizoaffective disorder. Individuals with major depressive disorders do not have hypomanic or manic episodes. A history of repeated depressions interspersed with normal functioning will often suffice to differentiate schizophrenia from a major psychotic depressive disorder.
Schizoaffective disorder	In individuals with schizoaffective disorder, the symptoms of a mood disorder coexist with those of schizophrenia for prolonged periods of time. DSM-IV posits that in such individuals, a major depressive, manic, or mixed episode occurs at the same time as the active-phase symptoms of schizophrenia.
Schizophreniform disorders	The positive symptoms of schizophreniform disorders are the same as those found in brief psychotic disorder and the acute form of schizophrenia. Schizophreniform disorder usually does not have significant negative symptoms, which may or may not be present early in an individual with schizophrenia. The major difference between a brief psychotic disorder, a schizophreniform disorder, and schizophrenia, however, is the length of the prodromal plus the psychotic symptoms. The symptoms of schizophreniform disorder last for at least 1 month but less than 6 months. The time

Table 1.1 Continued

	criteria include those of prodrome, active psychosis, and residual symptoms.
Personality disorders	
Schizotypal personality disorder	An individual with schizotypal personality disorder has few, if any, close relationships, and those that do exist are highlighted by continuous deficits and acute discomfort. In addition, there are cognitive and/or perceptual distortions and often eccentric behaviors. There are not, however, persistent psychotic symptoms.
Schizoid personality disorder	In an individual with schizoid personality disorder, there is a continuous detachment from relationships with others, as well as a limited range of emotional expression. There are not, however, persistent psychotic symptoms.
Borderline personality disorder	Borderline personality disorder is characterized by continuous unstable relationships with others, an unstable self-image, and an unstable affect. There may be marked impulsivity in some situations. Although there may be paranoid illusions or ideas, these tend to be transient and are usually associated with interactions with other individuals and respond to external structuring. When paranoid illusions and ideas last for months or years, they are less fixed than delusions.
Factitious disorders with psychological symptoms, and malingering	An individual with a psychological factitious disorder or who is malingering self-induces or feigns symptoms. In factitious disorder, these symptoms serve the sole purpose of appearing sick; in malingering however, the individual has a specific goal in mind, usually the avoidance of an adverse situation. Although a factitious disorder rarely takes the form of schizophrenia, it is not uncommon for an individual attempting to avoid the consequences of criminal behavior to malinger a schizophrenic-like illness. Currently, it may be beyond the capacity of psychiatry to distinguish an accomplished malingerer from an individual with schizophrenia.
Pervasive developmental disorders	Individuals with pervasive developmental disorder have severe and continuous impairment in more than one area of development. These may include impaired reciprocal interactions with other individuals, impaired communication skills, the presence of stereotyped behavior, and limited interests and activities. These disorders become evident in the first few years of life and may be associated with decreased intellectual function. Individuals with childhood-onset schizophrenia differ from those with pervasive development disorders because their symptoms begin later and only after several years of normal or almost normal development.
Paranoid personality disorder	Paranoid personality disorder is characterized by interpersonal aloofness and pervasive distrust and suspiciousness of others, whose motives are considered malevolent. Individuals with paranoid personality disorder also tend to react to minor stimuli with anger. Unlike schizophrenia, however, there is an absence of persistent

Table 1.1 Continued

	psychotic symptoms. If the disorder precedes a subsequent diagnosis of schizophrenia, the diagnosis is noted on Axis II, followed by 'Premorbid' in parentheses.
Other psychiatric disorders to consider	
Adjustment disorders	Adjustment disorders include adjustment disorder with depressed mood, anxiety, mixed anxiety and depressed mood, disturbance of conduct, mixed disturbance of emotions and conduct, and unspecified. All are characterized by significant emotional or behavioral distress in response to identifiable stressors. By definition the disorders must resolve within 6 months of the termination of the stressor(s). As a diagnosis, it is usually given when an individual's symptoms do not meet criteria for another psychiatric disorder, and in such cases it is often given for administrative reasons.
Asperger's syndrome	Asperger's syndrome begins in childhood, although some of its symptoms are not apparent until later. It is characterized by severely impaired social interaction, as well as the development of repetitive patterns of behavior, interests, and activities. There are no significant delays in language or cognitive development, but functioning is impaired. Because motor delays, motor clumsiness, and difficulties in social interaction usually appear during childhood, and because of the absence of psychotic symptoms, a careful patient history can usually establish the correct diagnosis.
Delusional disorder	An individual with delusional disorder experiences one or more nonbizarre delusions that persist for at least 1 month and may be accompanied by nonprominent auditory and visual hallucinations, or prominent but delusion-related tactile or olfactory hallucinations. Ideas of reference are common. Social, marital, or work problems can result from the delusions. However, functioning is not significantly impaired, speech is not disorganized, negative symptoms are not present, and behavior is neither odd nor bizarre. There are seven subtypes of the disorder: erotomanic, grandiose, jealous, persecutory, somatic, mixed, and unspecified. The bizarreness of the delusions can be one aspect for distinguishing this disorder from schizophrenia; however, bizarreness may be difficult to judge, especially across cultures. A delusion is considered bizarre if it is clearly implausible or not drawn from ordinary life. In addition, age of onset is usually in middle or later life, rather than young adulthood.
Dissociative identity disorder	Formerly known as multiple personality disorder, the distinguishing feature of dissociative identity disorder is the presence of two or more distinct identities or personality states that recurrently take control of an individual's behavior, as well as an inability to recall important personal information. Episodic and continuous courses have both been described. Delusions, hallucinations, thought disorder, and other symptoms of schizophrenia are not present, but

Table 1.1 Continued

	because the presence of one or more dissociated personality states may be mistaken for a delusion, a careful patient history is needed to establish the diagnosis.
Post-traumatic stress disorder	Post-traumatic stress disorder occurs after an individual has been exposed to an extreme traumatic event, which causes persistent re-experiencing of the event, avoidance of stimuli associated with the trauma, and symptoms of increased arousal. Social and occupational functioning are impaired. Onset can be acute, chronic, or delayed. The presence of flashbacks, as well as the functional impairment that may accompany the diagnosis, may cause it to be misdiagnosed as schizophrenia. Post-traumatic stress disorder, however, can also often accompany schizophrenia.

Substance of abuse-induced toxic disorders

Substance of abuse-induced psychoses can usually be differentiated from schizophrenia by the presence of delirium (characterized by a fluctuating global impairment of memory, perception, consciousness, and attention). The diagnosis is usually confirmed by examining the urine or blood for the suspected offending agent. There is usually a history of substance abuse, but sometimes patients are unaware that they have taken the drug, or are too confused to appreciate the significance of what they have done. Symptoms of drug-induced toxic disorders may include disorientation and visual hallucinations, and sometimes tactile hallucinations. A number of people may develop sustained psychosis, usually after prolonged use of drugs. If prodromal signs were present before drug use began, schizophrenia is usually diagnosed, but if no previous prodromal symptoms existed, the diagnosis becomes more difficult. Except for phencyclidine and methamphetamine, it is rare for the drugs listed below to produce a psychosis lasting longer than the pharmacological activity of the drug. Most data indicate that with the exception of methamphetamine and phencyclidine, these drugs only produce a chronic psychosis in individuals who are otherwise prone to develop a psychosis. In practice, particularly in the acute state, treatment that alleviates the acute symptoms may have to begin before there is good information on the cause of the psychosis.

Alcohol-induced psychotic disorder and other alcohol-related disorders	Alcoholics having symptoms of severe withdrawal such as delirium tremens (DTs) go into a state of confusion sometimes accompanied by visual, tactile, or auditory hallucinations. The major symptom may be paranoia. An alcohol-induced psychotic disorder is a temporary psychotic disorder, characterized by auditory hallucinations and/or paranoid delusions in the absence of any obvious signs of withdrawal and usually occurs with a clear sensorium. There is always a history of previous alcohol abuse, which the individual may deny.
Amphetamine, cocaine, methamphetamine, and other stimulants	Amphetamines, cocaine, and other stimulants (including phenylpropylamine, which is present in many over-the-counter medications) can produce a paranoid psychosis. Paranoia is usually the most prominent symptom, although the thought disorder, affective flattening and hallucinations also present in schizophrenia are seen less frequently. The individual with amphetamine psychosis may have compulsive stereotypic behavior. In these patients, there is

Table 1.1 Continued	
	a history of stimulant abuse, and the stimulant can be found in the urine. Most stimulant-induced paranoid psychoses clear within hours to days if the individual does not continue to use the drug. However, a number of reports indicate that long-term cocaine abuse may cause paranoid ideation, and visual and auditory hallucinations, resembling alcoholic hallucinosis.
	Methamphetamine (MAP)-induced psychosis can produce ideas of reference, delusions of persecution, and auditory and visual hallucinations. Auditory hallucinations, with voices commenting on the individual's behavior, are more common than visual hallucinations. Following the psychotic episode, individuals tend to have a flattened affect, and an enduring personality change. Although a MAP-induced psychosis can occur after only one or two uses, psychosis usually occurs after MAP use lasting a few months to several years. Early on, there is often a decrease in the drug's euphoric effects. With time, suspiciousness increases. Until recently, when more potent forms of MAP became available, MAP psychoses developed only after intravenous use. Although MAP is not usually present in the urine for more than 3–5 days, about half of MAP-induced psychoses can take a week to clear. Eighty percent of patients recover within a month of discontinuing MAP, but in a small number the symptoms can take up to 5 years to clear. There is also a strong tendency for relapse when the individual is further exposed to even small doses of MAP, alcohol and, at times, to psychological stress. A history of MAP use, finding needle marks on the arm, or finding MAP in the urine should increase the level of suspicion that the psychosis is due to MAP.
Anticholinergics, including belladonna alkaloids	Large doses of anticholinergic drugs (or relatively small doses in sensitive individuals) can lead to anticholinergic syndrome. When fully developed, this syndrome is characterized by disturbances in concentration, orientation and immediate recall, coupled with agitation, ataxia, and confusion. There also may be choreoathetoid and picking movements. The pupils may become dilated, the skin and mucosa dry, and there may be an increased heart rate, elevated blood pressure, and elevated temperature.
LSD, mescaline, and similar hallucinogens	LSD-induced psychosis is marked by prominent visual-perceptual alterations (the hallucinations of an individual with schizophrenia are more likely to be auditory), little or no flattening of affect and the absence of fixed delusions. Individuals with LSD psychosis tend to be concerned with their inability to express their thoughts, while individuals with schizophrenia often have a thought disorder. During the LSD experience itself, particularly early, there is often dizziness, weakness, tremor, nausea, drowsiness, paresthesias, and blurred vision. The most common acute medical problem associated with LSD-like drugs is episodes of panic. The LSD psychosis terminates as

Table 1.1 Continued	
	the effect of the drug wears off. Flashbacks are common with LSD use, but are not usually confused with the symptoms of schizophrenia.
Marijuana and tetrahydrocannabinol (THC)	Marijuana can sometimes produce ideas of reference, fear, paranoia, agitation, confusion, and even depersonalization. Individuals using marijuana may have an elevated heart rate and inflamed conjunctivae. In active marijuana users, THC is present in the urine.
Opioid-induced disorders	Opioids such as morphine, codeine, and heroin can cause auditory, visual, or tactile hallucinations with intact reality testing. Euphoria, apathy, dysphoria, and impaired social or occupational functioning can also occur, particularly in chronic users. Symptoms usually disappear after opioids are stopped, but withdrawal symptoms such as anxiety, dysphoria, anhedonia, and insomnia can persist for weeks or months.
PCP (phencyclidine)	PCP can produce a psychosis which, during the acute stage, may be accompanied by a mood disturbance, memory loss, facial grimacing, nystagmus, and ataxia. History of PCP use, when a history is available, and a urine screen can help make the diagnosis. Both the acute and the more chronic form of PCP psychosis can be associated with unpredictable physical violence towards oneself and others.
	Neurologic-medical disorders
Acute intermittent porphyria (AIP)	AIP is a liver porphyria that usually develops after puberty, or about the same time as schizophrenia. It can be triggered by exposure to some drugs, including barbiturates and sulfonamide antibiotics. During an acute attack, individuals with AIP can have hallucinations and paranoia, usually with anxiety, insomnia, depression, and disorientation. The presence of seizures, intermittent abdominal pain, and occasionally distention and diarrhea help make the diagnosis. During an acute attack, γ-aminolevulinic acid (ALA) and porphobilinogen (PBG) are increased in the urine and blood.
Adrenoleukodystrophy (ALD)	An X-linked recessive disorder affecting males, ALD is characterized by, among other symptoms, progressive dementia and other intellectual and neurological disturbances due to myelin degeneration in the white matter of the brain.
Alzheimer's disease, early	Hallucinations, agitation, and suspicion can be early symptoms of Alzheimer's disease. Usually, however, Alzheimer's disease is accompanied by problems with recent memory, loss of spontaneity and initiative, and poor judgment. With time, there is disorientation to time and place. Generally, there is progressive cerebral atrophy on CT and MRI scans. Although Alzheimer's disease can occur before middle age, it usually presents after the age of greatest risk for schizophrenia.
Congenital adrenal hyperplasia and Cushing's syndrome	The symptoms of Cushing's syndrome and the congenital adrenal hyperplasias are associated with increased adrenocortical secretion of cortisol. These diseases, and Cushing's syndrome in particular, are

Table 1.1 Continued	
	often associated with psychiatric disturbances. However, they are also associated with centripetal obesity, moon face, acne, abdominal striae, hypertension, decreased carbohydrate tolerance, and amenorrhea and hirsutism in women.
Epilepsy, complex partial seizures	The psychoses associated with complex partial seizure epilepsy resemble that of paranoid schizophrenia. However, patients tend to be warm, friendlier, and more cooperative than patients with schizophrenia, who display a detached, blunted affect, and social awkwardness. Complex partial seizures are accompanied by a loss of consciousness, which usually makes it easy to differentiate from schizophrenia. In time, complex partial seizures can appear more like an organic disorder.
Epilepsy, simple partial seizures	Hallucinations can be associated with epilepsy; specifically, the hallucinations associated with simple partial seizures are structured, may be of any sensory system, and can be elaborate. Illusions of size such as micropsia and macropsia occur. There may be a poverty of speech, and the patient may perseverate. There may be déjà vu, jamais vu, and recollections of past experiences. Fear, depression, anger, and irritability may occur. A patient does not lose consciousness with simple partial seizures (when consciousness is lost, the seizure is considered a complex partial seizure). When clonus and other motor signs are found the diagnosis is fairly easy. But because electrical activity is often small, scalp EEG electrodes may not show the abnormality. Simple partial seizures most commonly affect the temporal and frontal lobes, but because they may have their origins in other brain areas, the term 'temporal lobe epilepsy' (TLE) is no longer used.
Friedreich's ataxia	Psychosis may be present before the onset of the abnormal movements of Friedreich's and other forms of hereditary ataxia. Friedreich's ataxia presents before age 25, usually with dysarthria and a progressive staggering gait, falling, and stumbling. On examination the patient has nystagmus, dysarthria, dysmetria, and ataxia of both the trunk and extremities. At times there is moderate mental retardation and cardiomegaly.
Huntington's disease (HD)	Schizophrenia is occasionally the initial diagnosis of patients with Huntington's disease, particularly in younger patients. In patients under 20, there is usually also rigidity and seizures. Abnormal movements, a family history of Huntington's disease, and often the results of a CT or MRI scan increase the level of suspicion. Diagnostic blood tests can be conducted to confirm the diagnosis.
Ischemia, stroke	Although psychotic symptoms may accompany a stroke, there are usually focal symptoms and signs to aid in the diagnosis. Multiple small ischemic episodes, however, can produce psychotic symptoms without focal symptoms. Other indications of ischemic illness, including age, may be helpful.

Table 1.1 Continued

Metachromatic leukodystrophy (MLD)	Patients with MLD, who develop their illness during their teens and twenties, or at about the same time as the peak risk period for developing schizophrenia, often have the positive symptoms of schizophrenia. In addition they may have a thought disorder. Forgetfulness also may be an early symptom. The onset may be slow, and in the earliest stages may be confused with schizophrenia, but the disease is progressive. It may not be until the appearance of abnormal movements that MLD is suspected. These can include mild cerebellar findings, masked facies, and strange postures. The diagnosis is made when diminished arylsulfatase A activity is found in white blood cells, and increased excretion of sulfatides is found in the urine.
Multiple sclerosis (MS)	The usual psychiatric symptoms of MS include euphoria and emotional lability, but at times there are ideas of reference, delusions, and hallucinations, which can occur with or without intellectual deterioration. When these symptoms occur by themselves early in the illness, it may be difficult to distinguish MS from a psychiatric disorder, although only rarely does the symptom cluster present as schizophrenia.
Narcolepsy	Hypnogogic and hypnopompic hallucinations, as well as cataplexy, are part of narcolepsy. When less was known about narcolepsy, that illness was confused with schizophrenia. The recurrent uncontrollable attacks of sleep and sleep paralysis, as well as findings from polysomnography, help make the diagnosis.
Niemann-Pick's disease	There are three subtypes of this disease: a childhood onset, a delayed onset which begins in early childhood but progresses slowly, and a late-onset form that appears in adolescence or early adulthood and is characterized by an even slower rate of progression. This final subtype is characterized by psychomotor retardation, cerebellar ataxia, and extrapyramidal manifestations, but in some cases a psychosis may be the only evidence of illness for several years.
Phenylketonuria (PKU)	Some of the first descriptions of phenylketonuria were in patients whose family members had a high rate of schizophrenia. And in the distant past, it was thought that schizophrenia might be related to phenylketonuria. Because phenylketonuria is now diagnosed and treated from birth, it is not likely that a patient with symptoms of schizophrenia will have undiagnosed phenylketonuria.
Sleep apnea	On rare occasions, sleep apnea has produced a paranoid psychosis. A careful history that includes questions about snoring and excessive daytime sleepiness can help. If the symptoms are suggestive, polysomnography is done to establish the diagnosis.
Subarachnoid hemorrhage and subdural hematoma	Patients with space-occupying lesions may present with psychiatric symptoms including delusions and hallucinations. Usually, however, the patients are also disoriented or confused and have symptoms of

Table 1.1 Continued

	a focal neurological nature. A careful history and neurological examination, including a clear view of the fundi, help make these diagnoses.
Systemic lupus erythematosus (SLE)	Patients with an SLE psychosis are usually disorientated and have memory loss. Other symptoms and signs of SLE are usually present, including an elevated erythrocyte sedimentation rate (ESR), and autoantibodies.
Trauma to the head	Trauma to the head is often associated with a variety of psychiatric symptoms, although delusions and hallucinations are less common than irritability and confusion. Usually, there is a history of trauma and other generalized (e.g., alterations of consciousness) or focal neurological symptoms and signs. A history of past injury to the head, including a brief loss of consciousness, may suggest a traumatic injury.
Tumors of the brain and metastatic tumors	The most common symptoms and signs of brain tumors are focal. Symptoms related to raised intracranial pressure and seizures may not appear until late in the course. Occipital tumors can be associated with simple visual hallucinations. Temporal lobe tumors can be associated with complex visual and auditory hallucinations. There may also be olfactory and gustatory hallucinations. Parietal lobe tumors are characterized by tactile and kinesthetic hallucinations. Brain tumors, particularly those of meninges, can present with changes in personality, but are also often accompanied by visual changes, particularly field deficits. Other symptoms such as headaches, vomiting, and drowsiness are common.
Turner's syndrome (XO karyotype; gonadal dysgenesis)	Psychotic symptoms can be associated with Turner's syndrome, but when the characteristic features are present the diagnosis is not difficult. In a late adolescent or adult, these features include undeveloped external female genitalia, sparse body hair, immature breasts, and primary amenorrhea. The individual is short, has multiple congenital anomalies including a webbing of the neck, low hairline, and a shield-like chest with spaced nipples. In phenotypic women there are bilateral streak gonads. Classically, there is only one X chromosome, but some patients are mosaics, or have a structurally abnormal X chromosome.
Variegate porphyria (VP)	The psychiatric and neurologic symptoms of VP are very similar to those of AIP. Like many other forms of porphyria, patients with VP have skin manifestations associated with photosensitivity. VP also can be triggered by the same drugs as AIP. During acute symptoms, fecal and urine protoporphyrin and coproporphyrin are elevated.
Wilson's disease (hepatolenticular degeneration)	Psychosis was prominent in 8 of Wilson's original 12 patients. Usually, however, there are neurologic symptoms, in addition to bizarre behavior, including resting and intention tremors, spasticity, rigidity, chorea, drooling, dysphagia, and dysarthria. Usually, there are also characteristic abnormal movements of the upper

Table 1.1 Continued

extremities, often described as 'wing beating'. Symptoms usually develop between the ages of 12 and 15. Commonly, some form of liver disease develops after the neurologic and psychiatric symptoms and the liver becomes enlarged. Diagnosis is made by the presence of Kayser–Fleischer rings (copper deposits in the Descemet's membrane of the cornea) and a low concentration of serum ceruloplasmin. Elevated concentration of copper in the urine is also common.

Other neurologic and medical disorders occasionally presenting with symptoms similar to those of schizophrenia

18q– (missing piece of long arm of chromosome 18)	Albinism	Hepatic encephalopathy
5,q11–q13 (triplication of this region of chromosome 5)	Aqueduct stenosis	Homocystinuria
22,q11.2 deletion syndrome	Brain embolism	Hypoglycemia
XXX karyotype	Congenital iodine deficiency	Migraine
XXY Klinefelter karyotype	Familial basal ganglia calcification	Uremia
XYY karyotype	G-6-PD deficiency (favism)	Vascular dementia
		Vasculitis

Infections

Bacterial infection and other infections	Bacterial infections that do not directly invade the brain can nevertheless produce dementia-like or delirious symptoms, often followed by depression. These symptoms appear to be produced by a toxic reaction to the infectious agent or the body's reaction to the agent. High temperatures can also produce delirious states. Diagnosis is made by taking a careful history and a full physical examination.
Creutzfeldt–Jacob	CJD is usually sporadic, but can also be transmitted from person to person by contaminated grafts, surgical instruments, and through impure human growth hormone. CJD usually presents with rapidly developing dementia associated with myoclonus. Early symptoms may include hallucinations, usually with changes in mood, and slowed thinking. There is poor concentration, impaired judgment, and memory loss. Parkinsonian symptoms are common in later forms of the disease. The EEG may show typical periodic short sharp wave discharges on a slowed background. The sharp waves may be accompanied by myoclonic jerks, provoked by a startle. The CSF usually does not show a protein or cell elevation, but two-dimensional isoelectric focusing may show abnormal proteins.
Encephalitis lethargica	During the 1918–1926 influenza pandemic, the acute phase of encephalitis produced schizophrenia-like states, but a psychosis also developed as a postencephalitic sequel, sometimes accompanied by Parkinsonism.

Table 1.1 Continued	
Herpes simplex virus (HSV)	HSV produces an encephalitis that can present as an acute psychotic illness. The acute onset of HSV encephalitis begins with a fever and focal temporal lobe symptoms. An EEG, characterized by a focal spike and slow waves localized to the infected temporal lobe, when present, can help make the diagnosis. HSV also can be diagnosed by polymerase chain reaction of HSV DNA from the CSF, which takes about 10 days to develop. There is elevated protein and cell count in the CSF.
Human immunodeficiency virus (HIV) disease	Early in HIV–dementia complex, also called HIV-associated cognitive/motor complex, there are difficulties with concentration, loss of memory, a slowing of thought, personality changes, depression, and apathy. Many patients also have motor dysfunction. CT and MRI scans indicate the presence of a diffuse cerebral atrophy. The patient is seropositive for HIV infection.
Neurocysticercosis	Cysticercosis will occasionally begin with psychotic symptoms, but most often starts with seizures. Symptoms associated with increased intracranial pressure are also common. Cysticercosis is rare in the United States, Canada, and Western Europe, but can be acquired from eating foods (often, uncooked pork) contaminated with *Taenia solium* larvae (also known as the pig tapeworm). It can be diagnosed by observing calcifications on a CT or MRI scan. In some patients, cysts can be seen on the retina.
Rheumatic encephalitis and Sydenham's chorea	The term *'chorea insaniens'* was used in the past to describe patients having a clear consciousness, but who were hallucinating and having abnormal movements that sometimes occurred in acute rheumatic fever. Like the choreiform movements of rheumatic fever, the hallucinations occasionally occur weeks or months after the acute illness. Other behavioral manifestations include withdrawal, irritability, and emotional lability. The behavioral symptoms may last long after the choreiform movements.
Subacute sclerosing panencephalitis (SSPE)	SSPE usually develops before age 15, and follows a measles infection 6–8 years earlier. SSPE may start out with a decrease in school performance, a change in affect, as well as in personality. With time there is intellectual deterioration, seizures, myoclonus, ataxia and visual disturbances. CSF protein is usually normal or slightly elevated, but gamma globulin is dramatically elevated. The EEG has characteristic bursts every 3–8 seconds of high-voltage, sharp, slow waves, followed by periods with a flat background.
Syphilis; general paresis	In its tertiary, parenchymatous, clinically symptomatic form, syphilis (infection with *Treponema pallidum*) produces general paresis and tabes dorsalis. General paresis is associated with Argyll Robertson pupil (the pupil reacts to accommodation, but not to light), as well as changes in affect and personality, hyperactive reflexes, illusions, delusions and hallucinations, difficulties with recent memory, orientation, calculation, judgment and insight, and dysarthria. The

Table 1.1 Continued	
Tuberculous meningitis	Venereal Disease Research Laboratory (VDRL) test of the CSF is probably the standard test for the detection of CNS syphilis. Tuberculous meningitis of the central nervous system is unusual in adults unless they have been infected with HIV. In many cases, evidence of old pulmonary lesions or a miliary pattern is found on a chest radiograph. Symptoms of headache and mental changes may develop slowly, or confusion, lethargy, an altered sensorium, and neck rigidity may develop suddenly. Typically, the disease evolves over 1 or 2 weeks. Paresis of the ocular nerves is frequent. White cell count is elevated in the CSF, and glucose is decreased. In most cases culturing the CSF is diagnostic.
	Nutritional
Folic acid (pteroylmonoglutamic acid) deficiency	With folic acid deficiency, irritability, apathy, somnolence, suspiciousness, psychosis, and intellectual deterioration can occur with or without anemia. If anemia is present, it is megaloblastic and the usual signs of anemia, including fatigue, rapid heart rate, shortness of breath and more serious cardiovascular symptoms appear. Because they are usually malnourished, patients with folic acid deficiency are apt to have a wasted appearance. Diarrhea, cheilosis and glossitis are sometimes present. It is questionable to what degree neurological symptoms occur from folic acid deficiency alone.
Pellagra or niacin deficiency	Pellagra's three 'Ds' – dermatitis, dementia, and diarrhea – are now rarely seen in developed countries because of grain supplementation with niacin. Nevertheless, with large numbers of refugees coming from parts of the world deprived of good nutrition, it is found from time to time. The psychological symptoms include fatigue, insomnia, and apathy in less severe cases. These are followed by confusion, disorientation, hallucinations, loss of memory, and, finally, dementia. Pellagra is likely to be noted because of generalized wasting suggesting malnutrition, and the presence of a photosensitivity dermatitis on areas exposed to sunlight.
Vitamin B_{12} (cobalamin) deficiency	Vitamin B_{12} deficiency without hematologic abnormalities (normal hematocrit and hemoglobin) is fairly common, especially in the elderly. Mild symptoms include irritability and forgetfulness and more severe symptoms include delusions and hallucinations. There may also be dementia. With severe symptoms there are also usually neurological symptoms including peripheral neuropathies, and a gait disturbance. Other signs and symptoms may include numbness and paresthesias in the extremities, weakness, and ataxia, and even loss of control over sphincter muscles. There may be a Babinski sign, and position and vibration senses are usually diminished. If anemia is present it is megaloblastic, and the usual signs of anemia, including fatigue, rapid heart rate, shortness of breath and more serious

Table 1.1 Continued	

cardiovascular symptoms appear. Usually, folic acid deficiency and vitamin B_{12} deficiency are found together. Serum levels of methylmalonic acid are almost always increased.

Heavy metals

Heavy metal poisoning may occasionally, but does not usually, cause symptoms that are likely to become confused with those of schizophrenia.

Lead	Lead poisoning can induce a psychosis with hallucinations, agitation, and nightmares. At higher concentrations lead can induce delirium, seizures, and even coma. In adults, organic lead poisoning comes from two sources: inhalation of leaded gasoline and industrial accidents. The psychotomimetic effects include visual, auditory, and tactile hallucinations as well as sensations of a change in color and shape. Inorganic lead poisoning appears to be much more common, and is also likely to be work related, affecting, for example, automobile radiator repair employees. It usually occurs with abdominal pain, constipation, anemia, and peripheral nervous system difficulties, including wrist extensor and sensory problems. While more complex testing may be required, in the acute state a history of exposure and blood lead levels can help make the diagnosis.
Mercury	Generally, mercury poisoning produces irritability, avoidant behavior, depression, fatigue, lassitude, and tremor. Individuals at risk for mercury poisoning include those who manufacture items containing mercury such as mercury vapor lamps, thermometers and barometers, and dental amalgams. Photographers, photoengravers, feltmakers, battery makers, tanners, and embalmers may also be at some risk. Mercury poisoning can be diagnosed by a history of exposure and a blood mercury level.

Medications

Below is a partial list of the great number of medications that can produce symptoms also present in schizophrenia, including hallucinations, delusions, and thought disorder. For the most part, however, symptoms caused by medications are more consistent with depression, dementia or delirium. Because alterations in mental status are a relatively common reaction to medications, the clinician has to be aware that a great many medications can have profound psychological effects and when such symptoms are found, think of the medication the patient is taking as a possible cause. Fortunately, these symptoms are usually reversible when the medication is discontinued.

Acyclovir	Atenolol
Alprazolam	Atorvastatin
Amantadine	Atropine
Amitriptyline	Azithromycin
Amlodipine	Baclofen
Amphetamine	Beclomethasone

Table 1.1 Continued

Benzonatate	Ketoprofen
Bisoprolol	Ketorolac
Bromide	Lamotrigine
Bromocriptine	Lansoprazole
Bupropion	Leuprolide
Buspirone	Levodopa
Carbamazepine	Levofloxacin
Carbidopa	Lidocaine
Cefaclor	Lithium
Cephalexin	Loratadine
Cimetidine	Meperidine
Ciprofloxacin	Mesalamine
Citalopram	Methylphenidate
Clarithomycin	Metoprolol
Clobetasol	Mirtazapine
Clomipramine	Misoprostol
Clonazepam	Morphine
Clonidine	Naloxone
Corticosteroids and ACTH	Nefazodone
Cromolyn sodium	Nortriptyline
Cyclobenzaprine	Ofloxacin
Dexfenfluramine	Olanzapine
Dextroamphetamine	Omeprazole
Diazepam	Orphenadrine
Dicyclomine	Oxybutyrin
Digitalis	Paroxetine
Diltiazem	Pemoline
Diphenhydramine	Pentazocine
Disulfiram	Phentermine
Divalproex	Piroxicam
Donepezil	Promethazine
Doxepin	Propanolol
Efavirenz	Propoxyphene
Erythromycin	Pseudoephedrine
Famotidine	Ranitidine
Fluconazole	Rimantadine
Fluoxetine	Selegiline
Fluticasone	St John's Wort
Fluvoxamine	Sulfamethoxazole
Guaifenesin with pseudoephedrine or	Sulfasalazine
hydrocodone	Sumatriptan
Haloperidol	Temazepam
Hydrochlorthiazide	Terazosin
Hydromorphone	Tizanidine
Hyoscyamine	Tramadol
Ibuprofen	Triazolam
Imipramine	Trimethoprim
Indomethacin	Trovafloxacin
Interferon beta 1b	Venlafaxine
Isocarboxazid	Zolpidem
Isosorbide	

Table 1.2 Components of a diagnostic evaluation of schizophrenia.

Test	Is test indicated?
Medical and psychiatric history	Yes
Physical examination (including neurological)	Yes
Mental status examination	Yes
Complete blood count (CBC); blood electrolytes; blood glucose; liver, renal and thyroid function	Yes
HIV and syphilis status	Possible
Computed tomography (CT) scan	Possible
Magnetic resonance imaging (MRI) scan	Possible
Serological tests of sera and CSF	Possible
Blood/urine screens for drug or alcohol abuse	Possible
Pregnancy test	Possible

treatment goals by evaluating the capabilities of a patient, but they are not usually helpful in making a diagnosis. Many patients with schizophrenia will have a variety of cognitive deficits, but these can often be elicited on a standard mental status examination and are rarely diagnostic.

Diagnosis

As mentioned above, there are two widely accepted diagnostic schemes – DSM-IV and ICD-10 – for making a psychiatric diagnosis. These schemes are quite similar, but nevertheless differ significantly for diagnosing schizophrenia. In DSM-IV, the American Psychiatric Association sets out specific criteria that must be met in order to diagnose any psychiatric disorder. The DSM-IV diagnosis of schizophrenia differs from the World Health Organization's ICD-10 diagnosis in three fundamental ways.

1. DSM-IV requires a 6-month duration of illness, while ICD-10 requires a duration of only 1 month. Because of these differences, ICD-10 does not set out criteria for schizophreniform disorder, instead placing it under the rubric of 'other schizophrenia; schizophreniform disorder, NOS (not otherwise stated)'.

2. DSM-IV requires a deterioration in social functioning, and ICD-10 does not.

3. The two systems also differ in the criteria used to diagnose schizoaffective disorder. If a mood disorder predates the onset of psychotic symptoms in ICD-10, a diagnosis of schizoaffective disorder is endorsed. In DSM-IV, on the other hand, it is the length of time mood disorder symptoms are present that determines whether a patient receives a diagnosis of schizophrenia or schizoaffective disorder. When mood disorder symptoms are brief, even if they predate psychotic symptoms, the individual receives the diagnosis of schizophrenia in DSM-IV. According to field studies, because of the differences in diagnostic criteria, not all of the patients diagnosed with schizophrenia using DSM-IV will receive the same diagnosis when ICD-10 is used, and vice versa; however, about the same number of patients will be given a diagnosis of schizophrenia using the two systems.[30]

One administrative rather than diagnostic difference between the two systems is that numbering is different; ICD-10 uses F20.xx (with the xxs referring to the subtype) for schizophrenia, and DSM-IV uses 295.xx (again with the xxs delineating the subtype).

Differential diagnosis

1. MEDICAL/DRUG EXCLUSION

The first step in diagnosing schizophrenia is to determine if the individual is currently or has ever been psychotic. If not, schizophrenia is not a consideration. If yes, the clinician then determines whether the psychotic symptoms were or are due to a medical condition or substance abuse (this is **Criterion E** in DSM-IV). How extensively to evaluate this is often a matter of experience, judgment, and available resources.

2. DSM-IV CRITERIA

Below are reformatted criteria used to diagnose schizophrenia as set out by DSM-IV. The patient must meet Criteria A through F to be diagnosed with schizophrenia.

Criterion A is characteristic symptoms that represent the active phase of schizophrenia. Criterion A is met if the patient experiences one or more of the following lasting for a 'significant' (not defined) portion of a month (or less when the patient has been successfully treated):

1. Bizarre delusions. (A bizarre delusion is one that is implausible in the patient's culture. Thus, in the United States, a nonbizarre delusion would be the patient's belief that he is being followed by the FBI; this is possible, but not likely. A bizarre delusion would be the belief that the FBI has placed a transmitter in the patient's head and was reading his thoughts, something that is not possible.)
2. Hallucinations of a voice that keeps a running commentary on the patient's behavior or thoughts.
3. Hearing two or more voices that converse with each other.
4. And/or having two or more of the following psychotic symptoms:
   a. delusions;
   b. hallucinations (throughout the day for several days or several times per week for several weeks, each hallucinatory experience not being limited to a few brief moments);
   c. disorganized speech (for example, derailment, incoherence, blocking);
   d. grossly disorganized or catatonic behavior;
   e. negative symptoms (that is, affective flattening, alogia, avolition, or anergia).

If the psychotic symptoms last less than 1 month, the patient cannot be diagnosed with schizophrenia. Some other diagnoses that may be considered include the prodromal symptoms of schizophrenia, a delusional disorder, psychotic disorder, not otherwise stated (NOS), a mood disorder with psychotic features, and brief reactive psychotic disorder.

Criterion B is met if there has been significant disruption in social/occupational function as indicated by one of the following:

1. Since the onset of the disturbance, one or more major areas of functioning, such as work, interpersonal relations, or self-care, has dropped markedly below the level achieved prior to the onset of the disorder.
2. When the patient is too young to have achieved his or her full potential, disruption is measured by the patient not having achieved the projected level of interpersonal, academic, or occupational achievement that would be expected in his or her culture for his or her age.

Criterion C is met when the disorder has gone on for a sufficient duration for it to be clear that it is not a transitory phenomenon. The patient must have had continuous symptoms and/or signs of the disturbance for at least 6 months. The 6-month period must include at least 1 month of symptoms (or less when the patient has been successfully treated) that meet Criterion A (that is, active-phase symptoms) and may include periods of prodromal or residual symptoms. During these prodromal or residual periods, the only symptoms and signs of the disturbance may be negative symptoms, or one or more symptoms listed in Criterion A may be present in attenuated form (for example, odd beliefs instead of delusions, and unusual perceptual experiences instead of hallucinations).

Criterion D excludes patients if they have a schizoaffective or mood disorder. For a diagnosis of schizophrenia to be made, the patient cannot have a schizoaffective disorder or mood disorder with psychotic features.

When a mood disorder occurs with active phase or psychotic features described in Criterion A, the total duration of the mood disorder must be brief compared with the total duration of the active and residual phases of the disorder. A major depressive, manic or mixed episode cannot have occurred concomitantly with the active-phase symptoms.

Criterion E excludes patients whose symptoms have been induced by substance abuse, medications, or general medical conditions.

Criterion F excludes disturbances that are caused by a pervasive developmental disorder unless there are prominent delusions or hallucinations lasting at least 1 month (or less if the patient has been successfully treated).

DSM-IV also provides the opportunity to describe the course of schizophrenia up to the time of the current diagnosis. It is suggested that the course not be classified until at least 1 year has passed after the onset of the active phase of schizophrenia. Thus, after a year, a patient could be described as having had a single episode and in full remission, or in partial remission; if the patient is in partial remission, there may or may not be prominent negative symptoms; or a patient's illness can have an episodic course, with re-emergent active-phase symptoms interspersed with residual symptoms (which may or may not be negative). A number of other courses are possible.

DSM-IV and ICD-10 recognize five subtypes of schizophrenia: paranoid, disorganized, catatonic, undifferentiated and residual, based on the predominant features associated with each one (see Table 1.3). The value of some of these subtypes of schizophrenia is not always clear because the treatment differs little. For treatment purposes, it might be more useful to consider associated symptoms such as depression, anxiety, and obsessive-compulsiveness.

Conclusion

We began with a comment on the importance of diagnosis in psychiatry. In the past, diagnosis was important for understanding prognosis. During the twentieth century, diagnosis has been particularly important for making choices between effective treatments. As we add to our understanding of the pathophysiology of psychiatric diseases, the next century will bring dramatic improvements in those treatments. More importantly, information about causation may help us prevent or at least attenuate the severity of these diseases.

Today, although correctly diagnosing schizophrenia remains important for ensuring proper treatment, treatments remain nonspecific. For example, although most forms of psychosis benefit from antipsychotic medications, these medications appear to treat only what is common to psychosis – primarily the positive or florid symptoms. The antipsychotic medications are not very effective in treating deficit and cognitive symptoms, which some believe are the essence of schizophrenia; in addition to affecting the course, they are the principal symptoms that differentiate schizophrenia from other forms of psychosis. Our understanding of schizophrenia is more comprehensive than it was 100 years ago, and our treatments far better, but in the next century we must discover and understand the diseases that make up schizophrenia rather than its symptoms. And in order to do this, diagnostic instruments must become far more precise than those available today. Ultimately, however, progress in diagnosing schizophrenia will come through our understanding of the genetic and nongenetic causes of schizophrenia. These, in turn, will lead to more objective diagnosing and, more importantly, preventive and improved treatments.

Acknowledgement

I am grateful to Dr Nicole van de Laar and Ken Morel for their thoughtful review of this draft, and to Ioline Henter for her invaluable research, organizational, and editorial assistance.

Table 1.3 Schizophrenia subtype codes.

Subtype	Defining features	DSM-IV code	ICD-10 code
Paranoid	Prominent delusions or auditory hallucinations, but without prominent disorganized speech or behavior, catatonic behavior, or flat or inappropriate affect	295.30	F20.0x[a]
Disorganized	Prominent disorganized speech or behavior and flat or inappropriate affect without catatonic behavior	295.10	F20.1x[a]
Catatonic	Immobility that may include catalepsy or stupor, or apparently purposeless excessive motor activity, extreme negativism or mutism, posturing, stereotyped movements, mannerisms or grimacing, and echolalia and echopraxia	295.20	F20.2x[a]
Undifferentiated	Active-phase symptoms without the prominent symptoms of the paranoid, disorganized or catatonic types	295.50	F20.3x[a]
Residual	No prominent active-phase symptoms, no gross disorganization or catatonia. Negative symptoms or attenuated active-phase symptoms may be present	295.60	F20.5x[a]

a: The fifth character 'x' describes the course of schizophrenia: 2 = episodic with interepisode residual symptoms (specify whether there are prominent negative symptoms); 3 = episodic with no interepisode residual symptoms; 0 = continuous (specify whether there are prominent negative symptoms); 4 = single episode in partial remission (specify whether there are prominent negative symptoms); 5 = single episode in full remission; 8 = other or unspecified pattern; 9 = less than 1 year since onset of initial active-phase symptoms.

References

1. Sullivan H, Tentative criteria of malignancy in schizophrenia, *Am J Psychiatry* (1928) **7**:659–782.

2. Bellak L, ed, *Schizophrenia: A Review of the Syndrome* (Logos: New York, 1958).

3. Bellak L, Loeb L, eds, *The Schizophrenia Syndrome* (Grune & Stratton: New York, 1969).

4. Bellak L, ed, *Disorders of the Schizophrenia Syndrome* (Basic Books: New York, 1969).

5. Bleuler E, *Dementia Praecox or the Group of Schizophrenias*, J Zinkin (International Universities Press: New York, 1950).

6. American Psychiatric Association, *The Diagnostic and Statistical Manual of Mental Disorders-IV*, 4th edn (The American Psychiatric Association: Washington DC, 1994).

7. American Psychiatric Association, *The Diagnostic and Statistical Manual of Mental Disorders-III*, 3rd edn (The American Psychiatric Association: Washington DC, 1980).

8. American Psychiatric Association, *The Diagnostic and Statistical Manual of Mental Disorders-IIIR*, 3rd edn revised (The American Psychiatric Association: Washington DC, 1987).

9. World Health Organization, *The ICD-10 Classification of Mental and Behavioral Disorders: Clinical Descriptions and Diagnostic Guidelines* (World Health Organization: Geneva, 1992).

10. Spitzer R, Endicott J, Medical and mental disorder: Proposed definition and criteria. In: Spitzer R, Klein D, eds, *Critical Issues in Psychiatric Diagnosis* (Raven Press: New York, 1978) 15–39.

11. McHugh P, Slavney P, *The Perspectives of Psychiatry* (Johns Hopkins University Press: Baltimore, 1986).

12. Klein D, A proposed definition of mental illness. In: Spitzer RL, Klein DF, eds, *Critical Issues in Psychiatric Diagnosis* (Raven Press: New York, 1978) 41–72.

13. Altschule M, *The Development of Traditional Psychopathology* (John Wiley & Sons: New York, 1976).

14. Kraepelin E, *Dementia Praecox and Paraphrenia* (1919), RM Barclay (Robert E. Krieger: Huntington, NY, 1971).

15. Schneider K, *Clinical Psychopathology*, MW Hamilton (Grune & Stratton: New York, 1959).

16. Carpenter WTJ, Strauss JS, Cross-cultural evaluation of Schneider's first-rank symptoms of schizophrenia: a report from the International Pilot Study of Schizophrenia, *Am J Psychiatry* (1974) **131**:682–7.

17. Langfeldt G, *Schizophrenic States* (Munksgaard: Copenhagen, 1939).

18. Strakowski SM, Diagnostic validity of schizophreniform disorder, *Am J Psychiatry* (1994) **151**:815–24.

19. Kasanin J, The acute schizoaffective psychoses, *Am J Psychiatry* (1933) **13**:97–123.

20. Kety SS, Wender PH, Jacobsen B et al, Mental illness in the biological and adoptive relatives of schizophrenic adoptees. Replication of the Copenhagen Study in the rest of Denmark, *Arch Gen Psychiatry* (1994) **51**:442–55.

21. Cooper JE, Kendell RE, Gurland BJ et al, *Psychiatric Diagnosis in New York and London* (Oxford University Press: London, 1972).

22. Wing JK, Cooper JE, Sartorius N, *Measurement and Classification of Psychiatric Symptoms: An Instructional Manual for the PSE and Catego Program* (Cambridge University Press: London, 1974).

23. Feighner JP, Robins E, Guze SB et al, Diagnostic criteria for use in psychiatric research, *Arch Gen Psychiatry* (1972) **26**:57–63.

24. Crow TJ, Molecular pathology of schizophrenia: more than one disease process? *BMJ* (1980) **280**:66–8.

25. Andreasen N, Positive and negative schizophrenia: a critical evaluation, *Schizophr Bull* (1985) **11**:380–9.

26. Buchanan RW, Breier A, Kirkpatrick B et al, Structural abnormalities in deficit and nondeficit schizophrenia, *Am J Psychiatry* (1993) **150**:59–65.

27. Wyatt RJ, Neuroleptics and the natural course of schizophrenia, *Schizophr Bull* (1991) **17**:325–51.

28. Herz MI, Liberman RP, Lieberman JA et al, Practice guidelines for the treatment of patients with schizophrenia, *Am J Psychiatry* (1997) **154**: Suppl.

29. Frances A, Docherty J, Kahn D, Treatment of schizophrenia, *J Clin Psychiatry* (1996) **27**, [Supplement 12B]:1–58.

30. Flaum M, Amador X, Gorman J et al, DSM-IV Field Trial for Schizophrenia and Other Psychotic Disorders. In: Widiger T, Frances A, Pincus H, eds, *DSM-IV Sourcebook* (American Psychiatric Association: Washington DC, 1998) 687–713.

2

Pathobiology of Schizophrenia: Implications for Clinical Management and Treatment

John L Waddington and Maria M Morgan

Contents • Introduction • The nature of structural brain pathology • The nature of functional brain abnormality • Neuronal network dysfunction • The origin(s) of cerebral abnormalities • Cerebral asymmetry • Heterogeneity or homogeneity? • Lifetime trajectory, clinical management and treatment • Acknowledgements

Introduction

While it can now be stated with some confidence that schizophrenia as defined using contemporary operational criteria is a disorder of abnormal brain structure and function, the nature of the underlying pathobiology at the level of neuronal dysfunction is considerably less clear; the disorder appears to involve not any unitary 'lesion' but, rather, structural and functional abnormalities in one or more neuronal *network(s)*, the nature of which is now beginning to be clarified and the origins of which remain more conjectural but the subject of evolving research and modelling.[1–3] There is particular uncertainty as to how such neuronal dysfunction(s) translate into symptoms, and how these symptoms respond to clinical management and treatment both with antipsychotic drugs (conventional and novel, second-generation agents) and in terms of psychosocial/cognitive-behavioural interventions. This chapter seeks firstly to outline the evidence for, and nature of, abnormalities of brain structure and function in schizophrenia. It then considers the origin(s) and evolution of these abnormalities, and whether schizophrenia is a heterogeneous disorder characterized by diverse origins and pathobiologies that

give rise to overlapping clinical syndromes, or a more homogeneous disorder of common pathobiology that is manifested in clinical diversity. Finally, it considers the interface between pathobiology, clinical management and treatment.

The nature of structural brain pathology

X-ray computed tomography (CT)

Though having by contemporary standards only limited anatomical resolution, the application to schizophrenia of CT as the first of the structural imaging technologies generated a series of landmark quantitative observations[4] that have endured over the emergence of a new generation of imaging modalities. The essential findings were of enlargement of the cerebral ventricles ('ventricular dilatation') with widening of the cerebral cortical sulci ('cortical atrophy'). While these findings had little specificity, they constituted the first 'hard' evidence for structural brain pathology in schizophrenia. Furthermore, within the findings were details whose import can only now be appreciated fully: meta-analysis indicated enlargement of the third ventricle, on the midline, to be more prominent than that of the lateral ventricles, while cortical sulcal widening appeared somewhat more prominent in anterior (frontotemporal) than in posterior (parieto-occipital) regions.[5]

Magnetic resonance imaging (MRI)

Findings deriving from use of CT have been confirmed and elaborated in terms of the substantially greater anatomical resolution of MRI, to identify more circumscribed regions of pathology. The essential profile is of slightly reduced brain size; reduced volume of the temporal lobe and of medial temporal lobe structures, particularly the hippocampus; reduced area of the corpus callosum; and increased volume of the ventricular system. Recent studies indicate also reduced volumes of the thalamus and, in a manner that appears reversed by long-term antipsychotic therapy, of the striatum (caudate nucleus). There is reduced grey matter volume which appears more prominent in frontotemporal than in parieto-occipital areas, while a related technique known as diffusion tensor imaging indicates white matter to evidence reduction not in volume but in integrity.[6–12]

Neuropathology

The most direct approach to clarifying abnormalities of brain structure in schizophrenia is at the neuropathological level, though such directness presents its own methodological problems. Over the same period as applies to the above neuroimaging studies, a new wave of neuropathological investigations indicates the following: morphometric structural studies generally confirm neuroimaging findings of ventricular enlargement, reduced size of medial temporal lobe structures and decreased parahippocampal cortical thickness; morphometric microscopic studies indicate alterations in neuronal density and decreased neuronal size in limbic, temporal, frontal and thalamic regions; further microscopic studies indicate abnormal dendritic spine densities and intrinsic innervations, with abnormalities in

cytoarchitecture, in limbic, temporal and frontal (particularly cingulate) cortices; these abnormalities occur in the absence of any conventional indices of neurodegenerative disease.[13–15]

Overview

These findings show some consistency in indicating structural brain pathology, particularly in temporal and frontal lobe regions, on a background of loss of cortical grey matter along an apparent anterior>posterior gradient and of ventricular enlargement; there is some evidence for abnormalities of the thalamus and striatum. However, the extent to which such structural pathology subserves functional impairment, and the question whether dysfunction can occur in the apparent absence of structural brain pathology, are not addressed by these approaches; that is the realm of functional imaging techniques.

The nature of functional brain abnormality

Positron emission tomography (PET)

This technique, together with the related procedure of single photon emission computed tomography (SPECT), allows visualization and quantification of regional cerebral activity at the levels of blood flow and of glucose metabolism. The most consistent PET findings indicate reduced activity in the frontal and temporolimbic areas on a background of an anterior–posterior gradient in general activation, with some evidence for abnormalities also in the thalamus, striatum and cerebellum.[16,17]

Magnetic resonance spectroscopy (MRS)

In a complementary manner, MRS allows quantification of localized neurochemical processes, focusing particularly on membrane phospholipids, cellular energy metabolism and neuronal integrity. The most consistent findings indicate alterations in frontal lobe phospholipid metabolism and reduced neuronal integrity in the temporal lobe, with a particular focus on abnormalities in the dorsolateral prefrontal and anterior cingulate cortices and hippocampus.[18,19]

Functional magnetic resonance imaging (fMRI)

The most recent of the functional imaging techniques quantitates changes in regional blood oxygenation related to neuronal activity. While in its relative infancy, fMRI is of substantial potential particularly for studying cortical responses in relation to aspects of psychopathology and cognition; for example patients with schizophrenia show abnormal temporal lobe function during speech, and during auditory hallucinations.[20]

Overview

Findings from functional imaging studies appear in some concordance with those deriving from structural imaging. They indicate neuronal dysfunction in the frontal and temporal lobes, particularly dorsolateral prefrontal and anterior cingulate cortices and hippocampus, with some involvement of the thalamus, striatum and cerebellum.

Neuronal network dysfunction

While these regional abnormalities of structure and function may appear superficially to implicate diverse brain regions, they involve important elements in well-recognized or putative neuronal circuits that perform integrative functions by which information is relayed, filtered, processed, stored, recalled, co-ordinated and responded to; it is these same functions, which subserve thinking and perception, and bestow individuality and self-direction, that appear to be disturbed in schizophrenia at phenomenological and neuropsychological levels. One of the major advantages of functional imaging techniques is their ability to relate biological abnormalities to aspects of psychopathology and cognition, not just during resting conditions but also in relation to changes

in symptomatological experiences and to cognitive tasks which place demand on specific neuropsychological functions and their cerebral substrates. To take one example:[21] psychomotor poverty (negative symptoms) appears to be associated with abnormal activity in the dorsolateral prefrontal and anterior cingulate cortex, in the striatum, and in the posterior association cortex; disorganization (thought disorder) with abnormal activity in the prefrontal and anterior cingulate cortex, and in the dorsomedial thalamus; reality distortion (hallucinations and delusions) with abnormal activity in the parahippocampal region and striatum. More specifically, synthesis of the findings to date implicates disordered connectivity in frontostriatopallidothalamocortical, frontotemporal, and/or frontocerebellar-thalamic neuronal networks.[21–23]

The origin(s) of cerebral abnormalities

Given the weight of evidence for such network abnormalities of brain structure and function in schizophrenia, a fundamental question then arises: do these abnormalities reflect a brain that was once normal but became subject to some later pathological process, or do they reflect a brain whose early development was compromised in some way so as to preclude the establishment of normal cerebral structure and function? It will be appreciated that these alternatives constitute radically different routes to those current cerebral abnormalities that are usually determined in adult patients having an established pattern of illness; furthermore, they have radically different implications for aetiology and for lifetime course of illness.

'Read-back' analysis

Construction of a reverse time-line for schizophrenia, in the manner of a 'read-back' analysis, indicates firstly that most if not all of the brain abnormalities commonly identified in patients having an established illness are already evident in individuals experiencing their first episode of illness, at the onset of psychotic symptoms;[24-26] it then proceeds through childhood psychosocial impairments to infant neurointegrative deficits, to terminate in the intrauterine period.[27-30] Neuropathological studies indicate that structural brain pathology, even with prominent negative (deficit) symptoms and marked cognitive impairment, occurs in the absence of abnormalities typical of any neurodegenerative process; rather, structural abnormalities appear to involve cytoarchitectural features more indicative of disruption in brain growth over fetal life.[13-15,23] Though recent studies have failed consistently to replicate what were offered initially as characteristic cytoarchitectural abnormalities in medial temporal lobe structures,[14,28] other findings, particularly those in the anterior cingulate cortex, have proved more robust.[21,22,28] While MRI cannot resolve cytoarchitecture, it does reveal some anatomical abnormalities that have their origin over fetal life, such as cavum septum pellucidum; this abnormality is indicative of disturbance in the early growth of midline structures, and occurs in association with reduced volume of the hippocampus.[31,32]

Main craniofacial dysmorphology

Taken together, epidemiological and biological findings sustain initial formulations of schizophrenia as a neurodevelopmental disorder,[33,34] and elaborate the disease as having its origin(s) in disturbance(s) of intrauterine brain development.[28] However, more accessible, direct indices of such events have been needed. Over early fetal life, cerebral morphogenesis proceeds in exquisite embryological intimacy with craniofacial morphogenesis, such that classic neurodevelopmental disorders (such as Down's syndrome) are well recognized to evidence dysmorphic features which involve the body in general and the craniofacies in particular; these can range in severity from major congenital malformations to minor physical anomalies (MPAs), and constitute biological markers of late first/early second trimester dysgenesis.[27]

Several studies now indicate MPAs to occur to excess in patients with schizophrenia, particularly very subtle dysmorphology of the craniofacial area. Though heightening of the palate is one of the most consistent findings, the topography of MPAs in schizophrenia has been poorly understood; yet such information is fundamental to understanding the timing and nature of the dysmorphic event(s).[27,28] Recently, on applying an anthropometric approach, patients with schizophrenia were found to show multiple minor quantitative abnormalities and qualitative anomalies of craniofacial and other structures.[35]

Cerebral asymmetry

A considerable body of evidence indicates that in schizophrenia the normal pattern of gender-related left–right structural and functional brain asymmetry is disturbed in the direction of reduced asymmetry, in a manner that interacts with gender and possibly age at onset; there is a particular focus on loss of asymmetry in the left posterior superior temporal lobe (planum temporale; Wernicke's area) and left frontal lobe (Broca's area) and its putative relationship to language processing and production.[36,37] Evidence now suggests that dorsal midline cells are fundamental in the embryology of left–right development, with these midline events dependent upon anterior–posterior level;[38] furthermore, it should be noted that lateralized behaviour in the human fetus can be noted as early as 10–12 weeks and reaches its peak by 15–18 weeks of gestation.[39] On this basis, cerebral dysmorphogenesis affecting particularly anterior and midline structures over weeks 9/10 through 14/15[27,28] would be predicted to result in disturbance(s) of cerebral asymmetry.

Heterogeneity or homogeneity?

It is self-evident that schizophrenia is characterized by diversity in phenomenology and outcome, with no known psychological or biological index pathognomonic of the disorder; such a perspective underpins the common presumption that schizophrenia is a heterogeneous, syndromic disorder whereby diverse aetiologies and pathophysiologies are associated with some commonality of dysfunction and psychopathology. However, there is now a substantial body of evidence to contradict the presumption that ventricular enlargement, the most robust biological finding in schizophrenia, is present in some but not all patients with this disease; on the contrary, ventricular size is characterized by a unimodal distributional shift to the right (increased ventricular size) in the disorder, with each patient, even those well within the control range, having ventricles that are larger than would have been the case had schizophrenia not emerged in that person.[40]

Proceeding again with the 'read-back' analysis outlined above, both premorbid IQ and childhood educational test scores appear characterized by a unimodal distributional shift to the left (poorer attainment) for those in whom schizophrenia emerged subsequently, relative to those in whom it did not.[41,42] Thus, the resultant profile in schizophrenia is one not of heterogeneity but, rather, of homogeneity of effect.[27,28]

Lifetime trajectory, clinical management and treatment

The prominence of developmental arguments in the origin(s) of schizophrenia has engendered much controversy in relation to how such early events might lead to the emergence of diagnostic symptoms of psychosis only some two decades later, and the extent to which the disorder might progress thereafter.[1–3,27,28] It is important that early cerebrocraniofacial dysmorphogenesis is not misinterpreted as precluding any role for later events in determining overall course of illness or any subsequent progressive process. A brain that has been already compromised in fetal life will still be subject to the normal endogenous programme of developmental, maturational and involutional processes on which a variety of exogenous biological insults and psychosocial

stressors can impact adversely through infancy and childhood, to maturation and into old age, to sculpt both the structure and the (dys)function of the brain; furthermore, the effects of such endogenous programmes and exogenous insults on a brain already compromised early in development may be different from their effects on a brain whose fetal life proceeded essentially undisturbed.[27,28]

On this basis, a lifetime trajectory for schizophrenia might be as follows:[27,28] cerebral dysmorphogenesis, particularly along the midline and having an anterior>posterior gradient, gives rise to neuronal network dysfunction; these early brain abnormalities are associated with evolving neurointegrative deficits over the (mal)developmental course of infancy and, sequentially, with evolving psychosocial impairments over the (mal)developmental course of childhood;[27–30] thereafter, increasing recognition of neurointegrative and psychosocial deficits over the later (mal)developmental course towards early adulthood leads to their reconceptualization as cognitive impairment, and particularly as negative symptoms which appear to precede and augur the onset of psychosis;[27,43] psychosis emerges only on the functional maturation of cerebral systems/processes necessary for the underlying neuronal network dysfunction to be so expressed,[27,34] with the threshold for onset being modulated also by exogenous biological factors and psychosocial stressors; the onset of psychosis appears to reflect crudescence of some active morbid process, increasing duration of which is associated, at least in part, with increasingly poor outcome;[44–46] subsequent course of illness may therefore be modulated, at least in part, by the timeliness and effectiveness of intervention with antipsychotics to ameliorate this process following the onset of psychosis, and of psychosocial interventions to rescue, conserve and promote functioning, over what appears to be a critically maleable phase of early psychotic illness;[27,47,48] both over this phase and thereafter, there is now evidence for some longitudinal progression in structural brain pathology beyond that determined in early fetal life, the distribution of which does not deviate from unimodality in a manner consistent with a variable though homogeneous process;[49–51] negative symptoms and cognitive impairment can accrue in severity and adverse prognostic weight over later phases of illness, the course of which may continue to be influenced by the long-term effectiveness of antipsychotic medication and psychosocial interventions, but on a background of interactions with maturational and involutional processes.[27]

Such lifetime trajectory perspectives[27,28,48,52–54] offer a more parsimonious way forward in conceptualizing the pathobiology of schizophrenia beyond its putative fragmentation into 'neurodevelopmental' *or* 'neuroprogressive' entities;[55] but how might such pathobiology account more specifically for the effects of treatment? Though all antipsychotic drugs utilized to date, including novel, second-generation agents, share at least some action to block brain dopamine (DA) receptors, primarily those of the D_2-like family, it has proved difficult to identify pathophysiology in either dopaminergic neurons or receptors. However, evidence has become available recently for increased release of subcortical DA in schizophrenia under conditions of stressor challenge and in association with heightening of psychotic symptoms.[56] Recent evidence indicates also that in studies involving both patients with schizophrenia and non-human primates with developmental lesions of the medial temporal lobe,[57] greater pathology in the dorsolateral prefrontal cortex as indexed by MRS is associated by SPECT with attenuated subcortical dopaminergic activity under basal conditions but enhanced dopaminergic activity, with accentuation of psychotic symptoms, following stressor challenge.

These findings suggest that developmental pathology in temporofrontal circuitry in schizophrenia could give rise to reduction in tonic but heightening of phasic subcortical dopaminergic activity in relation to psychopathology. Furthermore, such dysregulation of dopaminergic func-

tion might contribute through a process of 'neurochemical sensitization' to the emergence of psychosis which, if persistent or recurrent, might progress to enduring morbidity, treatment resistance and clinical deterioration;[58] it should be noted that DA can induce apoptosis, whereby a conserved cell suicide programme is activated, with resultant cellular condensation, fragmentation and elimination of cell fragments through phagocytosis, in the absence of substantive inflammatory or gliotic reaction.[27] Finally, as is self-evident, dopaminergic neurons do not function in isolation. In particular, much current interest focuses on the interactions between DA and glutamate to influence each other's function. This intimacy between these two transmitters, together with a body of evidence for pathology in glutamatergic systems and for clinical pharmacological effects of glutamatergic agents,[59] indicates broader avenues for exploring the pathobiology and treatment of schizophrenia.

Acknowledgements

The authors' studies are supported by the Stanley Foundation.

References

1. Waddington JL, Schizophrenia: developmental neuroscience and pathobiology, *Lancet* (1993) **341:** 531–6.

2. Weinberger DR, Schizophrenia: from neuropathology to neurodevelopment, *Lancet* (1995) **346:** 552–7.

3. Schultz K, Andreasen NC, Schizophrenia, *Lancet* (1999) **353:**1425–30.

4. Johnstone EC, Crow TJ, Frith CD et al, Cerebral ventricular size and cognitive impairment in chronic schizophrenia, *Lancet* (1976) **ii:**924–6.

5. Raz S, Raz N, Structural brain abnormalities in the major psychoses: a quantitative review of the evidence from computerized imaging, *Psychol Bull* (1990) **108:**93–108.

6. Woodruff PWR, McManus IC, David AS, Meta-

analysis of corpus callosum size in schizophrenia, *J Neurol Neurosurg Psychiatry* (1995) **58**:457–61.

7. Ward EK, Friedman L, Wise A, Schulz SC, Meta-analysis of brain and cranial size in schizophrenia, *Schizophr Res* (1996) **22**:197–213.

8. Lawrie SM, Abukmeil SS, Brain abnormality in schizophrenia: a systematic and quantitative review of volumetric magnetic resonance imaging studies, *Br J Psychiatry* (1998) **172**:110–20.

9. Nelson MD, Saykin AJ, Flashman LA, Riordan HF, Hippocampal volume reduction in schizophrenia as assessed by magnetic resonance imaging, *Arch Gen Psychiatry* (1998) **55**:433–40.

10. Sullivan EV, Lim KO, Mathalon D et al, A profile of cortical gray matter volume deficits characteristic of schizophrenia, *Cereb Cortex* (1998) **8**:117–24.

11. Keshavan MS, Rosenberg D, Sweeney JA, Pettegrew JW, Decreased caudate volume in neuroleptic-naive psychotic patients, *Am J Psychiatry* (1998) **155**:774–8.

12. Lim KO, Hedehus M, Moseley M et al, Compromised white matter tract integrity in schizophrenia inferred from diffusion tensor imaging, *Arch Gen Psychiatry* (1999) **56**:367–74.

13. Arnold SE, Trojanowski JQ, Recent advances in defining the neuropathology of schizophrenia, *Acta Neuropathol* (1996) **92**:217–31.

14. Dwork AJ, Postmortem studies of the hippocampal formation in schizophrenia, *Schizophr Bull* (1997) **23**: 385–402.

15. Heckers S, Neuropathology of schizophrenia: cortex, thalamus, basal ganglia and neurotransmitter-specific projection systems, *Schizophr Bull* (1997) **23**:403–21.

16. Andreasen NC, O'Leary DS, Cizadlo T et al, Schizophrenia and cognitive dysmetria: a positron-emission tomography study of dysfunctional prefrontal-thalamic-cerebellar circuitry, *Proc Natl Acad Sci USA* (1996) **93**:9985–90.

17. Buchsbaum MS, Hazlett EA, Positron emission tomography studies of abnormal glucose metabolism in schizophrenia, *Schizophr Bull* (1998) **24**:343–64.

18. Bertolino A, Nawroz S, Mattay VS et al, Regionally specific pattern of neurochemical pathology in schizophrenia as assessed by multislice proton magnetic resonance spectroscopic imaging, *Am J Psychiatry* (1996) **153**:1554–63.

19. Kegeles LS, Humaran TJ, Mann JJ, In vivo neurochemistry of the brain in schizophrenia as revealed by magnetic resonance spectroscopy, *Biol Psychiatry* (1998) **44**:382–98.

20. Woodruff PWR, Wright IC, Bullmore ET et al, Auditory hallucinations and the temporal cortical response to speech in schizophrenia: a functional magnetic resonance imaging study, *Am J Psychiatry* (1997) **154**:1676–82.

21. Liddle PF, Friston J, Frith CD et al, Patterns of cerebral blood flow in schizophrenia, *Br J Psychiatry* (1992) **160**:179–86.

22. Benes FM, What an archaeological dig can tell us about macro- and microcircuitry in brains of schizophrenia subjects, *Schizophr Bull* (1997) **23**:503–7.

23. Andreasen NC, Paradiso S, O'Leary DS, 'Cognitive dysmetria' as an integrative theory of schizophrenia: a dysfunction in cortical-subcortical-cerebellar circuitry? *Schizophr Bull* (1998) **24**:203–18.

24. Andreasen NC, O'Leary DS, Flaum M et al, Hypofrontality in schizophrenia: distributed dysfunctional circuits in neuroleptic-naive patients, *Lancet* (1997) **349**:1730–4.

25. Velakoulis D, Pantelis C, McGorry PD et al, Hippocampal volume in first-episode psychoses and chronic schizophrenia: a high-resolution magnetic resonance imaging study, *Arch Gen Psychiatry* (1999) **56**:133–40.

26. Cecil KM, Lenkinski RE, Gur RE, Gur RC, Proton magnetic resonance spectroscopy in the frontal and temporal lobes of neuroleptic naive patients with schizophrenia, *Neuropsychopharmacology* (1999) **20**: 131–40.

27. Waddington JL, Lane A, Scully PJ et al, Neurodevelopmental and neuroprogressive processes in schizophrenia, *Psychiatr Clin North Am* (1998) **21**:123–49.

28. Waddington JL, Lane A, Larkin C, O'Callaghan E, The neurodevelopmental basis of schizophrenia: clinical clues from cerebro-craniofacial dysmorphogenesis, and the roots of a lifetime trajectory of disease, *Biol Psychiatry* (1999) **46**:31–39.

29. Hultman CM, Sparen P, Takei N et al, Prenatal and perinatal risk factors for schizophrenia, affective psychosis, and reactive psychosis of early onset, *BMJ* (1999) **318**:421–6.

30. Mortensen PB, Pedersen CB, Westergaard T et al, Effects of family history and place and season of

birth on the risk of schizophrenia, *N Engl J Med* (1999) **340**:603–8.

31. Nopoulos P, Swayze V, Flaum M et al, Cavum septi pellucidi in normals and patients with schizophrenia as detected by magnetic resonance imaging, *Biol Psychiatry* (1997) **41**:1102–8.

32. Kwon JS, Shenton ME, Hirayasu Y et al, MRI study of cavum septi pellucidi in schizophrenia, affective disorder and schizotypal personality disorder, *Am J Psychiatry* (1998) **155**:509–15.

33. Murray RM, Lewis SW, Is schizophrenia a neurodevelopmental disorder? *BMJ* (1987) **295**:681–2.

34. Weinberger DR, Implications of normal brain development for the pathogenesis of schizophrenia, *Arch Gen Psychiatry* (1987) **44**:660–9.

35. Lane A, Kinsella A, Murphy P et al, The anthropometric assessment of dysmorphic features in schizophrenia as an index of its developmental origins, *Psychol Med* (1997) **27**:1155–64.

36. DeLisi LE, Sakuma M, Kushner M et al, Anomalous cerebral asymmetry and language processing in schizophrenia, *Schizophr Bull* (1997) **23**:255–271.

37. Petty RG, Structural asymmetries of the human brain and their disturbance in schizophrenia, *Schizophr Bull* (1999) **25**:121–39.

38. Yost HJ, Left–right development from embryos to brains, *Dev Genet* (1998) **23**:159–63.

39. McCartney G, Hepper P, Development of lateralized behaviour in the human fetus from 12 to 27 weeks gestation, *Dev Med Child Neurol* (1999) **41**:83–6.

40. Daniel DG, Goldberg TE, Gibbons RD, Weinberger DR, Lack of a bimodal distribution of ventricular size in schizophrenia: a Gaussian mixture analysis of 1056 cases and controls, *Biol Psychiatry* (1991) **30**:887–903.

41. Davis AS, Malmberg A, Brandt L et al, IQ and risk for schizophrenia: a population-based cohort study, *Psychol Med* (1997) **27**:1311–23.

42. Jones PB, Rogers B, Murray R, Marmot M, Child developmental risk factors for adult schizophrenia in the British 1946 birth cohort, *Lancet* (1994) **344**: 1398–1402.

43. Hafner H, an der Heiden W, Behrens S et al, Causes and consequences of the gender difference in age at onset of schizophrenia, *Schizophr Bull* (1998) **24**: 99–113.

44. Wyatt RJ, Neuroleptics and the natural course of schizophrenia, *Schizophr Bull* (1991) **17**:325–51.

45. Loebel AD, Lieberman JA, Alvir JMJ et al, Duration of psychosis and outcome in first-episode schizophrenia, *Am J Psychiatry* (1992) **149**:1183–8.

46. Scully PJ, Coakley G, Kinsella A, Waddington JL, Psychopathology, executive (frontal) and general cognitive impairment in relation to duration of initially untreated vs subsequently treated psychosis in chronic schizophrenia, *Psychol Med* (1997) **27**: 1303–10.

47. Birchwood M, McGorry P, Jackson H, Early intervention in schizophrenia, *Br J Psychiatry* (1997) **170**:2–5.

48. Waddington JL, Buckley PF, Scully PJ et al, Course of psychopathology, cognition and neurobiological abnormality in schizophrenia: developmental origins and amelioration by antipsychotics? *J Psychiatr Res* (1998) **32**:179–89.

49. DeLisi LE, Sakuma M, Tew W et al, Schizophrenia as a chronic active brain process: a study of progressive brain structural change subsequent to the onset of schizophrenia, *Psychiatry Res: Neuroimaging* (1997) **74**:129–40.

50. Grimson R, Hoff Al, DeLisi LE, Schizophrenia as a chronic active brain process, *Psychiatry Res: Neuroimaging* (1997) **76**:135–8.

51. Davis KL, Buchsbaum MS, Shihabuddin L et al, Ventricular enlargement in poor-outcome schizophrenia, *Biol Psychiatry* (1998) **43**:783–93.

52. DeLisi LE, Is schizophrenia a lifetime disorder of brain plasticity, growth and aging? *Schizophr Res* (1997) **23**:119–29.

53. Waddington JL, Scully PJ, Youssef HA, Developmental trajectory and disease progression in schizophrenia: the conundrum, and insights from a 12-year prospective study in the Monaghan 101, *Schizophr Res* (1997) **23**:107–18.

54. Woods BT, Is schizophrenia a progressive neurodevelopmental disorder? Toward a unitary pathogenetic mechanism, *Am J Psychiatry* (1998) **155**: 1661–70.

55. Knoll JL, Garver DL, Ramberg JE et al, Heterogeneity of the psychoses: is there a neurodegenerative psychosis? *Schizophr Bull* (1998) **24**:365–79.

56. Abi-Dargham A, Gil R, Krystal J et al, Increased striatal dopamine transmission in schizophrenia: confirmation in a second cohort, *Am J Psychiatry* (1998) **155**:761–7.

57. Bertolino A, Knable MB, Saunders RC et al, The

relationship between dorsolateral prefrontal *n*-acetyl-aspartate measures and striatal dopamine activity in schizophrenia, *Biol Psychiatry* (1999) **45:**660–7.

58. Lieberman JA, Sheitman BB, Kinon BJ, Neurochemical sensitization in the pathophysiology of schizo-phrenia: deficits and dysfunction in neuronal regulation and plasticity, *Neuropsychopharmacology* (1997) **17:**205–29.

59. Tamminga CA, Schizophrenia and glutamatergic transmission, *Crit Rev Neurobiol* (1998) **12:**21–36.

3

The Outcome of Psychotic Illness

Jane Kelly, Robin M Murray and Jim van Os

Contents • Introduction • Prognostic factors • An empirical model of outcome, symptom dimensions and risk factors for psychosis • Management implications • Conclusion

Introduction

'What will happen to our son? Will he be able to have a normal life? Will he get ill again? Will he end up in an institution?' All psychiatrists will be familiar with the questions asked by the relatives and partners of patients suffering their first episode of psychosis. And all psychiatrists will be familiar with the difficulty in giving an honest and yet reassuring answer or indeed in knowing themselves the likely outcome. What knowledge do we have that can help us formulate an answer?

Contribution of the early outcome studies

The early United States and European long-term follow-up studies made it possible for the first time to quantify the variability of outcome in schizophrenia and related psychoses. Although these studies defy simple summary because of differences in the length of follow-up and in the definition of terms such as 'recovery', 'relapse', and 'unimproved',[1,2] there is no doubt that the course and outcome of psychotic illness is extremely variable.[3,4] Table 3.1 summarizes data from key studies that recruited patients at diagnosis or first hospitalization. Most studies found that variation of clinical outcome could be described accurately in three or four categories of severity, both in the

short and longer term. Although finer distinctions have been offered, the general rule that the proportion of patients showing poor, intermediate and good outcome is each around 30% seems to fit the published data reasonably.

Another important finding of the early studies was that within the group of functional psychoses, patients with a diagnosis of schizophrenia have the poorest outcome, with schizoaffective patients occupying an intermediate position between schizophrenia and affective psychosis. For example, Tsuang and Dempsey,[5] in a 30- to 40-year longitudinal study, showed that outcome for a group of 85 patients exhibiting both affective and schizophrenic features was significantly poorer compared to a group of 325 patients with affective disorders, selected by the criteria of Feighner and colleagues,[6] and significantly better than in a group of 200 schizophrenic patients. Coryell and colleagues[7,8] showed that affective psychotic disorders have a less disabling course than schizoaffective disorders. Grossman and collaborators showed that, overall, schizophrenic patients had poorest outcome, followed by schizoaffective patients, bipolar manic, and unipolar depressive patients.[9] Similar findings were reported by Brockington and colleagues,[10,11] Marneros and collaborators[12,13] and Maj and Perris.[14] Longer-term retrospective studies have yielded similar

Table 3.1 Classic follow-up studies that recruited patients at diagnosis or first admission.

Ref.	Length of FU	Level of clinical outcome (percentages in rows do not always add up to 100%)		
		Poor	Intermediate	Good
Müller (1951)[15]	30	41% insidious chronic course	17% phasic recurrent course without change to chronicity	33% recovered or substantially improved; 16% recovered throughout follow-up
Stephens (1978)[2]	5–16	30% unimproved	46% improved	24% recovered
Bland and Orn (1978)[16]	14	25% were socially, psychiatrically and occupationally disabled	25% had moderate to marked disability	Half the patients were managing well with little or no disability
Ciompi (1980)[17]	37	18% severe chronic illness	46% slight to moderate residual states	27% remitted completely
Salokangas (1983)[18]	7.5–8	24% continuous psychotic symptoms	29% occasional mild psychotic symptoms, 21% neurotic symptoms	
Sartorius et al (1986)[19]	2	40% unremitting psychotic symptoms	21% periodic relapse	40% one episode of psychosis, no or minimal symptoms at follow-up
Rabiner et al (1986)[20]	1	22% continuous symptoms over follow-up	22% relapse	56% remission
SSRG (1989)[21]	2	38% showed schizophrenic symptoms at follow-up	47% had been readmitted to hospital at at some time over the 2 years	37% were well
Shepherd et al (1989)[22]	5	43% remained impaired over follow-up.	35% recurrent episodes with increasing impairment	22% no relapse

results.[23,24] Thus, rather than discrete qualitative differences in outcome, there appears to be a 'dose-response' relationship between degree of affective symptomatology and outcome. Kendell and Brockington[25] specifically tried to disprove the existence of such a linear relationship, but failed.

Another aspect that has been brought forward is that outcome is not measurable on a single scale. Rather, it is a multidimensional concept, with clinical and social domains of illness course and outcome.[26] For example, a factor analysis of 21 outcome measures from a large study of patients with recent-onset psychosis was carried out in one study, with the aim of identifying the underlying outcome dimensions. This technique identified six factors which were: (1) severity of psychotic symptoms over the follow-up period, (2) negative symptoms and social functioning, (3) employment, (4) time living independently, (5) vagrancy and imprisonment, (6) depression and self-harm.[27] More recently, need for care, subjective quality of life and satisfaction with services from the sufferer's perspective are increasingly included in outcome studies.[28]

Prediction of outcome varies as a function of length of follow-up. Some studies follow up patients for 1 or 2 years,[29-31] others do so for two or more decades.[17,32-35] There is evidence that the greatest variability in illness is to be found in the first 5–10 years of illness,[36,37] after which less fluctuation in course can be expected, although substantial changes very late in the course may not be infrequent.[32,38,39] Furthermore, with the progression of time, a large group of patients becomes increasingly impaired with each subsequent episode. More than a third of patients developed such states of increasing impairment in the first 5 years of illness in a carefully conducted study of a sample of 49 representative incident cases of schizophrenia.[22] Longer-term studies suggest that this percentage further increases over the next 10 years, but McGlashan[3] has pointed out that the deterioration then tends to 'bottom out', and is in fact not infrequently followed by a phase of late

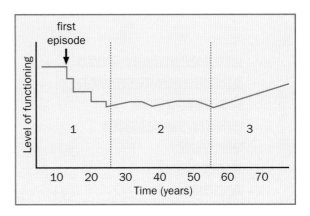

Figure 3.1 Hypothesized 'common' illness course trajectory showing initial stepwise decline with each episode (1), followed by a 'plateau' phase (2), and late improvement (3). (After Breier et al.[40])

improvement.[32,38,39,41,42] This state of affairs is depicted in Figure 3.1 after Breier and colleagues.[40] It follows that the stage of the illness is of crucial importance to the prediction that one is trying to make. For example, if one is trying to predict 5-year course during the 'plateau' phase, one may expect little fluctuation. Very late in the illness one may actually expect some degree of improvement. The greatest challenge for prediction lies in the early course of the illness, which some refer to as the 'critical period'.[43] It is hoped that altering the short-term course, for example by reducing the number of relapses, will reduce the overall level of deterioration.

Finally, there are some elements in the prediction of outcome that have clearly changed with time. For one outcome, namely discharge from the psychiatric hospital, there is a clear historical trend towards improvement (Figure 3.2). Another important historical trend is that related to diagnosis. A review of the literature, in which 320 follow-up studies from 1895 to 1992 were surveyed, found that outcome was significantly better in patients diagnosed according to systems with

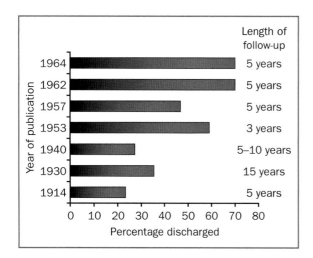

Figure 3.2 Percentage discharged at follow-up as a function of time.[44-50]

broad criteria or undefined criteria (46.5% and 41.0% were 'improved' respectively), as compared to systems with narrow criteria (27.3% improved). A decline in the reported rate of favourable outcomes over the past decade was also ascribed to shifts in diagnostic criteria.[51] This study highlights the fact that the results of all schizophrenia follow-up studies are highly dependent on the diagnostic construct used. For example, follow-up studies using 'intuitively' defined schizophrenia according to ICD-9 or the older 'broad' concept of DSM-II on average yield prognostically more favourable results than those using the more restrictive criteria of the later DSM series.[52]

Contribution of more recent studies
More recent studies have examined in great details and with methodological rigor, the influence of a range of demographic, social, psychological and biological prognostic factors (see below). The more recent studies also concur in having their focus on the years after the first episode of psychosis, and on mixing samples of patients with affective, schizoaffective, schizophrenic and atypical syndromes rather than a single diagnostic category. Indeed, an American commentator, reviewing the long-term outcome literature, concluded that 'until significant progress is made in reducing the heterogeneity of schizophrenia, its criteria should err in the direction of inclusiveness'.[3] For example, a recent study reported on 75 cases of possible psychotic illness whose symptomatology had been inadequate for the patients to enter a functional psychosis study, because the symptoms were partial or transient. These patients were compared at follow-up with those who fulfilled operational criteria for schizophrenic, affective or schizoaffective psychoses. Differences between the 'partial' cases and those fulfilling specific diagnostic criteria were few, but the transient cases had more favourable outcomes. Although the transient illnesses were recurrent, at 2.5-year follow-up they appeared to have a good social and psychopathological outcome.[53]

Although many outcome studies did establish that there are *mean* differences in outcome between patients with affective, non-affective and transient psychotic illness, the overall contribution of diagnosis to prediction is limited. For example, Johnstone and colleagues[54] found diagnostic classification only of limited value in predicting outcome in the functional psychoses, and similar results were reported from recent US studies.[55,56] Given the poor predictive validity of psychotic diagnoses, more recent studies have taken a different approach, in that they do not examine how different clusters of *cases* contribute to outcome variation, but rather how clusters of *symptoms* relate to course and outcome. Clusters of symptoms are referred to as symptom dimensions, and within the group of affective and non-affective psychoses, four or five main dimensions have been identified (Table 3.2). Thus, in dimensional studies, each patient is allocated a score on positive, negative, depressive and manic symptoms, and relationships between symptom scores and outcome are examined. Recent studies have proven this to be an effective approach with regard to prediction of outcome. In one study of

Table 3.2 Dimensions of psychosis – results of recent large studies.			
Kitamura et al (1995)[57]	van Os et al (1996)[27]	McGorry et al (1998)[58]	van Os et al (1999)[28]
Positive	Positive	Positive	Positive
Manic	Manic	Manic	Manic
Depressive	Depressive	Depressive	Depressive
Negative	Negative	Negative/	Negative
Catatonic	Catatonic/	Catatonic/	
	Disorganization	Disorganization	
(n = 584)	(n = 166)	(n = 509)	(n = 708)

166 patients with recent-onset psychotic illness, a dimensional representation of psychopathology proved to be a more informative predictor of 4-year social and clinical outcomes than the traditional categorical DSM and ICD classifications.[27] One reason for the superior predictive power of symptom dimensions is that they are more informative with regard to treatment needs at baseline. Thus, in a study of 708 patients with psychotic illness, a dimensional representation of psychopathology was more informative for clinicians with regard to the patients' treatment needs than DSM, RDC or ICD categories of psychotic illness such as affective psychosis, schizoaffective psychosis, unspecified psychosis, schizophreniform psychosis, delusional disorder and schizophrenia.[28] In a 2-year follow-up of this sample of 708 patients, it was shown that reductions in these psychopathological dimensions contributed to clinically significant reductions in a range of clinical and psychosocial treatment needs.[59]

Scope of this chapter

In the sections below, an attempt is made to combine the information from the early and more recent follow-up studies into a model of prediction based on prognostic risk factors across the most important dimensions of psychosis. Given that the recent work concentrates on these issues early in the course of psychotic illness, the focus of this chapter will be mainly on the first 5–10 years.

Prognostic factors

Prognostic significance of variables that are also known to increase the risk of onset of psychosis
Familial morbid risk
Having a first-degree relative with a psychotic illness is possibly the best established risk factor for schizophrenia,[60] but relatives of patients with schizophrenia also have an increased risk of depressive disorder.[61] There has been considerable interest in the relation between family history and outcome. Many studies have shown an association between a family history of affective psychosis and a good outcome in schizophrenia. Fowler and colleagues[62] compared 28 good- and 25 poor-prognosis schizophrenic patients and interviewed their relatives mostly blind to proband outcome status. Of the 126 first-degree relatives in the poor-prognosis group, 13 had schizophrenia; in the good-prognosis group the prevalence of schizophrenia was much lower (5 out of 137; risk ratio [RR] = 0.6; 95% CI = 0.5–0.9 – our calculations from the data provided). The risk for affective disorder (bipolar and unipolar depressive disorders) was lower in the poor outcome group, although this just failed

to reach statistical significance (RR = 0.4; 95% CI 0.2–1.1 – our calculations from the data provided). The largest study to date was by Kendler and Tsuang,[63] who examined outcome and familial psychopathology in a sample of 253 DSM-III schizophrenics and their 723 first-degree relatives. Morbid risk of non-affective psychotic disorder was higher in the relatives of poor-outcome probands, more so at short-term outcome than at long-term outcome, although for both periods this failed to reach statistical significance. Morbid risk of affective illness was significantly higher in relatives of good-outcome patients both at short-term and long-term follow-up.

A well-designed study by Verdoux and colleagues[64] looked for associations between familial loading (taking into account age, sex and number of relatives) and 4-year outcome in 150 patients with recent-onset functional psychotic disorder. They found that familial loading for psychotic disorder predicted persistent negative symptoms and was associated with more time in hospital and more social disability. The effect of familial loading for psychosis was greater in the group of patients with a diagnosis of schizophrenia than in patients with non-schizophrenic psychoses. Thus, there is some evidence to suggest that poor-outcome disorders with high levels of negative symptoms may breed true within families.[65]

Obstetric complications

There is good evidence that some cases of schizophrenia can be considered as the consequence of pre- and perinatal complications.[66,67] However, less is known about the relationship between obstetric complications and outcome of psychosis. One study did not find an association between presence of obstetric complications and poor treatment response, although the direction of the association was positive.[68] A 5-year follow-up of first-episode patients looked for a relationship between treatment response and obstetric complications in 59 people with their first episode of schizophrenia and schizoaffective disorder. Obstetric history was based on mothers' recall

alone in 44% of cases and supplemented with birth records in the rest of the sample. One-fifth of the sample had positive histories of 'clearly potentially harmful' events, such as early bleeding, very prolonged labour and asphyxia. This group had lower rates of treatment response over the follow-up (mean 225 weeks),[56,69] though obstetric complications did not predict relapse.[55] The effect of obstetric complications on treatment response was statistically independent of the effect of enlarged lateral ventricles and symptoms of disorganization. Two studies have suggested that there may be a link between obstetric complications, early onset of illness and poor outcome. Thus, patients with an early onset were more likely to have a history of obstetric complications in one study,[70,71] and additionally showed a poor response to antipsychotic treatment in another.[71] In the largest study to date, the medical histories of a group of 511 patients hospitalized for schizophrenia were examined for the occurrence of perinatal distress. In the context of a 40-year follow-up, 200 schizophrenia patients with a chronic illness course were compared with 311 cases with good prognosis. A history of perinatal distress was much more common in the poor prognosis group than in the good prognosis group.[72] The combined results of the above studies strongly suggest that fetal hypoxia is associated with treatment non-response, which is possibly mediated by permanent receptor or pathway damage.

Poor premorbid adjustment

Children who go on to develop a psychotic illness have more social deficits than control populations, more so than do children destined to develop affective disorder.[73–75] There is considerable evidence from retrospective studies that premorbid dysfunction is also one of the most important risk factors for poor outcome and a less favourable illness course.[76–78] Premorbid adjustment in most of the earlier studies was not assessed in a structured way, and information was derived from sources of widely varying reliability, and always retrospective. Later studies used better instruments, such as the Premorbid Adjustment Scale (PAS),[69] which assesses premorbid social and role functioning during childhood, early adolescence, late adolescence and adulthood in a more structured way, though still retrospectively. Better-designed prospective studies have also reported associations between premorbid dysfunction and a range of social and clinical outcomes.[20,55,80] Of the different symptom dimensions at follow-up, associations are clearly strongest with negative symptoms.[40,81–85] These findings are not restricted to schizophrenia in that poor premorbid function may also influence the outcome, though less consistently, of (schizo)affective psychosis.[86–89] Werry et al[90] carried out a study on representative incident cases of adolescent-onset psychosis (schizophrenia and bipolar disorder). Assessment of premorbid adjustment in this study was unusually accurate because of the availability of parent-informants. The authors found that abnormal premorbid adjustment (using DSM III-R major divisions of personality disorders on a 4-point scale of severity) was the best predictor of poor 5-year outcome in both schizophrenia and bipolar disorder, but more so in schizophrenia.

Cognitive dysfunction

Lower childhood IQ is a well-established risk factor for later schizophrenia,[74] and to a lesser degree for later affective disorder.[15] There is also strong evidence that cognitive function is also associated with outcome. Poorer cognitive functioning and lower IQ is associated with an unfavourable clinical and rehabilitation outcome.[91–94] It has been suggested that intact verbal memory and vigilance predict a favourable outcome in terms of community functioning and social problem-solving.[95] Similarly, there are data to suggest that negative symptoms are closely related to the primary cognitive deficit in schizophrenia.[42,63,96–98] In a 5-year follow-up study of 54 first-episode patients, changes in negative symptoms were correlated with changes in verbal IQ and full-scale IQ but not performance IQ.

Improvement in verbal cognition was observed when negative symptoms improved.[99] However, some aspects of cognitive functioning, for example reaction time, may be associated with positive symptoms of psychosis.[97,100,101]

Structural brain changes

Enlarged cerebral ventricles are a risk factor for schizophrenia and, to a lesser degree, for affective disorder.[102,103] There have been four prospective studies of outcome in relation to structural cerebral measures.[30,104–106] These studies concurred in the general finding that larger intracerebral cerebrospinal fluid spaces at baseline were predictive of poorer outcome. For example, in the largest of these studies,[105] a cohort of 140 patients with functional psychoses of recent onset were interviewed 4 years after baseline computed tomographic (CT)-scanning and assessed on six dimensions of course and outcome of illness. Analytical methods were used to adjust for possible confounding by age, gender, diagnosis, ethnic group, social class, head size, age at onset and duration of illness. It was found that left and right sylvian fissure volumes and, to a lesser extent, third ventricular volume predicted negative symptoms and unemployment over the course of the follow-up period, the latter association being mediated by poor cognitive functioning. No associations were found with global illness severity, duration of hospitalization, homelessness or affective symptomatology. The findings were true outcome findings and not simply repetitions of baseline associations. The findings were stronger in but not specific to the DSM-III-R category of schizophrenia.

A recent structural magnetic resonance imaging (MRI) study[107] found that the parahippocampal gyrus and the hippocampus were reduced in volume in 27 people with chronic (never recovered) schizophrenia compared to first-episode schizophrenia, schizoaffective and schizotypal disorders, and to controls. This suggests that the reduction in volume is a marker for an active degenerative process that is the cause of the chronicity. Alternatively, the volume reduction could be the result of being chronically ill, e.g. the effects of medication and/or poor diet. In a recent prospective study, 53 patients with DSM-III-R diagnoses of chronic schizophrenia were subdivided into a 'Kraepelinian' and 'non-Kraepelinian' subtype on the basis of longitudinal criteria. The cerebral ventricles showed a bilateral increase in size over the 4-year interval in the Kraepelinian subgroup. By contrast, neither the non-Kraepelinian subgroup nor the normal volunteers showed significant CT changes from scan 1 to scan 2.[108] In another study, cerebral structures were measured in a series of MRI scans taken over a 4-year period in 20 patients and five controls. Total volume reduction was noted in both hemispheres to a greater degree in patients than controls. When adjusted for total brain size, left ventricular enlargement occurred in patients, but not controls, over time.[109] Although these studies suggested a cerebral degenerative process, other studies have suggested no progress of cognitive decline or volume reduction of cerebral structural measures.[110]

Male sex

Although over the lifetime the risk for schizophrenia is said to be equal in men and women, this is so because the rate of older women with symptoms of schizophrenia compensates for the higher rate of schizophrenia in men before the age of 60 years.[111] If one accepts that psychotic illness in the elderly may not be continuous with earlier-onset syndromes,[112] the incidence of schizophrenia appears to be higher in men.[113,114] Many first- or recent-onset psychosis studies with follow-up durations of between 1 and 8 years have shown that women have a better outcome.[115] This holds across cultures.[116] Women are more likely to live independently, are admitted less frequently, spend more time in remission and overall suffer less social impairment, whereas men are three times more likely to have a non-remitting illness course.[117–121] In chronic schizophrenia, however, sex differences are less likely to be seen.[115,122]

It has been suggested that the effect of gender on outcome may be explained by a third variable that has a confounding effect on outcome. A likely confounder is brain abnormality, as there is some evidence that the male brain is more vulnerable to pre-, peri- and postnatal damage, and that male schizophrenic patients have more structural brain abnormalities than their female counterparts.[111] However, Navarro et al[119] found that adjusting for cerebral ventricle size (a frequent finding in cerebral damage) and obstetric complications had little effect in diminishing the differences in outcome between men and women with a psychotic illness. Similarly adjusting for family history had only a small effect. Adjusting for the variables age at onset, type of onset and diagnosis reduced the association between female sex and good outcome substantially but did not nullify it. It may be that women have less severe forms of psychosis or that they are protected against its effects. Some claim that oestrogen has such an effect, and that the prognosis for women whose schizophrenic symtoms have their onset after the menopause is worse.[123,124]

There have been consistent reports of both more and more severe negative symptoms in men as compared to women,[125–129] although not all studies concur.[130] The pathological processes resulting in negative symptoms may mediate part of the association between male sex and poor outcome.

Younger age

The likelihood to develop delusional thinking greatly increases after puberty and has its peak in early adulthood.[131–133] It is therefore no surprise that schizophrenia is mostly a disease of young individuals.[134] *Within* the group of individuals with a diagnosis of schizophrenia, younger age has clinical and prognostic significance. Like male sex, early age of onset is associated with higher levels of negative symptoms.[83,135–137] Earlier age of onset of psychosis is also associated with a more deteriorated course of schizophrenia, particularly in the case of psychosis becoming apparent before the age of 18 years.[29,68,138] The effect of early age of onset is not diagnosis-specific, similar findings transpiring in investigations of samples with schizoaffective disorder,[86,87] and affective disorder.[138,139] The association between age of onset and prognosis has face validity, as the impact of illness is much more damaging in an individual who has not completed the task of social and physical maturation, especially in illnesses which often run a chronic course, such as psychotic disorders. Although it is particularly difficult to distinguish between different diagnostic categories at presentation in the age group below 18 years old, it is possible, however, to identify patients who have an illness that is qualitatively the same as adult-onset DSM-III-R schizophrenia. Werry listed the quantitative differences between this and adult-onset schizophrenia as being: (1) male predominance; (2) higher rate of insidious onset; (3) more neurodevelopmental abnormalities; (4) more maladaptively 'odd' premorbid personalities; (5) greater resistance to antipsychotic drug treatment; (6) less differentiated symptomatology, such as well-formed delusions; and (7) increased family history of schizophrenia. These factors are likely to mediate the poor outcome seen in this group. Werry traced 30 subjects with early-onset schizophrenia and found that only 17% were well at follow-up (mean of 4.3 years after diagnosis).[90,140]

Psychosocial stress

An excess of life events has been found in the months preceding onset and relapse of schizophrenia.[141,142] The association between life events and illness onset is not specific to any particular diagnostic category within the functional psychoses, but there is evidence that the effect sizes are greater in affective illness than in schizophrenia.[141–144] Traditionally, it is held that psychosis that follows stressful life events has a better outcome,[145,146] and the available evidence supports this assertion. In the Camberwell Collaborative Psychosis study, a sample of 59 recent-onset psychotic patients with datable onset of illness,

half of whom had experienced a life event (LE+) prior to the episode, were assessed with the contextual rating of threat technique developed by Brown and Harris, and followed up for 4 years blind to exposure status. Analyses were adjusted for possible confounding variables, including sex and diagnosis. LE+ patients were nearly ten times more likely to have a symptom severity of *mild* or *recovered* over most of the follow-up period, and had accordingly spent less time in hospital over the follow-up period. There was an interaction with diagnosis, in that the association was stronger in (but not confined to) the affective psychoses than in schizophrenia.[147] Other forms of psychosocial stress, such as the level of 'expressed emotions' also predict relapse in psychotic illness,[148] although expressed emotion in the relatives is likely to be at least in part a reflection of more severe illness in the patient.[149,150] Other forms of adversity associated with depressive symptoms include subjective reactions to the experience of psychotic decompensation. It has been suggested that the high level of depressive symptoms seen in patients experiencing their first episode of schizophrenia may not only represent a core part of the acute illness but may also be in part a subjective reaction to the experience of psychotic decompensation.[151]

Society and ethnic minority status

Outcome of psychotic disorders seems to be better in developing countries. The international WHO-DOS study which followed up 80% of 1379 incident cases found differences in type of onset did not contribute to differences in outcome, therefore providing evidence that the better outcome seen in the developing countries is not a confound of age of onset.[29] Using the WHO-DOS data, Susser and Wanderling showed that the incidence of non-affective remitting psychosis in developing countries was ten-fold that in industrialized countries.[120]

It has also been found that immigrants to Western countries from the developing countries who develop schizophrenia have a better outcome than other patients with such a diagnosis.[152–154] For example, a 4-year follow-up study of consecutive admissions with recent-onset psychosis in south London compared course and outcome of psychotic illness between 53 African-Caribbeans and 60 British-born Whites.[154] African-Caribbeans were more often admitted involuntarily, and more often imprisoned over the follow-up period. They received antidepressant and psychotherapeutic treatment less often than their White counterparts. However, with regard to clinical outcome, the Caribbeans were less likely to have had a continuous unremitting illness course (adjusted OR = 3). The effect of ethnic group tended to be stronger in the group of non-schizophrenic, affective psychoses.[4] This is interesting, given the fact that in a recent comparative study of the symptomatology of White and African-Caribbean patients, the only difference between the two ethnic groups was seen on a mixed mania–catatonia dimension on which the African-Caribbean group was overrepresented.[155] Similarly, the incidence of schizomanic illness in African-Caribbeans living in the UK was found to be much higher than that of the White population.[156] These results suggest that the high incidence observed in UK African-Caribbeans is coupled with a less deteriorated illness course in this ethnic group. Excess exposure to precipitants in the social environment, resulting in good-prognosis 'reactive' illness with affective symptoms, may be one explanation.[27] More recent studies on psychotic patients with outcome comparisons contrasting African-Caribbean and White British groups have reported findings in the same direction of decreased likelihood of a continuous illness course in African-Caribbean patients, but the differences between the African-Caribbean and White patients were more attenuated, with an effect size of less than 2.[157,158]

In the United States, the increase in the use of involuntary admission of African-Americans with psychosis has been well documented.[159,160] A 1-year follow-up of the sample of the Epidemiologic Catchment Area Program revealed that African-

Americans, Hispanics and other minorities were much less likely to have consulted with a professional in the specialized mental health care sector than Whites. The odds of consultation in African-Americans, adjusted for other factors such as sex and diagnosis, were less than one-fourth of that in Whites.[161] Differences between United States ethnic groups are also apparent in populations with identical insurance coverage.[162] Therefore, these findings suggest low permeability of filters on the pathway to mental health care for ethnic minorities and therefore lower levels of service use. In comparisons to all other ethnic groups, African-Americans make more use of emergency rooms for routine psychiatric care.[163,164] In spite of the low permeability of the filters on the pathway to care for many ethnic minority groups, there is an important overrepresentation of African-Americans at the level of hospital-based psychiatric services, which may be increasing.[165] More work is needed on how these factors affect clinical and service-related outcomes in different ethnic groups in the United States.[166]

Prognostic significance of variables that are risk-neutral
Socioeconomic status

It remains uncertain whether lower socioeconomic status increases the risk for onset of psychotic disorder.[167] However, socioeconomic status is an important determinant of outcome in many medical situations, and psychiatric disorders are no exception. People of lower social class have a worse outcome of a psychotic illness. A study of 219 first-admission patients from a defined geographical area examined several measures of course and outcome in relation to social class. A linear trend was seen in the association between social class and time spent in hospital in the first 2 and 5 years of illness. Patients of lower social class were less likely to recover, less likely to respond to rehabilitation and more likely to be readmitted.[168] Similar findings emerged from a large study in the United States,[169] and these findings have since been confirmed.[170,171] The Camberwell Collaborative Psychosis Study investigated the outcome of illness in 166 people with recent-onset psychosis. Over three levels of socioeconomic status the risk of non-remitting illness during the 4 years of follow-up increased multiplicatively by a factor of 2.4 and the risk of non-recovery by a factor of 2 for each level of lower social class.[154] In this study, the association between social class and outcome was not diagnosis-specific within the functional psychoses. Indeed, similar findings have been reported in a sample of 248 bipolar patients.[172]

Duration of untreated illness

Before treatment is initiated, patients with psychotic illness already display psychotic symptoms for a period of around 12 months.[173,174] The possible adverse clinical effect of untreated psychosis in schizophrenic patients, particularly early in the course of illness, has been a topic of considerable interest in recent years. Several studies have found an association between duration of untreated psychosis (DUP) and poor outcome in terms of relapse and level of remission achieved. Crow et al[175] followed up 120 first-admission patients with schizophrenia. They were all treated with antipsychotics and then entered into a randomized controlled trial of maintenance antipsychotics. Duration of illness prior to the start of antipsychotic medication was the most important determinant of relapse. Jablensky and colleagues[29] found duration of illness between onset and initial examination was associated with 4 out of 7 outcome variables in the WHO-DOS study. This still held after adjusting for setting and type of onset. Loebel et al[176] followed up 70 first-admission patients with schizophrenia and schizoaffective disorder for up to 3 years. Duration of illness before treatment was significantly associated with time to and level of remission after adjusting for sex and diagnosis.[176] In another study, patients with 1 or more years of untreated psychosis prior to their first antipsychotic treatment displayed a more severe poverty syndrome at the time of admission and discharge and a more severe reality distortion syndrome at discharge from the index hospitalization. These findings were not related to age, premorbid functioning, duration of illness or first- vs multiple-episodes status.[177]

All the above studies have demonstrated an association between DUP and outcome but this does not prove causality. There might have been confounding factors, such as ethnic group, socioeconomic status, high levels of negative symptoms, abnormal personality, or a form of illness with insidious onset and poor prognosis. For example, Verdoux and colleagues[178] found that duration of untreated psychosis in a sample of first-episode patients was associated with low educational level, poor adjustment in the previous year, and greater illness severity at admission.[178] These are all factors that are known to be associated with poor outcome. In another study DUP was associated with male sex and unemployment, also known to affect outcome negatively.[179] Randomized studies are designed to control for known and unknown confounding factors. May and colleagues[180] randomly assigned 228 first-admission schizophrenic patients to one of five treatment groups. Patients who were initially treated with antipsychotics had improved outcome over the subsequent 3 years compared with those initially not treated with antipsychotics. This would seem to constitute good evidence that delayed treatment leads to a worse outcome, but randomization with small groups may not be entirely successful and it is remotely possible that the psychotherapy that those not initially treated with antipsychotics received led to their worse outcome. A more recent randomized trial involving 105 patients found that a 4-week delay in initiating active treatment in patients with functional psychosis had no long-term adverse effects over a period of 2.5 years.[181]

Drug use

The relationship between drug use and pathogenesis in psychosis is extremely complex and underinvestigated. This is partly because drug use has, until recently, been difficult to assess accurately. It is possible that drug use increases the chance of a vulnerable person developing schizophrenia who might otherwise not have done so,[182,183] but there is no conclusive evidence at present that drug use in itself is a risk factor for subsequent psychotic illness. However, there is no doubt that drug use adversely affects outcome. Patients presenting with psychosis and drug use tend to do so persistently over time, make more use of psychiatric services and spend more time in hospital.[184,185] Linzsen and collaborators[186] carried out a study into cannabis use and outcome in schizophrenia. It was carried out in a country where cannabis use was not restricted by legislation and not associated with stigma. They took account of various confounding factors such as gender, use of alcohol and other drugs. They found that cannabis use is associated with more and earlier relapse in recent-onset schizophrenia. In addition, there was an interaction with intensity of cannabis use, heavy users having a 3.4-fold risk of relapse (our calculation from the data provided; similar data were reported from the United Kingdom by Grech and colleagues).[187] The two main hypotheses relating drug use and schizophrenia are the 'self-medication hypothesis' and the 'comorbid addiction vulnerability hypothesis',[188] and more research is needed to clarify these issues. Is is clear that comorbid drug use in patients with schizophrenia will have severe consequences in terms of rehospitalization, homelessness, risk of other medical illness, disruption of social and vocational function, exacerbation of symptoms, suicide, and increased health care expenses.[189]

An empirical model of outcome, symptom dimensions and risk factors for psychosis

The data reviewed above are compatible with an empirical model of psychosis outcome based partly on risk factors for onset of psychosis and partly on prevailing symptom dimensions. It was observed that:

- There is evidence that some of the risk factors that increase the risk of *developing* psychotic illness also modify *course and outcome* of psychotic illness. Thus, familial morbid risk for schizophrenia, cerebral ventricle enlargement, cognitive dysfunction, premorbid social dysfunction, obstetric complications, psychosocial stress and ethnic minority status not only affect the risk for onset of illness, but also have prognostic relevance.

- Whereas indicators of *psychosocial stress* such as life events and ethnic minority status tend to be associated with good outcome and have larger effect sizes at the affective side of the spectrum of psychosis, the reverse holds for the risk factors associated with *impaired neurodevelopment*. Thus, cerebral ventricle enlargement, younger age, male sex, premorbid cognitive and social dysfunction, familial morbid risk of schizophrenia and obstetric complications tend to be associated with poorer outcome and
  - have larger effect sizes at the non-affective side of the spectrum of psychotic illness; and/or
  - have particularly strong associations with negative symptoms.

- Other variables such as lower social class, longer duration of untreated psychosis and drug use are not well-established risk factors for onset of psychosis and not associated with any particular symptom dimension, but there is evidence that they do influence course and outcome both in affective and non-affective psychosis.

These issues have been summarized in Figure 3.3. We propose a psychopathological continuum, with discrete effects of clusters of (a) psychosocial and (b) developmental/familial risk factors working preferentially, though not exclusively, at opposite ends of the continuum. We suggest that there is a *gradient*, both in terms of severity/prognosis and the magnitude of the effect of risk factors, along dimensions of the continuum, rather than qualitative distinctions between cat-

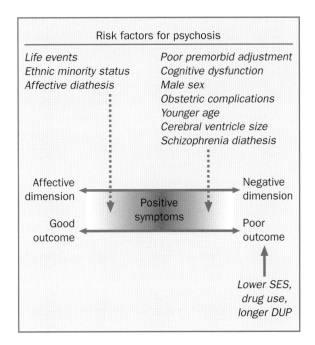

Figure 3.3 Model of prognostic, psychopathological and aetiological heterogeneity in psychosis. Psychosis includes variation in various symptom dimensions, that are differentially, though not exclusively, associated with clusters of risk factors and variation in outcome.

egories. Developmental and familial factors, for example low childhood cognitive ability, increased cerebral ventricle size and familial morbid risk of schizophrenia, operate preferentially, though *not* specifically, at that end of the psychopathological spectrum characterized by a preponderance of negative features and poor outcome. On the other hand, adverse life events have a larger impact at the end associated with predominance of affective features and better outcome. This dimensional model based on risk factors for onset and persistence of psychosis can be seen as an extension of previously proposed models for good-outcome and bad-outcome schizophrenia, the most influential one being that proposed by Robins and Guze.[190]

Management implications

With the advent of evidence-based medicine, it is likely that more research will be carried out to answer questions about patient management. Should a first-episode psychotic patient with poor premorbid social adjustment and enlarged ventricles be treated for longer than one without these features? Should resources be targeted at improving the environment for ethnic minorities with psychotic illness? Should patients with signs of neurodevelopmental impairment receive treatments aimed specifically at reducing and preventing negative and cognitive symptoms? Should scarce resources be directed towards early detection of individuals with psychotic illness in order to reduce the duration of untreated psychosis?

While many questions remain to be answered, there are already some indications that it is possible to provide specific treatments to individuals with a specific risk factor profile. For example, some forms of treatment, such as intensive case management, have been shown to be particularly effective for individuals with the highest degree of cognitive impairment,[191] and there is evidence that patient–therapist ethnic matching can have a beneficial effect in delivering psychiatric treatments.[192] Treatment with typical antipsychotics often controls positive symptoms but there is little evidence that it alters the long-term progression once the disease is established; however, it is not clear whether this is due to limited effectiveness or poor compliance. It is too soon to know whether the newer atypicals have an effect on subsequent prognosis, although they may be more effective in controlling negative and cognitive symptoms associated with psychosis.[193–195] Negative symptoms may be reduced by cognitive-behavioural activity scheduling techniques, and cognitive remediation may be effective in the case of neuropsychological dysfunction.[196,197] Two studies suggest that an early intervention model may improve outcome by reducing duration of untreated psychosis, but the evidence from these before-vs-after comparisons remains circumstantial.[198,199] High rates of affective symptoms associated with psychosocial adversity may warrant treatment with mood stabilizers or antidepressants. There is evidence supporting adjunctive antidepressant treatment for schizophrenic and schizoaffective patients who develop a major depressive syndrome after remission of acute psychosis, although there are mixed results for treatment of subsyndromal depression.[200] There is some evidence that atypical antipsychotics may be more effective in the treatment of affective symptoms.[201]

Conclusion

By breaking down psychotic syndromes into their underlying symptom dimensions which each tend to be differentially associated with clusters of risk factors, a useful model for the prediction of outcome can be created. As the newer treatments that are being developed increasingly target specific symptom dimensions and individuals at risk, such a model may provide patients with opportunities for better care than the traditional Kraepelinian dichotomy.

References

1. Falloon IR, Relapse: a reappraisal of assessment of outcome in schizophrenia, *Schizophr Bull* (1984) **10**:293–9.
2. Stephens JH, Long-term prognosis and followup in schizophrenia, *Schizophr Bull* (1978) **4**:25–47.
3. McGlashan TH, A selective review of recent North American long-term followup studies of schizophrenia, *Schizophr Bull* (1988) **14**:515–42.
4. van Os' J, Wright P, Murray RM, Risk factors for the emergence and persistence of psychosis. In: Weller M, Kammen Dv, eds, *Progress in Clinical Psychiatry* (Saunders: London, 1997) 152–206.
5. Tsuang MT, Dempsey GM, Long-term outcome of major psychoses. II. Schizoaffective disorder compared with schizophrenia, affective disorders, and a surgical control group, *Arch Gen Psychiatry* (1979) **36**:1302–4.
6. Feighner JP, Robins E, Guze SB et al, Diagnostic criteria for use in psychiatric research, *Arch Gen Psychiatry* (1972) **26**:57–63.
7. Coryell W, Keller M, Lavori P, Endicott J, Affective syndromes, psychotic features, and prognosis. I. Depression, *Arch Gen Psychiatry* (1990) **47**:651–7.
8. Coryell W, Keller M Lavori P, Endicott J, Affective syndromes, psychotic features, and prognosis. II. Mania, *Arch Gen Psychiatry* (1990) **47**:658–62.
9. Grossman LS, Harrow M, Goldberg JF, Fichtner CG, Outcome of schizoaffective disorder at two long-term follow-ups: comparisons with outcome of schizophrenia and affective disorders, *Am J Psychiatry* (1991) **148**:1359–65.
10. Brockington IF, Kendell RE, Wainwright S, Depressed patients with schizophrenic or paranoid symptoms, *Psychol Med* (1980) **10**:665–75.
11. Brockington IF, Wainwright S, Kendell RE, Manic patients with schizophrenic or paranoid symptoms, *Psychol Med* (1980) **10**:73–83.
12. Marneros A, Deister A, Rohde A et al, Long-term outcome of schizoaffective and schizophrenic disorders: a comparative study. I. Definitions, methods, psychopathological and social outcome, *Eur Arch Psychiatry Neurol Sci* (1989) **238**:118–25.
13. Marneros A, Deister A, Rohde A, Psychopathological and social status of patients with affective, schizophrenic and schizoaffective disorders after long-term course, *Acta Psychiatr Scand* (1990) **82**:352–8.
14. Maj M, Perris C, Patterns of course in patients with a cross-sectional diagnosis of schizoaffective disorder, *J Affect Disord* (1990) **20**:71–7.
15. Müller V, Katamnestische Errhebungen Uber der Spontanverlauf der Schizophrenie, *Monatsschrift fur Psychiatrie-Neurologie* (1951) **122**:257–76.
16. Bland RC, Orn H, 14-year outcome in early schizophrenia, *Acta Psychiatr Scand* (1978) **58**:327–58.
17. Ciompi L, The natural history of schizophrenia in the long term, *Br J Psychiatry* (1980) **136**: 413–20.
18. Salokangas RK, Prognostic implications of the sex of schizophrenic patients, *Br J Psychiatry* (1983) **142**:145–51.
19. Sartorius N, Jablensky A, Korten A et al, Early manifestations and first-contact incidence of schizophrenia in different cultures. A preliminary report on the initial evaluation phase of the WHO Collaborative Study on determinants of outcome of severe mental disorders, *Psychol Med* (1986) **16**:909–28.

20. Rabiner CJ, Wegner JT, Kane JM, Outcome study of first-episode psychosis. I. Relapse rates after 1 year, *Am J Psychiatry* (1986) **143:**1155–8.

21. McCreadie RG, Wiles D, Grant S et al, The Scottish first episode schizophrenia study VII. Two-year follow-up. Scottish Schizophrenia Research Group. *Acta Psychiatrica Scandinavia* (1989) **80:**597–602.

22. Shepherd M, Watt D, Falloon I, Smeeton N, The natural history of schizophrenia: a five-year follow-up study of outcome and prediction in a representative sample of schizophrenics, *Psychol Med Monogr Suppl* (1989) **15:**1–46.

23. Harrow M, Grossman LS, Outcome in schizoaffective disorders: a critical review and reevaluation of the literature, *Schizophr Bull* (1984) **10:** 87–108.

24. Samson JA, Simpson JC, Tsuang MT, Outcome studies of schizoaffective disorders, *Schizophr Bull* (1988) **14:**543–54.

25. Kendell RE, Brockington IF, The identification of disease entities and the relationship between schizophrenic and affective psychoses, *Br J Psychiatry* (1980) **137:**324–31.

26. Strauss JS, Carpenter WT Jr, The prognosis of schizophrenia: rationale for a multidimensional concept, *Schizophr Bull* (1978) **4:**56–67.

27. van Os J, Fahy TA, Jones P et al, Psychopathological syndromes in the functional psychoses: associations with course and outcome, *Psychol Med* (1996) **26:**161–76.

28. van Os J, Gilvarry C, Bale R et al, A comparison of the utility of dimensional and categorical representations of psychosis. UK700 Group, *Psychol Med* (1999) **29:**595–606.

29. Jablensky A, Sartorius N, Ernberg G et al, Schizophrenia: manifestations, incidence and course in different cultures, A World Health Organization ten-country study [published erratum appears in *Psychol Med Monogr Suppl* (1992) **22:**following 1092], *Psychol Med Monogr Suppl* (1992) **20:**1–97.

30. Lieberman J, Jody D, Geisler S et al, Time course and biologic correlates of treatment response in first-episode schizophrenia, *Arch Gen Psychiatry* (1993) **50:**369–76.

31. Johnstone EC, Macmillan JF, Frith CD et al, Further investigation of the predictors of outcome following first schizophrenic episodes, *Br J Psychiatry* (1990) **157:**182–9.

32. Ciompi L, Muller C, [Lifestyle and age of schizophrenics, A catamnestic long-term study into old age], *Monogr Gesamtgeb Psychiatr Psychiatry Ser* (1976) **12:**1–242.

33. Harding CM, Brooks GW, Ashikaga T et al, The Vermont longitudinal study of persons with severe mental illness. II. Long-term outcome of subjects who retrospectively met DSM-III criteria for schizophrenia, *Am J Psychiatry* (1987) **144:**727–35.

34. Huber G, Gross G, Schuttler R, Linz M, Longitudinal studies of schizophrenic patients, *Schizophr Bull* (1980) **6:**592–605.

35. McGlashan TH, The Chestnut Lodge follow-up study. II. Long-term outcome of schizophrenia and the affective disorders, *Arch Gen Psychiatry* (1984) **41:**586–601.

36. Bleuler M, The long-term course of the schizophrenic psychoses, *Psychol Med* (1974) **4:**244–54.

37. Strauss JS, Carpenter WT Jr, Prediction of outcome in schizophrenia. III. Five-year outcome and its predictors, *Arch Gen Psychiatry* (1977) **34:** 159–63.

38. Bleuler M, *The Schizophrenic Disorders: Long Term Patient and Family Studies* (Yale University: New Haven, 1978).

39. Harding CM, Brooks GW, Ashikaga T et al, The Vermont longitudinal study of persons with severe mental illness. I. Methodology, study sample, and overall status 32 years later, *Am J Psychiatry* (1987) **144:**718–26.

40. Breier A, Schreiber JL, Dyer J, Pickar D, Course of illness and predictors of outcome in chronic schizophrenia: implications for pathophysiology, *Br J Psychiatry Suppl* (1992) **18:**38–43.

41. Engelhardt DM, Rosen B, Feldman J et al, A 15-year followup of 646 schizophrenic outpatients, *Schizophr Bull* (1982) **8:**493–503.

42. Vaillant GE, Prognosis and the course of schizophrenia, *Schizophr Bull* (1978) **4:**20–4.

43. Birchwood M, Todd P, Jackson C, Early intervention in psychosis, The critical period hypothesis, *Br J Psychiatry Suppl* (1998) **172:**53–9.

44. Rosanoff AJ, A statistical study of prognosis in insanity, *J Am Med Assoc* (1914) **62:**3–6.

45. Fuller RG, Expectation of hospital life and outcome for mental patients on first admission, *Psychiatr Q* (1930) **4:**295–323.

46. Rupp C, Fletcher EK, A five to ten year follow up

study of 641 schizophrenic cases, *Am J Psychiatry* (1940) **96:**877–88.

47. Malzberg B, Rates of discharge and rates of mortality among first admissions to the New York civil state hospitals (3rd paper), *Mental Hygiene* (1953) **37:**619–54.

48. Shepherd M, *A Study of the Major Psychoses in an English County* (Oxford University Press: London, 1957).

49. Locke BZ, Outcome of first hospitalisation of patients with schizophrenia, *Publ Health Rep* (1962) **77:**801–5.

50. Peterson DB, Olsen GW, First admitted schizophrenics in drug era, *Arch Gen Psychiatry* (1964) **11:**137–44.

51. Hegarty JD, Baldessarini RJ, Tohen M et al, One hundred years of schizophrenia: a meta-analysis of the outcome literature, *Am J Psychiatry* (1994) **151:**1409–16.

52. Westermeyer JF, Harrow M, Prognosis and outcome using broad (DSM-II) and narrow (DSM-III) concepts of schizophrenia, *Schizophr Bull* (1984) **10:**624–37.

53. Johnstone EC, Connelly J, Frith CD et al, The nature of 'transient' and 'partial' psychoses: findings from the Northwick Park 'Functional' Psychosis Study, *Psychol Med* (1996) **26:**361–9.

54. Johnstone EC, Frith CD, Crow TJ et al, The Northwick Park 'Functional' Psychosis Study: diagnosis and outcome, *Psychol Med* (1992) **22:**331–46.

55. Robinson D, Woerner MG, Alvir JM et al, Predictors of relapse following response from a first episode of schizophrenia or schizoaffective disorder, *Arch Gen Psychiatry* (1999) **56:**241–7.

56. Robinson DG, Woerner MG, Alvir JM et al, Predictors of treatment response from a first episode of schizophrenia or schizoaffective disorder, *Am J Psychiatry* (1999) **156:**544–9.

57. Kitamura T, Okazaki Y, Fujinawa A et al, Symptoms of psychoses, A factor-analytic study, *Br J Psychiatry* (1995) **166:**236–40.

58. McGorry PD, Bell RC, Dudgeon PL, Jackson HJ, The dimensional structure of first episode psychosis: an exploratory factor analysis, *Psychol Med* (1998) **28:**935–47.

59. van Os J, Gilvarry C, Bale R et al, To what extent does symptomatic improvement result in better outcomes in psychotic illness? *Psychol Med* (1999).

60. Kendler KS, McGuire M, Gruenberg AM et al, The Roscommon Family Study. I. Methods, diagnosis of probands, and risk of schizophrenia in relatives, *Arch Gen Psychiatry* (1993) **50:**527–40.

61. Maier W, Lichtermann D, Minges J et al, Continuity and discontinuity of affective disorders and schizophrenia. Results of a controlled family study, *Arch Gen Psychiatry* (1993) **50:**871–83.

62. Fowler RC, McCabe MS, Cadoret, RJ, Winokur G, The validity of good prognosis schizophrenia, *Arch Gen Psychiatry* (1972) **26:**182–5.

63. Kendler KS, Tsuang MT, Outcome and familial psychopathology in schizophrenia, *Arch Gen Psychiatry* (1988) **45:**338–46.

64. Verdoux H, van Os J, Sham P et al, Does familiality predispose to both emergence and persistence of psychosis? A follow-up study [published erratum appears in *Br J Psychiatry* (1996) **169:**116], *Br J Psychiatry* (1996) **168:**620–6.

65. Kay SR, Opler LA, Fiszbein A, Significance of positive and negative syndromes in chronic schizophrenia, *Br J Psychiatry* (1986) **149:**439–48.

66. Jones PB, Rantakallio P, Hartikainen AL et al, Schizophrenia as a long-term outcome of pregnancy, delivery, and perinatal complications: a 28-year follow-up of the 1966 north Finland general population birth cohort, *Am J Psychiatry* (1999) **155:**355–64.

67. Verdoux H, Geddes JR, Takei N et al, Obstetric complications and age at onset in schizophrenia: an international collaborative meta-analysis of individual patient data, *Am J Psychiatry* (1997) **154:**1220–7.

68. Nimgaonkar VL, Wessely S, Tune LE, Murray RM, Response to drugs in schizophrenia: the influence of family history, obstetric complications and ventricular enlargement, *Psychol Med* (1988) **18:**583–92.

69. Alvir JM, Woerner MG, Gunduz H et al, Obstetric complications predict treatment response in first-episode schizophrenia, *Psychol Med* (1999) **29:**621–7.

70. Kirov G, Jones PB, Harvey I et al, Do obstetric complications cause the earlier age at onset in male than female schizophrenics? *Schizophr Res* (1996) **20:**117–24.

71. Smith GN, Kopala LC, Lapointe JS et al, Obstetric complications, treatment response and brain

morphology in adult-onset and early-onset males with schizophrenia, *Psychol Med* (1998) **28**:645–53.

72. Wilcox JA, Nasrallah HA, Perinatal distress and prognosis of psychotic illness, *Neuropsychobiology* (1987) **17**:173–5.

73. Done DJ, Crow TJ, Johnstone EC, Sacker A, Childhood antecedents of schizophrenia and affective illness: social adjustment at ages 7 and 11, *BMJ* (1994) **309**:699–703.

74. Jones P, Rodgers B, Murray R, Marmot M, Child developmental risk factors for adult schizophrenia in the British 1946 birth cohort, *Lancet* (1994) **344**:1398–402.

75. van Os J, Jones P, Lewis G et al, Developmental precursors of affective illness in a general population birth cohort, *Arch Gen Psychiatry* (1997) **54**:625–31.

76. Bromet E, Harrow M, Kasl S, Premorbid functioning and outcome in schizophrenics and non-schizophrenics, *Arch Gen Psychiatry* (1974) **30**:203–7.

77. Ciompi L, Catamnestic long-term study on the course of life and aging of schizophrenics, *Schizophr Bull* (1980) **6**:606–18.

78. Gittelman-Klein R, Klein DF, Premorbid asocial adjustment and prognosis in schizophrenia, *J Psychiatr Res* (1969) **7**:35–53.

79. Cannon Spoor HE, Potkin SG, Wyatt RJ, Measurement of premorbid adjustment in chronic schizophrenia, *Schizophr Bull* (1982) **8**:470–84.

80. Bailer J, Brauer W, Rey ER, Premorbid adjustment as predictor of outcome in schizophrenia: results of a prospective study, *Acta Psychiatr Scand* (1996) **93**:368–77.

81. Fennig S, Putnam K, Bromet EJ, Galambos N, Gender, premorbid characteristics and negative symptoms in schizophrenia, *Acta Psychiatr Scand* (1995) **92**:173–7.

82. Fenton WS, McGlashan TH, Natural history of schizophrenia subtypes. II. Positive and negative symptoms and long-term course, *Arch Gen Psychiatry* (1991) **48**:978–86.

83 Gupta S, Rajaprabhakaran R, Arndt S et al, Premorbid adjustment as a predictor of phenomenological and neurobiological indices in schizophrenia, *Schizophr Res* (1995) **16**:189–97.

84. Larsen TK, Johannessen JO, Opjordsmoen S, First-episode schizophrenia with long duration of untreated psychosis. Pathways to care, *Br J Psychiatry Suppl* (1998) **172**:45–52.

85. Peralta V, Cuesta MJ, de Leon J, Positive and negative symptoms/syndromes in schizophrenia: reliability and validity of different diagnostic systems, *Psychol Med* (1995) **25**:43–50.

86. del Rio Vega JM, Ayuso-Gutierrez JL, Course of schizoaffective psychosis: a retrospective study, *Acta Psychiatr Scand* (1990) **81**:534–7.

87. Marneros A, Deister A, Rohde A et al, Long-term course of schizoaffective disorders. Part I. Definitions, methods, frequency of episodes and cycles, *Eur Arch Psychiatry Neurol Sci* (1988) **237**:264–75.

88. McGlashan TH, Williams PV, Predicting outcome in schizoaffective psychosis, *J Nerv Ment Dis* (1990) **178**:518–20.

89. Opjordsmoen S, Long-term course and outcome in unipolar affective and schizoaffective psychoses, *Acta Psychiatr Scand* (1989) **79**:317–26.

90. Werry JS, McClellan JM, Chard L, Childhood and adolescent schizophrenic, bipolar, and schizoaffective disorders: a clinical and outcome study, *J Am Acad Child Adolesc Psychiatry* (1991) **30**:457–65.

91. Aylward E, Walker E, Bettes B, Intelligence in schizophrenia: meta-analysis of the research, *Schizophr Bull* (1984) **10**:430–59.

92. Goldman RS, Axelrod BN, Tandon R et al, Neuropsychological prediction of treatment efficacy and one-year outcome in schizophrenia, *Psychopathology* (1993) **26**:122–6.

93. Harvey PD, Howanitz E, Parrella M et al, Symptoms, cognitive functioning, and adaptive skills in geriatric patients with lifelong schizophrenia: a comparison across treatment sites, *Am J Psychiatry* (1998) **155**:1080–6.

94. Silverstein ML, Harrow M, Mavrolefteros G, Close D, Neuropsychological dysfunction and clinical outcome in psychiatric disorders: a two-year follow-up study, *J Nerv Ment Dis* (1997) **185**:722–9.

95. Green MF, What are the functional consequences of neurocognitive deficits in schizophrenia? *Am J Psychiatry* (1996) **153**:321–30.

96. Addington J, Addington D, Premorbid functioning, cognitive functioning, symptoms and outcome in schizophrenia, *J Psychiatry Neurosci* (1993) **18**:18–23.

97. Addington J, Addington D, Maticka-Tyndale E,

Cognitive functioning and positive and negative symptoms in schizophrenia, *Schizophr Res* (1991) **5(2):**123–34.

98. Wong AH, Voruganti LN, Heslegrave RJ, Awad AG, Neurocognitive deficits and neurological signs in schizophrenia, *Schizophr Res* (1997) **23:**139–46.

99. Gold S, Arndt S, Nopoulos P et al, Longitudinal study of cognitive function in first-episode and recent-onset schizophrenia, *Am J Psychiatry* (1999) **156:**1342–8.

100. Hoff AL, Sakuma M, Wieneke M et al, Longitudinal neuropsychological follow-up study of patients with first-episode schizophrenia, *Am J Psychiatry* (1999) **156:**1336–41.

101. Lieh-Mak F, Lee PW, Cognitive deficit measures in schizophrenia: factor structure and clinical correlates, *Am J Psychiatry* (1997) **154(Suppl 6):**39–46.

102. Elkis H, Friedman L, Wise A, Meltzer HY, Meta-analyses of studies of ventricular enlargement and cortical sulcal prominence in mood disorders, Comparisons with controls or patients with schizophrenia, *Arch Gen Psychiatry* (1995) **52:** 735–46.

103. Jones PB, Harvey I, Lewis SW et al, Cerebral ventricle dimensions as risk factors for schizophrenia and affective psychosis: an epidemiological approach to analysis, *Psychol Med* (1994) **24:**995–1011.

104. DeLisi LE, Stritzke P, Riordan H et al, The timing of brain morphological changes in schizophrenia and their relationship to clinical outcome [published erratum appears in *Biol Psychiatry* (1992) **31:**1172], *Biol Psychiatry* (1992) **31:**241–54.

105. van Os J, Fahy TA, Jones P et al, Increased intra-cerebral cerebrospinal fluid spaces predict unemployment and negative symptoms in psychotic illness, A prospective study, *Br J Psychiatry* (1995) **166:**750–8.

106. Vita A, Dieci M, Giobbio GM et al, CT scan abnormalities and outcome of chronic schizophrenia, *Am J Psychiatry* (1991) **148:**1577–9.

107. Razi K, Greene KP, Sakuma M et al, Reduction of the parahippocampal gyrus and the hippocampus in patients with chronic schizophrenia *Br J Psychiatry* (1999) **174:**512–19.

108. Davis KL, Buchsbaum MS, Shihabuddin L et al,

Ventricular enlargement in poor-outcome schizophrenia, *Biol Psychiatry* (1998) **43:**783–93.

109. DeLisi LE, Tew W, Xie S, et al, A prospective follow-up study of brain morphology and cognition in first-episode schizophrenic patients: preliminary findings, *Biol Psychiatry* (1995) **38:** 349–60.

110. Goldberg TE, Hyde TM, Kleinman JE, Weinberger DR, Course of schizophrenia: neuropsychological evidence for a static encephalopathy, *Schizophr Bull* (1993) **19:**797–804.

111. Castle DJ, Murray RM, The neurodevelopmental basis of sex differences in schizophrenia [editorial], *Psychol Med* (1991) **21:**565–75.

112. Van Os J, Howard R, Tokei N, Murray R, Increasing age is a risk factor for psychosis in the elderly. *Soc Psychiatry Psychiatr Epidemiol* (1995) **30:**161–4.

113. Castle DJ, Wessely S, Murray RM, Sex and schizophrenia: effects of diagnostic stringency, and associations with and premorbid variables, *Br J Psychiatry* (1993) **162:**658–64.

114. Iacono WG, Beiser M, Are males more likely than females to develop schizophrenia? *Am J Psychiatry* (1992) **149:**1070–4.

115. Bardenstein KK, McGlashan TH, Gender differences in affective, schizoaffective, and schizophrenic disorders. A review, *Schizophr Res* (1990) **3:**159–72.

116. Hambrecht M, Maurer K, Hafner H, Sartorius N, Transnational stability of gender differences in schizophrenia? An analysis based on the WHO study on determinants of outcome of severe mental disorders, *Eur Arch Psychiatry Clin Neurosci* (1992) **242:**6–12.

117. Angermeyer MC, Kuhn L, Goldstein JM, Gender and the course of schizophrenia: differences in treated outcomes, *Schizophr Bull* (1990) **16:** 293–307.

118. Goldstein JM, Gender differences in the course of schizophrenia, *Am J Psychiatry* (1988) **145:** 684–9.

119. Navarro F, van Os J, Jones P, Murray R, Explaining sex differences in course and outcome in the functional psychoses, *Schizophr Res* (1996) **21:** 161–70.

120. Susser E, Wanderling J, Epidemiology of nonaffective acute remitting psychosis vs schizophrenia. Sex and sociocultural setting, *Arch Gen Psychiatry* (1994) **51:**294–301.

121. Szymanski S, Lieberman JA, Alvir JM et al, Gender differences in onset of illness, treatment response, course, and biologic indexes in first-episode schizophrenic patients, *Am J Psychiatry* (1995) **152**:698–703.

122. Kendler KS, Walsh D, Gender and schizophrenia, Results of an epidemiologically-based family study, *Br J Psychiatry* (1995) **167**:184–92.

123. Hafner H, Behrens S, De Vry J, Gattaz WF, Oestradiol enhances the vulnerability threshold for schizophrenia in women by an early effect on dopaminergic neurotransmission, Evidence from an epidemiological study and from animal experiments, *Eur Arch Psychiatry Clin Neurosci* (1991) **241**:65–8.

124. Seeman MV, Current outcome in schizophrenia: women vs men, *Acta Psychiatr Scand* (1986) **73**:609–17.

125. Johnstone EC, Frith CD, Lang FH, Owens DG, Determinants of the extremes of outcome in schizophrenia, *Br J Psychiatry* (1995) **167**:604–9.

126. Larsen TK, McGlashan TH, Johannessen JO, Vibe Hansen L, First-episode schizophrenia. II. Premorbid patterns by gender, *Schizophr Bull* (1996) **22**:257–69.

127. Ring N, Tantam D, Montague L et al, Gender differences in the incidence of definite schizophrenia and atypical psychosis—focus on negative symptoms of schizophrenia, *Acta Psychiatr Scand* (1991) **84**:489–96.

128. Schultz SK, Miller DD, Oliver SE et al, The life course of schizophrenia: age and symptom dimensions, *Schizophr Res* (1997) **23**:15–23.

129. Shtasel DL, Gur RE, Gallacher F et al, Gender differences in the clinical expression of schizophrenia, *Schizophr Res* (1992) **7**:225–31.

130. Hafner H, Loffler W, Maurer K et al, Depression, negative symptoms, social stagnation and social decline in the early course of schizophrenia, *Acta Psychiatr Scand* (1999) **100**:105–18.

131. Galdos P, van Os J, Gender, psychopathology, and development: from puberty to early adulthood, *Schizophr Res* (1995) **14**:105–12.

132. Peters ER, Joseph SA, Garety PA, The measurement of delusional ideation in the normal population: introducing the PDI (Peters et al Delusions Inventory), *Schizophr Bull* (1999) **25**:553–76.

133. Verdoux H, van Os J, MauriceTison S et al, Is early adulthood a critical developmental stage for psychosis proneness? A survey of delusional ideation in normal subjects, *Schizophr Res* (1999) **29**:247–54.

134. Galdos PM, van Os JJ, Murray RM, Puberty and the onset of psychosis, *Schizophr Res* (1993) **10**:7–14.

135. Andreasen NC, Flaum M, Swayze VWd et al, Positive and negative symptoms in schizophrenia. A critical reappraisal, *Arch Gen Psychiatry* (1990) **47**:615–21.

136. Hoff AL, Harris D, Faustman WO et al, A neuropsychological study of early onset schizophrenia, *Schizophr Res* (1996) **20**:21–8.

137. Yang PC, Liu CY, Chiang SQ et al, Comparison of adult manifestations of schizophrenia with onset before and after 15 years of age, *Acta Psychiatr Scand* (1995) **91**:209–12.

138. Johnstone EC, Owens DG, Bydder GM et al, The spectrum of structural brain changes in schizophrenia: age of onset as a predictor of cognitive and clinical impairments and their cerebral correlates, *Psychol Med* (1989) **19**:91–103.

139. Winokur G, Coryell W, Keller M et al, A prospective follow-up of patients with bipolar and primary unipolar affective disorder, *Arch Gen Psychiatry* (1993) **50**:457–65.

140. Werry JS, Child and adolescent (early onset) schizophrenia: a review in light of DSM-III-R, *J Autism Dev Disord* (1992) **22**:601–24.

141. Bebbington P, Wilkins S, Jones P et al, Life events and psychosis. Initial results from the Camberwell Collaborative Psychosis Study, *Br J Psychiatry* (1993) **162**:72–9.

142. Ventura J, Nuechterlein KH, Lukoff D, Hardesty JP, A prospective study of stressful life events and schizophrenic relapse, *J Abnorm Psychol* (1989) **98**:407–11.

143. Paykel ES, Contribution of life events to causation of psychiatric illness, *Psychol Med* (1978) **8**:245–53.

144. Dohrenwend BP, A psychosocial perspective on the past and future of psychiatric epidemiology, *Am J Epidemiol* (1998) **147**:222–31.

145. Stephens JH, Astrup C, Mangrum JC, Prognostic factors in recovered and deteriorated schizophrenics, *Am J Psychiatry* (1996) **122**:1116–21.

146. Vaillant GE, The prediction of recovery in schizophrenia, *Int J Psychiatry* (1966) **2**:617–27.

147. van Os J, Fahy TA, Bebbington P et al, The influence of life events on the subsequent course of psychotic illness, A prospective follow-up of the Camberwell Collaborative Psychosis Study, *Psychol Med* (1994) **24:**503–13.

148. Bebbington P, Kuipers L, The clinical utility of expressed emotion in schizophrenia, *Acta Psychiatr Scand Suppl* (1994) **382:**46–53.

149. Glynn SM, Randolph ET, Eth S et al, Patient psychopathology and expressed emotion in schizophrenia, *Br J Psychiatry* (1990) **157:**877–80.

150. Schreiber JL, Breier A, Pickar D, Expressed emotion. Trait or state? *Br J Psychiatry* (1995) **166:**647–9.

151. Koreen AR, Siris SG, Chakos M et al, Depression in first-episode schizophrenia, *Am J Psychiatry* (1993) **150:**1643–8.

152. Callan AF, Schizophrenia in Afro-Caribbean immigrants, *J R Soc Med* (1999) **89:**253–6.

153. Holloway J, Carson J, Intensive case management: does it work? *European Psychiatry* (1996) **11:**263–4.

154. McKenzie K, van Os J, Fahy T et al, Psychosis with good prognosis in Afro-Caribbean people now living in the United Kingdom, *BMJ* (1995) **311:**1325–8.

155. Hutchinson G, Takei N, Sham P et al, Factor analysis of symptoms in schizophrenia: differences between White and Caribbean patients in Camberwell, *Psychol Med* (1999) **29:**607–12.

156. van Os J, Takei N, Castle DJ et al, The incidence of mania: time trends in relation to gender and ethnicity, *Soc Psychiatry Psychiatr Epidemiol* (1996) **31:**129–36.

157. Harrison G, Outcome of psychosis in people of African-Caribbean family origin, *Br J Psychiatry* (1999) **175:**43–9.

158. McKenzie K, Samele C, Van Horn E et al, A comparison of the outcome and treatment of psychosis in people of Caribbean origin living in the UK and British Whites, submitted.

159. Sanguineti VR, Samuel SE, Schwartz SL, Robeson MR, Retrospective study of 2,200 involuntary psychiatric admissions and readmissions, *Am J Psychiatry* (1999) **153:**392–6.

160. Tomelleri CJ, Lakshminarayanan N, Herjanic M, Who are the 'committed'? *J Nerv Ment Dis* (1977) **165:**288–93.

161. Gallo JJ, Marino S, Ford D, Anthony JC, Filters on the pathway to mental health care. II. Sociodemographic factors, *Psychol Med* (1995) **25:**1149–60.

162. Scheffler RM, Miller AB, Demand analysis of mental health service use among ethnic subpopulations, *Inquiry* (1989) **26:**202–15.

163. Hu TW, Snowden LR, Jerrell JM, Nguyen TD, Ethnic populations in public mental health: services choice and level of use, *Am J Public Health* (1991) **81:**1429–34.

164. Klinkenberg WD, Calsyn RJ, The moderating effects of race on return visits to the psychiatric emergency room, *Psychiatr Serv* (1997) **48:**942–5.

165. Thompson JW, Belcher JR, DeForge BR et al, Changing characteristics of schizophrenic patients admitted to state hospitals, *Hosp Community Psychiatry* (1993) **44:**231–5.

166. Dassori AM, Miller AL, Saldana D, Schizophrenia among Hispanics: epidemiology, phenomenology, course, and outcome, *Schizophr Bull* (1995) **21:**303–12.

167. van Os J, McKenzie K, Jones P, Cultural differences in pathways to care, service use and treated outcomes, *Current Opinion in Psychiatry* (1997) **10:**178–82.

168. Cooper B, Social class and prognosis in schizophrenia, *Br J Prevent Soc Med* (1961) **15:**17–41.

169. Myers JK, Bean LL, *A Decade Later: A Follow-up of Social Class and Mental Illness* (Wiley: New York, 1968).

170. Eaton WW, Social class and chronicity of schizophrenia, *J Chronic Dis* (1975) **28:**191–8.

171. Gift TE, Harder DW, The severity of psychiatric disorder: a replication, *Psychiatry Res* (1985) **14:**163–73.

172. O'Connell RA, Mayo JA, Flatow L et al, Outcome of bipolar disorder on long-term treatment with lithium, *Br J Psychiatry* (1991) **159:**123–9.

173. Hafner H, Maurer K, Loffler W et al, The epidemiology of early schizophrenia. Influence of age and gender on onset and early course, *Br J Psychiatry Suppl* (1994) **23:**29–38.

174. Larsen TK, Johannessen JO, Opjordsmoen S, First-episode schizophrenia with long duration of untreated psychosis. Pathways to care, *Br J Psychiatry Suppl* (1998) **172:**45–52.

175. Crow TJ, MacMillan JF, Johnson AL, Johnstone

EC, A randomised controlled trial of prophylactic neuroleptic treatment, *Br J Psychiatry* (1986) **148:**120–7.

176. Loebel AD, Lieberman JA, Alvir JM et al, Duration of psychosis and outcome in first-episode schizophrenia, *Am J Psychiatry* (1992) **149:**1183–8.

177. Haas GL, Garratt LS, Sweeney JA, Delay to first antipsychotic medication in schizophrenia: impact on symptomatology and clinical course of illness, *J Psychiatr Res* (1998) **32:**151–9.

178. Verdoux H, Bergey C, Assens F et al, Prediction of duration of psychosis before admission, *European Psychiatry* (1998) **13:**346–52.

179. Johannessen JO, Larsen TK, McGlashan T, Duration of untreated psychosis: an important target for intervention in schizophrenia? *Nordic Journal of Psychiatry* (1999) **53:**275–283.

180. May PR, Tuma AH, Dixon WJ et al, Schizophrenia. A follow-up study of the results of five forms of treatment, *Arch Gen Psychiatry* (1981) **38:**776–84.

181. Johnstone EC, Owens DG, Crow TJ, Davis JM, Does a four-week delay in the introduction of medication alter the course of functional psychosis? *J Psychopharmacol* (1999) **13:**238–44.

182. Andreasson S, Allebeck P, Engstrom A, Rydberg U, Cannabis and schizophrenia. A longitudinal study of Swedish conscripts, *Lancet* (1987) **2:**1483–6.

183. McGuire PK, Jones P, Harvey I et al, Cannabis and acute psychosis, *Schizophr Res* (1994) **13:**161–7.

184. Bartels SJ, Drake RE, Wallach MA, Long-term course of substance use disorders among patients with severe mental illness, *Psychiatr Serv* (1995) **46:**248–51.

185. Regier DA, Farmer ME, Rae DS et al, Comorbidity of mental disorders with alcohol and other drug abuse, Results from the Epidemiologic Catchment Area (ECA) Study, *JAMA* (1990) **264:**2511–18.

186. Linszen DH, Dingemans PM, Lenior ME, Cannabis abuse and the course of recent-onset schizophrenic disorders, *Arch Gen Psychiatry* (1994) **51:**273–9.

187. Grech A, van Os J, Murray RM, Influence of cannabis on the outcome of psychosis, *Schizophr Res* (1999) **36:**41.

188. Krystal JH, D'Souza DC, Madonick S, Petrakis IL, Toward a rational pharmacotherapy of comorbid substance abuse in schizophrenic patients, *Schizophr Res* (1999) **35(Suppl):**S35–49.

189. Turner WM, Tsuang MT, Impact of substance abuse on the course and outcome of schizophrenia, *Schizophr Bull* (1990) **16:**87–95.

190. Robins E, Guze SB, Establishment of diagnostic validity in psychiatric illness: its applications to schizophrenia, *Am J Psychiatry* (1970) **126:**983–7.

191. Tyrer P, Hassiotis A, Ukoumunne O et al, Intensive case management for psychotic patients with borderline intelligence. UK 700 Group [letter], *Lancet* (1999) **354:**999–1000.

192. Snowden LR, Hu TW, Jerrell JM, Emergency care avoidance: ethnic matching and participation in minority-serving programs, *Community Ment Health J* (1995) **31:**463–73.

193. Moller HJ, Muller H, Borison RL et al, A path-analytical approach to differentiate between direct and indirect drug effects on negative symptoms in schizophrenic patients, A re-evaluation of the North American risperidone study, *Eur Arch Psychiatry Clin Neurosci* (1995) **245:**45–9.

194. Purdon SE, Cognitive improvement in schizophrenia with novel antipsychotic medications, *Schizophr Res* (1999) **35(Suppl):**S51–60.

195. Tollefson GD, Sanger TM, Negative symptoms: a path analytic approach to a double-blind, placebo- and haloperidol-controlled clinical trial with olanzapine, *Am J Psychiatry* (1997) **154:**466–74.

196. Rund BR, Borg NE, Cognitive deficits and cognitive training in schizophrenic patients: a review, *Acta Psychiatr Scand* (1999) **100:**85–95.

197. Wykes T, Reeder C, Corner J et al, The effects of neurocognitive remediation on executive processing in patients with schizophrenia, *Schizophr Bull* (1999) **25:**291–307.

198. Carbone S, Harrigan S, McGorry PD et al, Duration of untreated psychosis and 12-month outcome in first-episode psychosis: the impact of treatment approach, *Acta Psychiatr Scand* (1999) **100:**96–104.

199. Johannessen JO, Early intervention and prevention in schizophrenia – experiences from a study in Stavanger, Norway, *Seishin Shinkeigaku Zasshi* (1998) **100:**511–22.

200. Levinson DF, Umapathy C, Musthaq M, Treatment of schizoaffective disorder and schizophrenia with mood symptoms, *Am J Psychiatry* (1999) **156:**1138–48.

201. Tollefson GD, Sanger TM, Lu Y, Thieme ME, Depressive signs and symptoms in schizophrenia: a prospective blinded trial of olanzapine and haloperidol, *Arch Gen Psychiatry* (1998) **55:**250–8.

4

Pharmacological Treatment of Schizophrenia

Susan L Siegfreid, Wolfgang Fleischhacker and Jeffrey A Lieberman

Contents • Introduction • History • Classification and terminology • Chemistry • Pharmacodynamics • Pharmacokinetics • Indications for use of antipsychotic drugs • Selection and dosing of an antipsychotic agent • Combination antipsychotic therapy • Adjunctive treatments • Switching antipsychotics • Electroconvulsive therapy • Adverse effects • Conclusions

Introduction

The modern era of psychopharmacology of schizophrenia started with the recognition of the unique properties of chlorpromazine in the early 1950s. Chlorpromazine and its congeners were effective in treating psychotic symptoms and allowed many institutionalized patients to live and be treated in a community setting. The introduction of chlorpromazine also provided resurgence of interest in the pathogenesis and treatment of schizophrenia. It is clear that over the second half of the twentieth century, antipsychotic medications had a profound impact on the treatment of psychotic symptoms and have now become the cornerstone of treatment for schizophrenia. Antipsychotic drugs have also provided a platform on which to use adjunctive treatments, both pharmacological and psychosocial, to augment the effects of these drugs and treat residual and comorbid symptoms of schizophrenia. This chapter reviews the pharmacology, use, and side effects of antipsychotic agents and describes other drugs that are used in association with them.

History

Phenothiazines were first developed in the late nineteenth century and initially used as urinary antiseptics. Charpentier synthesized chlorpromazine as a potential antihistamine for use with anesthetics in 1950. While using the agent to potentiate anesthetics, a French surgeon, Henri Laborit, recognized a unique property of chlorpromazine to produce a certain disinterest (*désintéressement*) in the environment and an 'artificial hibernation'.[1] Laborit reported on the results of his experience using chlorpromazine, speculating: 'These findings allow one to anticipate certain indications for the use of this compound in psychiatry. . . '.[1] Delay and Deniker soon followed with their report on its use in psychiatric patients.[2] Chlorpromazine was subsequently found to have antipsychotic properties that produced dramatic improvements in schizophrenic patients. Chlorpromazine was the first drug in psychiatry to effectively treat the symptoms of schizophrenia and related psychotic disorders. Thus, it became the prototypic antipsychotic agent.

Chlorpromazine, and the antipsychotic drugs that followed, initiated a pharmacological revolution in psychiatry. These compounds greatly improved the ability to treat psychotic illness and produced a dramatic shift in psychiatric practice. The introduction of chlorpromazine marked the beginnings of modern psychopharmacology.

Classification and terminology

Historically, antipsychotic medications were referred to as 'major tranquilizers' for the observed effects on agitation and anxiety. The term is a misnomer, since it refers to a side effect and not a therapeutic effect of the medication. It is no longer in common use.

The term 'neuroleptic' was originally used to describe the psychomotor slowing and other neurological side effects (extrapyramidal syndrome or EPS) characteristic of older antipsychotic medications. Alternatively, 'neuroleptic' has also been applied to describe medications with both experimentally and clinically significant antagonism of dopamine receptors. Since the introduction of clozapine and other newer agents that possess antipsychotic effects with a low liability for EPS, continued use of this term is not an adequate descriptor of these compounds. The term has been largely replaced by the broader term 'antipsychotic'.

The term 'atypical' was first used to describe clozapine, since its pharmacological properties were found to be very different from those of older, conventional 'neuroleptics' or 'typical' antipsychotic drugs. Many of the properties of clozapine were used to define an 'atypical' antipsychotic drug. As other novel antipsychotic drugs have been introduced over time, the meaning of the term 'atypical' has created a great deal of debate. At present, there is no consensus on the criteria that define an antipsychotic drug as 'atypical', but features based on both preclinical and clinical data have been commonly used.[3–5] In general, an 'atypical' antipsychotic drug can be characterized by the following criteria: (a) low propensity to cause acute EPS or tardive dyskinesia; (b) both superior and broader spectrum of antipsychotic efficacy; (c) minimal elevation of prolactin levels; (d) low potential to cause catalepsy in preclinical animal studies; and (e) lower dopamine (D_2) receptor affinity and higher serotonin (5-HT) receptor affinity.[3–5] When these criteria are applied to all currently available antipsychotic medications, it becomes apparent that there exists a continuum of 'typical' and 'atypical' agents, rather than two distinct groups. As no meaningful distinction can be made using these terms, the compounds may be more correctly described as 'second generation' or 'novel' antipsychotics. In this chapter, the newer antipsychotic drugs will be referred to interchangeably as novel or atypical.

Chemistry

Antipsychotic drugs can be classified by their chemical structures, but this is simplistic and provides little meaningful distinction between agents. These structurally dissimilar compounds, however, do share many pharmacological properties.

All phenothiazines share the same three-ring structure and can be subdivided by their different side chain moieties into three groups: (a) aliphatic (such as chlorpromazine); (b) piperazine (such as fluphenazine); and (c) piperidine (such as thioridazine). Thioxanthenes (such as thiothixene, flupenthixol) are another group of antipsychotic agents structurally similar to phenothiazines.

Dibenzepines, a group of tricyclic antipsychotic compounds, are also based on the phenothiazine ring structure with a seven-member center ring. Dibenzepine derivatives include loxapine (a dibenzoxazepine) and clozapine (a dibenzodiazepine). Both olanzapine (a thienobenzodiazepine) and quetiapine (a benzothiazepine) are structurally related to clozapine.

Heterocyclic compounds include several chemical classes: (a) butyrophenones (such as haloperidol) and structurally similar diphenylbutylpiperidines (such as pimozide); (b) dihydroindole derivatives (such as molindone); (c) benzisoxazole derivatives (such as risperidone); (d) benzisothiazole derivatives (such as ziprasidone); and (e) benzamides (such as amisulpride and sulpiride). The structure–activity relationships of antipsychotic drugs are beyond the scope of this chapter and have been reviewed elsewhere.[6]

Pharmacodynamics

Relative potency

Based on the belief that both the antipsychotic and extrapyramidal side effects were the result of dopamine receptor antagonism, the older antipsychotic medications have been classified by drug potency. Potency can be defined in terms of the minimum amount of antipsychotic drug in milligrams to achieve an antipsychotic effect. Antipsychotic drug potency is correlated with its binding affinity for dopamine D_2 receptors.[7] Potency can also be expressed in terms of chlorpromazine equivalents, that is, the ratio of an antipsychotic drug's potency compared to a standard dose of chlorpromazine. A useful generalization is that high-potency drugs (such as haloperidol) have a chlorpromazine equivalent dose of less than 5 mg and have a greater tendency to cause EPS. Low-potency drugs (such as thioridazine) have a chlorpromazine equivalent dose of more than 40 mg and have a greater propensity to cause sedation, hypotension, and anticholinergic side effects.

Receptor pharmacology

Research in molecular pharmacology over the past few decades has provided new insight into the mechanisms involved in both the therapeutic benefits and side effects of antipsychotic drugs. This new information has also provided a basis for new hypotheses regarding the pathophysiology of schizophrenia. Identification of specific neurotransmitter systems and receptors provides a rationale for the development of novel compounds with more specific pharmacological properties.

Both in vitro studies and, more recently, in vivo radioligand studies of receptor binding using positron emission tomography (PET) have demonstrated that antipsychotic drugs bind to various neurotransmitter receptors. Generally, antipsychotic drugs act as antagonists at these receptor sites. The profiles of receptor binding affinities for various antipsychotic drugs in clinical use are shown in Table 4.1.

The first evidence that antipsychotic drugs blocked dopamine receptors came from the work of Carlsson and Lindquist, who reported that administration of chlorpromazine or haloperidol to mice resulted in the accumulation of dopamine metabolites in dopaminergic brain regions.[8] As reported by both Seeman et al and Creese et al, the observed correlation between the binding affinity of conventional antipsychotics for the D_2 receptors and their effective clinical dose provided strong evidence that one mechanism of action of typical antipsychotic drugs includes D_2 receptor blockade.[9–11] PET radioligand binding studies have further elucidated the importance of dopamine receptor occupancy as a predictor of antipsychotic response and adverse effects. Prospective studies have suggested that antipsychotic effects are associated with approximately 60% D_2 receptor antagonism, but that occupancy greater than 80% significantly increases the risk of EPS.[11–13] These studies indicate that there is a narrow therapeutic–toxic index for most conventional antipsychotics.[14]

Antagonism of dopamine-mediated neurotransmission within the striatum occurs within hours of administration of an antipsychotic drug, but it may take several weeks to manifest a clinical effect.[11–13] It has been proposed that, acutely, these drugs act to block postsynaptic dopamine receptors.[15] Subsequent increases in presynaptic dopamine activity manifested by increased metabolism and firing rates of dopaminergic neurons is termed 'depolarization activation'.[15] These early responses are later replaced by depression of presynaptic dopamine activity and seem to correlate with the time course to clinical response, which is described as 'depolarization inactivation'.[15]

Dopamine receptor antagonism may have direct effects, depend on second messenger systems, or initiate a cascade of 'downstream' receptor activity. The long-term reduction in dopaminergic function may be evident by its

Table 4.1 Antipsychotic drugs: in vitro receptor binding (affinity values K_i in nmol).						
	Haloperidol	Clozapine	Risperidone	Olanzapine	Quetiapine	Ziprasidone
D_1	210	85	430	31	460	525
D_2	1	160	2	44	580	4
D_3	2	170	10	50	940	7
D_4	3	50	10	50	1900	32
$5HT_{1A}$	1100	200	210	>10000	720	3
$5HT_{1D}$	>10000	1900	170	800	6200	2
$5HT_{2A}$	45	16	0.5	5	300	0.4
$5HT_{2C}$	>10000	10	25	11	5100	1
$5HT_6$	9600	14	2200	10	33	130
$5HT_7$	1200	100	2	150	130	23
5HT reuptake	1700	5000	1300	–	–	50
NE reuptake	4700	500	>10000	–	–	50
$NE_{\alpha1}$	6	7	1	19	7	10
$NE_{\alpha2}$	360	8	1	230	90	200
H_1	440	1	20	3	11	50
Muscarinic	5500	2	>1000	2	>1000	>1000

The lower the number, the stronger the affinity for the specific neuroreceptor.
K_i, inhibitory constant; NE, norepinephrine.

effects on major dopamine pathways in the brain. These effects may include a reduction in the positive symptoms of schizophrenia thought to be mediated by the mesolimbic pathway and the appearance of EPS via the nigrostriatal pathway. The clinical significance of antagonism of other dopamine receptor subtypes (D_1, D_3, D_4 and D_5) is unclear.

Some degree of D_2 receptor occupancy by antipsychotic drugs appears to be necessary for their therapeutic effects but it is not always sufficient. Many patients do not respond to medication, despite adequate D_2 occupancy.[11] The broader pharmacological spectrum of atypical antipsychotic agents, with a lower affinity for D_2 receptors in combination with higher serotonin (5-HT_2) receptor antagonism, has modified previous hypotheses to explain the mechanism of action of these compounds. Clozapine, the proto-

typical 'atypical antipsychotic', has a low affinity for the D_2 receptor, with studies reporting occupancy in the range of 20–67%.[12,13,16] It does, however, have significant 5-HT_{2A} receptor antagonism, with occupancy between 85–90%.[16] Serotonin is thought to modulate dopamine activity, although it may also play a more direct role in the pathophysiology of schizophrenia.[17]

Serotonergic blockade may be the underlying mechanism for the apparent efficacy of atypical antipsychotic drugs in treating the positive symptoms and possibly the negative symptoms of schizophrenia.[12,13] A reduction in serotonergic tone increases dopamine levels in the nigrostriatal pathway, which could reduce the propensity of these agents to produce EPS.[17] Antagonism of 5-HT_2 receptors in the mesocortical pathway, especially in the prefrontal cortex, may enhance dopamine activity in this area, which is postulated to mediate some of the negative signs and symptoms of schizophrenia.[17] It has been argued that the ratio of relative affinity of antipsychotic agents for 5-HT$_2$ receptors to D$_2$ receptors may also have some value in classifying these drugs as atypical antipsychotics.[4,5] Other putative atypical antipsychotic agents also possess significant 5-HT$_2$ antagonism (often greater than 80% receptor occupancy), which is seen in conjunction with a lower affinity (usually less than 80% occupancy) for D$_2$ receptors.[13]

Antagonism at other neurotransmitter receptors, such as muscarinic cholinergic, histaminic (H$_1$), and alpha-adrenergic receptors, may contribute to both therapeutic and adverse effects seen with antipsychotic agents.[14] Figure 4.1 describes the binding affinities of antipsychotic drugs at these neurotransmitter receptors.

Effects of age on pharmacodynamics

There is evidence to suggest that pharmacodynamic effects altered by aging may be responsible for the increase in side effects seen in geriatric patients given antipsychotic medication.[18] Decreases in dopamine and acetylcholine in the brain may predispose this population to increased risk of EPS, and greater sensitivity to the central effects of medications possessing anticholinergic activity, respectively.[18] It is unclear, however, whether these pharmacodynamic changes with aging have clinically significant effects on the therapeutic efficacy of antipsychotic medications.

Pharmacokinetics

Absorption and distribution

Antipsychotic drugs tend to be rapidly absorbed from the gastrointestinal tract and undergo varying degrees of presystemic or first-pass hepatic metabolism.[6] Since they are highly lipid-soluble and protein-bound, antipsychotics have a rapid distribution phase and are easily transported across the blood–brain barrier.[6] In addition, significant amounts of these drugs are stored in tissues with a large blood supply. Consequently,

tissue concentrations often exceed plasma concentrations and this is reflected in a relatively large volume of distribution.[6]

The average half-life of most antipsychotic drugs administered orally is greater than 20 hours, allowing for a single daily dose to be given.[6] Among the newer atypical antipsychotic agents, risperidone, clozapine, and quetiapine have relatively shorter half-lives and are usually administered in divided doses. Their therapeutic effects, however, may extend beyond the time period predicted by their half-life with repeated dosing and/or the presence of active metabolites.[19] With most antipsychotics given orally, the time to steady state concentrations is approximately 3–7 days, or four to five times the individual drug's half-life.[19] Older age, concurrent medications, hepatic disease or slow absorption may increase the half-life of an antipsychotic drug and the time required to attain steady state concentrations.[6]

Hepatic metabolism

Antipsychotics vary in the extent to which they are metabolized in the liver. This variability is often attributed to heterogeneity of bioavailability and drug metabolism. Other factors that may contribute to variability are drug–drug interactions, cigarette smoking, and comorbid medical conditions.[19] Patients on a stable dose of medication may need dosage adjustments whenever other medications are started or discontinued. In addition, drug interactions must be considered in clinical situations involving the combination of two or more antipsychotic agents or when adjunctive medications are added to a treatment regimen.

Most antipsychotics are metabolized by hepatic microsomal oxidases (cytochrome P450 system). The major isoenzyme systems involved are CYP1A2, CYP2C19, CYP2D6, and CYP3A4.[19] Several of the antipsychotic medications are metabolized into active metabolites (for instance, norclozapine).[20] These active metabolites can accumulate to a steady state concentration in relation to their own half-life independent of the

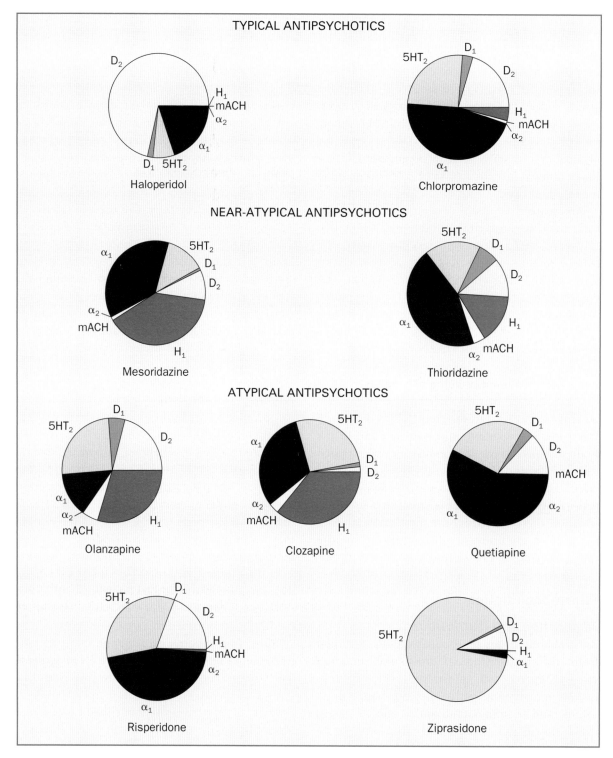

Figure 4.1 Relative neuroreceptor binding affinities of antipsychotic drugs. *m*ACH, Muscarinic acetylcholine. Reproduced with permission from *Psychiatric Drugs*, Lieberman, Tasman, eds. (Saunders: Philadelphia, 2000).

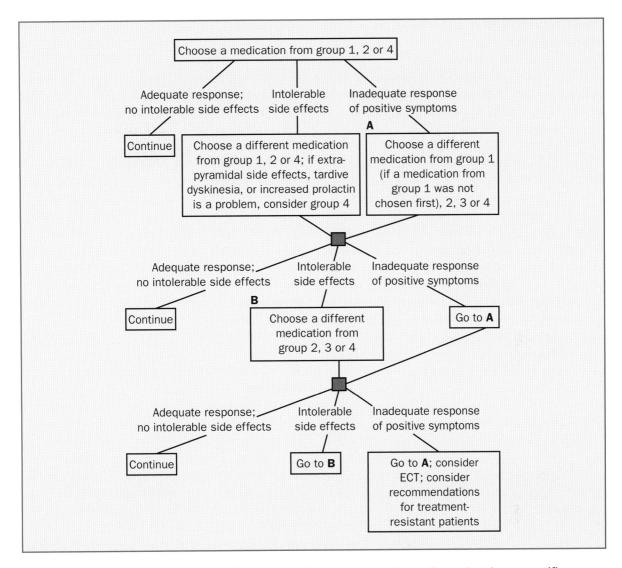

Figure 4.2 Pharmacologic treatment of schizophrenia in the acute phase. If a patient has a specific contra-indication to any medication, remove that medication from the possibilities for that patient. At each point in the algorithm, medications are chosen on the basis of (1) past response, (2) side effects, (3) patient preference, and (4) planned route of administration. Group 1: Conventional antipsychotic medications. Group 2: Risperidone. Group 3: Clozapine. Group 4: New antipsychotic medications: olanzapine, ziprasidone, quetiapine. (Ziprasidone has not yet obtained FDA approval.) (Adapted from *Practice Guidelines for the Treatment of Patients with Schizophrenia*, American Psychiatric Association, 1997.)

parent compound.[6] Active metabolites may have equivalent or greater potency as antipsychotic agents compared to the parent compound (for example, 9-hydroxyrisperidone).[20]

Elimination

Antipsychotic drugs and their metabolites ultimately undergo conjugation or glucuronidation and are excreted mainly in the urine.

Pharmacokinetics of parenteral administration

Several of the antipsychotic drugs are also available in a short-acting parenteral form. The main indication for parenteral administration of antipsychotic medication in the acute setting is to treat severely agitated patients. The bioavailability of these agents may increase significantly, mainly due to their ability to bypass most of the first-pass metabolism that occurs with oral administration.[6,21] Parenteral forms tend to have rapid onset of action with respect to sedation and may reach peak plasma concentration within one-half to 1 hour.[6] Since the bioavailability of parenteral antipsychotics may increase up to tenfold, the initial dose should be decreased three- to fourfold compared to the usual oral dose.[6] At the time of publication, there is no atypical antipsychotic agent commercially available in parenteral form.

Long-acting repository, or 'depot' preparations of antipsychotic drugs are administered as esters dissolved in an oil vehicle.[21] Several antipsychotic drugs (for instance, haloperidol or fluphenazine) are available in these long-acting or 'depot' forms. In various European countries and other parts of the world, long-acting drugs including flupenthixol decanoate, perphenazine enanthate, and zuclopenthixol decanoate are also available.

These agents are designed to be absorbed slowly but continually over the time interval between injections, typically 2–4 weeks.[22] The rate-limiting step in absorption is diffusion into surrounding tissues. Once these drugs are absorbed, they are rapidly hydrolyzed into the parent compound.[21] A relatively constant plasma level can be achieved, since these drugs bypass presystemic metabolism.[6,21] It can take from 3 to 6 months to reach steady state plasma level and elimination is very slow.[6]

Long-acting preparations are often used for maintenance treatment of schizophrenia and are particularly advantageous in patients demonstrating repeated noncompliance with oral medications.[21] Guidelines for the use of depot antipsychotic medications can be found elsewhere.[23] None of the newer, atypical antipsychotic agents are currently available in a long-acting parenteral form. Several atypical drugs are being developed in long-acting forms. The atypical drug furthest along in development is a long-acting microsphere preparation of risperidone.

Variables affecting pharmacokinetics

Several clinically significant factors can affect antipsychotic drug metabolism including: (a) age; (b) substance use, especially alcohol and nicotine; (c) hepatic disease; and (d) concurrent medications that either induce or inhibit hepatic microsomal enzymes. Other variables that may be of significance in certain clinical situations include genetic polymorphisms, ethnic differences in microsomal enzymes, gender, and changes in binding proteins.[6,19]

Pharmacokinetic considerations in children

The metabolism of medications in children is much higher and consequently the pharmacokinetics of psychotropic drugs is different in children than in adults. As children mature, their metabolism changes, requiring adjustments and dosing changes throughout childhood and adolescence.[22] Children have a larger reservoir for lipophilic drugs because they have more body fat, which may prolong the half-life of antipsychotic medication.[22] Prepubertal children have a much higher hepatic clearance rate relative to their body weight compared to adults.[24] Larger or more frequent dosing is often required to achieve therapeutic blood levels.[24] In general, younger patients also tend to be more sensitive to the pharmacological effects of drugs.

Pharmacokinetic considerations in the elderly

Pharmacokinetic differences in geriatric populations must be taken into account when using psychotropic agents in this group. Aging, in general, can affect any relevant pharmacokinetic factor.

With age, there is a decrease in lean muscle mass and an increase in body fat, which can affect the distribution and half-life of lipophilic drugs. As the volume of drug distribution increases, a longer period of time is required to reach steady-state concentrations.[18] Hepatic metabolism is also affected by changes in microsomal enzyme structure and activity, decreasing the rate of medication clearance.[18]

Drug–drug interactions

Enzyme induction

Cigarette smoking has been shown to induce cytochrome CYP1A2 and increases drug clearance for many antipsychotic drugs. Inhaled smoke can decrease the plasma concentrations of high-potency typical antipsychotics by 10–50%.[20] The clearance rates of clozapine and olanzapine are similarly increased by 20–50%.[19] Other enzyme inducers include anticonvulsants (carbamazepine, phenobarbital, and phenytoin) and subchronic alcohol use. Coadministration of anticonvulsants with typical antipsychotic medications can increase their clearance rate more than twofold.[25] Anticonvulsants may not have a significant effect on the metabolic clearance of olanzapine or risperidone.[19]

Enzyme inhibition

Many medications can inhibit microsomal enzymes and decrease the clearance of antipsychotic drugs, possibly leading to toxicity. Conventional antipsychotic drug clearance can be decreased by 50% with concurrent administration of antidepressants, beta-blockers, some antibiotic/antifungal agents, and cimetidine.[19,25] Elevations in clozapine levels, potentially leading to toxicity, have been reported with coadministration of fluvoxamine.[26] Refer to Table 4.2 for clinically significant interactions with specific cytochrome P450 isoenzymes.

Plasma levels

The use of blood levels as a guide for dosing or determining lack of response to an antipsychotic medication is not common in clinical settings and remains controversial. There is a wide interindividual variation in blood levels and a narrow dose range between therapeutic efficacy and increasing risk of side effects.[27,28] Plasma levels among typical antipsychotic agents have been established for several compounds, but there is at best a moderate correlation between these levels and clinical response.[28,29] Haloperidol and perphenazine levels of 15 ng/ml and 1.5–2 ng/ml, respectively, have been suggested as optimal.[30]

It may be helpful to measure the plasma level of conventional antipsychotics under certain circumstances. Before deciding that an antipsychotic medication is ineffective despite an adequate trial at a sufficient dose, it is important to determine whether it may be due to alterations in the pharmacokinetics of the drug.[27] A low plasma level may necessitate increasing the dose or addressing compliance issues. Significantly elevated plasma levels may require a decrease in the dose because medication side effects may be overshadowing therapeutic effects. Other instances when plasma level monitoring may be indicated include: (a) special patient populations (children and the elderly); (b) suspected pharmacokinetic interactions in combination with other psychotropic agents, and (c) when decreasing medication dosage during maintenance therapy, since low plasma levels may indicate an increased risk of relapse.

Some researchers have proposed using the plasma level of clozapine as a guide to dose titration. Since there are dosing discrepancies in terms of mean dose used of up to twofold between the United States and many European countries, higher plasma levels have been recommended in the United States.[31] Vander Zwaag et al has proposed that target plasma levels should be between 200 and 250 ng/ml, although many patients will respond at lower plasma levels.[32] A plasma level below 100 ng/ml is viewed by some as too low, and conversely, levels above 500 ng/ml as high.[33] Whether plasma levels of clozapine correlate with therapeutic efficacy, however, is unclear.[34] Clozapine plasma levels do correlate with some of the drug's side effects including

Table 4.2 Antipsychotic drugs: substrates, inhibitors, and inducers for selected cytochrome P450 isoenzymes.

Isoenzyme	Substrates	Inhibitors	Inducers
CYP1A2	Clozapine		
	Olanzapine		
CYP2C9	(None)	(None)	
CYP2C19	Clozapine		
CYP2E1	(None)	(None)	
CYP2D6	Clozapine	Haloperidol	
	Fluphenazine	Thioridazine	
	Haloperidol		
	Olanzapine		
	Perphenazine		
	Risperidone		
	Thioridazine		
CYP3A4	Clozapine	Fluoxetine	
	Haloperidol		
	Pimozide		
	Quetiapine		
	Ziprasidone		

Specific cytochrome P450 enzymes that metabolize some of the older drugs were not determined since clozapine was the first antipsychotic drug for which that was required in its New Drug Application by the U.S. Food and Drug Administration.

electroencephalogram (EEG) alterations, seizures, and confusion.[31,35]

Indications for use of antipsychotic drugs

Antipsychotic drugs are effective for treatment of psychotic symptoms. They are the mainstay in the treatment of acute psychotic episodes and the maintenance of symptom remission in patients with schizophrenia. The strategies and goals of treatment vary with the severity and course of illness.

Acute treatment

An acute psychotic episode or relapse is characterized by severe psychotic symptoms, including hallucinations, delusions, and disorganized speech and thinking. The specific goals of treatment include reducing or resolving these acute psychotic symptoms. All antipsychotic medications have demonstrated efficacy in treating the positive symptoms of schizophrenia. They are indicated for almost all acute episodes of the illness, including both first-episode psychosis and recurrence in chronic schizophrenia.[36] Antipsychotic medications should be instituted without undue delay because early intervention has been shown to improve the chances of therapeutic response and decrease long-term morbidity.[37–39]

Conventional antipsychotic medications have been found to be effective for positive symptoms associated with acute psychosis. Typical antipsychotic agents are much less effective against negative symptoms, cognitive impairment, or mood symptoms associated with schizophrenia. With the introduction of atypical antipsychotics, it has been suggested that these agents may have a broader spectrum of activity against negative symptoms, as well as other symptom dimensions in schizophrenia. To date, only amisulpride has demonstrated efficacy against primary negative symptoms/deficit states.[40] Sharif has reviewed the clinical issues and common goals in the management of an acute exacerbation of schizophrenia.[41]

Maintenance treatment

During this phase, the acute psychotic symptoms have decreased in severity but the patient is at risk for relapse. Risk factors for relapse include psychosocial stressors, substance abuse, premature lowering or discontinuation of the antipsychotic medication, or the nature of the illness itself. The goals of maintenance treatment are to maintain or improve symptom remission, improve quality of life, achieve psychosocial reintegration, and prevent relapse.

Symptoms, if present during this phase, tend to be relatively stable and less severe than during the acute episode. The clinical presentation may be predominantly negative symptomatology or attenuated positive and negative symptoms. The value of long-term maintenance treatment in preventing relapse has now been demonstrated in a large number of studies.[42] Furthermore, those patients who do relapse while taking medication seem to have milder symptoms and a greater rate of improvement compared with patients who discontinue antipsychotic medication.[43]

Guidelines developed for relapse prevention in schizophrenia recommend maintenance therapy for 1–2 years following a first episode of psychosis and at least 5 years of maintenance treatment for chronic patients with multiple episodes of illness.[33,44–47]

First-episode schizophrenia

In general, first-episode patients are more responsive to treatment and require a lower dose of medication than chronic patients.[38,48] This group of patients tends to have a greater rate of recovery from an acute psychotic episode and lower rates of relapse during maintenance treatment.[38] Maintenance treatment for first-episode psychosis can present a clinical dilemma. A small minority of these patients will not have a recurrence of psychotic illness.[44] Most first-episode patients, however, will have a recurrence of psychotic symptoms within 3 years following their initial episode.[48] Since the small subgroup of patients that do not have a recurrence cannot be identified on an a priori basis, it is generally accepted that, time-limited maintenance treatment is indicated.

Treatment-resistant schizophrenia

The definition of treatment resistance continues to evolve over time and there is no current consensus on its criteria. Patients considered to be treatment-resistant, in the broadest terms, include those with: (a) failure to respond to two previous antipsychotic trials; (b) intolerable side effects, such as severe EPS or tardive dyskinesia; (c) persistent psychotic symptoms despite treatment; or (d) violent behavior unresponsive to antipsychotic medications.[33] Treatment resistance is present in approximately 10–15% of patients at the onset of schizophrenia. During the course of the illness, 30–60% of patients become only partially responsive or completely unresponsive to treatment.[48,49] Serious medication-induced side effects may occur in almost half of patients.[50] Currently, clozapine is regarded as the treatment of choice in refractory patients. However, recent studies have shown that other atypical drugs (e.g. olanzapine, risperidone) may also be effective in refractory patients and thus obviate the need for clozapine and associated hematologic monitorings[50a,b] the only medication that has been shown to be effective in this patient population is clozapine. It is possible that other novel antipsychotic agents may be useful in treatment-resistant patients.

Patients with tardive dyskinesia

Patients who develop tardive dyskinesia (TD) or have preexisting TD as a result of exposure to antipsychotic medication and still require treatment present a clinical dilemma. The American Psychiatric Association Task Force on Tardive Dyskinesia recommendations include using the lowest effective dose of antipsychotic medication for patients who respond to treatment.[51] Clozapine has been shown to improve TD symptoms in several studies.[52,53] The mechanism by which clozapine mitigates or reverses tardive dyskinesia is unknown. Although other novel antipsychotic agents have not been systematically evaluated for effects on TD, it is reasonable to use these agents prior to a trial with clozapine.[54]

Childhood-onset schizophrenia

Few studies of antipsychotic drugs have been conducted in children and adolescents, but most have supported the use of these drugs in childhood-onset schizophrenia.[55,56] Typical antipsychotic drugs, olanzapine and risperidone have been recommended as first-line treatment for psychosis in children and adolescents.[55–58] A clozapine trial is indicated after failure of two adequate antipsychotic drug trials.[56] The reader is referred to 'Practice Parameters for the Assessment and Treatment of Children and Adolescents with Schizophrenia' published by the American Academy of Child and Adolescent Psychiatry[59] for further information.

Late-onset schizophrenia

Approximately 10% of all cases of first-episode schizophrenia occur in individuals over the age of 45.[60] Late-onset psychosis is similar in many respects to schizophrenia presenting in late adolescence or early adulthood with regard to positive symptomatology, chronic course, response to typical antipsychotic drugs, and family history. The clinical presentation of late-onset schizophrenia has fewer negative symptoms, female predominance, less severe cognitive impairment, and therapeutic effects at lower doses of antipsychotic medication.[61] There is also a general tendency for greater susceptibility to EPS, and females, in particular, seem more vulnerable to developing tardive dyskinesia with typical antipsychotics.[62] As with children, few studies have examined the efficacy of antipsychotics in older populations. Pertinent clinical issues related to the use of antipsychotic drugs in the elderly are reviewed elsewhere.[62]

Pregnancy and lactation

Because of the high lipophilicity of most antipsychotic drugs, they readily cross the placental barrier and are secreted in breast milk.[6] A meta-analysis by Altshuler et al on the effects of low-potency typical antipsychotic drugs during the first trimester of pregnancy reported that there was a very small increase in the relative risk for congenital abnormalities.[63] No evidence to date suggests that high-potency conventional antipsychotic agents increase the risk to the fetus.[63] It has been suggested that fetal exposure over the course of the pregnancy may affect development of the dopamine system. If possible, antipsychotic drugs should be avoided, at least during the first trimester, unless the risk to the mother/fetus outweighs the risk of using the medication.[33] Antipsychotic medications may be relatively safe during the second and third trimesters of pregnancy. If a typical antipsychotic agent is used, high-potency compounds are preferred because they have a lower propensity to cause orthostatic hypotension.[33] Low doses should be given and antipsychotic medication should be discontinued 5–10 days prior to delivery.[33] Anticholinergic agents should be avoided during pregnancy if at all possible.[33] Infants should not be breastfed if the mother resumes taking antipsychotic medication post partum.[64,65]

Selection and dosing of an antipsychotic agent

Pretreatment assessment

Prior to selecting a pharmacologic intervention, patients should have a thorough initial evaluation. This assessment will aid the clinician in establishing a baseline of symptoms and may be used to rule out medical or neurological causes of psychotic symptoms. The evaluation should include a complete psychiatric and medical history, physical examination, and an assessment for preexisting movement disorders using an instrument such as the Abnormal Involuntary Movement Scale (AIMS).[33,66] Baseline laboratory tests including a complete blood count, blood chemistries, urine drug screen, and evaluation of liver, renal, and thyroid function should be performed.[33] An electrocardiogram (ECG) should be obtained at baseline. Depending on the antipsychotic medication used for treatment, patients may require additional periodic monitoring for ECG abnormalities. Other diagnostic tests, such as an electroencephalogram (EEG), magnetic resonance imaging (MRI) of the brain, or neuropsychological tests, should be performed as indicated by the initial examination.

An equally important component of the initial assessment should include education of the patient and their family regarding the nature of the illness, its course, prognosis, and treatment.

Initial drug selection

Selection of an appropriate antipsychotic agent should be based on prior therapeutic response, tolerability, side effect profile, intended route of administration, patient preference, and the long-term treatment plan. Atypical antipsychotic drugs may be considered as first-line treatment for many patients, including those who are being treated for the first time. The treatment algorithm from the American Psychiatric Association *Practice Guidelines for the Treatment of Schizophrenia* may be helpful in choosing an appropriate antipsychotic drug (Figure 4.2).[33]

Treatment initiation and dose titration

It is important when initiating an antipsychotic medication to select a target dose that maximizes therapeutic benefit, while minimizing side effects. All typical antipsychotic drugs are equally efficacious, although they do vary in potency and side effect profiles. The effective daily dose range based on a meta-analysis of studies of typical antipsychotics is generally between 100 mg chlorpromazine (or 5 mg haloperidol) equivalents and 700 mg chlorpromazine (or 20 mg haloperidol) equivalents.[67]

When using a low-potency typical antipsychotic, the initial dose should be low (25–50 mg twice daily) and titrated upward over several days in order to minimize side effects such as orthostatic hypotension and sedation. When starting a high-potency typical antipsychotic such as haloperidol, slow titration is rarely necessary.

Among the atypical antipsychotics, risperidone can be started at a dose of 1–2 mg per day. This initial dose is increased over the next 3–7 days to a target daily dose range of 3–4 mg per day. If there is no treatment response after 2 weeks, the dose of risperidone can be increased to at least 6 mg per day. Kopala et al have demonstrated that lower doses of risperidone, especially in first-episode patients, may reduce the risk for motor side effects.[68] Olanzapine is usually started at a dose of 5–10 mg at bedtime to minimize sedation. A dose range for olanzapine is generally between 10–20 mg per day. Quetiapine can be started at 25 mg twice a day. The dose can be increased by 25–50 mg per day as tolerated until a target dose of 400–500 mg per day is achieved. Quetiapine has been shown to be effective at doses of 300–750 mg per day. Atypical antipsychotic drugs may have less of a sedative effect and the addition of a sedative-hypnotic agent during the acute phases of treatment may be required for agitation and insomnia.

If the patient can tolerate a dose of medication in the clinical dose range, it should be maintained for at least 3 weeks. The time course to response can be gradual.

Treatment evaluation

If a patient has failed to respond to a 3-week trial of an antipsychotic medication at an adequate dose, several factors should be evaluated. Plasma levels may be helpful to determine whether pharmacokinetic factors or noncompliance can explain a lack of response. Low plasma levels can be the cause of apparent lack of improvement in some patients. Adjusting the dose of medication so that a therapeutic plasma level is attained may lead to response.[27]

If the patient has been compliant with medication, assessment of whether there has been a partial response to treatment or no response to a drug trial should guide subsequent interventions.

When a patient has had a partial response to a conventional antipsychotic drug, a common clinical intervention is to increase the dose, although this practice is often not beneficial and may result in more side effects. The dose–response relationships of the newer atypical drugs have not been as well studied and increasing the dose may convert a partial responder into a full responder. Alternatively, medication side effects may be overshadowing antipsychotic effects and a dose reduction may be warranted. Adjunctive agents, as described below, have been used to augment antipsychotic efficacy in partially responsive patients.

A second trial of an antipsychotic medication may be indicated for patients who have not or have only partially responded to one antipsychotic drug. This practice of switching patients to another drug remains controversial.[69–71] If a conventional antipsychotic drug was used for the initial drug trial with poor response, it is likely to predict poor response with other typical agents.[72] One of the newer, atypical antipsychotic agents should be chosen for use in a second drug trial.

If poor compliance is the reason for lack of therapeutic response, a trial with a depot antipsychotic medication should be considered. The optimal dosage and interval between administrations must be tailored to the individual patient. Patients should be treated with the oral form of the antipsychotic drug first in order to determine approximate dosing requirements and drug tolerability. Common dosage conversions for fluphenazine and haloperidol are based on a 10 mg per day oral dose of either drug. This oral dose is roughly equivalent to 12.5–25 mg fluphenazine decanoate every 2 weeks or 100–200 mg haloperidol decanoate every 4 weeks. A reasonable starting dose is 12.5 mg fluphenazine decanoate or 25 mg haloperidol decanoate. Zuclopenthixol decanoate is given in doses of 100–400 mg every 4 weeks and flupenthixol decanoate is given in doses of 50–200 mg once a month. Ideally, patients should be switched from the oral to depot form of administration. Supplemental oral medication may be required during the first few months for symptom management until a therapeutic dose has been established.

Maintenance treatment

Individuals who experience acute symptomatic relief with a particular antipsychotic drug should be continued on it for a minimum of 1 year to prevent relapse. Emphasis should be placed on continuous risk–benefit assessment and the involvement of patients' significant others in all treatment efforts to ensure optimal treatment during maintenance therapy.

A general principle for maintenance treatment is to use the same dose of antipsychotic medication that was efficacious during acute treatment. If dose reduction is desired, it has been recommended that medication doses in stable patients be slowly reduced by increments not greater than 20% of the previous maintenance dose. Since there can be a significant lag in time to relapse, the time interval between dose reductions should be between 3 and 6 months.[73]

In patients on long-acting preparations, a recent study by Carpenter et al has suggested that drug exposure itself can be reduced by extending the interval between administration of standard doses of fluphenazine decanoate.[74] This study demonstrated that maintenance treatment could be administered every 6 weeks, as opposed to every 2 weeks, without increasing the risk of side effects or relapse.[74]

Intermittent or targeted therapy, as opposed to continuous treatment, has been shown to have at least a twofold higher risk for relapse in most studies and is not a feasible alternative for most patients.[75] Continuous treatment with an antipsychotic medication, therefore, is recommended.[33]

Treating refractory patients

Clozapine is the only medication with proven efficacy in treatment-resistant schizophrenia.[76] Current United States guidelines regarding the use of this medication reserve it for severely ill schizophrenic patients who fail to show clinical response to adequate trials, in terms of dosage and duration of treatment, of at least two different standard antipsychotic medications. Clozapine is available only through a central distribution system that ensures the appropriate laboratory monitoring of the white blood cell count prior to dispensing the medication.

Treatment with clozapine requires a baseline and weekly white blood cell count and differential for between 18 weeks for some European countries and 24 weeks in the United States. After the initial period of blood monitoring, patients must continue to have a white blood cell count and differential every other week in the United States and monthly in many European countries.

Clozapine dosing also differs significantly between the United States and Europe. A usual initial dose of clozapine in the United States is 12.5 mg per day and the dose is titrated in 25 mg increments every other day, as tolerated. In contrast, a test dose strategy giving 25 or 50 mg of clozapine at bedtime is often employed in European countries. If the test dose is well tolerated, titration is much quicker than that recommended in the United States.

The target or mean dose range in the United States (400–600 mg per day) is almost twice that used in many European countries.[77] Consequently, the recommended plasma levels of the parent compound that may be useful for dose titration are also considerably higher in the United States.[30] The most recent United States plasma level response study by VanderZwaag et al recommends optimal plasma levels between 200 and 250 ng/ml.[32] These differences between countries are of clinical relevance, since many of clozapine's side effects are dose- and plasma level-dependent.[78]

Long-term (up to 1 year) clozapine treatment trials have shown that the proportion of patients that responded to clozapine continued to increase over the duration of the trial.[79,80] These results suggest that the time to response with clozapine in treatment-refractory patient populations may be longer than previously thought. A clozapine trial should last a minimum of 12 weeks and improvement may continue over months to years.

Combination antipsychotic therapy

Combination therapy refers to the simultaneous use of two or more antipsychotic medications. Clinical research data are lacking in regard to the indications for and efficacy of this alternative treatment strategy. There are only a few empirically based indications for long-term combination therapy. Combination treatment may be disadvantageous, especially in the case of drug–drug interactions and potentiation of side effects.

Generally, combining antipsychotic drugs provides no added benefit over a single antipsychotic, with few exceptions. Patients who are partial responders to clozapine or a long-acting depot medication may benefit from the addition of an agent from a different class.[81,82] Clozapine-responsive patients who have limited tolerance to its side effects have been successfully augmented with sulpiride in a double-blind trial.[83] When a patient has failed sequential trials of all atypical antipsychotics and refuses clozapine, combination therapy may also be a reasonable strategy.

Adjunctive treatments

Adding another class of psychiatric medication may

be attempted to enhance therapeutic efficacy when there has only been a partial response to an antipsychotic drug or to treat residual or other nonpsychotic symptoms. Most of these agents have been found to have limited benefit and require further study.

Benzodiazepines

Benzodiazepines have commonly been used as adjunctive therapy in schizophrenia. As monotherapy, benzodiazepines only have mild efficacy compared to typical antipsychotic medications.[33] A review by Wolkowitz and Pickar of benzodiazepine use in the treatment of schizophrenia found a 33–50% response rate when a benzodiazepine was added to an antipsychotic medication.[84] As adjunctive treatment, benzodiazepines have been found to be most effective for anxiety and psychotic agitation and are commonly used in the initial stages of treatment.[33] Patients with motor disturbances including akathisia and catatonia may benefit from benzodiazepines. Other indications for the addition of a benzodiazepine to antipsychotic medication include general augmentation, treatment of anxiety, and short-term treatment of psychotic agitation or insomnia.[84] Although there is no clear difference in efficacy between benzodiazepines, lorazepam, diazepam, and clonazepam have been used most frequently. Most likely these benzodiazepines are favored for availability in parenteral form and increased potency. Wassef et al have extensively reviewed the role of GABAergic drugs, including benzodiazepines and valproic acid in the treatment of schizophrenia.[85]

Lithium

Lithium has been studied both as monotherapy as an adjunctive agent in schizophrenia. As the sole agent used to treat psychotic symptoms, lithium appears to have limited efficacy and may worsen symptoms in some individuals.[33] Several studies using lithium as an adjunct in treatment-resistant patients suggest that it may enhance the efficacy of antipsychotic medication.[33] Additionally, it may be beneficial for affective symptoms, impulsivity, or violent behavior.[33,81] Lithium is usually added to the ongoing antipsychotic treatment regimen and titrated to a dose that produces a therapeutic serum level (0.8–1.2 mEq/l). Treatment-emergent problems associated with lithium include worsening of preexisting EPS, additive cognitive side effects, and possibly increased risk of neurotoxicity, in addition to lithium's usual side effect profile.[86]

Anticonvulsants

Unlike bipolar mood disorders, anticonvulsants have no current indication as monotherapy in schizophrenia. They have been found to augment the efficacy of antipsychotic medications in some studies.[87] Anticonvulsants may be most useful for specific subgroups of patients.[88] Manic, impulsive, or violent behavior may respond well to the addition of carbamazepine or valproic acid.[33,89,90] Patients with concurrent seizure disorder or who have had a clozapine-related seizure may also benefit from the addition of an anticonvulsant.[50] Valproic acid is usually preferred over carbamazepine due to greater metabolic interactions and blood dyscrasias associated with the latter agent. Titration to a dose range that produces therapeutic serum levels is recommended.

Antidepressants

Depression is common in schizophrenia. Addition of an antidepressant is indicated when symptoms of depression are present. Both selective serotonin reuptake inhibitors (SSRIs) and tricyclic antidepressants (TCAs) have been used to treat depression in schizophrenic populations.[33,91,92] Residual negative symptoms, obsessive-compulsive symptoms, and other anxiety symptoms may also respond to SSRIs.[93] Drug–drug interactions can occur when either SSRIs or TCAs are administered concurrently with antipsychotic medications. Increased plasma levels of either the antidepressant or antipsychotic medication may result from pharmacokinetic interactions.[19] In particular, fluvoxamine, which is metabolized via the CYP1A2 system, can substantially increase clozapine levels.[19,26]

Beta-blockers

High-dose propranolol (in doses up to 1200 mg per day) has been shown to augment antipsychotic efficacy in treatment-refractory schizophrenia.[88] Propranolol may produce its beneficial effect through its ability to treat EPS (akathisia), by increasing antipsychotic serum levels decreasing anxiety symptoms, or through potential anticonvulsant effects.[88]

Glycine and D-cycloserine

Recently, much interest has surrounded the use of glycine and partial agonists (for instance, D-cycloserine) acting through the glycine site on N-methyl-D-aspartate (NMDA) receptors in the treatment of negative symptoms in schizophrenia. Early trials with low-dose glycine produced mixed results. More recent studies with higher doses of glycine (30–60 mg per day) have shown improvement in negative symptoms when added to antipsychotic medication.[94,95] Trials with D-cycloserine have also demonstrated improvement in negative symptoms when added to ongoing typical antipsychotic treatment.[95,96] Although these agents warrant further study, the current consensus is that adjunctive glycine or glycine partial agonists provide some benefit as adjunctive treatment for negative symptoms.

Switching antipsychotics

With the introduction of more novel antipsychotic compounds, clinicians will be faced with the issue of determining when it is appropriate to switch medications. If a patient has discontinued medication, a new treatment can be initiated as described previously. When a patient is currently maintained on an antipsychotic drug and the decision is made to switch to another agent, there is little agreement regarding the most effective technique. The most common method for switching is by cross-tapering of the old and new medications. The dosage of the current drug is continued, and the new antipsychotic is added. The doses of the old and new drugs are then decreased, and increased, respectively, over a specific time interval. The rate of cross-taper usually depends on the medications being switched. Antiparkinsonian agents used concurrently with typical antipsychotic medication should be continued for some time when switching from a typical to an atypical antipsychotic drug. Due to the intrinsic anticholinergic properties of clozapine, when switching from clozapine to another antipsychotic drug cholinergic rebound symptoms may occur. Clinical issues and management of switching antipsychotic medications are beyond the scope of this chapter and have been reviewed elsewhere.[97,98]

Electroconvulsive therapy

The role of electroconvulsive therapy (ECT) in the treatment of schizophrenia is controversial. A trial of ECT in an acute psychotic episode may be warranted in catatonic patients who do not respond to a benzodiazepine trial.[33] Several open trials in treatment-refractory patients, including those with refractory positive symptoms, have shown enhancement of antipsychotic efficacy with the addition of ECT.[99] Some treatment-resistant patients with only partial response to clozapine treatment have also responded favorably to the combination of clozapine and ECT.[100] Other patients with refractory symptoms who cannot tolerate or do not respond to clozapine may be candidates for ECT.[101] There are no controlled studies evaluating whether ECT is effective as a maintenance treatment or in preventing relapse, but it can be useful in ECT-responders who are intolerant of or unresponsive to any pharmacologic treatment. Krueger and Sackeim have extensively reviewed studies examining the role of ECT in schizophrenia.[102]

Adverse effects

Antipsychotic medication, in general, has a wide range of potential side effects. Conventional and atypical antipsychotic drugs differ markedly in their side effect profiles, which reflects their different pharmacologic properties. The most common side effects encountered in clinical practice are reviewed along with treatment options.

Central nervous system effects
Medication-induced movement disorders

The most common medication-induced movement disorders in psychiatry are those related to antipsychotic drugs. Onset of these syndromes can occur acutely or after prolonged exposure to antipsychotic medications.

Acute extrapyramidal syndromes (EPS), including parkinsonism, dystonia, akathisia, and acute dyskinesias develop early in the course of treatment.[103] These disorders are reversible and dose-dependent.[103] Tardive or latent forms of EPS, especially tardive dyskinesia (TD), occur after chronic exposure to antipsychotic drugs.[103]

It has been estimated that some 50–90% of patients who receive conventional antipsychotic medications acutely develop some form of extrapyramidal side effect.[33,103,104] A prospective study by Chakos et al of first-episode schizophrenic patients treated with typical antipsychotic medications reported that EPS had occurred in 62% of the patients during the first 2 months of treatment.[105] In this study, 36% of patients developed acute dystonia, parkinsonism was found in 34% of patients and akathisia occurred in 18% of patients.[105] All antipsychotic medications are capable of producing these side effects; however, clozapine and other novel antipsychotic compounds appear less likely to cause EPS. Extrapyramidal side effects are a major reason for discontinuation of antipsychotic drugs.[104]

Initial management should consist of lowering the dose or discontinuing the antipsychotic medication. If this is not clinically feasible, other treatment options should be considered, as reviewed below.

DYSTONIAS

Acute dystonia presents as sustained muscular rigidity, spastic contraction of discrete muscle groups, or abnormal postures.[106] Dystonic reactions occur soon after starting antipsychotic

therapy or after rapidly raising the antipsychotic dose.[106] Approximately 90% of cases occur within the first 3 days of treatment.[104] Dystonic reactions tend to be sudden in onset, often dramatic in appearance, and extremely distressing to patients. Dystonias can occur in various body regions, most commonly the eyes, neck, and trunk.[107] The most serious and potentially fatal dystonic reaction is laryngeal-pharyngeal spasm, which can compromise the individual's airway. The majority of reactions are short-lived, usually lasting only a few hours.

Risk factors for an acute dystonic reaction include: a history of prior dystonic reaction, young age, male gender, use of a high-potency antipsychotic drug, high dose of medication, and parenteral administration.[33]

Acute dystonic reactions respond rapidly to intravenous or intramuscular administration of an anticholinergic agent or antihistamine. Treatment is usually initiated with benztropine 2 mg or diphenhydramine 50 mg administered IM or IV push. If there is no response after 10–15 minutes, the dose should be repeated. After reversal of the dystonia, an oral regimen of an antiparkinsonian agent should be continued for at least 2 weeks.[108]

Tardive dystonia occurs with a mean prevalence of 3% of patients treated with antipsychotics and is frequently misdiagnosed as other involuntary movement disorders including tardive dyskinesia.[109] Approximately one-half of cases occur within the first 5 years of exposure to antipsychotic agents, with one-fifth of cases occurring in the first year.[110] Tardive dystonia is distinct from tardive dyskinesia in that it lacks a female predominance, has an earlier age of onset, and can be alleviated by anticholinergic agents.[109] Although it can affect any body area, the muscle groups most often affected are in the face and neck.[111,112]

Tardive dystonia is difficult to treat. If an antipsychotic drug must be continued, the minimum dose required should be used or switching to a novel antipsychotic agent should be considered. Clozapine is the only atypical antipsychotic drug that has been reported to improve dystonic movements.[109] Benzodiazepines, dopamine-depleting agents, and anticholinergic drugs have also been used to treat this disorder.[50,109] For focal dystonias, botulinum toxin may be considered as an alternative treatment.[33,109] If the dystonia fails to remit, the individual should be considered for treatment with clozapine or another novel antipsychotic drug.[33]

PARKINSONISM

This form of EPS is so named because it is phenomenologically similar to the symptoms of Parkinson's disease including rigidity, tremor, akinesia, and bradykinesia. The pathophysiology involved is thought to be an alteration in the balance between dopamine and acetylcholine in the basal ganglia. Since dopaminergic antagonism is thought to be at least in part responsible for the therapeutic efficacy of antipsychotic drugs, most treatments target acetylcholine. Restoration of the balance between these neurotransmitters is thought to occur by reducing the levels of acetylcholine.

Medication-induced parkinsonism is estimated to occur in at least 50% of patients treated with antipsychotic drugs and up to 90% of cases occur within the first 10 weeks of treatment.[113] Elderly patients appear to be at greater risk for parkinsonism.[114] At times, it can be difficult to distinguish depression or negative symptoms from parkinsonism.[114] In addition to a careful clinical assessment, response to either dose reduction of the antipsychotic medication or addition of an antiparkinsonian medication may distinguish parkinsonism from depression or negative symptoms. Depression, however, can occur in over half of cases of akinesia and may therefore coexist with parkinsonism[114,33] In severe cases, parkinsonism must be differentiated from catatonia.[33,113]

Initial treatment strategies should include dose reduction and considering switching to an atypical or a low-potency typical antipsychotic drug.[106] When conservative measures are ineffective, the treatment of choice for parkinsonism is an antiparkinsonian drug.[33,108] The most commonly used drugs are anticholinergic agents. These medications are tertiary amine congeners of atropine that are lipophilic and able to cross the blood–brain barrier. All anticholinergic agents are equally effective, but they vary in potency, duration of action, and available route(s) of administration. In general, benztropine tends to be one of the most potent agents and also the most frequently used parenteral anticholinergic. Less potent but equally effective drugs include trihexyphenidyl, biperiden, and procyclidine. If the patient is unable to tolerate an anticholinergic agent or symptoms persist, alternative medications include amantadine or diphenhydramine.[33] Amantadine is a weak dopamine agonist and may be used in doses of 100–300 mg per day.[33,50] Diphenhydramine is typically dosed at 25–100 mg per day.[50]

AKATHISIA

Akathisia is the subjective experience of restlessness, inner tension, and discomfort. Characteristic motor features include psychomotor agitation, such as pacing, rocking from foot to foot, or the inability to sit still.[33,115] Akathisia usually occurs within days or a few weeks of initiating treatment with an antipsychotic medication or raising the dose.[33,115,116] Akathisia may also manifest after reducing the dose of an anticholinergic agent used to treat other symptoms of EPS. This side effect occurs in up to 20–25% of patients and is often very distressing to the patient.[33] Akathisia is a frequent cause of poor drug compliance in patients. At its extremes, akathisia may be so distressful that the patient becomes dysphoric, aggressive, or suicidal.[33] If a decrease in the dose of antipsychotic medication does not improve symptoms, the treatment of choice is a lipophilic beta-blocker such as propranolol.[33,116] A typical dose of propranolol usually ranges from 30 to 90 mg per day given in divided doses.[33,116] If other symptoms of EPS are also present, an anticholinergic agent is preferred.[33] Benzodiazepines, such as lorazepam and clonazepam, are considered second-line agents.[33]

Akathisia can be a persistent side effect in a subgroup of patients.[117] Two studies of chronic schizophrenic patients estimated a prevalence rate of 35% for tardive akathisia.[50] Treatment studies with various agents have produced inconsistent results. Tardive akathisia may respond to the same medications used to treat acute akathisia. Reserpine has also been used with some success.[118]

DYSKINESIAS

Dyskinetic movements can be divided into four types: spontaneous, withdrawal, acute, and tardive. Spontaneous dyskinesias have been observed in greater than 20% of drug-naïve schizophrenic patients.[119] Withdrawal dyskinesias occur upon dose reduction or withdrawal of an antipsychotic medication, but usually resolve within 1–2 months and generally do not require treatment.[33]

Rabbit syndrome, named for the fine rapid perioral movements that resemble the chewing motions of a rabbit, is often considered a form of dyskinesia.[120] It tends to occur with prolonged treatment and may be present in up to 4% of patients not treated concurrently with an anticholinergic agent.[121] The treatment of choice is an anticholinergic drug.

Tardive dyskinesia is a late-onset disorder of repetitive, involuntary choreoathetoid and dyskinetic buccolinguomasticatory, limb or trunk movements caused by sustained exposure to antipsychotic medication.[51]

The exact mechanism that underlies tardive dyskinesia is unknown. Several hypotheses have been generated to explain this movement disorder. The most common hypothesis is that prolonged dopamine receptor blockade produces postsynaptic dopamine receptor supersensitivity.[122] Another idea is that tardive dyskinesia may be understood as part of the pathophysiology of schizophrenia.[52]

The estimated prevalence of tardive dyskinesia (TD) is in part a function of age, with prevalence rates of 5–10% in those less than 40 years old.[52] The estimated prevalence of TD in adults may be greater than 50% in high-risk groups.[52,123] Many risk factors have been proposed for tardive dyskinesia. The most consistent predictors for the development of TD include: (a) age; (b) gender; (c) presence of EPS; (d) presence of an affective disorder; (e) dose and duration of antipsychotic medication; (f) diabetes mellitus.[52,124,125] A review of risk factors for the development of TD can be found in a report by Casey.[52]

The APA Task Force on Tardive Dyskinesia outlined diagnostic criteria for tardive dyskinesia.[51] These criteria include that the movements are decreased during relaxation or sleep and can be suppressed volitionally.[51] Dyskinetic movements are increased by movements of unaffected areas of the body and by emotional arousal.[51] The abnormal movements are moderate in one body area or mild in at least two body areas.[51] The dyskinetic movements must have been present for at least 4 weeks and there has been at least 3 months' total cumulative antipsychotic drug exposure.[51] It is important to rule out potential idiopathic causes for abnormal movements. With mild cases, the patient may be unaware of the movements, whereas with severe dyskinesias they may have difficulty with eating and other activities of daily living.

For most patients, the dyskinetic movements are not progressive.[51] The onset of TD tends to be insidious with a fluctuating course.[51] Over time, it stabilizes or improves despite continued antipsychotic treatment.[126] The movements may be temporarily masked by an increase in dose of antipsychotic medication, followed by reemergence of symptoms that are often more severe. After discontinuation of antipsychotic medication, at least a 50% reduction in severity occurs in most patients within 18 months.[127] When antipsychotic medication is discontinued a significant proportion of patients will have remission of symptoms, especially if the TD is of recent onset or the patient is young.

There is no definitive treatment for tardive dyskinesia. Dose reduction may cause a temporary worsening of symptoms, and then the dyskinetic movements should improve. Discontinuation of antipsychotic medication should only be considered if the patient is in full remission and very stable or on patient request.[33,52] Tardive dyskinesia in elderly patients is less likely to remit once antipsychotic medication is stopped.[51] When medication cannot be discontinued, the clinician should reduce the medication to the lowest effective dose.[33,52] Other interventions should be tried if substantial improvement in the dyskinesias is not observed within 3–6 months of dose reduction or discontinuation. Casey and Egan et al provide more complete reviews of medications used to treat tardive dyskinesia.[52,128]

Several studies have suggested that atypical antipsychotic agents may have a lower propensity to cause EPS, and possibly tardive dyskinesia. Clozapine has been shown to reduce the severity of TD and may even produce remission in some cases.[53,128] Casey argues that atypical antipsychotics be used as first-line treatment for patients with TD and those individuals at high risk.[52] If the patient has severe dyskinetic movements or is extremely distressed, switching to clozapine remains the preferred option.[33]

EPS PROPHYLAXIS

In the past, anticholinergic agents were routinely given concurrently with high-potency typical antipsychotic agents to prevent EPS. More recently, prophylactic use of anticholinergic medications has become controversial. Miller has suggested that lower doses and slow titration of antipsychotic dose may prevent the development of EPS.[115] Novel antipsychotic use may become one of the most important forms of prophylaxis for EPS.

The prophylactic use of antiparkinsonian medications should be determined by clinical and patient factors.[33] A prior history of EPS/acute dystonic reaction, other risk factors for EPS, and patient preference should be weighed against the consequences of anticholinergic side effects. The World Health Organization consensus statement on anticholinergic prophylaxis suggests that these agents should only be used if parkinsonism develops.[129] Anticholinergic drugs should then be discontinued later in the course of treatment to determine whether their continued use is warranted.[129]

Thermoregulatory side effects

NEUROLEPTIC MALIGNANT SYNDROME (NMS)

This severe medication-induced movement disorder is of sudden onset, usually occurring early in the course of antipsychotic treatment, and can be fatal in 5–20% of untreated cases.[33] DSM-IV criteria for diagnosis specify that muscle rigidity and hyperthermia (101–104 °F) must be present in association with the use of an antipsychotic medication.[112] Other symptoms most commonly associated with NMS include autonomic instability, leukocytosis (greater than 15 000 mm^3), change in level of consciousness, and elevation of creatine kinase (greater than 300 U/ml).[112]

NMS can occur with any antipsychotic medication, including atypical antipsychotics.[130,131] It can occur at any time during antipsychotic treatment. The incidence of NMS varies from 0.02% to 3.23%, reflecting differences in criteria.[132] Prevalence rates are unknown, but are estimated to vary from 0.001% to 1% of patients treated with antipsychotic medication.[133] Proposed risk factors include: (a) prior episode of NMS; (b) younger age; (c) use of high-potency antipsychotics; (d) rapid dose titration; (e) parenteral (IM) preparations; (f) dehydration; (g) agitation; (h) concurrent use of certain medications, such as lithium; and (i) preexisting neurological or mood disorder.[33,132]

If NMS is suspected, the patient should have a thorough medical work-up to rule out other causes for the symptoms. Treatment of neuroleptic malignant syndrome is mainly supportive.[134] The offending agent is immediately discontinued and secondary complications such as acute renal failure must be addressed. Both dantrolene and dopamine agonists such as bromocriptine have also been used in the treatment of NMS.[132,135] These agents, however, have not shown greater efficacy than supportive treatment.[132,136] Some evidence suggests that early administration of electroconvulsive therapy (ECT) may be helpful, especially when there is diagnostic uncertainty and catatonia cannot be ruled out.[132,137] Since hemodynamic alterations can be associated with ECT, it should generally be reserved as a second-line therapy for NMS.[33]

The usual course of treatment is 5–10 days. Long-acting depot preparations will prolong recovery time. After several weeks of recovery, the patient may be cautiously rechallenged with an antipsychotic from a different class.

HYPERTHERMIA

Benign hyperthermia occurs in about 5% of patients during the first few weeks of clozapine treatment.[138] Hyperthermia is also seen with other antipsychotic agents. It is usually a transient phenomenon and body temperature rarely exceeds 100 °F (38 °C).[138]

Hyperthermia during the summer months may predispose individuals to heat stroke, catatonia, and neuroleptic malignant syndrome. Heat stroke can occur under conditions of high temperatures and high humidity. Anticholinergic or antihistaminic effects of antipsychotic agents can also impair heat loss.[50]

A persistent elevation of body temperature or a fever above 100 °F (38 °C), in the absence of other symptoms, should be investigated to rule out infection, blood dyscrasia, and neuroleptic malignant syndrome.[50] Persistent hyperthermia, in the absence of other causes, can be treated with antipyretics.

HYPOTHERMIA

Hypothermia is defined as a core body temperature below 95 °F (35 °C). Mild hypothermia has occurred in patients treated with phenothiazine antipsychotics.[139] It has no known clinical significance, although it has been implicated in sudden unexplained death attributed to antipsychotic medications.[139,140]

EEG alterations and seizures

All antipsychotic medications decrease the seizure threshold to some degree.[50] Low-potency typical antipsychotic medications and clozapine are associated with the greatest risk of seizures.[33] Other risk factors include: (a) personal or family history of seizure disorder; (b) high dose of medication; (c) rapid titration of dose; (d) parenteral administration; (e) concurrent medications that lower the seizure threshold; (f) recent benzodiazepine discontinuation; (g) concurrent alcohol use disorder; and (h) prior head injury.[141] For typical antipsychotic drugs, the incidence is less than 1% at therapeutic doses and the frequency of seizures appears to be dose-related.[142] Seizure risk is dose- and plasma level-dependent with clozapine.[31,35] The risk of seizure with clozapine ranges from 2% with doses below 300 mg to 4–6% with doses above 600 mg per day.[138]

If a seizure occurs while a patient is on an antipsychotic medication, an EEG and neurological consultation should be considered. With typical antipsychotic medications, discontinuation of the offending agent or reduction to at least half of the preseizure dose is recommended.[33] After a clozapine-induced seizure, the medication should be held for no more than a few days and then restarted at approximately half the preseizure dose.[143] If clozapine must be discontinued for more than a few days, it is advisable to restart at the initial dose and titrate slowly to the lowest effective dose.

A clozapine-induced seizure is not an absolute contraindication for continuing to use the agent. In one study, over three-quarters of patients who had a seizure while taking clozapine were able to continue treatment after reduction of the dose, modifying the dose titration or adding an anticonvulsant.[138]

Seizure risk may be related to peak blood levels of clozapine and it has been suggested that dividing the dose may be prophylactic.[138] An anticonvulsant should be considered for prophylaxis.[138] Valproic acid is less likely to interfere with the metabolism of antipsychotic drugs than either phenytoin or carbamazepine. Carbamazepine is relatively contraindicated in combination with clozapine since both drugs have a propensity for blood dyscrasias.[138]

Central anticholinergic toxicity

Central anticholinergic toxicity can present as a change in mental status with memory impairment, confusion, bizarre behavior, hallucinations, somnolence, or delirium.[33,114] Physical signs and symptoms include dry skin and mucous membranes, tachycardia, flushing, and hyperthermia.[144] Treatment is generally symptomatic. Medications possessing anticholinergic properties should be discontinued.

In an emergency room setting, when there is uncertainty regarding the diagnosis or the symptoms are severe, intravenous physostigmine can both confirm the diagnosis and treat the anticholinergic symptoms.[33,144] Physostigmine itself can potentially produce cholinomimetic toxicity, which can be reversed with atropine.[144] Physostigmine should not be administered to individuals with autonomic instability, asthma, or history of cardiac abnormalities.

Sedation

Sedation is a common side effect.[33,138] It should be distinguished from akinesia and hypotension. This side effect occurs early in the course of treatment and most patients usually develop tolerance over the subsequent 4–6 weeks. While sedation may initially be beneficial for agitated patients, it can impair functioning over time. Initial conservative management for persistent sedation includes shifting the majority of dose to evening, reducing the dose, or changing to a less sedating medication.[33,145]

Cardiovascular side effects
Orthostatic hypotension

Orthostatic hypotension is the most common cardiovascular side effect of antipsychotic drugs. It is usually seen with conventional antipsychotic agents, risperidone, quetiapine, zotepine, olanzapine and clozapine. Orthostasis is most likely to occur during the first few days after initiation of treatment or when increasing the medication

dose. Most patients develop tolerance to this effect in the ensuing 4–6 weeks.[138] In the elderly, orthostatic hypotension may predispose them, for example, to falls.[33] The mechanism by which antipsychotic medication causes orthostatic hypotension and compensatory tachycardia is through alpha-adrenergic antagonism.

Patients should be instructed to move gradually from a lying or sitting position to standing, especially on awakening. Other management strategies include increases in fluid and salt intake or the use of support stockings.

When conservative measures fail, several medications have proven useful in treating persistent orthostasis. Fludrocortisone, ephedrine, and dihydroergotamine have all been used to treat orthostatic hypotension.[146-148] Epinephrine paradoxically worsens antipsychotic-induced orthostatic hypotension through stimulation of beta-adrenergic receptors and is therefore contraindicated.[113]

Tachycardia

Tachycardia may be due to the anticholinergic effect on vagal inhibition or secondary to orthostatic hypotension. With clozapine, approximately 25% of patients will have a sinus tachycardia with an increase of about 10–15 beats per minute.[145] Most patients will develop tolerance to this side effect over time.

If tachycardia is sustained or becomes symptomatic, an electrocardiogram (ECG) should be obtained. Additional conservative management of patients should include either lowering the dose or slowing the titration of the medication. Beta-blockers, such as propranolol and atenolol, have been used to treat medication-induced tachycardia.[138,145] Atenolol is often preferred because it avoids the central nervous system effects often seen with propranolol.[138]

Electrocardiogram changes

Electrocardiogram (ECG) changes are observed with many antipsychotic drugs. Both high- and low-potency typical antipsychotic medications have been associated with changes in the Q–T interval.[14]

Changes in the Q–T interval have been associated with the potentially fatal arrhythmia 'Torsade des pointes'.[113] The pathophysiological mechanism is thought to be mediated by alteration in cardiac ion channels.[149] Sertindole is an atypical antipsychotic drug that was approved by the FDA but not marketed in the United States because it more commonly produces prolongation of the Q–T interval. Moreover, it was also withdrawn from use worldwide for fear that this effect may have been associated with a small number of cases of sudden death in patients receiving the drug. Ziprasidone, a drug recently approved in the US and parts of Europe, has also been found to produce Q–T prolongation that is greater than other atypical drugs (except sertindole) but less than thioridazine.[149a] However, the clinical significance of this is unclear. Studies in the wake of the increased concern about drug effects on Q–T parameters have revealed that thioridazine produces increased Q–T prolongation relative to the other conventional and atypical antipsychotic drugs which has resulted in increased restrictions in its use in the United States.[149a] Other ECG changes include prolongation of the P–R interval, ST depression, and T wave blunting. These changes must be evaluated in the context of the individual patient's clinical history.

Sudden death and cardiotoxicity

Unexplained sudden death may be a rare side effect of antipsychotic medication and has been attributed to cardiac arrhythmias in the absence of another explanation.[150] There is currently no evidence that antipsychotic medications are causally linked to sudden death. This topic has been reviewed in depth elsewhere.[151]

Hematologic side effects

Blood dyscrasias, most notably neutropenia, leukopenia, and agranulocytosis have been associated with many typical antipsychotics and clozapine. The most serious of these hematologic side effects, agranulocytosis, is also the most concerning aspect in the use of clozapine.

Neutropenia

Benign or transient neutropenia has been described with phenothiazines and clozapine.[152] It occurs in up to 22% of patients treated with clozapine.[152] Neutropenia usually resolves over time without treatment.

Leukopenia

Antipsychotic drugs may cause blood dyscrasias, including leukopenia and agranulocytosis. Leukopenia is the more common of the two disorders. It is usually transient and resolves spontaneously. Chlorpromazine has been most commonly associated with leukopenia, which occurs in up to 10% of patients.[33,50] Leukopenia can also be a harbinger of impending agranulocytosis.

Agranulocytosis

Agranulocytosis (granulocyte count below $500/mm^3$) is a life-threatening side effect of antipsychotics. It can occur with both conventional and atypical antipsychotic drugs. Approximately 0.32% of patients treated with chlorpromazine and 1% treated with clozapine will develop agranulocytosis.[33,50,152,153] This disorder carries a mortality rate of approximately 3%.[154] It tends to occur slightly more often in women, the elderly, and young patients (less than 21 years old).[152,153] The risk of agranulocytosis with clozapine is highest in the first 5 months of treatment.[152,153]

Before initiating treatment with clozapine, patients are entered into a national registry. Patients must have weekly white blood cell (WBC) counts during the first six months of treatment with clozapine. After the first 6 months, patient WBC counts are then monitored biweekly as long as the patients continue on clozapine in the United States. White blood cell count monitoring may vary from country to country.

If the WBC count falls below $3000/mm^3$ or the absolute neutrophil count (ANC) drops below $1500/mm^3$, clozapine should be discontinued and daily WBC counts with differential should be drawn, along with close monitoring of the patient for signs or symptoms of infection.[153]

If the WBC count falls below 2000/mm^3 or the ANC is less than 1000/mm^3, clozapine should be discontinued, daily WBC counts with differential should be drawn, and a hematologist should be consulted.

Agranulocytosis constitutes a medical emergency and management includes hospitalization, reverse isolation, and prophylactic antibiotics. Granulocyte colony-stimulating factor or granulocyte-macrophage colony-stimulating factor may be required.[145] Use of these agents has shown to decrease morbidity and may shorten the course of illness.[138] Once a patient has developed clozapine-induced agranulocytosis, they should not be treated in the future with drugs that have a propensity to produce blood dyscrasias.[152,155]

Gastrointestinal side effects
Xerostomia
Dry mouth is a common complaint and can lead to oral infections, dental caries, or polydipsia.[113] Patients should be advised to rinse their mouths frequently, chew sugarless gum or candy, and have regular dental care.[113]

Sialorrhea
This side effect occurs in almost all patients treated with clozapine.[138,156] Tolerance does not appear to develop over time.[138,156] Sialorrhea is generally benign, but can be a source of great distress to patients. Hypersalivation is most pronounced during sleep. Since both cholinergic and adrenergic mechanisms are involved in the production of saliva, the pathophysiology of this side effect is unclear.

Placing a towel on the pillow at night can be helpful. Pharmacologic treatments that have been used include anticholinergic agents and adrenergic agonists. Although both low doses of amitriptyline and benztropine control hypersalivation, these agents also add to the intrinsic anticholinergic effects of clozapine itself and are generally not recommended.[20] Pirenzepine, a selective muscarinic type 1 receptor antagonist, and clonidine have been used successfully to treat sialorrhea.[138]

Constipation
This side effect is commonly encountered with the low-potency typical antipsychotic medications and clozapine, suggesting that it is most likely due to muscarinic receptor antagonism. Conservative measures such as increasing dietary fiber, exercise, and fluid intake may be helpful for mild constipation.[50] Stool softeners and laxatives can be used for more severe symptoms. Stimulant cathartics may be used on a short-term basis for severe constipation. In rare cases, constipation may progress to paralytic ileus.

Hepatotoxicity
ELEVATION OF LIVER ENZYMES

Transient increases in liver enzymes are common among all antipsychotics.[14] Mild to moderate elevations in transaminase levels can occur in up to 70% of patients treated with antipsychotic drugs.[157] It appears to be a direct effect of the drug on the liver. Liver function tests often return to normal over time. Rare cases of hepatotoxicity have been reported in clozapine and risperidone.[157,158]

CHOLESTATIC JAUNDICE

With typical antipsychotic agents, especially phenothiazines, obstructive or cholestatic jaundice occurs infrequently. Approximately 0.1–0.5% of patients treated with chlorpromazine develop cholestatic jaundice, usually within the first month of treatment.[113] In these cases, the offending medication should be discontinued. Recovery occurs in up to 75% of patients within 2 months and 90% recover within 1 year.[50]

Patients who present with symptoms such as nausea, fever, abdominal pain, and rash should have tests of their liver function performed to rule out hepatotoxicity. In most cases of cholestatic jaundice, the laboratory features are consistent with a picture of obstruction including elevation of direct bilirubin, alkaline phosphatase, and aminotransferases.[113] Eosinophilia is seen on peripheral blood smear.[113]

Ophthalmologic side effects

Anticholinergic effects

Cycloplegia and difficulties with accommodation may result in blurred vision. Patients with narrow-angle glaucoma should avoid antipsychotic agents with anticholinergic side effects.

Drug-specific effects

Long-term treatment with phenothiazines, especially high doses of thioridazine or chlorpromazine, can lead to changes in the cornea, lens, and retina.

Chlorpromazine has been shown to cause granular deposits in the anterior lens or posterior cornea along with benign pigment deposition in the lens.[113] These conditions are usually reversible upon discontinuation of chlorpromazine.

Thioridazine, usually in doses exceeding 800 mg per day, has been associated with a pigmentary retinopathy that can lead to blindness and may not be reversible upon drug discontinuation.[113]

Quetiapine has been associated with the development of cataracts in animal studies.[159] It is recommended that patients should have an ophthalmologic examination every 6 months while taking quetiapine.[159]

Since these conditions are preventable and probably reversible if detected early, the American Psychiatric Association *Practice Guidelines for the Treatment of Schizophrenia* (1997) recommend periodic ophthalmologic examinations (approximately every 2 years) in patients taking phenothiazines.[33]

Neuroendocrine side effects

Hyperprolactinemia

Prior to the introduction of clozapine, hyperprolactinemia was thought to be a consequence of treatment with typical antipsychotics. Hyperprolactinemia is defined as prolactin levels above 20 µg/ml. The excessive prolactin secretion, as seen with prolactinomas, is not found commonly even with conventional antipsychotics. Although one of the criteria used to define 'atypical' antipsychotic drugs is little or no elevation of prolactin, both risperidone and amisulpride increase prolactin levels to a degree comparable to conventional antipsychotic drugs.[160,161]

INFERTILITY AND MENSTRUAL DISTURBANCES

Hyperprolactinemia can cause amenorrhea and other menstrual irregularities such as menorrhagia and anovulatory cycles. Amenorrhea was estimated to be present in 15–91% of females in one large study.[162] In males, hyperprolactinemia may lead to azoospermia.[158]

GALACTORRHEA

Inappropriate production of breast milk associated with hyperprolactinemia may occur in both sexes, although it is more commonly seen in females.[163] Windgassen et al found that galactorrhea was present in 14% of 150 schizophrenic patients on various antipsychotic drugs.[163]

GYNECOMASTIA

Gynecomastia has been reported to occur in 3% of females and 6% of males during antipsychotic drug treatment.[158,162] An increase in the nonfatty breast tissue in males has not been directly correlated with hyperprolactinemia.[162] Abnormally high levels of prolactin can decrease testosterone and there appears to be a relationship between increases in the estrogen-to-androgen ratio in males and breast enlargement.[164] Patients may not spontaneously disclose symptoms such as galactorrhea and gynecomastia due to embarrassment and therefore clinicians must ask about these side effects.

OTHER EFFECTS

There are several other clinical effects of hyperprolactinemia. Estrogen deficiency resulting from excessive prolactin secretion can have negative effects on cognitive function and may contribute to exacerbations of psychotic illness.[165]

Hyperprolactinemia has been implicated but not established as a risk factor for breast cancer, decreased bone density, osteoporosis, and cardiovascular disease.[165] Two other side-effects related to hyper PRL, sexual dysfunction and weight gain are discussed elsewhere in this chapter.

Decreasing the dose of antipsychotic medication can treat symptoms caused by elevated prolactin levels.[33] It has been suggested that antipsychotic doses should be adjusted to maintain prolactin levels below 50 mg/ml.[165] An alternative method of treating hyperprolactinemia is to change antipsychotic medications. If dosage adjustment or switching antipsychotic medication are not feasible options, dopaminergic agents have been used to suppress prolactin secretion.[33]

Sexual dysfunction

Several neurotransmitter systems that mediate sexual function are affected by antipsychotic drugs. Different mechanisms may be contributing to antipsychotic-induced sexual dysfunction including prolactin levels, cholinergic stimulation, and activation of the sympathetic nervous system.[162,166]

Few studies have rigorously investigated sexual dysfunction during antipsychotic treatment. It is therefore important for clinicians to obtain a baseline sexual history prior to starting treatment with antipsychotic drugs. Those few studies evaluating the frequency of sexual side effects in patients report prevalence rates of up to 60% in men and up to 30% in women.[166–168]

Conventional antipsychotic medications, with their propensity to raise prolactin levels, were thought to result in an increased incidence of sexual dysfunction. This assumption has not been confirmed in two recent studies. Hummer et al found that there was no difference in frequency of sexual side effects in men treated with either clozapine or haloperidol.[166] No correlation was found between prolactin levels and prolactin-related side effects by Kleinberg et al in both men and women treated with risperidone.[160] These side effects may also be dose-dependent and transient disturbances.[160,168]

ERECTILE DYSFUNCTION

Disorders ranging from impotence to priapism have been reported in 23–54% of males and occur most often with typical antipsychotic drugs.[33] Reports of priapism have been most frequently associated with the low-potency antipsychotics chlorpromazine and thioridazine, although they may occur with any antipsychotic.[162] Priapism is not dose-dependent and can occur at any time during treatment. It seems to occur most frequently in men between the ages of 30 and 50 years old.[162] The mechanism by which antipsychotic medications cause erectile difficulties is unclear, but may involve antagonism of cholinergic receptors or stimulation of the sympathetic nervous system.[158]

Treatment for erectile dysfunction, other than adjusting the medication dosage or changing medications, includes the use of yohimbine, benztropine, diphenhydramine or cyproheptadine.[33,50] Sildenafil (Viagra) has been reported successfully to treat erectile dysfunction of various etiologies. Although there are no reports on its use with antipsychotic-induced impotence, a case report has described the use of sildenafil to treat fluvoxamine-induced erectile dysfunction.[169] Further study of this medication to treat erectile dysfunction associated with psychiatric medication is warranted.

EJACULATORY DYSFUNCTION

Ejaculatory disorders have been well documented with phenothiazines and are likely to occur to some extent with all antipsychotic medications.[162] Thioridazine has been most frequently associated with delayed or retrograde ejaculation.[113] The incidence of ejaculatory dysfunction in male patients has been reported to range from 18.7 to 58%.[162] Several theories regarding its pathophysiology have been suggested, including blockade of cholinergic receptors, alpha-1-adrenergic antagonism, or calcium channel blockade.[162] Initial treatment is to decrease the dose of medication or change medications. Pharmacologic strategies to manage this side effect have included low-dose imipramine (25–50 mg a day), yohimbine, sympathomimetics or antihistamines such as cyproheptadine or brompheniramine.[33,170]

ORGASMIC DYSFUNCTION AND LOSS OF LIBIDO

Reduced sexual desire has been estimated to occur in approximately 36% of patients between the ages of 20 and 60 years old treated with antipsychotic drugs.[162] After age 60, the incidence rises to almost 50% of patients.[162] Loss of libido seems to be equally common among males and females. Orgasmic dysfunction occurs in approximately 28.5% of patients, with females reporting anorgasmia more often than males.[162] In one open study, sildenafil was used to successfully treat women with antidepressant-induced anorgasmia or delayed orgasm.[171] This drug has not been evaluated in the treatment of antipsychotic-induced orgasmic dysfunction and further study is necessary before it can be recommended as a treatment option.

FERTILITY

Hyperprolactinemia secondary to antipsychotic medication is known to affect fertility, but this is a reversible condition.[161] Normalization of prolactin secretion by switching to so-called 'prolactin-sparing' antipsychotic medications can result in unplanned pregnancies.[161] Counseling in family planning and contraceptive methods should occur prior to switching both male and female patients to 'prolactin-sparing' atypical antipsychotic agents.[161,162]

Weight gain

This side effect is a common problem with most antipsychotic medications. It is an important issue in the management of patients because drug-induced increases in weight can have significant medical and psychosocial consequences.

Different antipsychotic drugs seem to vary in their ability to induce weight gain. A recent meta-analysis by Allison et al demonstrated that both typical and novel antipsychotic drugs are associated with weight gain.[172] With respect to the newer atypical drugs, clozapine and olanzapine appear to have the greatest liability to cause weight gain, while ziprasidone is associated with little or no weight gain.[172] It is unclear whether this side effect is dose-dependent or whether it may stabilize with ongoing treatment.[172] The endocrine mechanism by which weight gain occurs has not been established, but several neuro-transmitter systems, including serotonin and histamine, have been implicated.[158]

Weight gain may predispose individuals to certain medical illnesses, such as diabetes and cardiovascular disease. At the same time, weight gain may also play a significant emerging factor in noncompliance.

Current management includes: (a) patient education prior to initiating treatment; (b) decreasing the dose of antipsychotic medication; (c) discontinuing other agents used concurrently that may be contributing to weight gain. Dietary education should be provided and regular exercise encouraged in all patients receiving antipsychotic medication.

Glucose and lipid metabolism

Elevations of glucose, cholesterol, and triglycerides have been associated with atypical antipsychotic drugs. In addition, several studies have suggested an association between treatment with antipsychotic medications and impaired glucose tolerance and insulin resistance.[173] In recent years, case reports have implicated both clozapine and olanzapine in the emergence of non-insulin dependent (type II) diabetes mellitus.[174] No clear mechanism of action has been established. Significant weight gain or antagonism of specific serotonin receptor subtypes may contribute to the development of these abnormalities.[174]

It has been suggested that atypical antipsychotic drugs may hasten the development of the diabetes in patients at risk.[174] Management of new-onset type II diabetes includes early diagnosis, dietary modifications and, if necessary, treatment with oral hypoglycemic agents.[174]

A recent retrospective study reported increased serum triglycerides in patients treated with clozapine compared to patients given haloperidol.[175] This report replicates findings in other research groups.[175]

Genitourinary side effects
Urinary incontinence

Both phenothiazines and clozapine can cause urinary incontinence.[176,177] The pathophysiologic mechanism underlying clozapine-induced enuresis is unknown, but it has been speculated to be related to alpha-adrenergic antagonism or anticholinergic-induced urinary retention with subsequent overflow incontinence.[145,178]

Management strategies include avoiding fluids during evening hours, voiding before going to bed and scheduled awakenings to void during the night. Pharmacologic interventions include: (a) ephedrine, starting at 25 mg and titrated to a maximum dose of 150 mg; (b) desmopressin (DDAVP) as an intranasal spray, 20–40 μg at bedtime; (c) oxybutynin at doses of 5–15 mg per day.[140,178,179]

Anticholinergic effects

Antipsychotic agents with potent anticholinergic effects can produce urinary difficulties ranging from hesitancy to urinary retention. These agents should be avoided in patients with benign prostatic hypertrophy and other conditions that predispose to urinary retention. Bethanechol has been used to treat recurrent urinary retention in some patients.[180]

Dermatologic side effects

Allergic reactions

As with most medications, antipsychotic drugs may produce allergic rashes. Exfoliative dermatitis is rare. Treatment includes discontinuing the offending agent and providing an antihistamine for symptomatic relief.

Photosensitivity reactions

Low-potency typical antipsychotic medications may cause photosensitivity reactions that resemble a sunburn or rash. Patients should be instructed to avoid excessive sun exposure and to use sunscreen on exposed areas of skin.[33] Phenothiazines, especially chlorpromazine, uncommonly may also cause a blue-gray discoloration of the skin in areas exposed to the sun, especially the head and neck.[113]

Conclusions

Significant advances have been made in the treatment of schizophrenia since the introduction of chlorpromazine in 1952. Combined with psychosocial interventions, pharmacological treatments have been able to make a significant impact in the lives of schizophrenic patients in terms of relapse prevention, quality of life and resocialization. Although pharmacologic agents have substantially advanced the treatment of schizophrenia much remains to be done to develop novel and more effective compounds. In addition, although pharmacotherapy provides the foundation, optimal treatment should also include appropriate psychosocial therapies.

References

1. Laborit H, Hugenard P, Alluaume R, Un nouveau stabilisateur végétatif (le 4560 RP), *Presse Médicale* 1952; **60:**206–8.
2. Delay J, Deniker P, Harl J-M, Utilisation en thérapeutique psychiatrique d'une phénothiazine d'action centrale elective (4560 RP), *Ann Med Psychol (Paris)* (1952) **110:**112–17.
3. Kinon BJ, Lieberman JA, Mechanisms of action of atypical antipsychotic drugs: a critical analysis, *Neuropsychopharmacology* (1996) **124:**2–34.
4. Meltzer HY, Matsubara S, Lee JC, Classification of typical and atypical antipsychotic drugs on the basis of dopamine D-1, D-2 and serotonin₂ pKi values, *J Pharmacol Exp Ther* (1989) **251:**238–46.
5. Meltzer HY, Matsubara S, Lee JC, The ratio of serotonin-2 and dopamine-2 affinities differentiate atypical and typical antipsychotic drugs, *Psychopharmacol Bull* (1989) **25:**390–2.
6. Baldessarini RJ, Drugs and the treatment of psychiatric disorders: psychosis and anxiety. In: Hardman JG, Limbird LE, Molinoff PB et al, eds, *Goodman & Gilman's The Pharmacological Basis of Therapeutics* (McGraw-Hill: New York, 1996) 399–420.
7. Hirsch SR, Barnes TRE, The clinical treatment of schizophrenia with antipsychotic medication. In: Hirsch SR, Weinberger DR, eds, *Schizophrenia* (Blackwell Science: Oxford, 1995, 443–68).

8. Carlsson A, Lindquist M, Effect of chlorpromazine or haloperidol on the formation of 3-methoxytyramine and normetanephrine in mouse brain, *Acta Pharmacol Toxicol* (1963) **20:**140–4.

9. Seeman P, Lee T, Chau-Wong M et al, Antipsychotic drug doses and neuroleptic/dopamine receptors, *Nature* (1976) **261:**717–19.

10. Creese I, Burt DR, Snyder SH, Dopamine receptor binding predicts clinical and pharmacologic potencies of antischizophrenic drugs, *Science* (1976) **192:**481–3.

11. Nordström AL, Farde L, Wiesel FA et al, Central D2–dopamine receptor occupancy in relation to antipsychotic drug effects: a double blind PET study of schizophrenic patients, *Biol Psychiatry* (1993) **33:**227–35.

12. Farde L, Nordström AL, Wiesel FA et al, Positron emission tomographic analysis of central D1 and D2 dopamine receptor occupancy in patients treated with classical neuroleptics and clozapine: relation to extrapyramidal side effects, *Arch Gen Psychiatry* (1992) **49:**538–44.

13. Kapur S, Zipursky RB, Remington G, Clinical and theoretical implications of 5-HT2 and D2 receptor occupancy of clozapine, risperidone and olanzapine in schizophrenia, *Am J Psychiatry* (1999) **156:**286–93.

14. Casey DE, The relationship of pharmacology to side effects, *J Clin Psychiatry* (1997) **58(Suppl 10):**55–62.

15. Chiodo LA, Bunney BS, Population response of midbrain dopaminergic neurons to neuroleptics: further studies on time course and nondopaminergic neuronal influences, *J Neurosci* (1987) **7:**629–33.

16. Nordström A-L, Farde L, Nyberg S et al, D_1, D_2 and 5-HT$_2$ receptor occupancy in relation to clozapine serum concentration: a PET study of schizophrenic patients, *Am J Psychiatry* (1995) **152:**1444–9.

17. Lieberman JA, Mailman RB, Duncan G et al, Serotonergic basis of antipsychotic drug effects in schizophrenia, *Biol Psychiatry* (1998) **44:**1099–117.

18. Satlin A, Wasserman C, Overview of geriatric psychopharmacology. In: McElroy S, ed. *Psychopharmacology Across the Life Span* (American Psychiatric Press: Washington, DC, 1997) IV-143–6.

19. Ereshefsky L, Drug interactions: update for new antipsychotics, *J Clin Psychiatry* (1996) **57(Suppl 11):**12–25.

20. Lieberman JA, Kane JM, Johns CA, Clozapine: guidelines for clinical management, *J Clin Psychiatry* (1989) **50:**329–38.

21. Marder SR, Hubbard JW, Van Putten T, Midha KK, The pharmacokinetics of long-acting injectable neuroleptic drugs: clinical implications, *Psychopharmacology* (1989) **98:**433–9.

22. Hughes CW, Preskorn SH, Pharmacokinetics in child/adolescent psychotic disorders, *Psychiatr Annals* (1994) **24:**76–82.

23. Kane JM, Aguglia E, Altamura AC et al, Guidelines for depot antipsychotic treatment in schizophrenia. European Neuropsychopharmacology Consensus Conference in Siena, Italy, *Eur Neuropsychopharmacol* (1998) **8:**55–66.

24. Briant RH, An introduction to clinical pharmacology. In: Werry JS, ed. *Pediatric Psychopharmacology: The Use of Behavior Modifying Drugs in Children* (Brunner/Mazel: New York, 1978) 3–28.

25. Ciraulo DA, Shader RI, Greenblatt DJ, Creelman WL, eds, *Drug Interactions in Psychiatry* (Williams & Wilkins: Baltimore, 1995) 129–74.

26. Hiemke C, Weigmann H, Hartter S et al, Elevated serum levels of clozapine after addition of fluvoxamine, *J Clin Psychopharmacol* (1994) **14:**279–81.

27. Van Putten T, Marder SR, Wirshing WC et al, Neuroleptic plasma levels, *Schizophr Bull* (1991) **17:**197–216.

28. Kane JM, Marder SR, Psychopharmacologic treatment of schizophrenia, *Schizophr Bull* (1993) **19:**287–302.

29. Shriqui CL, Neuroleptic dosing and neuroleptic plasma levels in schizophrenia: determining the optimal regimen, *Can J Psychiatry* (1995) **40(suppl 2):**S38–48.

30. Fleischhacker WW, Pharmacological treatment of schizophrenia: a review. In: Maj M, Sartorius N, eds, *WPA Series Evidence and Experience in Psychiatry*, vol 2, *Schizophrenia* (John Wiley & Sons: Chichester, 1999) 75–107.

31. Fleischhacker WW, Hummer M, Kurz M et al, Clozapine dose in the United States and Europe: implications for therapeutic and adverse effects, *J Clin Psychiatry* (1994) **55(Suppl B):**78–81.

32. VanderZwaag C, McGee M, McEvoy JP et al, Response of patients with treatment refractory schizophrenia to clozapine within three serum level ranges, *Am J Psychiatry* (1996) **153:**1579–84.

33. American Psychiatric Association, Practice Guidelines for the Treatment of Schizophrenia, (American Psychiatric Press: Washington, DC, 1997).

34. Zarin DA, Pincus HA: Diagnostic tests with multiple possible thresholds: the case of plasma clozapine levels, *J Prac Psychiatry Behav Health* (1996) **2:**183–5.

35. Haring C, Neudorfer C, Schwitzer J et al, EEG alterations in patients treated with clozapine in relation to plasma levels, *Psychopharmacology* (1994) **114:**97–100.

36. Dixon LB, Lehman AF, Levine J, Conventional antipsychotic medications for schizophrenia, *Schizophr Bull* (1995) **21:**567–77.

37. Wyatt RJ, Neuroleptics and the natural course of schizophrenia, *Schizophr Bull* (1991) **17:**325–51.

38. Lieberman JA, Koreen AR, Chakos M et al, Factors influencing treatment response and outcome in first-episode schizophrenia: implications for understanding the pathophysiology of schizophrenia, *J Clin Psychiatry* (1996) **57(suppl 9):**5–9.

39. Loebel AD, Lieberman JA, Alvir JMJ et al, Duration of psychosis and outcome in first-episode schizophrenia, *Am J Psychiatry* (1992) **149:**1183–8.

40. Loo H, Poirier-Littre M-F, Theron M et al, Amisulpride versus placebo in the medium-term treatment of the negative symptoms of schizophrenia, *Br J Psychiatry* (1997) **170:**18–22.

41. Sharif ZA, Common treatment goals of antipsychotics: acute treatment, *J Clin Psychiatry* (1998) **59(Suppl 19):**5–8.

42. Davis JM, Overview: maintenance therapy in psychiatry I: schizophrenia, *Am J Psychiatry* (1975) **132:**1237–45.

43. Bartko G, Maylath E, Herczeg I, Comparative study of schizophrenic patients relapsed on and off medication, *Psychiatry Res* (1987) **22:**221–7.

44. Kissling W, Kane JM, Barnes TRE et al, Guidelines for neuroleptic relapse prevention in schizophrenia: towards a consensus view. In: Kissling W, ed, *Guidelines for Neuroleptic Relapse Prevention in Schizophrenia* (Springer-Verlag: Berlin, 1991) 155–63.

45. Lehman AF, Steinwachs DM, and the Survey Co-Investigators of the PORT Project: Patterns of usual care for schizophrenia: initial results from the Schizophrenia Patient Outcomes Research Team (PORT) client survey, *Schizophr Bull* (1998) **24:**11–20.

46. Gaebel W, Falkai P: *Praxisleitlinien in Psychiatrie und Psychotherapie*, Band 1. *Behandlungsleitlinie Schizophrenie* (Steinkopff Darmstadt, 1998).

47. McEvoy JP, Scheifler PL, Frances A et al, The Expert Consensus Guideline Series. Treatment of schizophrenia, *J Clin Psychiatry* (1999) **60(Suppl 11):**1–80.

48. Lieberman J, Jody D, Geisler S et al, Time course and biological correlates of treatment response in first-episode schizophrenia, *Arch Gen Psychiatry* (1993) **50:**369–76.

49. Lieberman JA, Pathophysiologic mechanisms in the pathogenesis and clinical course of schizophrenia, *J Clin Psychiatry* (1999) **60(Suppl 12):**9–12.

50. Kane JM, Lieberman JA, eds, *Adverse Effects of Psychotropic Drugs* (Guilford: New York, 1992).

50a. Breier A, Hamilton S, Comparative efficacy of olanzapine and haloperidol for patients with resistant schizophrenia. *Biol Psych* (1999) **45:**403–11.

50b. Bondolfi G, Dufour H, Patris M et al: Risperidone versus clozapine in treatment resistant schizophrenia. *Am J Psychiatry* (1998) **155:**499–504.

51. Kane JM, Jeste DV, Barnes TRE et al, *Tardive Dyskinesia: A Task Force Report of the American Psychiatric Association.* (American Psychiatric Association: Washington, DC, 1992).

52. Casey DE, Tardive dyskinesia and atypical antipsychotic drugs, *Schizophr Res* (1999) **35(Suppl):**S61– 6.

53. Lieberman JA, Saltz BL, Johns CA et al, The effect of clozapine on tardive dyskinesia, *Br J Psychiatry* (1991) **158:**503–10.

54. Beasley CM, Dellva MA, Tamura RN et al, Randomised double-blind comparison of the incidence of tardive dyskinesia in patients with schizophrenia during long-term treatment with olanzapine or haloperidol, *Br J Psychiatry* (1999) **174:**23–30.

55. Schultz SC, Findling RL, Friedman L, Treatment and outcomes in adolescents with schizophrenia, *J Clin Psychiatry* (1998) **(Suppl 1):**50–4.

56. Kumra S, Children and adolescent psychotic disorders. In: Walsh BT, ed. *Child Psychopharmacology*

(American Psychiatric Press: Washington, DC, 1998) 65–89.

57. Mandoki MW, Risperidone treatment of children and adolescents: increased risk of extrapyramidal side effects? *J Child Adolesc Psychopharmacol* (1995) **5**:49–67.

58. Sternlicht HC, Wells SR, Risperidone in childhood schizophrenia, *J Am Acad Child Adolesc Psychiatry* (1995) **34**:5.

59. McClellan J, Werry JS, Practice parameters for the assessment and treatment of children and adolescents with schizophrenia, *J Am Acad Child Adolesc Psychiatry* (1997) **36(Suppl)**:177S-193S.

60. Larco JP, Jeste DV, Geriatric psychosis, *Psychiatr Q* (1997) **68**:247–60.

61. Woerner MG, Alvir JMJ, Saltz BL et al, Prospective study of tardive dyskinesia in the elderly: rates and risk factors, *Am J Psychiatry* (1998) **155**:1521–8.

62. Maixner SM, Mellow AM, Tandon R, The efficacy, safety, and tolerability of antipsychotics in the elderly, *J Clin Psychiatry* (1999) **60(Suppl 8)**:29–41.

63. Altshuler LL, Cohen L, Szuba MP et al, Pharmacologic management of psychiatric illness during pregnancy: dilemmas and guidelines, *Am J Psychiatry* (1996) **153**:592–606.

64. Barnas C, Bergant A, Hummer M et al, Clozapine concentrations in maternal and fetal plasma, amniotic fluid, and breast milk [letter], *Am J Psychiatry* (1994) **151**:945.

65. Buist A, Norman TR, Dennerstein L, Breastfeeding and the use of psychotropic medication: a review, *J Affect Disord* (1990) **19**:197–206.

66. Guy W, ed, *ECDEU Assessment Manual for Psychopharmacology: Publication ADM 76–338* (US Department of Health, Education, and Welfare: Washington, DC, 1976) 534–7.

67. Baldessarini RJ, Cohen BM, Teicher MH, Significance of neuroleptic dose and plasma level in the pharmacological treatment of psychoses, *Arch Gen Psychiatry* (1988) **45**:79–91.

68. Kopala LC, Fredrikson D, Good KP et al, Symptoms in neuroleptic-naïve, first-episode schizophrenia: response to risperidone, *Biol Psychiatry* (1996) **39**:296–8.

69. Kinon BJ, Kane JM, Johns C et al, Treatment of neuroleptic-resistant schizophrenic relapse, *Psychopharmacol Bull* (1993) **29**:309–14.

70. Shalev A, Hermesh H, Rothberg J, Munitz H, Poor neuroleptic response in acutely exacerbated schizophrenic patients, *Acta Psychiatr Scand* (1993) **87**:86–91.

71. Kolakowska T, Williams AO, Ardern M et al, Schizophrenia with good and poor outcome. I: early clinical features, response to neuroleptics and signs of organic dysfunction, *Br J Psychiatry* (1985) **146**:229–39.

72. Kane JM, Lieberman JA, Maintenance pharmacotherapy in schizophrenia. In: Meltzer HY, ed, *Psychopharmacology: The Third Generation of Progress* (Raven: New York, 1987) 1103–9.

73. Johnson DAW, Further observations on the duration of depot neuroleptic maintenance therapy in schizophrenia, *Br J Psychiatry* (1979) **135**:524–30.

74. Carpenter WT, Buchanan RW, Kirkpatrick B et al, Comparative effectiveness of fluphenazine decanoate injections every 2 weeks versus every 6 weeks, *Am J Psychiatry* (1999) **156**:412–18.

75. Kane JM, Management strategies for the treatment of schizophrenia, *J Clin Psychiatry* (1999) **60(suppl 12)**:13–17.

76. Kane JM, Honigfel G, Singer J, Meltzer HY, The Clozaril Collaborative Study Group: Clozapine for the treatment-resistant schizophrenic, *Arch Gen Psychiatry* (1988) **45**:789–96.

77. Fleischhacker WW, Hummer M, Kurz M et al, Clozapine dose in the United States and Europe: implications for therapeutic and adverse effects, *J Clin Psychiatry* (1994) **55(Suppl B)**:78–81.

78. Haring C, Neudorfer C, Schwitzer J et al, EEG alterations in patients treated with clozapine in relation to plasma levels, *Psychopharmacology* (1994) **114**:97–100.

79. Rosenheck R, Cramer J, Xu W et al, A comparison of clozapine and haloperidol in hospitalized patients with refractory schizophrenia, *N Engl J Med* (1997) **337**:809–15.

80. Kane JM, Marder SR, Schooler NR et al, Clozapine and haloperidol in moderately refractory schizophrenia: a six month double-blind comparison, *Arch Gen Psychiatry*, submitted.

81. Marder SR, Management of treatment-resistant patients with schizophrenia, *J Clin Psychiatry* (1996) **57(suppl 11)**:26–30.

82. Naber D, Optimizing clozapine treatment, *J Clin Psychiatry* (1999) **60(Suppl 12)**:35–8.

83. Shiloh R, Zemishlany Z, Aizenberg D et al, Sulpiride augmentation in people with schizophrenia partially responsive to clozapine: a double-blind, placebo-controlled study, *Br J Psychiatry* (1997) **171**:569–73.

84. Wolkowitz DM, Pickar D, Benzodiazepines in the treatment of schizophrenia: a review and reappraisal, *Am J Psychiatry* (1991) **148**:714–26.

85. Wassef AA, Dott SG, Harris A et al, Critical review of GABA-ergic drugs in the treatment of schizophrenia, *J Clin Psychopharmacol* (1999) **19**:222–32.

86. Freeman M, Stoll A, Mood stabilizer combinations: a review of safety and efficacy, *Am J Psychiatry* (1998) **155**:12–21.

87. Fein S, Treatment of drug-refractory schizophrenia, *Psychiatr Annals* (1998) **28**:215–19.

88. Johns C, Thompson J, Adjunctive treatments in schizophrenia: pharmacotherapies and electroconvulsive therapy, *Schizophr Bull* (1995) **21**:607–619.

89. Okuma T, Yamashitu I, Tahaharhi R et al, A double blind study of adjunctive carbamazepine versus placebo on excited states of schizophrenia and schizoaffective disorders, *Acta Psychiatr Scand* (1989) **80**:250–9.

90. Luchin DJ, Carbamazepine in violent nonepileptic schizophrenia, *Psychopharmacol Bull* (1984) **20**:569–71.

91. Siris SG, Depression in schizophrenia. In: Hirsch SR, Weinberger DR, eds, *Schizophrenia* (Blackwell Science: Oxford, 1995) 128–45.

92. Goff DC, Kamal KM, Sarid-Segal O et al, A placebo-controlled trial of fluoxetine added to neuroleptics in patients with schizophrenia, *Psychopharmacol* (1995) **117**:417–23.

93. Sussman N, Augmentation of antipsychotic drugs with selective serotonin reuptake inhibitors, *Primary Psychiatry* (1997) **4**:24–31.

94. Heresco-Levy U, Javitt DC, Ermilov M et al, Efficacy of high-dose glycine in the treatment of enduring negative symptoms of schizophrenia, *Arch Gen Psychiatry* (1999) **56**:29–36.

95. Farber NB, Newcomer JW, Olney W, Glycine agonists: what can they teach us about schizophrenia? *Arch Gen Psychiatry* (1999) **56**:13–17.

96. Goff DC, Guochuan T, Levitt J et al, A placebo-controlled trial of D-cycloserine added to conventional neuroleptics in patients with schizophrenia, *Arch Gen Psychiatry* (1999) **56**:21–7.

97. Weiden PJ, Aquila R, Dalheim L, Standard JM, Switching antipsychotic medications, *J Clin Psychiatry* (1997) **58(Suppl 10)**:63–72.

98. Weiden PJ, Aquila R, Emanuel M, Zygmunt A, Long-term considerations after switching antipsychotics, *J Clin Psychiatry* (1998) **59(Suppl 19)**:36–49.

99. Friedel RO, The combined use of neuroleptics and ECT in drug resistant schizophrenic patients, *Psychopharmacol Bull* (1986) **22**:928–30.

100. Safferman AZ, Munne R, Combining clozapine with ECT, *Convulsive Ther* (1992) **8**:141–3.

101. Meltzer HY, Treatment of the neuroleptic-nonresponsive schizophrenic patient, *Schizophr Bull* (1992) **18**:515–42.

102. Krueger RB, Sackeim HA, Electroconvulsive therapy and schizophrenia. In: Hirsch SR, Weinberger DR, eds, *Schizophrenia* (Blackwell Science: Oxford, 1995) 503–45.

103. Casey DE, Neuroleptic drug-induced extrapyramidal syndromes and tardive dyskinesia, *Schizophr Res* (1991) **4**:109–20.

104. Casey DE, Tardive dyskinesia and atypical antipsychotic drugs, *Schizophr Res* (1999) **35(Suppl)**:S61–6.

105. Chakos MH, Mayerhoff DI, Loebel AD et al, Incidence and correlates of acute extrapyramidal symptoms in first episode of schizophrenia, *Psychopharmacol Bull* (1992) **28**:81–6.

106. Casey DE, Extrapyramidal syndromes: epidemiology, pathophysiology and the diagnostic dilemma, *CNS Drugs* (1996) **5(Suppl 1)**:1–12.

107. Rupniak NM, Jenner P, Marsden CD, Acute dystonia induced by neuroleptic drugs, *Psychopharmacology (Berl)* (1986) **88**:403–19.

108. Casey DE, Keepers GA, Neuroleptic side effects: acute extrapyramidal syndromes and tardive dyskinesia. In: Casey DE, Christensen AV, eds, *Psychopharmacology: Current Trends* (Springer-Verlag: Berlin, 1988).

109. VanHarten PN, Kahn RS, Tardive dystonia, *Schizophr Bull* (1999) **25**:741–8.

110. Kang UJ, Burke RE, Fahn S, Tardive dystonia. In: Fahn S, Marsden CD, Calne DB, eds, *Advances in Neurology*, vol 50. *Dystonia 2* (Raven: New York, 1988) 415–29.

111. Burke RE, Fahn S, Jankovic J et al, Tardive dystonia: late-onset and persistent dystonia caused by antipsychotic drugs, *Neurology* (1982) **32**:1335–46.

112. American Psychiatric Association, *Diagnostic and Statistical Manual of Mental Disorders*, 4th edn (DSM-IV) (American Psychiatric Association: Washington, DC, 1994).

113. Janicak PG, Davis JM, Preskorn SH, Ayd FJ Jr, *Principles and Practice of Psychopharmacotherapy*, 2nd edn (Williams & Wilkins: Baltimore, 1997).

114. Van Putten T, May PRA, Akinetic depression in schizophrenia, *Arch Gen Psychiatry* (1978) **35**:1101–7.

115. Miller CH, Hummer M, Oberbauer et al, Risk factors for the development of neuroleptic-induced akathisia, *Eur Neuropsychopharmacol* (1997) **7**:51–5.

116. Fleischhacker WW, Roth SD, Kane JM, The pharmacologic treatment of neuroleptic-induced akathisia, *J Clin Psychopharmacol* (1990) **10**:12–21.

117. Burke RE, Kang UJ, Jankovic J et al, Tardive akathisia: an analysis of clinical features and response to open therapeutic trials, *Mov Disord* (1989) **4**:157–75.

118. Yassa R, Nair V, Iskandar H, A comparison of severe tardive dystonia and severe tardive akathisia, *Acta Psychiatr Scand* (1989) **80**:155–9.

119. Fenton WS, Wyatt RJ, McGlashan TH, Risk factors for spontaneous dyskinesias in schizophrenia, *Arch Gen Psychiatry* (1994) **51**:643–50.

120. Casey DE, The rabbit syndrome. In: Joseph AB, Young R, eds, *Movement Disorders in Neurology and Neuropsychiatry* (Blackwell: Boston, 1992) 139–42.

121. Yassa R, Lal S, Prevalence of the rabbit syndrome, *Am J Psychiatry* (1986) **143**:656–7.

122. Tarsy D, Baldessarini RJ, Behavioral supersensitivity to apomorphine following chronic treatment with drugs which interfere with the synaptic function of catecholamines, *Neuropsychopharmacology* (1974) **13**:927–40.

123. Jeste DV, Caligiuri MP, Paulsen JS, et al, Risk of tardive dyskinesia in older patients, *Arch Gen Psychiatry* (1995) **52**:756–65.

124. Kane JM, Woerner M, Lieberman J, Tardive dyskinesia: prevalence, incidence, and risk factors, *J Clin Psychopharmacol* (1988) **8**:525–65.

125. Jeste DV, Caligiuri MP, Tardive dyskinesia, *Schizophr Bull* (1993) **19**:303–15.

126. Gardos G, Casey DE, Cole JO et al, Ten-year outcome of tardive dyskinesia, *Am J Psychiatry* (1994) **151**:836–41.

127. Glazer WM, Moore DC, Schooler NR et al, Tardive dyskinesia: a discontinuation study, *Arch Gen Psychiatry* (1984) **41**:623–7.

128. Egan MF, Apud J, Wyatt RJ, Treatment of tardive dyskinesia, *Schizophr Bull* (1997) **23**:583–609.

129. World Health Organization, Prophylactic use of anticholinergics in patients on long-term neuroleptic treatment, *Br J Psychiatry* (1990) **156**:412–14.

130. Hasan S, Buckley P, Novel antipsychotics and the neuroleptic malignant syndrome: a review and critique, *Am J Psychiatry* (1998) **155**:1113–16.

131. Filice GA, McDougall BC, Ercan-Fang N, Billington CJ, Neuroleptic malignant syndrome associated with olanzapine, *Ann Pharmacother* (1998) **32**:1158–9.

132. Caroff SN, Mann SC, Neuroleptic malignant syndrome, *Med Clin North Am* (1993) **77**:185–202.

133. Keck PE Jr, Pope HG Jr, McElroy SL, Frequency and presentation of neuroleptic malignant syndrome: a prospective study, *Am J Psychiatry* (1987) **144**:1344–6.

134. Kusumi I, Koyana T, Algorithms for the treatment of acute side effects induced by neuroleptics, *Psychiatry Clin Neurosci* (1999) **53**:19–22.

135. Tsutsumi Y, Yamamoto K, Matsura S et al, The treatment of neuroleptic malignant syndrome using dantrolene sodium, *Psychiatry Clin Neurosci* (1998) **52**:433–8.

136. Levenson JL, Neuroleptic malignant syndrome, *Am J Psychiatry* (1985) **142**:1137–45.

137. Hermesch H, Aizenberg D, Weizman A, A successful electroconvulsive treatment of neuroleptic malignant syndrome, *Acta Psychiatr Scand* (1987) **75**:237–9.

138. Young CR, Bowers MB Jr, Mazure CM, Management of the adverse effects of clozapine, *Schizophr Bull* (1998) **24**:381–90.

139. Young DM, Risk factors for hypothermia in psychiatric patients, *Ann Clin Psychiatry* (1996) **8**:93–7.

140. Maier U, Aigner JM, Klein HE, Hypothermia caused by neuroleptics: 2 case reports and review of the literature, *Nervenarzt* (1994) **65**:488–91.

141. Buckley PF, Meltzer HY, Treatment of schizophrenia. In: Schatzberg AF, Nemeroff CB, eds, *The American Psychiatric Press Textbook of Psychopharmacology* (American Psychiatric Press: Washington, DC, 1995) 615–39.

142. Devinsky O, Pacia SV, Seizures during clozapine therapy, *J Clin Psychiatry* (1994) **55(Suppl B):**153–6.

143. Pacia SV, Devinsky O, Clozapine-related seizures: experience with 5,629 patients, *Neurology* (1994) **44:**2247–9.

144. Arana GW, Santos AB, Anticholinergics and amantadine. In: Kaplan HI, Sadock BJ, eds, *Comprehensive Textbook of Psychiatry/VI* (Williams & Wilkins: Baltimore, 1995) 1919–23.

145. Lieberman JA, Maximizing clozapine therapy: managing side effects, *J Clin Psychiatry* (1998) **59(Suppl 3):**38–43.

146. Patterson T, Sedation. In: Yesavage J, ed. *Clozapine: A Compendium of Selected Readings* (Sandoz Pharmaceuticals Corporation: Stanford, CA, 1992) 136–8.

147. Davies IB, Barrister PS, Wilcox CS, Fludrocortisone in the treatment of postural hypotension, *Br J Clin Pharmacol* (1978) **6:**444–5.

148. Whitworth AB, Fleishhacker WW, Adverse effects of antipsychotic drugs, *Int Clin Psychopharmacol* (1995); **9:**21–7.

149. Casey DE, Side effect profiles of new antipsychotic agents, *J Clin Psychiatry* (1996) **57(Suppl 11):**40–5.

149a. Schneider L, A funny thing happened on the way to the FDA Forum, *Primary Psychiatry* (2000) **79:**24–25.

150. Brown RP, Kocsis JH, Sudden death and antipsychotic drugs, *Hosp Community Psychiatry* (1984) **35:**486–91.

151. American Psychiatric Association Task Force Report 27, Sudden Death in Psychiatric Patients: The Role of Neuroleptic Drugs (American Psychiatric Association: Washington, DC, 1987).

152. Hummer M, Kurz M, Barnas C et al, Clozapine-induced transient white blood count disorders, *J Clin Psychiatry* (1994) **55:**429–32.

153. Alvir JMJ, Lieberman, JA, Safferman AZ et al, Clozapine-induced agranulocytosis: incidence and risk factors in the United States, *N Engl J Med* (1993) **329:**162–7.

154. Honigfeld G, The Clozaril National Registry System: forty years of risk management, *J Clin Psychiatry* (1996) **14:**29–32.

155. Honigfeld G, Arellano F, Sethi J et al, Reducing clozapine-related morbidity and mortality: 5 years of experience with the clozaril national registry, *J Clin Psychiatry* (1998) **59(Suppl 3):**3–7.

156. Lieberman JA, Safferman AZ, Clinical profile of clozapine: adverse reactions and agranulocytosis, *Psychiatr Q* (1992) **63:**51–70.

157. Hummer M, Kurz M, Kurzthaler I et al, Hepatotoxicity of clozapine, *J Clin Psychopharmacol* (1997) **17:**314–17.

158. Hummer M, Fleischhacker WW: Non-motor side effects of novel antipsychotics, *Arch Gen Psychiatry*, in press.

159. Seroquel. In: Abramowicz M, ed. *The Medical Letter On Drugs and Therapeutics* (Medical Letter Inc: New Rochelle, NY, 1997) **39:**117.

160. Kleinberg DL, Davis JM, DeCoster R et al, Prolactin levels and adverse events in patients treated with risperidone, *J Clin Psychopharmacol* (1999) **19:**57–61.

161. Grunder G, Wetzel H, Schlosser R et al, Neuroendocrine response to antipsychotics: effects of drug type and gender, *Biol Psychiatry* (1999) **45:**89–97.

162. Crenshaw TL, Goldberg JP, *Sexual Pharmacology: Drugs that Affect Sexual Function* (W.W. Norton: New York, 1996) 307–16.

163. Windgassen K, Wesselmann U, Schulze-Mönking H, Galactorrhea and hyperprolactinemia in schizophrenic patients on neuroleptics: frequency and etiology, *Neuropsychobiology* (1996) **33:**142–6.

164. Bartke A, Suare BB, Doherty MS et al, Effects of hyperprolactinemia on male reproductive functions. In: Negro-Vilar A, ed. *Reproduction and Andrology* (Raven: New York, 1983) 1–11.

165. Dickson RA, Glazer WM, Neuroleptic-induced hyperprolactinemia, *Schizophr Res* (1999) **35(Suppl):**S75–86.

166. Hummer M, Kemmler G, Kurz M et al, Sexual disturbances during clozapine and haloperidol treatment for schizophrenia, *Am J Psychiatry* (1999) **156:**631–3.

167. Mitchell JE, Popkin MK, Antipsychotic drug therapy and sexual dysfunction in men, *Am J Psychiatry* (1982) **139:**633–7.

168. Ghadirian A, Chouinard G, Annable L, Sexual dysfunction and plasma prolactin levels in neuroleptic-treated outpatients, *J Nerv Ment Dis* (1982) **170:**463–7.

169. Balon R, Fluvoxamine-induced erectile dysfunc-

tion responding to sildenafil, *J Sex Marital Ther* (1998) **24:**313–17.

170. Aizenberg D, Shiloh R, Zemishlany Z, Weizman A, Low-dose imipramine for thioridazine-induced male orgasmic disorder, *J Sex Marital Ther* (1996) **22:**225–9.

171. Nurnberg HG, Hensley PL, Lauriello J et al, Sildenafil for women patients with antidepressant-induced sexual dysfunction, *Psychiatr Serv* (1999) **50:**1076–8.

172. Allison DB, Mentore JL, Moonseong H, Antipsychotic-induced weight gain: a comprehensive research synthesis, *Am J Psychiatry* (1999) **156:**1686–96.

173. Schultz SK, Arndt S, Ho B-C et al, Impaired glucose tolerance and abnormal movements in patients with schizophrenia, *Am J Psychiatry* (1999) **156:**640–2.

174. Wirshing DA, Spellberg BJ, Erhart SM et al, Novel antipsychotics and new onset diabetes, *Biol Psychiatry* (1998) **44:**778–83.

175. Gaulin BD, Markowitz JS, Caley CF, Clozapine-associated elevation in serum triglycerides, *Am J Psychiatry* (1999) **156:**1270–2.

176. Fuller MA, Borovicka MC, Jaskiw GE et al, Clozapine-induced urinary incontinence: incidence and treatment with ephedrine, *J Clin Psychiatry* (1996) **57:**514–18.

177. Van Putten T, Malkin MD, Weiss MS, Phenothiazine-induced stress incontinence, *J Urol* (1973) **109:**625–6.

178. Aronowitz JS, Safferman AZ, Lieberman JA, Management of clozapine-induced enuresis [letter], *Am J Psychiatry* (1995) **152:**472.

179. Steingard S, Use of desmopressin to treat clozapine-induced nocturnal enuresis [letter], *J Clin Psychiatry* (1994) **55:**325–6.

180. Tueth MJ, DeVane CL, Evans DL, Treatment of psychiatric emergencies. In: Schatzberg AF, Nemeroff CB, eds, *The American Psychiatric Press Textbook of Psychopharmacology* (American Psychiatric Press: Washington, DC, 1995) 917–29.

5

Cognitive-behavioural Therapy

Philippa A Garety, David Fowler and Elizabeth Kuipers

Introduction

In recent years, particularly in the United Kingdom, there has been a growing interest in developing cognitive-behavioural therapy for those people with psychosis who continue to experience psychotic symptoms, despite efforts to treat these symptoms with antipsychotic medication. It can be estimated that between one-quarter and one-half of people with a diagnosis of schizophrenia experience medication-resistant persistent symptoms such as delusions and hallucinations, which cause distress and interference with functioning.[1] The need for an effective psychological intervention for psychotic symptoms also arises from the reluctance of many patients to take long-term medication, with its unpleasant and even disabling side-effects, and the fact that relapse occurs commonly even in patients who do adhere to medication regimes.[2] A recent promising development has been the research application of cognitive-behavioural approaches with younger people with a first episode of psychosis[3] and with people in the acute phases of their illness.[4] Here the focus is more on enhancing the resolution of symptoms and recovery from the acute episode, on improving insight, mood and social functioning and on preventing relapse. In this chapter, we will give an overview of the theory and practice of cognitive-behav-ioural therapy for psychosis, briefly review the outcome data, and consider the application of this approach in the clinical setting.

What is cognitive-behavioural therapy for psychosis?

Unlike certain other psychological interventions for people with schizophrenia spectrum disorders (hereafter referred to as 'psychosis'), such as social skills training or cognitive remediation approaches, cognitive-behavioural therapy takes as its central focus the experiences of psychosis (that is the symptoms) and the person's attempts to understand them. In recent years, three books have been published providing detailed descriptions of cognitive-behavioural therapy for people with psychosis.[1,5,6] Although there are some differences of emphasis, there is agreement concerning the goals and main methods of therapy; indeed there has been a fruitful cross-fertilization of ideas. The principal aim of cognitive-behavioural therapy for psychosis is to reduce the distress and interference with functioning caused by psychotic symptoms. The thoughts, beliefs and images experienced by people are the core material with which cognitive-behavioural therapists work. The approach draws extensively on the cognitive therapy of Beck and colleagues.[7] This is both in terms of therapeutic style and of content. In terms of style, the therapist works collaboratively, setting agendas and agreeing therapy goals, and takes an actively enquiring stance towards the clients' accounts of their experiences. The content of therapy involves identifying thoughts and beliefs, reviewing evidence for these, self-monitoring of cognitions, relating thoughts to mood and behaviour and identifying thinking biases. However, the standard cognitive therapy approach must be modified to address effectively the particular problems of psychosis. These include the special difficulties of establishing a therapeutic relationship; the complexity and severity of the problems presented; the need to take account of neurocognitive deficits; and the importance of working on the subjective understanding of psychosis.

Theoretical background

A number of theoretical models and hypotheses provide a theoretical underpinning to cognitive-behavioural therapy for psychosis. In general, psychoses are viewed as heterogeneous and multifactorial, and as best understood within a biopsychosocial framework. It is assumed that there are different degrees to which biological vulnerability, psychological processes and the social environment have contributed in the individual case to the expression of psychosis.[1,8] This is consistent with widely accepted 'stress-vulnerability' models.[9,10] These posit that the individual has an enduring vulnerability to psychosis, possibly but not necessarily of genetic or neurodevelopmental origin, a vulnerability which may be heightened by childhood experiences, whether social, psychological or biological. The psychosis becomes manifest on subsequent exposure to a range of additional stresses, which again may be social, psychological or biological, such as adverse environments, major life transitions or drug misuse. A further set of factors may be important in maintaining the illness in the longer term (such as the meaning attributed to psychotic experiences, loss of social roles or the use of medication). In apply-

ing the stress-vulnerability framework in the context of cognitive-behavioural therapy, the key implication is that there are different factors exerting their influence in different cases and at different times. The therapist aims to develop an individual account of a person's vulnerabilities, stresses and responses, and to help the person to modify cognitions and behaviour accordingly.[11] 'Personal therapy', an approach developed and evaluated in the United States by Hogarty and colleagues, also draws on the stress-vulnerability framework, and in some respects is similar to the cognitive-behavioural approaches developed in the United Kingdom.[12,13] Personal therapy emphasizes working on the identification of the experience of stress and its modification, with a clear focus on enhancing personal and social adjustment and on relapse prevention; this is shared by cognitive-behavioural therapy. However, personal therapy has less of an emphasis on direct work on symptoms of psychosis, which is a key characteristic of cognitive-behavioural therapy. This aspect of cognitive-behavioural therapy is grounded in cognitive models of psychotic symptoms.

The core symptoms and experiences of psychosis are manifest as disturbances of cognition, both in basic cognitive processes concerned with information-processing, resulting in anomalies of perception and experience of the self (for example hallucinations), and in conscious appraisals and judgements leading to unusual beliefs (delusions). Cognitive psychology, applying an understanding of cognitive processes involved in the general population, has found evidence of disruptions and biases in processes which are thought to contribute to the development and persistence of psychotic symptoms (see Garety and Freeman[14] for a review).

There are several competing cognitive theories to explain psychotic symptoms.[15] Theorists such as Hemsley[16] and Frith[17] have suggested that some of the primary anomalous experiences associated with delusions result from cognitive neuropsychological deficits and probably a brain dysfunction.

For example, Frith[17] has proposed that a deficit in the self-monitoring of thoughts and intentions to act (a cognitive process occurring outside conscious awareness) gives rise to the symptoms of thought insertion and alien control. Others have suggested that delusions may arise as reasonable attempts to explain puzzling anomalous experiences,[18] while Garety and Hemsley[8] have identified that delusions are associated with a 'jumping to conclusions' style of reasoning which may play a role in their formation or persistence. Still other theorists have suggested that delusions are motivational in origin and may serve the function of defending a person against threats to self-esteem.[19,20] It is probable that there is no single pathway to delusions or other psychotic symptoms. In some cases, careful assessment may suggest that one type of process may satisfactorily explain the presence of the symptom, but in other cases symptoms appear to be the product or final common pathway of several interacting processes, be they biological, psychological or social.

Cognitive accounts have also considered how psychotic experiences, however they arise, may be negatively appraised by individuals. For example, the delusional belief that one is being persecuted or the experience of an abusive voice is likely to result in emotional disturbance, such as depression, or anxiety, or in negative evaluations of the self. This disturbance then contributes further to the development and maintenance of the symptoms and distress.[21,22] The hypothesized role of emotional processes such as depression and anxiety in the maintenance and the onset of psychosis leads to the direct application of cognitive therapy techniques for these problems.[23,24]

The central assumption of cognitive-behavioural therapy is that people with psychosis, like all of us, are attempting to make sense of the world and their experiences. The meanings attributed to their experiences and the way they process them, together with their earlier personality development, will influence the expression and development of symptoms, emotional responses and behaviour. Helping people to become aware of the processes which influence their thoughts and emotions and to re-evaluate their views of themselves and the psychosis is therefore central to therapy. Cognitive-behavioural therapy combines approaches based on these cognitive models with interventions grounded in the stress-vulnerability model.

However, in placing cognitive accounts of psychosis within broader stress-vulnerability models, it is clear that there is a role for a range of different interventions with people with psychosis. Individual cognitive therapy is only one approach in a wide array of potentially beneficial methods of treatment and support. These include biological treatments, that is antipsychotic medication, as well as a wide range of psychosocial interventions, which are described elsewhere in this book.

The therapeutic approach

The broad aims of cognitive-behavioural therapy for people with psychosis are threefold.[1] They are:

1. To reduce the distress and disability caused by psychotic symptoms.
2. To reduce emotional disturbance.
3. To help the person to arrive at an understanding of psychosis in order to promote the active participation of the individual in reducing the risk of relapse and levels of social disability.

The general approach is concerned with understanding and making sense, working to achieve collaboration between the person with psychosis and the therapist, rather than didactic, interpretative or confrontational styles. It is important to note that cognitive-behavioural therapy differs, in goals and methods, from psychodynamically oriented therapies. These latter have not been demonstrated to be effective for people with schizophrenia in well-controlled trials; one possible reason for this is that traditional psychodynamic approaches are too emotionally intense for at least some patients.[25,26]

We have conceptualized therapy as a series of

six components or stages, although we do not intend that they should be viewed as an inflexible linear sequence.[11] In practice, engagement issues (the first 'stage') may be readdressed at various times as required, while the work described in the final 'stage' may be considered earlier. The six stages should therefore be seen as a guiding framework to be applied flexibly. In describing the therapeutic techniques, we also highlight the particular adaptations of cognitive-behavioural therapy required by working with this client group.

Building and maintaining a therapeutic relationship: engagement and assessment

Cognitive-behavioural therapy begins with a period of building and establishing a collaborative therapeutic relationship in which enabling the client to feel understood is of paramount importance. While establishing a therapeutic alliance is an important predictor of therapy success in general,[27] it is of particular relevance to working with people with psychosis. In the initial stages of therapy people with psychosis may be suspicious, may be angry with mental health services or may deny the relevance of therapy for their problems. If attention is not paid to these issues, early drop-out is likely. Our solution is a flexible approach to therapy which is accepting of the client's beliefs and emotions and starts by working from the client's own perspective. Particularly at this stage, we emphasize checking and discussing carefully with the client how they experience the sessions and their thoughts about the therapist's role. If the client finds sessions arousing or disturbing, we recommend shortening sessions or changing the topic to a less distressing subject. The primary aim is to ensure that the sessions are tolerable, always explicitly discussing this with the client. The occurrence of psychotic symptoms during the session, such as hallucinations or paranoid ideas, is acknowledged and very gently discussed. Gradually, the therapist moves from empathic listening to more structured assessment interviewing, in which the therapist attempts to clarify the particular life circumstances, events and

experiences which provided the context for the onset of psychosis and makes a detailed analysis of specific distressing symptoms and other problems. Over a period of approximately six sessions (although this can be longer or shorter) the therapist carries out a detailed assessment, covering past history and present circumstances, while also aiming to develop rapport and trust. By the end of this period, some preliminary shared goals for therapy should be developed. These must be relevant to the client and expressed in their own terms, while being compatible with what the therapy can hope to achieve. For example, goals might be: 'to feel less paranoid while out of the house', 'to cope better with the voices when at the day centre' or 'to feel less upset and angry with myself if the day goes badly'. Such quite limited goals can be elaborated or changed as therapy progresses. The intervention which follows will be individualized and will focus on problems identified in collaboration with the client.

Cognitive-behavioural coping strategies

Work on coping strategies follows directly from the assessment, in which current distressing symptoms and experiences have been identified, such as episodes of hearing voices and feeling anxious or suspicious when out. A range of cognitive and behavioural strategies has been shown to reduce the occurrence or duration of such problems, including activity scheduling, anxiety reduction or attention control techniques (see Tarrier 1992[28]). Yusupoff and Tarrier[29] describe these methods as essentially pragmatic and emphasize identifying what works in the individual case by undertaking a detailed assessment of existing strategies and of the antecedents and consequences of current symptoms. The goal is to manipulate any factors which contribute to symptom maintenance. Finding an approach which is helpful generally requires trial and error. Developing an effective coping strategy can bring particular relief in cases where symptoms are experienced as overwhelming and uncontrollable, resulting, for example, in self-harm or disturbed behaviour. The aim is to foster feelings of control and hope and to provide practical help in the early stages of therapy.

Implementing a new coping strategy may involve asking the client to undertake a homework task, such as keeping a record of the occurrence of the target symptom. Here adjustments to standard cognitive-behavioural practice may be needed. Clients with low IQ, literacy problems or the specific neurocognitive deficits found in psychosis (such as deficits in memory or planning) may have difficulties with such tasks. Our approach is to take account of the client's cognitive abilities and to tailor tasks accordingly. For example, self-monitoring diaries can be set up to minimize literacy demands by use of prepared recordings sheets with individualized multiple-choice questions, while memory for use of a self-instruction strategy can be aided by the use of prompt cards.

Developing a new understanding of the experience of psychosis

Discussion of the experience and meaning of psychosis is an important element of cognitive-behavioural therapy. Even though most people, at this stage in therapy, maintain strong conviction in their delusions, and may lack good insight as defined formally, it is our experience that the experience of psychosis is recognized by most as some kind of personal dysfunction, however caused. A key first step in helping people to re-evaluate their beliefs is constructing a new model of events, which is acceptable and makes sense to the client. This can provide the foundation for the re-evaluation of more specific ideas and beliefs subsequently. This work is similar to the 'psychoeducation' component of other psychosocial approaches to psychosis, such as family work (reviewed by Penn and Mueser[30]). However, in cognitive-behavioural therapy, the focus is not so much on 'education about schizophrenia' as on developing an individualized account, drawing on knowledge of psychosis, but which aims to make sense of the particular history and perspective of

the client. Constructing a new model of psychosis therefore starts with exploring the clients' current understanding of their predicament, building on the acknowledgement, however tentative, of the experience of personal dysfunction. We explore the questions of whether the clients see themselves as ill, stressed or, perhaps, suffering from schizophrenia. We discuss their views of what caused their problems and what helps them. We ask how they view the future. Building on the client's views and the information gained from the assessment, the therapist will aim tentatively to offer an individualized formulation, within a broad stress-vulnerability framework, but emphasizing an explanation of the person's subjective experience of psychosis. The formulation will make links between the person's life history and any identified vulnerability factors, stressful events which may have been precipitating factors at the onset of psychosis and processes which may be maintaining the symptoms. Evidence that psychotic experiences occur in the general population under certain stressful conditions (such as sensory and sleep deprivation) is used to 'normalize' psychosis.[5] Depending on the ability and interest of the client, we discuss biopsychosocial theories of psychosis and cognitive models of symptoms. The possible mechanisms of antipsychotic medication are often usefully discussed and set within the broader stress-vulnerability framework. In fostering a new or fuller understanding of the experience of psychosis, the therapist aims to reduce the guilt or denial associated with it and to provide a rationale for engaging in behaviours which reduce the risk of relapse and enhance functioning.

Working on delusions and hallucinations

It is not assumed that simply discussing a formulation will lead to delusional belief change. Where delusions and beliefs about voices are well established, they are typically maintained by repeated misinterpretations of specific events, by ongoing anomalous experiences and by cognitive and behavioural patterns which preferentially seek out confirmation and prevent disconfirmation of existing beliefs.[8] For example, there is strong evidence that some people with delusions 'jump to conclusions' on the basis of little evidence and that they have a biased attributional style in which other people are blamed for negative events.[14] The beliefs may also serve the function of protecting self-esteem, and at the least, will have made subjective sense of disturbing or puzzling experiences. Therefore, the emotional consequences of changing strongly held beliefs need to be explored. After discussing in general terms how events may be misinterpreted as a result of cognitive biases and how inner experiences (thoughts or images) may be misattributed to external sources, a detailed analysis of day-to-day experiences and judgements is made. In each session, over a number of weeks or months, these are reviewed and alternatives generated. Chadwick et al.[6] have provided a full account of this work with delusional beliefs, while Chadwick and Birchwood[21] have developed approaches to auditory hallucinations which show that changing the beliefs held about voices (for example, about their identity or powerfulness) will reduce distress.

This central work of identifying and changing the distressing and disabling delusions and hallucinations, by a systematic process of reviewing the evidence and generating alternatives, draws on standard cognitive approaches. However, there are some differences of method. First, as will have been noted, we only undertake this work once the therapeutic relationship is firmly established. It may often be that this detailed discussion of delusions and hallucinations will take place in the second half of therapy. Secondly, the approach is gentle and non-confrontative; the therapist must carefully judge whether and how far to challenge the client's interpretations. Also, perhaps more commonly than in standard cognitive therapy, the therapist may supply alternative interpretations rather than always seek to ensure the client generates them. This helps to compensate for the cognitive inflexibility or impairment of some clients. Thirdly, despite our best efforts, some clients

firmly resist re-evaluating their beliefs; in these cases, we aim to 'work within' the delusions, identifying possible ways of reducing distress and disability despite the continuance of the belief. For example, one of us worked with a person who believed that the voice of God commanded her to jump out of the window. She had, in fact, more than once jumped out of an upstairs window, causing serious harm. However, she was not willing or able to re-evaluate the evidence for the belief that she had a special relationship with God and heard his voice. Instead, it was possible to retain the belief that God talked to her in this way, but to discuss whether a benevolent God would wish her to do herself harm. The consequences of acting and not acting on such commands were explored, together with anxiety reduction strategies to manage the high levels of arousal experienced at such times.

Addressing negative self-evaluations, anxiety and depression

Low self-esteem is common in people with medication-resistant symptoms of psychosis.[31] Furthermore, links between the content of delusions or hallucinations and the characteristics of threatening and traumatic events in earlier life may have been identified in the assessment and formulation stages. These may indicate that there are long-standing unresolved difficulties and associated negative self-evaluations (for example, believing oneself to be evil or worthless). Such self-evaluations are likely to be factors in the maintenance of delusions and voices, for example, by being congruent with and thereby appearing to confirm the accuracy of abusive voices.[22] Having identified negative evaluations, standard cognitive therapy approaches are often applicable, reviewing the history of the development of these ideas over the lifespan and re-evaluating the evidence. Many people with psychosis have experienced very adverse life events and circumstances, including the psychosis itself and its consequences. In such cases, reappraisal may take the form of assisting the client to view him-

/herself as not, for example, 'a total failure' or 'a worthless person', but as someone who has struggled heroically with adversity.

The impact of the experience of psychosis is also relevant not only to specific evaluations, but also more generally to depression and anxiety. Birchwood et al[32] have documented how people experience demoralization and feelings of loss of control as a result of the onset of psychosis, while McGorry et al[33] have identified traumatic reactions to onset. Anxiety is often severe in people with psychosis, but is often overlooked.[24] Standard cognitive approaches of identifying automatic thoughts and dysfunctional assumptions and exploring alternative appraisals are recommended.

Managing risk of relapse and social disability

The final stage of therapy involves reviewing the work done and looking to the future. The understanding clients have of psychosis (discussed earlier) influences their engagement with services and supports and their attitudes to medication. This is reviewed and discussed further as appropriate. Although aspects of social functioning will have been discussed throughout therapy (for example, difficulties in social and family relationships, work or other activities), short- and medium-term plans are discussed further, in the light of what has been learned in therapy. The approach is not didactic, but aims to help the person to weigh up the advantages and disadvantages of different strategies and plans. At this stage, if the client is vulnerable to symptom exacerbations or relapses, it is helpful to review what has been learned about the specific individual precursors of relapse and to discuss again strategies to reduce the risk of relapse.[34]

Outcome research

Over the past 10 years there has been a growing number of published reports of evaluations of cognitive-behavioural therapy with people with medication-resistant symptoms. Some have focused on working with a particular symptom, such as delusions[35,36] or hallucinations.[37,38] Some also use a more restrictive range of therapeutic techniques than described above, such as the earlier coping strategy enhancement work of Tarrier and colleagues.[39] In general, these more specific approaches are increasingly being integrated into a more comprehensive therapeutic approach, along the lines of the description of the therapy above. Bouchard et al[40] reviewed 15 studies of 'cognitive restructuring' in the treatment of schizophrenia, most of which were individual case studies or small case series using cognitive-behavioural approaches with medication-resistant delusions or hallucinations. Of these, they considered 5 studies, including 1 small controlled trial,[41] to be both methodologically rigorous and also performed with people with schizophrenia. Bouchard et al[40] focused on changes in positive symptoms as the main measure of outcome. They concluded that these studies suggest that cognitive approaches are effective to reduce or eliminate delusions and hallucinations in people with schizophrenia. In a detailed examination of the studies, however, they found that the effect may be greater on delusions than hallucinations, the former reliably showing substantial changes.

Randomized controlled trials, despite having limitations (such as generalizing from research to clinical settings) are more conclusive than case reports or case series as valid tests of the efficacy of various forms of therapy. Two randomized controlled trials with people with medication-resistant psychosis have recently been completed.[42,43]

Table 5.1 shows details of these trials, together with two earlier controlled trials undertaken by the same two research groups. The most consistent finding is that there are significant benefits in terms of symptom reduction, particularly in positive symptoms, as a result of cognitive-behavioural therapy. This is found in all cases where the cognitive-behavioural therapy plus standard treatment group is compared to a standard treatment-only control group. These benefits are

Table 5.1 Controlled trials of cognitive-behavioural therapy with medication-resistant psychosis.

Study	Diagnosis (n) Duration of illness	Design	Treatment conditions	Treatment duration (mean no. of sessions) and follow-up	Outcome
1. Kuipers et al (1997, 1998)[42,44]	Schizophrenia-spectrum psychoses (60) Duration 13.1 yrs (range 1–33)	RCT	1. CBT + standard treatment 2. Standard treatment	9 months (18 sessions) Follow-up at 9 months	1. Significant improvement in CBT group of standard treatment in: – total symptoms (BPRS) – delusions (distress) – hallucinations (frequency) 2. Economic evaluation indicates cost of CBT offset by reduced use of services, partic. in-patient days.
2. Tarrier et al (1998, 1999)[43,45]	Schizophrenia (87) Duration 14.2 yrs (SD 9.9)	RCT	1. CBT + standard treatment 2. Supportive counselling + standard treatment 3. Standard treatment	10 weeks (20 sessions) Follow-up at 12 months	1. CBT and supportive counselling showed significant improvement of standard treatment in: – positive symptoms – negative symptoms 2. CBT showed significant improvements maintained at 12 months' follow-up, for positive symptoms. 3. Some advantages for CBT cf supportive counselling at end of treatment, but not at follow-up.
3. Garety et al (1994)[41]	Schizophrenia and schizoaffective disorder (20) i. CBT group – 16.5 yrs (range 6–30) ii. Control group–10.9 yrs (range 5–20)	Waiting list, non-random allocation	1. CBT + standard treatment 2. Standard treatment waiting list.	6 months (15 sessions) No follow-up	Significant improvements in CBT group in: – total symptoms (BPRS) – delusions (conviction and action) – depression – subjective appraisal of problems
4. Tarrier et al (1993)[39]	Schizophrenia (27) Duration 12.2 yrs. (SD 9.2)	Controlled trial (non-random allocation)	1. Cognitive-behavioural coping strategy enhancement + standard treatment 2. Problem-solving + standard treatment 3. Standard treatment waiting list	5 weeks (7 sessions) 6 months follow-up	1. Both treatment groups significantly improved in total symptoms, cf. standard treatment group. 2. CB coping strategy group greater improvements in: – delusions – anxiety

CBT, cognitive-behavioural therapy; RCT, randomized controlled trial; BPRS, Brief Psychiatric Rating Scale.

sustained at follow-up, up to 1 year after treatment. In one study,[44] there was some evidence of further improvement in the cognitive-behavioural therapy group after treatment, while the control group reverted to baseline. There is also a preliminary indication that cognitive-behavioural therapy may reduce days in hospital. Effects are not only apparent in positive symptoms although these findings are less consistent: Tarrier et al[45] showed a reduction in negative symptoms, while Garety et al[41] found reductions in depression scores. Overall, therefore, there is good evidence, from controlled trials, that cognitive-behavioural therapy is effective in terms of psychotic symptom reduction, and preliminary evidence that it may contribute to relapse reduction. These same conclusions are drawn by Jones et al[46] in a recent systematic review of cognitive-behavioural therapy for schizophrenia, which also includes two trials of therapy in the acute episodes. However, social functioning has not been found to improve, despite its being targeted in therapy. Furthermore, in the study where cognitive-behavioural therapy was compared with another psychosocial intervention, supportive counselling,[45] there were only few advantages, particularly at follow-up, over cognitive-behavioural therapy.

It is a truism, but noteworthy nonetheless, that statistical significance does not equate to clinical significance. Both Kuipers et al[42] and Tarrier et al[43] examined clinically significant changes. Kuipers et al defined a reliable clinical change as a change of five points or greater on the Brief Psychiatric Rating Scale (BPRS). (This equates to an improvement of at least 20% on the total scale score.) At 9 months post therapy, 15/23 in the cognitive-behavioural therapy (CBT) group showed a reliable clinical improvement compared with 4/24 of the control group.[44] Tarrier et al[43] found a significant advantage of the CBT group over the other two groups (supportive counselling and standard treatment) at the end of treatment in terms of 50% or greater improvement in positive symptoms, with supportive counselling in an intermediate position.

Cognitive-behavioural therapy for acute and early psychosis

Although most of the work in cognitive-behavioural therapy for psychosis has been targeted at people with medication-resistant positive symptoms, an innovation has been the application of this approach to the acute episodes of psychosis.[4] The aims of this are to hasten the resolution of positive symptoms and to promote full recovery, reducing the severity of residual symptoms. It is also hoped that by reducing the distress associated with the psychotic episode itself, subsequent traumatic responses and depression may be lessened. Drury et al[4] report a randomized controlled trial of an intensive psychosocial intervention, including individual cognitive-behavioural therapy combined with cognitive group therapy and a brief family intervention, delivered during approximately 12 weeks of an inpatient admission for an acute episode. About one-third of the patients were experiencing a first episode of psychosis. The results are impressive. The people in the cognitive therapy condition showed a significantly faster and more complete recovery from their psychotic episodes. At 9-month follow-up 95% of the cognitive therapy group and 44% of the activity control group reported no or only minor hallucinations or delusions. The cognitive therapy group also had a significantly shorter stay in hospital. This is an exciting study which indicates that intensive multimodality cognitive-behavioural work with people during their acute episodes may be beneficial and cost-effective. Further research is now being conducted, particularly targeting people in the early stages of psychosis.[3]

Applying cognitive-behavioural therapy in the clinical setting

A number of questions arise when considering how to offer cognitive-behavioural therapy to people in the setting of ordinary clinical services. These concern the selection of suitable patients, the frequency and duration of therapy, the integration of therapy with other interventions and the decision about which components of therapy are important.

It is apparent that cognitive-behavioural therapy for medication-resistant psychosis is most effective for the key targets of therapy: persistent positive symptoms. In order to engage patients, we have found it helpful to identify with them how their symptoms are distressing or interfere with their own goals. In the clinical setting, we therefore focus our resources on those people who report distress or interference with achieving their goals as a result of experiencing positive symptoms. Those patients who report no distress or personal difficulties may not engage well with therapy. An example of such patients is those whose delusions are mainly grandiose in content, especially if they also deny that there are any problems which arise from their beliefs or experiences. Clinically, it is likely that a good time to offer therapy is when a person expresses some interest in having some further help. This is consistent with the findings from a study which attempted to identify predictors of a positive response to cognitive-behavioural therapy.[47] We found that people who had a certain cognitive flexibility concerning their delusions, which we have called a 'chink of insight', did better. However, it is important to emphasize that this does not mean that the therapy does not work effectively with people who are fully convinced of their delusions or who are formally rated as having poor insight. In addition, we found that IQ or cognitive impairment does not predict therapy outcome; it appears entirely possible to work successfully with people with a wide range of IQ, including people with impairments in cognitive functions, such as planning and memory, sometimes present in people with psychosis. In such cases, however, it is important to tailor the therapy to match the ability of the patient, as described above.

In terms of the duration and frequency of therapy, although the duration of therapy in the research studies has varied, most have offered a median of approximately 20 sessions. In clinical settings, it is our experience that therapy is best delivered over between 6 months and 1 year, preferably starting weekly and reducing to fortnightly for the greater part of the period. However, monthly sessions may be offered towards the end and continued for selected patients for a much longer period, if resources allow. Although there is no research to back this, it is possible that people with a vulnerability to relapse or very unstable belief systems may be helped by such continued contact. Alternatively, it may be practicable to make a full and careful transition to another mental health worker, who is in regular contact with the patient, who can offer cognitively informed ongoing support.

As we have noted, cognitive-behavioural therapy is normally offered alongside a range of other treatments and services, such as medication, day or vocational services and case management. Indeed, optimal care requires the integration of such interventions.[48] However, engagement in services is variable. Cognitive-behavioural therapy can be offered to people who do not engage in other services or who do not take medication. Nonetheless, many patients do take antipsychotic medications concurrently with therapy. An area yet to be researched is how cognitive-behavioural therapy interacts with medication or with other forms of psychosocial intervention. In practice, it seems that cognitive-behavioural therapy can be helpful in facilitating patients' engagement with other services, such as vocational or social programmes; it may also enhance medication or other treatment adherence in individual cases (although this has not been demonstrated). Of particular interest for patients living with families is whether the outcome is improved when this individual approach is offered in addition to a family intervention, which has previously been shown to be beneficial.[30] This has not been systematically studied. Especially with younger patients whose psychosis is of recent onset, a combined individual cognitive-behavioural and family approach may be beneficial.

As we have emphasized, given the heterogeneity of the problems presented by people with psychosis, cognitive-behavioural therapy involves a detailed assessment, an individualized formulation and individually selected therapy goals. It follows that for each person the therapy will focus on specific elements of the six 'stages' listed above. Although it is clear that the first stage, of developing a therapeutic relationship, is common to all, it is not known which of the other elements are necessary or most effective in particular cases. In practice, we find that, for medication-resistant symptoms, the stages of developing an understanding of psychosis and working on delusions and hallucinations form the core of the work, while developing coping strategies and work on negative self-evaluations or mood disturbance may be less relevant to certain patients. Nonetheless, the disappointing lack of clear benefits in the studies in reducing depression suggests that further work is needed to improve the therapeutic approach to achieve this. For people with a more favourable response to medication, but a relapsing course, there will be a stronger emphasis on the specific issues described above in the sixth stage: working on relapse prevention and enhancing social functioning.

Conclusions

Cognitive-behavioural therapy is emerging as an effective approach for the relief of symptoms which are not optimally helped by antipsychotic medication. It has been shown to reduce positive psychotic symptoms and there is evidence that it may contribute to relapse reduction.[46] One study has shown that improvements were sustained or even increased at follow-up, suggesting that the approach can transmit skills of self-management.[44] It is also likely to prove cost effective, especially if the evidence that it delays relapse proves robust. Finally, there is some evidence that cognitive approaches can help people with acute and early psychosis. Indeed, an intervention which focuses on the beliefs and the understanding a person develops in the context of the experience of psychosis is very likely to be more helpful if offered early. However, given the complexity and heterogeneity of psychosis, optimal care will require that a range of interventions as described in this handbook is offered, as desired by the patients and their carers and as judged appropriate to need. Cognitive-behavioural therapy should be considered as one possible component of a comprehensive treatment plan.

References

1. Fowler D, Garety P, Kuipers E, *Cognitive Behaviour Therapy for People with Psychosis* (John Wiley & Sons: Chichester, 1995).

2. Roth A, Fonagy P, Schizophrenia. In: Roth A, Fonagy P, eds, *What Works for Whom? A Critical Review of Psychotherapy Research* (Guildford Press: New York, 1996).

3. McGorry P, ed, *Verging on Reality*. Vol 172 Suppl. 33rd edn. (Royal College of Psychiatrists: Dorchester, 1998, 1–136).

4. Drury V, Birchwood M, Cochrane R, MacMillan F, Cognitive therapy and recovery from acute psychosis: a controlled trial. I. Impact on psychotic symptoms, *Br J Psychiatry* (1996) **169:**593–601.

5. Kingdon D, Turkington D, *Cognitive-Behavioural Therapy for Schizophrenia* (Lawrence Erlbaum Associates: Hove, 1994).

6. Chadwick PDJ, Birchwood M, Trower P, *Cognitive Therapy for Delusions, Voices and Paranoia* (John Wiley & Sons: Chichester, 1996).

7. Beck AT, Rush AJ, Shaw BF, Emery G, *Cognitive Therapy of Depression* (Guilford: New York, 1979).

8. Garety PA, Hemsley DR, *Delusions: Investigations into the Psychology of Delusional Reasoning*. Maudsley Monograph (Oxford University Press: Oxford, 1994).

9. Zubin J, Spring B, Vulnerability – a new view on schizophrenia, *J Abnorm Psychol* (1977) **86:**103–26.

10. Strauss JS, Carpenter WT, *Schizophrenia* (Plenum: New York, 1981).

11. Garety PA, Fowler D, Kuipers E, Cognitive-behavioural therapy for medication-resistant symptoms *Schizophr Bull* in press.

12. Hogarty GE, Kornblith SJ, Greenwald D et al,

Personal therapy: a disorder-relevant psychotherapy for schizophrenia, *Schizophr Bull* (1995) **21**:379–93.

13. Hogarty GE, Kornblith SJ, Greenwald D et al, Three-year trials of personal therapy among schizophrenic patients living with or independent of family, I: Description of study and effects on relapse rates, *Am J Psychiatry* (1997) **154**:1504–13.

14. Garety PA, Freeman D, Cognitive approaches to delusions: a critical review of theories and evidence, *Br J Clin Psychol* (1999) **38**:113–54.

15. Nuechterlein KH, Subotnik KL, The cognitive origins of schizophrenia and prospects for intervention. In: Wykes T, Tarrier N, Lewis S, eds, *Outcome and Innovation in Psychological Treatment of Schizophrenia* (John Wiley & Sons: Chichester, 1998) 17–43.

16. Hemsley DR. Perceptual and cognitive abnormalities as the bases for schizophrenic symptoms. In: David AS, Cutting JC, eds, *The Neuropsychology of Schizophrenia* (Lawrence Erlbaum: Hove, 1994) 97–116.

17. Frith CD, *The Cognitive Neuropsychology of Schizophrenia* (Lawrence Erlbaum: Hove, 1992).

18. Maher BA, Anomalous experience and delusional thinking: the logic of explanations. In: Oltmanns TF, Maher BA, eds, *Delusional Beliefs* (Wiley & Sons: New York, 1988).

19. Freud S, *A Case of Paranoia Running Counter to the Psychoanalytic Theory of Disease* (Hogarth: London, 1915/1956).

20. Bentall R, Kinderman P, Kaney S, The self, attributional processes and abnormal beliefs: towards a model of persecutory delusions, *Behav Res Ther* (1994) **32**:331–41.

21. Chadwick P, Birchwood M, The omnipotence of voices: a cognitive approach to auditory hallucinations, *Br J Psychiatry* (1994) **164**:190–201.

22. Close H, Garety PA, Cognitive assessment of voices: further developments in understanding the emotional impact of voices, *Br J Clin Psychol* (1998) **37**:173–88.

23. Birchwood M, Iqbal Z, Depression and suicidal thinking in psychosis: a cognitive approach. In: Wykes T, Tarrier N, Lewis S, eds, *Outcome and Innovation in Psychological Treatment of Schizophrenia* (John Wiley & Sons: Chichester, 1998).

24. Freeman D, Garety PA, Worry, worry processes and dimensions of delusions: an exploratory investigation of a role for anxiety processes in the mainte-

nance of delusional distress *Behavioural and Cognitive Psychotherapy* (1999) **27**:47–62.

25. Mueser KT, Berenbaum H, Psychodynamic treatment of schizophrenia: is there a future? *Psychol Med* (1990) **20**:253–62.

26. Gunderson JG, Frank AF, Katz HM et al, Effects of psychotherapy in schizophrenia. II. Comparative outcome of two forms of treatment, *Schizophr Bull* (1984) **10**:564–98.

27. Horvath AO, Symonds BD, Relationship between working alliance and outcome in psychotherapy: a meta-analysis, *J Consult Clin Psychol* (1991) **38**:139–49.

28. Tarrier N, Management and modification of residual positive psychotic symptoms. In: Birchwood M, Tarrier N, eds, *Innovations in the Psychological Management of Schizophrenia* (John Wiley & Sons: Chichester, 1992).

29. Yusupoff L, Tarrier N, Coping strategy enhancement for persistent hallucinations and delusions. In: Haddock G, Slade PD, eds, *Cognitive-Behavioural Interventions with Psychotic Disorders* (London: Routledge, 1996).

30. Penn DL, Mueser KT, Research update on the psychosocial treatment of schizophrenia, *Am J Psychiatry* (1996) **153**:607–17.

31. Freeman D, Garety PA, Fowler D et al, The London–East Anglia randomized controlled trial of cognitive-behavioural therapy for psychosis IV: Self esteem and persecutory delusions, *Br J Clin Psychol* (1998) **37**:415–30.

32. Birchwood M, Mason R, MacMillan F, Healy J, Depression, demoralisation and control over psychotic illness: a comparison of depressed and non-depressed patients with a chronic psychosis, *Psychol Med* (1998) **23**:387–95.

33. McGorry PD, Chanen A, McCarthy E. Post-traumatic stress disorder following recent onset psychosis. An unrecognised postpsychotic syndrome, *J Nerv Ment Dis* (1991) **179**:253–8.

34. Birchwood M. Early interventions in psychotic relapse: cognitive approaches to detection and management. In: Haddock G, Slade P, eds, *Cognitive-Behavioural Interventions with Psychotic Disorders* (Routledge: London, 1996).

35. Chadwick PDJ, Lowe CF, Measurement and modification of delusional beliefs, *J Consult Clin Psychol* (1990) **58**:225–32.

36. Alford BA, Beck AT, Cognitive therapy of delusional beliefs, *Behav Res Ther* (1994) **32:**369–80.

37. Morrison AP, Cognitive behaviour therapy for auditory hallucinations without concurrent medication: a single case, *Behavioural and Cognitive Psychotherapy* (1994) **22:**259–64.

38. Haddock G, Bentall RP, Slade PD, Psychological treatment of auditory hallucinations: focusing or distraction? In: Haddock G, Slade PD, eds, *Cognitive-Behavioural Interventions with Psychotic Disorders* (Routledge: London, 1996) 45–70.

39. Tarrier N, Beckett R, Harwood S et al, A trial of two cognitive-behavioural methods of treating drug-resistant residual symptoms in schizophrenic patients. I. Outcome, *Br J Psychiatry* (1993) **162:** 524–32.

40. Bouchard S, Vallières A, Roy M-A, Maziade M, Cognitive restructuring in the treatment of psychotic symptoms in schizophrenia: a critical analysis, *Behavior Therapy* (1996) **27:**257–77.

41. Garety PA, Kuipers E, Fowler D et al, Cognitive behavioural therapy for drug-resistant psychosis, *Br J Med Psychol* (1994) **67:**259–71.

42. Kuipers E, Garety P, Fowler D et al, London–East Anglia Randomised Controlled Trial of Cognitive-Behavioural Therapy for Psychosis. I: Effects of the treatment phase, *Br J Psychiatry* (1997) **171:**319–27.

43. Tarrier N, Yusupoff L, Kinney C et al. Randomised controlled trial of intensive cognitive behaviour therapy for chronic schizophrenia, *BMJ* (1998) **317:**303–7.

44. Kuipers E, Fowler D, Garety P et al, London–East Anglia Randomised Controlled Trial of Cognitive-Behavioural Therapy for Psychosis. III: Follow-up and Economic Evaluation at 18 Months, *Br J Psychiatry* (1998) **173:**61–8.

45. Tarrier N, Wittowski A, Kinney C et al, The durability of the effects of cognitive-behaviour therapy in the treatment of chronic schizophrenia: twelve months follow-up, *Br J Psychiatry* (1999) **174:**500–4.

46. Jones C, Cormac I, Mota J, Campbell C, Cognitive behaviour therapy for schizophrenia (Cochrane Review). In: The Cochrane Library (Update Software: Oxford, 1999).

47. Garety P, Fowler D, Kuipers E et al, London–East Anglia Randomised Controlled Trial of Cognitive-Behavioural Therapy for Psychosis. II: Predictors of Outcome, *Br J Psychiatry* (1997) **171:**420–6.

48. Fenton W, McGlashan TH, We can talk: individual psychotherapy for schizophrenia, *Am J Psychiatry* (1997) **154:**1493–5

6

Rehabilitative Treatment of Schizophrenia

Alan S Bellack

Contents • Issues in the design of psychosocial interventions • Rehabilitation strategies • Summary and conclusions

The accumulated evidence over the past several decades has led to a general consensus that schizophrenia is a brain disease (or set of diseases) caused by genetic and/or prenatal and perinatal insult.[1,2] Even in the absence of the discovery of specific biological markers for the illness, this consensus opinion is consistent with the conclusion that treatment for schizophrenia must generally be based on effective biological/ medical intervention. However, there is little question that psychosocial factors have a significant impact on the course and outcome of the illness, and a compelling case can be made that psychosocial treatment is a necessary and valuable component of a multifactorial treatment approach. This conclusion is supported by a series of consensus treatment guidelines developed in the latter half of the 1990s.[3–5]

In considering the case for psychosocial treatment it is important to be clear about the goals of the intervention. If the goal is narrowly defined in terms of the reduction of primary psychopathology (for example, positive and negative symptoms) and/or the prevention of relapse, available techniques fall well short of the mark and doubts may be raised (see below) about the prospects for psychosocial approaches. Chapters 5 and 8 in this volume attest to the benefits of several innovative psychosocial approaches for dealing with positive

symptoms and relapse, but even the most promising trials have produced only modest effect sizes on these domains. Core symptoms and the recurrence of symptom exacerbation appear to be closely tied to the neurobiology of the illness and, as such, are apt to be less responsive to psychosocial interventions than they are to pharmacological treatments.

A more optimistic picture of the role of psychosocial treatment emerges if one adopts a broader view of outcomes that takes into account the complex, chronic, and multiply handicapping nature of schizophrenia. The illness is marked by poor social role performance, chronic unemployment (or underemployment), excess medical morbidity and mortality, shortened life expectancy (including a markedly elevated risk for suicide), high levels of substance abuse, and increased risk for criminal victimization. Despite the dramatic benefits provided by antipsychotic medication, including the new atypicals, medication alone generally does not, and arguably cannot, restore premorbid levels of functioning, lead to normative role performance, or substantially improve quality of life for most patients. Schizophrenia strikes in late adolescence or young adulthood, thereby disrupting a critical period for socialization and development of adult life skills (for example, dating and sexuality, work skills). The illness then results in increasing social isolation, failure and frustration in attempts at fulfilling requisite social roles, demoralization, anxiety, and maladaptive ways of coping with symptoms (such as substance use, avoidance and social isolation). It can be assumed that these various problems become more severe and entrenched as the duration of illness increases. Even if medications were 100% successful at eliminating core symptoms, which they are not, the hoped for Rip van Winkle effect would be a rare event. Most patients would still be left with a residue of psychosocial symptoms and skill deficits. For the majority of patients who experience continued symptoms despite *effective* pharmacotherapy, the level and breadth of functional impairments is magnified. Consequently, the long-term management of schizophrenia requires a multidimensional approach,[3,6] and it is doubtful whether significant improvements in overall level of functioning can be achieved without psychosocial interventions.

Issues in the design of psychosocial interventions

The potential benefits of psychosocial treatment are often not achieved in the community owing to poor understanding of the special needs and liabilities of schizophrenia patients. Five factors need to be taken into account when implementing psychotherapeutic interventions and evaluating the results: (1) the need to base interventions on a compensatory model; (2) the need for long-term treatment; (3) individual differences in treatment needs; (4) the role of the patient in treatment; and (5) the limitations imposed by impairments in information-processing.

Adoption of a compensatory model
As indicated above, schizophrenia is a multiply handicapping disorder. It impacts on: ability to perform activities of daily living (ADLs) and ability to fulfil social roles, including worker, homemaker, student, parent, and spouse; it

increases the risk of substance abuse and disease, including HIV; and it interferes with performance of appropriate health care behaviors, including compliance with both medical and psychiatric treatment. A large proportion of patients also have residual psychotic symptoms and periodic exacerbations, and they experience high levels of depression and anxiety. Overall, they suffer from poor quality of life. In light of this panoply of impairments, no single treatment is likely to have a sufficiently broad-based impact. This circumstance stands in marked contrast to less severe disorders, such as unipolar depression, panic, and eating disorders, in which a single intervention may be expected to produce substantial amelioration of the condition. Nevertheless, psychosocial treatments have often been held to this same standard, leading to the conclusion that they are not effective for schizophrenia.

A rehabilitation model, the primary focus of this chapter, is more appropriate than the standard treatment model as it: (a) implies a narrower focus on specific skills and behaviors, and (b) aims to improve functioning in specific areas, rather than eliminating or *curing* an entire condition. Another common aspect of the rehabilitation approach that is particularly germane for schizophrenia is its use of a *compensatory* model rather than the *restorative or reparative* model typical of treatment approaches. For example, rehabilitation for people with visual impairments involves teaching them to rely more on other senses, to use special appliances, such as Braille keyboards, to use aides, such as canes and guide dogs, and to systematically arrange their environment to minimize the need for sight. Success is achieved by improving independence, role functioning, and quality of life, not by restoring vision. Comparable rehabilitation programming is provided for stroke patients, individuals with paralysis, and amputees. Robert P. Liberman (personal communication) decries this use of physical disabilities as a metaphor for schizophrenia as he contends it implies an overly pessimistic stance. While it is pessimistic to the extent that it presumes we cannot *cure* schizophrenia, it is, in fact, a very optimistic perspective in that we have well-developed technologies for several of the specific dysfunctions experienced by schizophrenia patients. Moreover, we are much more likely to develop effective new focal techniques for other problems than we are to reverse the neurodevelopmental insult that underlies schizophrenia and restore normative functioning.

The need for long-term treatment

Although longitudinal data have challenged the assumption that schizophrenia necessarily has a deteriorating course,[7,8] the illness characteristically is life-long and severe. The net result is that patients often need assistance meeting a wide variety of needs, ranging from learning how to handle the tasks of day-to-day living to the management of psychotic symptoms, and they require help over an extended period of time.[9,10] Nevertheless, much research on psychosocial interventions has focused on short-term, time-limited strategies. Brief treatments, such as 3 to 6 months of social skills training, may be useful for reducing stress or teaching patients how to cope with specific problems (for example, discussing medication side effects with a physician). Research indicates that gains from brief treatment can be maintained over time.[11,12] However, it is unlikely that any brief intervention can produce broad-based improvement in overall functioning, or enduring changes in vulnerability to symptom exacerbations and relapse. Moreover, most patients will require intermittent booster treatment even for circumscribed skills training programs, while others will need continuing support throughout their lives.

Individual differences in treatment needs

Schizophrenia, sometimes referred to as the schizophrenias, is a heterogeneous disorder, with wide variability in symptom presentation, severity, course, and treatment response. This heterogeneity has been interpreted as reflecting either multiple etiologies or multiple disease entities.[13,14] It

may also reflect the variable input of the environment and individual differences unrelated to the core illness (for example, comorbid vulnerability to depression or substance abuse).

Evidence of heterogeneity in areas commonly assumed to be impaired in schizophrenia underscores the importance of individual differences in treatment planning. For example, Mueser and colleagues[15] found that 50% of schizophrenia patients had persistent deficits in social skills over a 1-year period, while 11% did not differ from nonpatient controls, and the remainder showed variable performance. Thus, the common assumption that patients with schizophrenia have deficits in their social skills is true for many but not all patients. Similar evidence of heterogeneity exists in regard to neuropsychological deficits. Schizophrenia patients have repeatedly been found to perform more poorly than normal controls on the Wisconsin Card Sorting Test (WCST),[16] a measure of prefrontal cortical functioning.[17,18] However, the performance of many patients (up to 20%) is in the normal range.[19,20] There is also considerable variability in the extent to which patients can be taught to improve their performance,[21] and in the extent to which performance improvements generalize to other tasks.[22]

In addition to the variability between patients, significant changes occur within patients over time that have a bearing on their treatment needs. Young patients need special help in dealing with the fact that they have a serious illness which may interfere with their personal goals and their ability to achieve independence, a problem which may contribute to their high vulnerability to suicide and substance abuse.[23,24] Older patients may adjust to the difficulties of the illness through withdrawal or positive coping strategies,[10,25] but they face unique problems of their own. For example, parents are unable to continue caring for an offspring with schizophrenia as the patient grows older, necessitating a shift in caretaking responsibility to either siblings[26] or the mental health system. A survey of the needs of schizophrenia patients in regular contact with their families indicated that concern over what happens when a parent dies was ranked fourth highest out of 45 topics (parents ranked this concern fifth).[27]

Despite this well-recognized heterogeneity, there is relative homogeneity in psychosocial treatment programming. Most agencies employ a 'one size fits all' approach to treatment, with the primary interpatient variability resulting ad hoc from patient noncompliance and clinician idiosyncracies. This approach has serious clinical limitations, and also leads to nihilistic views of the potential impact of psychosocial programs. Empirical trials of new interventions tend to recruit subjects based on diagnostic criteria rather than on patients' needs or motivation for the particular approach. The consequence is often high dropout rates and small effect sizes.

In order for psychosocial interventions to meet the real needs of patients, between-patient differences and changes over time need to be taken into account. Research is sorely needed that addresses issues of patient–treatment matching. An example comes from a project I am conducting to develop a treatment for substance use in schizophrenia. The intervention is based on a rehabilitative model.[28] Preliminary outcome data revealed a bimodal distribution: half of the subjects did very well, providing clean urine samples in 90.79% of the treatment sessions. The remaining half did very poorly, either dropping out of treatment or continuing to use drugs throughout (mean % clean urines = 22.33). Of note, there were marked pretreatment differences in readiness to change on two measures from the Transtheoretical Model of Change:[29] the University of Rhode Island Change Assessment (URICA)[30] and decisional balance.[31] The good-outcome subjects had a mean readiness score on the URICA of 11.72 (SD = 1.65), compared to a mean of 7.47 (SD = 3.25) for the poor performers. This difference was highly significant. There was a similar effect for perceived cons of drug use (reasons not to use) on the decisional balance scale: means

were 3.95 (SD = 0.61) and 2.57 (SD = 1.19) for the good- and poor-outcome groups, respectively. These data, which suggest that treatment might best be initiated when subjects are *ready* (for example, motivated) to reduce drug use, underscore the importance of patient–treatment matching.

The role of the patient
The combination of thought disorder and negative symptoms (such as apathy, anhedonia) often lead to the false assumption that patients are not capable of being active participants in their own treatment. Indeed, many patients seem unmotivated and are noncompliant. However, such apparent disinterest and passivity should not be interpreted as immutable traits. Negative symptoms are not always stable, and they may be secondary to demoralization, psychotic symptoms, medication side effects, and other factors that vary over time.[32,33] Paul and Lentz[34] have shown that even extremely withdrawn, chronic schizophrenia patients can be motivated by a systematic incentive program.

As cogently argued by Strauss,[25] schizophrenia patients have an active *will*. Much of their behavior is goal-directed and reflects an attempt to cope with the illness as best they can. Consequently, it is essential to view the patient as a potentially active partner, and involve him or her in goal-setting and treatment-planning. Too often, treatments are imposed on patients by the treatment team and family members, with little consideration of the patient's own desires. It should not be surprising in such circumstances that the patient fails to adhere to treatment recommendations, increasing the risk of relapse and creating tensions in relationships with family members and treatment providers. To be sure, engaging the patient to establish treatment goals can be a long, arduous process, but failure to do so courts the larger risk of undermining the very purpose of the intervention.

Impairments in information processing

It is now well established that impaired information-processing represents one of the most significant areas of dysfunction in schizophrenia. The illness is marked by neuropsychological deficits in multiple domains, including memory (especially working memory), attention, speed of processing, abstract reasoning, and sensorimotor integration.[35,36] As summarized in a seminal paper by Michael Green,[37] a number of studies document a relationship between these impairments and both social functioning and performance in skills training programs. For example, Mueser and colleagues[38] found that poor memory had a deleterious effect on learning in social skills training, but that pretreatment symptomatology was unrelated to social skill acquisition. Kern and colleagues[39] also found that memory impairment, as well as poor sustained attention (on the Continuous Performance Test), was associated with decreased learning in social skills training.

A related issue concerns the impact of neurocognitive deficits on the generalization of treatment effects. A basic assumption of all psychotherapies is that skills acquired in treatment sessions must be transferred or generalized to the patient's natural environment. Yet, such generalization is contingent upon cognitive processes that are often disrupted in schizophrenia, especially including executive functions mediated by the dorsolateral prefrontal cortex.[1] Several analog studies suggest that generalization is limited at best, even when explicitly programmed.[22,40]

Unfortunately, clinical rehabilitation programs have lagged behind the experimental literature in this arena, and neurocognitive deficits have not been addressed in a systematic manner. To be sure, most sophisticated rehabilitation programs do adjust the rate at which information is presented and the amount of detail or nuance provided. Allowance is also generally made for the need for repetition and regular review. However, these adjustments do not necessarily compensate for deficits in working memory and higher-level

executive processes. For example, there are impairments in the ability to perceive the continuity of experience over time and to plan behavior accordingly: that is, to see how past experiences relate to current circumstances, or how what is currently being discussed can be applied in the future.[41] This problem would interfere with the ability to utilize newly acquired skills at appropriate times, to pursue goals in a systematic manner, or to use past experience to problem solve. While there are strong data to document that rehabilitation programs are effective in teaching new behavior,[42] the literature does not document that newly acquired skills are applied in the community. Even in cases where interventions result in better clinical outcomes the data do not support the face valid assumption that changes are due to what has been taught. This point was amply illustrated in the Treatment Strategies in Schizophrenia project, in which family treatment was associated with reduced relapse rates despite an absence of any change in communication patterns, the purported mechanism of change.[43] Determination of the mechanisms that mediate behavior change in the community is perhaps the greatest challenge facing the field over the next decade if we are to develop more effective treatments.

Rehabilitation strategies

In the following sections we will briefly describe and evaluate the two types of rehabilitation programs that have had the greatest clinical and heuristic impact on the field in the 1990s and promise to play a similar role in the first decade of the new millenium: social skills training and cognitive rehabilitation.

Social skills training

Social dysfunction is a defining characteristic of schizophrenia that is semi-independent of other domains of the illness.[44,45] Social functioning is also predictive of the course and outcome of the illness.[46,47] The most useful perspective for understanding social functioning and social dysfunction in the illness has been the *social skills model*.[48,49] Social skills are specific response capabilities necessary for effective performance. They include verbal response skills (for example, the ability to start a conversation or to say 'No' when needed), paralinguistic skills (for example, use of appropriate voice volume and intonation), and nonverbal skills (such as, appropriate use of gaze, hand gestures, and facial expressions). These skills tend to be stable over time and make a unique contribution to the performance of social roles and quality of life.[15,50] Increasing social competence and improving social role functioning has been a major focus of rehabilitation efforts for the past 25 years, and a well-developed technology for teaching social skills has been developed and empirically tested: Social Skills Training (SST).[51]

The basic technology for training social skills was developed in the 1970s and has not changed substantially in the intervening years. It is a highly structured educational procedure that is generally conducted in small groups. Trainers are more like teachers than traditional therapists. They first model appropriate behavior, and then engage patients in role-playing social encounters as a vehicle for practicing new skills. The therapists provide social reinforcement after each role-played response and shape improved performance. Complex social repertoires, such as making friends and dating, are broken down into component elements, such as maintaining eye contact and asking questions. Patients are first taught to perform the elements, and then gradually learn smoothly to combine them.

A large number of single case studies and small group designs have demonstrated the efficacy of SST for teaching a wide range of skills, including conversational skill, assertiveness, and medication management.[52,53] Over the past decade, six larger group studies have been conducted.[11,12,54–57] The findings have been consistent with those of the smaller trials, and indicate that effects of SST are maintained for at least 6–12 months.

Four of the six studies examined the effects of

SST on symptoms, relapse, and social adjustment with mixed results. Bellack et al[11] compared 3 months of group SST in a day hospital with day hospital treatment alone. At the 6-month follow-up, patients who received SST were less symptomatic and had better social adjustment, but there were no differences in relapse at the 1-year follow-up. Liberman et al[56] compared 2 months of intensive SST with 'holistic health' treatment for long-term residents of a state hospital awaiting discharge. At the 2-year follow-up, the SST patients were better on several symptom measures and social adjustment, but relapse rates did not differ significantly. Eckman et al[12,58] compared 1 year of intensive group SST with a supportive group. At the 2-year follow-up, patients who had received SST had better social adjustment, although their relapse rates did not differ from the control group.

In the only study to examine individual SST, Hogarty et al[57,59] compared SST, family psychoeducation, SST plus family psychoeducation, and medication only. All patients were living with or in contact with high expressed emotion (EE) family members. SST, alone and in combination with family therapy, was associated with reduced relapse rates throughout the first 21 months of the study. By the twenty-fourth month, however, the effect of SST was no longer significant, due to several relapses in the last 3 months for this group. Follow-up data on social adjustment were only collected for nonrelapsed patients, so the effect of SST on social functioning in this study is unclear.

Several trends emerge from these studies. SST is clearly effective in increasing the use of specific behaviors (such as gaze) and improving functioning in the specific domains that are the primary focus of the treatment. However, it is unclear whether other, more diffuse, dimensions of social functioning are affected, or the extent to which learning in the clinic translates into improved role functioning in the community. The effects of SST on relapse rate and symptoms appear to be negligible, although this is not surprising given the narrow focus of the intervention. SST is widely employed in clinical settings and is often considered to be among the most effective psychosocial treatments for schizophrenia. However, many questions remain about the clinical utility of SST. Several recent reviews of empirically supported treatments rated SST as no more than *promising*, a somewhat disappointing evaluation after 25 years of study. SST is clearly an effective teaching technology that is well received by both patients and clinicians. It provides an excellent model for conducting other rehabilitation programming with this population. Nevertheless, it may well be that no time-limited, compartmentalized, office-based treatment can have broad-based effects. As discussed earlier in this chapter, it may be necessary to employ longer-term treatments that extend into the community and that are integrated with an array of intervention strategies.

Cognitive rehabilitation

Recognition of the importance of neurocognitive deficits has stimulated increasing interest in the prospects for cognitive remediation. It is difficult to trace the history of interest in this topic, but it certainly goes back at least as far as Meichenbaum's seminal work in the early 1970s.[60] He generated considerable interest in the possibility of teaching patients to use self-talk to guide problem-solving in a pair of provocative studies. Platt and Spivack[61,62] provided some thought-provoking data on problem-solving during that period that also pointed to a role for cognitive rehabilitation. However, these somewhat anomalous studies were not replicated, and interest in cognitive training languished as the emphasis of psychosocial treatment shifted to more promising interventions that were more consistent with the increasingly sophisticated neurobiological models of schizophrenia.

Two studies in the late 1980s rekindled interest in the possibility of cognitive rehabilitation. Brenner and his colleagues[63] described Integrated Psychological Therapy (IPT), a comprehensive program to improve social competence by first enhancing basic cognitive skills. The Brenner results were not particularly robust, but the work has had tremendous heuristic value, and still serves as the most systematic test of the feasibility of cognitive rehabilitation to date (see below). Goldberg and colleagues at NIH[21] reported that patients with schizophrenia were unable to benefit from explicit instructions and practice on the Wisconsin Card Sorting Test (WCST), a putative neuropsychological marker of prefrontal function. This failure to benefit from training, combined with data on diminished blood flow, was interpreted as evidence of an unmodifiable abnormality of the dorsolateral prefrontal cortex. Curiously, the first of these reports held out the promise for effective cognitive rehabilitation, while the second implied that a basic neurophysiological impairment made such rehabilitation impossible. The NIH work stimulated a spate of mostly successful demonstrations that WCST performance deficits, albeit widespread, are neither endemic to the illness nor immutable.

In one of the first studies designed to challenge this pessimistic conclusion my colleagues and I demonstrated that performance on the WCST can be improved by reinforcement and specific instructions.[19] Other laboratories have been able to produce comparable effects using our training strategy[64,65] and slightly different variations, with improvements lasting from several weeks[39,66] to 1 month.[67]

There have been a handful of published studies in which cognitive training strategies have been employed to improve performance on other measures of information-processing as well. Benedict and colleagues[68] employed a computer-based training program that had been developed to enhance attention in brain-injured patients. While subjects improved their performance on the computerized tasks, there was no associated improvement on Asarnow and Nuechterlein's Span of Apprehension Test or degraded stimulus Continuous Performance Test. In a recent study by Wexler et al,[69] subjects were given extensive practice on a motor dexterity task and either a visual reading task or a dot spatial memory task. Improved performance was gradually shaped over 10 weeks. A majority of subjects reached normative levels on the reading and dot tasks, and most showed improvement on the dexterity task as well. These results are consistent with other studies[70,71] that demonstrate that modest improvements can be observed on a variety of tasks with practice alone, or practice supplemented by incentives.

The accumulated findings provide clear evidence that it is possible to achieve enhanced performance on a range of cognitive tasks through practice, instruction, and provision of incentives. However, these practice-related changes typically fall short of full normalization of performance, and may not be long-lived. Such results do suggest that the deficits present on formal testing likely represent a combination of stable as well as more plastic factors (such as demoralization and lack of motivation). However, the more important issue remains that the gains achieved in these studies do not appear to have had large clinical effects on other aspects of functioning.

Unfortunately, there has been a dearth of new data on clinical applications of cognitive rehabilitation strategies. The most comprehensive program for cognitive rehabilitation is Integrated Psychological Therapy.[63] This program first focuses on the remediation of basic cognitive capacities (for example, concept formation, memory) before training in problem-solving and social skills. Cognitive training proceeds on tasks adapted from neuropsychological test procedures (for example, a card-sorting task) and word games (for example, finding synonyms and antonyms). Brenner and his colleagues have conducted several small sample studies on IPT.[72] This sophisticated, multilayered program was 'state of the art' when first described at scientific meetings in the late 1980s, and it remains the most ambitious effort to date. The program has considerable face validity and has had great heuristic value. However, the results have been modest, at best. There have been improvements on several

of the neuropsychological tasks targeted in training, akin to the practice effects reported in several of the analog studies referred to above. However, there has not been evidence of widespread improvements in cognitive functioning, or generalization to higher-level domains (such as social skills).

Spaulding and colleagues[73,74] have translated the Brenner materials into English and have been engaged in a replication trial at a long-term hospital for chronic patients in Nebraska. The preliminary results appear to be no better than the results of the Brenner trial. There were modest improvements on a few tests from a comprehensive neuropsychological assessment, but these results could have been due to chance given the number of statistical tests conducted. Spaulding et al[74] also conclude that the modest changes are little different from what is seen in normal subjects who practice unfamiliar tasks, and that there are no indications that 'such changes confer ecologically significant benefits in personal or social functioning.'

A somewhat different approach to cognitive rehabilitation has been developed by Wykes and colleagues in the United Kingdom.[75] Their intervention is conducted individually, as opposed to the group format employed for IPT. It focuses exclusively on neurocognitive processes, including executive functioning (for example, cognitive flexibility, working memory, and planning). In contrast to the numerous reports that provide little more than extended practice on neuropsychological tests, this approach employs a sophisticated training model that is based on principles of errorless learning, targeted reinforcement, and massed practice. A preliminary trial yielded promising results on several neuropsychological measures. This approach warrants further study.

As previously indicated, judging the potential for cognitive rehabilitation based on existing trials (analog or clinical) is difficult due to the risk of type II error. It may be safe to conclude that a particular strategy is not effective, but one cannot extrapolate from any single trial or group of trials to the broader domain. For example, a particular technique that fails to produce an effect in 10 training sessions might be effective after 50. Ten sessions of practice on computerized memory tasks may not be sufficient to produce a generalizable increase in processing capacity, but meaningful changes might begin to occur after 100 sessions. Alternatively, an innovative program based on a different conceptual model could produce results that the simpler practice/rehearsal strategies currently in vogue do not. Nevertheless, the current literature does not provide strong grounds for optimism.

A limitation of the work on cognitive rehabilitation is that the role of information-processing deficits in producing functional impairments in schizophrenia remains unknown. Since patients tend to have a broad array of cognitive deficits, the selection of which deficits to target for rehabilitation is somewhat arbitrary. In addition, the primary methods employed to improve performance rely primarily on repeatedly practicing cognitive skills and on the use of complex mnemonics, although neither approach has been successful in producing significant gains in brain-injured patients.[76–78] A more fruitful avenue to explore for the management of cognitive deficits may be to focus on environmental change, compensatory strategies, and coping skills until there is a better understanding of the factors underlying the poor role performance of schizophrenia patients.

Summary and conclusions

This chapter has provided an overview of issues involved in providing effective rehabilitation programming for people with schizophrenia. Interest in psychosocial treatment, including rehabilitation, has waxed and waned over the past several decades. Psychosocial treatments have never achieved their most optimistic aims, but neither have pharmacotherapies. Even the new atypicals leave patients with considerable residual deficits, especially including problems in information-pro-

cessing and ability to fulfil social roles. Hence, there is at least as much need for effective psychosocial treatments now as there was prior to the modern era. That being said, we discussed a number of critical factors that must be addressed if psychosocial treatments are to be effective, including: (1) the need to base interventions on a compensatory model; (2) the need for long-term treatment; (3) individual differences in treatment needs; (4) the role of the patient in treatment; and (5) the limitations imposed by information-processing deficits. We then reviewed work on two rehabilitation strategies that have received considerable attention: social skills training and cognitive rehabilitation. Both approaches have been the subject of extensive study over a number of years but questions remain about the clinical utility of both. SST is an effective teaching/training strategy, but it is not clear that the intervention can produce meaningful changes in community performance unless it is embedded in a comprehensive, community-oriented intervention program. The potential for cognitive rehabilitation is less clear. Current approaches seem to be based on an overly simplistic model of neurocognitive functioning and rely primarily on a naïve *exercise* model that attempts to alter brain function by repeated practice. This approach is not supported by the existing literature, which may be overly optimistic about the potential for neurocognitive repair or restoration of function. A compensatory model which structures the environment and shapes behavior to minimize demands on higher-level cognitive processes may ultimately be more effective.

References

1. Weinberger DR, Implications of normal brain development for the pathogenesis of schizophrenia, *Arch Gen Psychiatry* (1987) **44**:660–9.

2. Roberts GW, Schizophrenia: a neuropathological perspective, *Br J Psychiatry* (1991) **158**:8–17.

3. American Psychiatric Association, *Practice Guideline for the Treatment of Patients with Schizophrenia*

(American Psychiatric Association: Washington, DC, 1997).

4. Lehman AF, Steinwachs DM, Translating research into practice: the schizophrenia patient outcomes research team (PORT) treatment recommendations, *Schizophr Bull* (1998) **24:**1–10.

5. McEvoy JP, Scheifler PL, Frances A, Treatment of schizophrenia 1999, *J Clin Psychiatry* (1999) **60(Suppl. 11).**

6. Bellack AS, A comprehensive model for the treatment of schizophrenia, In: Bellack AS, ed, *A Clinical Guide for the Treatment of Schizophrenia* (Plenum: New York, 1989) 1–22.

7. Harding CM, Brooks GW, Ashikaga T et al, The Vermont longitudinal study of persons with severe mental illness. I: Methodology, study sample, and overall status 32 years later, *Am J Psychiatry* (1987) **144:**718–26.

8. Harding CM, Brooks GW, Ashikaga T et al, The Vermont longitudinal study of persons with severe mental illness. II: Long-term outcome of subjects who retrospectively met DSM-III criteria for schizophrenia, *Am J Psychiatry* (1987) **144:**727–35.

9. Ciompi L, Toward a coherent multidimensional understanding and therapy of schizophrenia: converging new concepts. In: Strauss JS, Boker W, Brenner HD, eds, *Psychosocial Treatment of Schizophrenia: Multidimensional Concepts, Psychological, Family, and Self-help Perspectives* (Hans Huber: Toronto, 1987) 48–62.

10. Wing JK, Psychosocial factors affecting the long-term course of schizophrenia. In: Strauss JS, Boker W, Brenner HD, eds, *Psychosocial Treatment of Schizophrenia* (Hans Huber: Toronto, Canada, 1987) 13–29.

11. Bellack AS, Turner SM, Hersen M, Luber RF, An examination of the efficacy of social skills training for chronic schizophrenic patients, *Hosp Community Psychiatry* (1984) **35:**1023–8.

12. Eckman TA, Wirshing WC, Marder SR, Technology for training schizophrenics in illness self-management: a controlled trial, *Am J Psychiatry* (1992) **149:**1549–55.

13. Tsuang MT, Lyons MJ, Faraone SV, Heterogeneity of schizophrenia: conceptual models and analytic strategies, *Br J Psychiatry* (1990) **156:**17–26.

14. Carpenter WT, Buchanan RW, Kirkpatrick B et al, Strong interence, theory testing, and the neuro-anatomy of schizophrenia, *Arch Gen Psychiatry* (1993) **50:**825–31.

15. Mueser KT, Bellack AS, Douglas MS, Morrison RL, Prevalence and stability of social skill deficits in schizophrenia, *Schizophr Res* (1991) **5:**167–76.

16. Heaton RK, *Wisconsin Card Sorting Test Manual* (Psychological Assessment Resources: Odessa, FL, 1981).

17. Berman KF, Zec RF, Weinberger DR, Physiologic dysfunction of dorsolateralprefrontal cortex in schizophrenia. II. Role of neuroleptic treatment, attention, and mental effort, *Arch Gen Psychiatry* (1986) **43:**126–35.

18. Weinberger DR, Berman KF, Zec RF, Physiologic dysfunction of dorsolateral prefrontal cortex in schizophrenia. I. Regional cerebral blood flow evidence, *Arch Gen Psychiatry* (1986) **43:**114–24.

19. Bellack AS, Mueser KT, Morrison RL et al, Remediation of cognitive deficits in schizophrenia, *Am J Psychiatry* (1990) **147:**1650–5.

20. Braff DL, Heaton R, Kuck J et al, The generalized pattern of neuropsychological deficits in outpatients with chronic schizophrenia with heterogeneous Wisconsin Card Sorting Test results, *Arch Gen Psychiatry* (1991) **48:**891–8.

21. Goldberg TE, Weinberger DR, Berman KF et al, Further evidence for dementia of the prefrontal type in schizophrenia? *Arch Gen Psychiatry* (1987) **44:**1008–14.

22. Bellack AS, Weinhardt LS, Gold JM, Gearon JS, *Generalization of Training Effects in Schizophrenia* submitted.

23. Test MA, Wallisch LS, Allness DJ, Ripp K, Substance use in young adults with schizophrenic disorders, *Schizophr Bull* (1989) **15:**465–476.

24. Caldwell CB, Gottesman II, Schizophrenics kill themselves too: a review of risk factors for suicide, *Schizophr Bull* (1990) **16:**571–89.

25. Strauss JS, Subjective experiences of schizophrenia: toward a new dynamic psychiatry. II, *Schizophr Bull* (1989) **15:**179–87.

26. Horwitz AV, Tessler RC, Fisher GA, Gamache GM, The role of adult siblings in providing social support to the severely mentally impaired, *Journal of Marriage and the Family* (1992) **54:**233–41.

27. Mueser KT, Bellack AS, Wade JH et al, An assessment of the educational needs of chronic psychiatric patients and their relatives, *Br J Psychiatry* (1992) **160:**674–80.

28. Bellack AS, DiClemente CC, Treating substance

abuse among patients with schizophrenia, *Psychiatr Serv* (1999) **50:**75–80.

29. Prochaska JO, DiClemente CC, *The Transtheoretical Approach: Crossing the Traditional Boundaries of Therapy* (Krieger: Malabar, FL, 1984).

30. DiClemente CC, Hughes SO, Stages of change profiles in outpatient alcoholism treatment, *J Subst Abuse* (1990) **2:**217–35.

31. Carbonari JP, DiClemente CC, Aweben A, A readiness to change scale: its development, validation and usefulness. Discussion symposium: assessing critical dimensions for alcoholism treatment. Presented at the annual meeting of the AABT, San Diego, CA.

32. Carpenter WT, Heinrichs DW, Wagman AMI, Deficit and nondeficit forms of schizophrenia: the concept, *Am J Psychiatry* (1988) **145:**578–83.

33. McGlashan TH, Fenton WS, The positive–negative distinction in schizophrenia: review of natural history validators, *Arch Gen Psychiatry* (1992) **49:** 63–72.

34. Paul GL, Lentz RJ, *Psychosocial Treatment of Chronic Mental Patients: Milieu Versus Social-Learning Programs* (Harvard University Press: Cambridge, MA, 1997).

35. Braff DL, Information processing and attentional abnormalities in the schizophrenia disorders. In: Magaro PA, ed, *Cognitive Bases of Mental Disorders* (Sage: Newbury Park, CA, 1991) 262–307.

36. Green MF, Nuechterlein KH, Should schizophrenia be treated as a neurocognitive disorder? *Schizophr Bull* (1999) **25:**309–18.

37. Green MF, What are the functional consequences of neurocognitive deficits in schizophrenia? *Am J Psychiatry* (1996) **154:**321–30.

38. Mueser KT, Bellack AS, Douglas MS, Wade JH, Prediction of social skill acquisition in schizophrenic and major affective disorder patients from memory and symptomatology, *Psychiatry Res* (1991) **37:** 281–96.

39. Kern RS, Green MF, Satz P, Neuropsychological predictors of skills training for chronic psychiatric patients, *Psychiatry Research* (1992) **43:**223–30.

40. Bellack AS, Blanchard JJ, Murphy P, Podell K, Generalization effects of training on the Wisconsin Card Sorting Test for schizophrenia patients, *Schizophr Res* (1996) **19:**189–94

41. Hemsley DR, A cognitive model and its implications for psychological intervention, *Behavior Modification* (1996) **20:**139–69.

42. Smith TE, Bellack AS, Liberman RP, Social skills training for schizophrenia: review and future directions, *Clin Psychol Rev* (1996) **16:**599–617.

43. Bellack AS, Haas GL, Schooler NR, Flory JD, *The effects of behavioral family treatment on family communication and patient outcomes in schizophrenia,* submitted.

44. Strauss JS, Carpenter WT Jr, Bartko JJ, The diagnosis and understanding of schizophrenia. Part III. Speculations on the processes that underlie schizophrenic symptoms and signs, *Schizophr Bull* (1974) **11:**61–9.

45. Lenzenweger MF, Dworkin RH, Wethington E, Examining the underlying structure of schizophrenic phenomenology: evidence for a three-process model, *Schizophr Bull* (1991) **17:**515–24.

46. McGlashan TH, The prediction of outcome in chronic schizophrenia, IV. The Chestnut Lodge follow-up study, *Arch Gen Psychiatry* (1986) **43:**167–75.

47. Johnstone EC, Macmillan JF, Frith CD et al, Further investigation of the predictors of outcome following first schizophrenic episodes, *Br J Psychiatry* (1990) **157:**182–9.

48. Meir VJ, Hope DA, Assessment of social skills. In: Bellack AS, Hersen M, eds, *Behavioral Assessment*, 4th edn (Allyn & Bacon: Needham Heights, MA 1998) 232–55.

49. Morrison RL, Bellack AS, Social skills training. In: Bellack AS, ed, *Schizophrenia: Treatment, Management, and Rehabilitation* (Grune & Stratton: Orlando, FL, 1984) 247–79.

50. Bellack AS, Morrison RL, Wixted JT, Mueser KT, An analysis of social competence in schizophrenia, *Br J Psychiatry* (1990) **156:**809–18.

51. Bellack AS, Mueser KT, Gingerich S, Agresta J, *Social Skills Training for Schizophrenia: A Step-by-Step Guide* (The Guilford Press: New York, 1997).

52. Benton MK, Schroeder HE, Social skills training with schizophrenics: a meta-analytic evaluation, *J Consult Clin Psychol* (1990) **58:**741–7.

53. Halford WK, Hayes R, Psychological rehabilitation of chronic schizophrenic patients: recent findings on social skills training and family psychoeducation, *Clin Psychol Rev* (1991) **11:**23–44.

54. Brown MA, Munford AM, Life skills training for chronic schizophrenics, *J Nerv Ment Dis* (1983) **17:**466–70.

55. Spencer PG, Gillespie CR, Ekisa EG, A controlled comparison of the effects of social skills training and remedial drama on the conversational skills of

chronic schizophrenic inpatients, *Br J Psychiatry* (1983) **143:**165–72.

56. Liberman RP, Mueser KT, Wallace CJ, Social skills training for schizophrenic individuals at risk for relapse, *Am J Psychiatry* (1986) **143:**523–6.

57. Hogarty GE, Anderson CM, Reiss DJ et al, Family psychoeducation, social skills training, and maintenance chemotherapy in the aftercare treatment of schizophrenia. I. One-year effects of a controlled study on relapse and expressed emotion, *Arch Gen Psychiatry* (1986) **43:**633–42.

58. Marder SR, Wirshing WC, Eckman T et al, Psychosocial and pharmacological strategies for maintenance therapy: effects on two-year outcome, *Schizophr Res* (1993) **9:**260.

59. Hogarty GE, Anderson CM, Reiss DJ et al, Family psychoeducation, social skills training, and maintenance chemotherapy in the aftercare treatment of schizophrenia. II. Two-year effects of a controlled study on relapse and adjustment, *Arch Gen Psychiatry* (1991) **48:**340–7.

60. Meichenbaum DH, Cameron R, Training schizophrenics to talk to themselves: a means of developing attentional controls, *Behavior Therapy* (1973) **4:**515–34.

61. Platt JJ, Spivack G, Problem-solving thinking of psychiatric patients, *J Consult Clin Psychol* (1972) **39:**148–51.

62. Platt JJ, Spivack G, Social competence and effective problem-solving thinking in psychiatric patients, *J Clin Psychol* (1972) **28:**3–5.

63. Brenner HD, Kraemer S, Hermanutz M, Hodel B, Cognitive treatment in schizophrenia. In: Straube E, Hahlweg K, eds, *Schizophrenia: Models and Interventions* (Springer Verlag: New York, 1990) 161–91.

64. Nisbet H, Siegert R, Hunt M, Fairley N, Improving Wisconsin card-sorting performance, *Br J Clin Psychol* (1996) **35:**631–3.

65. Vollema MG, Geurtsen GJ, van Voorst AJP, Durable improvements in Wisconsin Card Sorting Test performance in schizophrenic patients, *Schizophr Res* (1994) **16:**209–15.

66. Metz JT, Johnson MD, Pliskin NH, Luchins DJ, Maintenance of training effects on the Wisconsin Card Sorting Test by patients with schizophrenia or affective disorders, *Am J Psychiatry* (1994) **151:**120–2.

67. Young DA, Freyslinger MG, Scaffolded instruction and the remediation of Wisconsin Card Sorting Test deficits in chronic schizophrenia, *Schizophr Res* (1995) **16:**199–207.

68. Benedict RHB, Harris AE, Markow T et al, Effects of attention training on information processing in schizophrenia, *Schizophr Bull* (1994) **20:**537–46.

69. Wexler BE, Hawkins KA, Rounsaville B et al, Normal neurocognitive performance after extended practice in patients with schizophrenia, *Schizophr Res* (1997) **26:**173–80.

70. Goldman RS, Axelrod BN, Tompkins LM, Effect of instructional cues on schizophrenic patients' performance on the Wisconsin Card Sorting Test, *Am J Psychiatry* (1992) **149:**1718–22.

71. Stratta P, Mancini F, Mattei P et al, Information processing strategy to remediate Wisconsin Card Sorting Test performance in schizophrenia: a pilot study, *Am J Psychiatry* (1994) **151:**915–18.

72. Brenner HD, Roder V, Hodel B et al, *Integrated Psychological Therapy for Schizophrenia Patients* (Hogrefe & Hogrefe: Toronto, 1994).

73. Spaulding W, Reed D, Elting D et al, Cognitive changes in the course of rehabilitation. In: Brenner HD, Boker W, Genner R, eds, *Towards a Comprehensive Therapy for Schizophrenia* (Hogrefe & Huber: Seattle, WA, 1997) 106–17.

74. Spaulding WD, Fleming SK, Reed D et al, Cognitive functioning in schizophrenia: implications for psychiatric rehabilitation, *Schizophr Bull* (1999) **25:**275–89.

75. Wykes T, Reeder C, Corner J et al, The effects of neurocognitive remediation on executive processing in patients with schizophrenia, *Schizophr Bull* (1999) **25:**291–307.

76. Schacter DL, Glisky EL, Memory remediation: restoration, alleviation, and the acquisition of domain-specific knowledge. In: Uzzell BP, Gross Y, eds, *Clinical Neuropsychology of Intervention* (Martinus Nijhoff: Boston, MA, 1986) 257–82.

77. Butler RW, Namerow NS, Cognitive retraining in brain-injury rehabilitation: a critical review, *J Neuropsychology and Rehabilitation* (1988) **2:**97–101.

78. Benedict RH, The effectiveness of cognitive remediation strategies for victims of traumatic head-injury: a review of the literature, *Clin Psychol Rev* (1989) **9:**605–26.

7

Clinician Interactions with Patients and Families

Diana O Perkins, Jennifer Nieri and Janet Kazmer

Introduction

A variety of treatment modalities is needed for the comprehensive care of individuals with schizophrenia. Antipsychotic medications are the cornerstone of treatment, used to minimize symptom severity with as few side effects as possible. However, to achieve and maintain maximal symptomatic and functional recovery usually requires other types of interventions, including individual and group psychotherapy, family therapy, case management, inpatient treatment, supervised housing, and social and vocational rehabilitative services. Decisions regarding the optimal therapeutic interventions should be based on the patient's needs. These needs will vary with the stage and severity of illness, and with the patient's individual goals. In addition, the resources available to the patient will necessarily influence treatment options. Treatment is thus highly individualized, and will change as the patient's condition and available resources change.

Schizophrenia can be conceived of having premorbid, prodromal, first-episode, deteriorating, and chronic residual stages, with treatment interventions varying considerably depending on the stage of illness.[1] Premorbidly there may be subtle alterations in thinking and behavior but most individuals who develop schizophrenia are indistinguishable from their peers in childhood. The prodromal stage is marked by the onset of changes in thinking, perception, mood, and behavior. The severity of symptoms worsens, until frank psychosis in a form such as delusional ideation or hallucinations emerges. With treatment individuals often recover from the first psychotic episode. Relapse is very common, however, occurring in 80% of patients who recover from a first episode, and is usually associated with medication discontinuation.[2] With repeated relapses there is often a limited period of symptomatic worsening and functional decline, and the severity of illness and disability usually stabilizes after 5–10 years of illness. The following sections discuss general principles of clinician–patient interactions in the treatment of schizophrenia, followed by principles specific to the premorbid, prodromal, first-episode, and chronic stages of illness.

General principles

While each stage of schizophrenia poses unique challenges, there are general principles that apply to, and may enhance, interactions with patients and their families regardless of stage or level of acceptance of illness. First, therapy is optimized when the clinician and patient work as partners, and share common therapeutic goals.[3] When poor insight limits the ability of the patient to engage in treatment, it is still helpful for the clinician to understand the patient's conception of the illness and perceived benefits and costs of treatment.[4] The therapeutic alliance is greatly strengthened when there is one or more agreed treatment goals. For example, while the patient may not recognize their ideas about being spied upon as delusional, he or she may agree that 'anxiety' and 'poor sleep' are appropriate treatment goals.

Patient confidentiality and the involvement of family in treatment-planning are critical clinical issues that need to be defined and addressed throughout the stages of schizophrenia. While families are often involved in treatment and indeed desire involvement in treatment-planning, patients may refuse to consent for clinicians to actively inform or involve family members in clinical decision-making. Thus, confidentiality can be a source of contention for clinicians, involved family members, and patients. The three Rs of confidentiality, 'respect, refer, and revisit', provide a useful clinical guideline when family is involved in the care of the patient or desires information about the patient's clinical status, but the patient refuses consent to involve the family. First, while it is critical to *respect* patients' confidentiality, it is possible to include families in treatment without disclosing specific clinical information. For example, the clinician may listen to family members' concerns and reports about the patient's behavior, and provide general education without violating clinician–patient confidentiality.[5] Similarly, the clinician may *refer* family members to appropriate educational material and other treatment providers or organizations as sources of support and further education. As the therapeutic relationship strengthens, and as the patient's insight and clinical condition improve, the issue of confidentiality may be *revisited*. Patients may eventually agree that certain specific information be provided to family members. The patient may benefit from discussions of how important information will be shared with family members by enhancing their ownership of treatment, especially when they themselves relay important information.

Several factors may hamper communication with patients and families, including the impact of schizophrenia on cognitive function, and the fact that many clinician–patient interactions occur during times of crisis. Key concepts in presenting information include knowing and using the patient/family member's way of describing symptoms (for example, patients may refer to auditory hallucinations as 'the spirits'), using nonjudgmental terms, and respecting the patient/family as 'experts' on the illness as it affects them. Information is best presented in a graduated, concise manner. Care should be taken to not overwhelm patients and families with too much information at once. Repetition is often needed, as it is difficult for both patients and families to hear and integrate information about the illness or treatment, especially during a crisis. It is also important to be sensitive to where the patient/family are in the process of treatment and recovery. For example, a family new to treatment, with a daughter in her first episode of psychosis, described how on initial contact with the hospital social worker they were told they should begin to 'grieve the loss of their daughter as they knew her', and that 'she would never be able to hold a job, or return to school'. These premature and inaccurate statements caused this family unnecessary alarm and hopelessness, and impaired their ability to trust mental health clinicians. Fostering a sense of hope in the context of providing realistic information is a critical balancing act for the clinician.

The diagnosis of schizophrenia continues to carry significant stigma that has an impact on both patients and their families, and may interfere with functional recovery.[6] It is often of use for clinicians to address both self-stigma and stigma from others directly. Self-stigma will affect the patient's confidence and self-esteem and impede rehabilitative efforts. Cognitive-behavioral techniques may be useful in challenging self-stigmatizing ideas. In addition, it may be helpful to discuss the patient's experience of stigma from friends and family members and from society. Clinical interventions should focus on countering myths and stigmas. In addition, clinicians involved in the treatment of schizophrenia may want to assume greater effort to combat stigma, for example through education of the larger public about the realities of mental illness and as advocates for social and political change.[7]

Patient–clinician interactions in the premorbid stage

Individuals with a personal or family history of schizophrenia may be concerned about the risk of illness in themselves or in other relatives, and may seek information and counseling from mental health professionals about their concerns or to inform family planning. Often referred to as 'genetic counseling', the clinical intervention is individualized, but typically includes general information about the prevalence and course of schizophrenia, and a discussion about the risk of a psychotic illness to family members. Information about the genetics of schizophrenia and possible environmental factors that may affect risk is often useful as well.[8]

For example, it may be useful to inform individuals seeking such counseling that in the general population, approximately 1/100 individuals will be affected by schizophrenia. The risk is increased to tenfold to about 1/10 individuals who have a first-degree relative (parent, sibling, or offspring) with schizophrenia. The risk is further increased to about 4–5/10 individuals who have both parents or a monozygotic twin with schizophrenia. The risk of schizophrenia is only slightly elevated (2–3/100)

from the general population risk when a second-degree relative (for example, aunt, uncle, grandparent) is affected.[9]

It is often useful for individuals seeking genetic counseling to understand that while genetic factors are thought to contribute to risk, the genetics of the illness is complex and environmental factors are also thought to play a role in risk of illness. It is most likely that a specific grouping of genes and/or environmental factors, that individually do not cause disease, in combination cause schizophrenia. Certain environmental factors have been associated with increased risk of illness. Individuals seeking genetic counseling as part of family planning may find it helpful to know that schizophrenia has been associated with stressful environmental events during fetal life, such as maternal infectious disease, maternal starvation, and perinatal complications.[10] Thus, individuals concerned about family planning can be advised that good prenatal care, while not a guarantee of a healthy child, may influence risk of illness. Individuals concerned about their own risk or risk to a family member may find it useful to know that heavy use of marijuana and other drugs is more common premorbidly in individuals with schizophrenia than in control subjects. Thus, while not a guarantee of good health, it may be that abstinence from marijuana, amphetamines, and other illegal drugs may decrease risk of illness.

Finally, with individuals concerned about personal risk or risk in close family members, it may be helpful to discuss the early warning signs of psychosis and to develop a help-seeking plan should symptoms occur. It may also be valuable to point out that the symptoms of schizophrenia are often treatable, and that early intervention may influence the severity and course of illness, and often results in symptom remission.

Patient–clinician interactions in the prodromal stage

Retrospective studies indicate that most individuals with schizophrenia experience prodromal changes in thinking, mood, and perception for an average of 1–2 years prior to developing psychotic symptoms.[11] Prodromal symptoms include perceptual abnormalities, distortions of thinking (for example, ideas of reference, suspiciousness), negative symptoms (such as decreased drive and motivation), subjective cognitive complaints (such as distractibility), affective disturbances (affective lability; depressed, irritable, or anxious mood). These symptoms are often accompanied by behavioral disturbances such as decline in functioning at school or work, social withdrawal, impaired hygiene, aggressive behaviors, or suicidal ideation.

The symptoms that occur in the prodromal stages of schizophrenia are nonspecific, and may be symptoms of disorders other than schizophrenia. Preliminary data suggest that between 40% and 60% of individuals with marked prodromal symptoms will develop a psychotic disorder.[12,13] While these initial research efforts suggest that criteria can be developed to describe a clinical state at high risk for development of a subsequent psychotic illness, many individuals with prodromal symptoms are not at risk for psychosis. In addition to the early stages of a psychotic disorder, diagnoses that should be considered in patients experiencing prodromal symptoms include: a mood disorder (bipolar disorder, major depression, or an anxiety disorder), a reaction to overwhelmingly stressful life events, a difficult but normal adolescence, a substance use disorder, or a metabolic or other disorder that affects brain function (for example, thyroid disease, seizure disorder). Regrettably, to date little is known about factors that differentiate individuals that are in the prodromal stages of a psychotic disorder from individuals who are experiencing self-limiting symptoms or who have symptoms due to other clinical syndromes.

Patients and families will seek help due to the emotional distress caused by prodromal symptoms, or due to decline in social, occupational, or school functioning. Patients may not volunteer more specific symptoms, such as perceptual abnormalities or thought disturbances. Retrospective descriptions of treatment of individuals prior to development of a psychotic disorder suggest that multiple nonpsychotic diagnoses are common.[14] Thus, it is likely that when patients present with prodromal symptoms, clinicians may not consider the early stages of a psychotic disorder as part of the differential diagnosis, and may include specific questions about other prodromal symptoms in their clinical evaluation. Also, concern over possible stigmatization may lead some clinicians to hesitate to include a psychotic disorder in the differential diagnosis of prodromal symptoms. However, the consequences of overlooking a psychotic disorder are potentially serious, including maintenance of inappropriate treatment (for example, misdiagnosis as attention deficit disorder and treatment with a psychostimulant), and lack of monitoring for emergence of frank psychosis, with risk of aggressive behaviors, suicide, or involuntary hospitalization.

When a patient presents with vague disturbances in mood, cognition, perception, or decline in function and does not clearly meet criteria for a psychiatric syndrome (such as major depression or post-traumatic stress disorder), then the prodromal stages of a psychotic disorder should be considered in the differential diagnosis. Here, the patient evaluation should include a thorough review of psychiatric symptoms that includes perceptual abnormalities, thought disturbances, cognitive impairments, and mood symptoms. In many cases, patients may be embarrassed or anxious when revealing their recent unusual experiences. The clinician can help reduce feelings of anxiety and isolation with careful questioning and empathetic responses.

Patients and families appreciate information about the symptoms and are usually able to understand the uncertain prognosis. It may be useful, for example, for the clinician to explain that while these symptoms are often self-limiting, there is a risk that the symptoms will worsen, with the development of a more serious mental illness such as bipolar disorder or schizophrenia. In addition, it may be useful to call these symptoms 'basic symptoms'[15] rather than 'prodromal symptoms', in order to make clear that the symptoms may not be the early 'prodromal' stages of a psychotic disorder, and thus to minimize the risk of unnecessary stigmatization. Finally, the treatment plan should also include education about recognizing and intervening appropriately should psychotic symptoms emerge.

There are no established guidelines for the treatment of prodromal symptoms. Depending on symptom presentation and family history, the clinician and patient may elect to 'watch and wait'. or to intervene with psychotherapy (for example, supportive, stress-management, or cognitive-behavioral therapy), and/or initiate a medication trial (with an antipsychotic, antidepressant, anxiolytic, or mood stabilizer drug). There are few empirical data to guide clinical interventions, and in making treatment decisions patients will need to know about the lack of established guidelines for treating prodromal symptoms. The preliminary study suggests that low-dose antipsychotic treatment may improve prodromal symptoms and reduce risk of development of a psychotic disorder.[16] It was of interest that in this pilot study antidepressant treatment did not alter risk of development of a psychotic disorder. Many patients and their families may be reluctant to take medication, especially given the lack of proven efficacy for any pharmacological treatment. In addition, cognitive-behavioral interventions may be of value. For example, with a patient who is experiencing ideas of reference, the clinician might discuss how all humans, especially when stressed or fatigued, may be overly sensitive and misinterpret ordinary events or interactions. If this patient describes feeling suspicious of and threatened by a friend who passes without a greeting, the therapist could then discuss alternative explanations (for instance that the friend may not have seen him or her, or had a lot on their mind) and strategies to check out their interpretations of others' behavior.

There is renewed interest in investigating strategies to identify and treat individuals in the prodromal stages of schizophrenia.[17] These efforts may well lead to improved outcomes, and possibly even the prevention of schizophrenia in high-risk individuals.

Patient–clinician interactions in the first episode

The first episode of schizophrenia, characterized by the onset of positive symptoms such as hallucinations, delusions, and disorganized thinking or behavior, is an enormous challenge to the affected individual. Such symptoms usually cause great distress to patients and their families, and often a crisis will have precipitated initial treatment contact.

Retrospective studies indicate that many patients with schizophrenia and related psychotic disorders experience active symptoms for a considerable period of time before receiving appropriate medical treatment, possibly increasing the likelihood of poor treatment response and a more severe illness course.[18] Psychotic symptoms will have occurred on average for 1 year and some symptoms of illness have persisted 2–3 years before antipsychotic treatment is obtained.[19] Studies suggest that patients and their families recognize significant changes in the patient's mood, thinking and behavior, but do not identify these symptoms as part of an illness, and have difficulties obtaining appropriate clinical care. Delays result primarily from the patient, family, law enforcement authorities, and mental health care providers not recognizing the presence and/or seriousness of active symptoms.[14,20] Preliminary data suggest that educational efforts directed at clinicians and the general public may reduce treatment delays.[21,22]

Patients in the early stages of a psychotic illness have special needs that are not readily addressed by traditional treatment approaches used for patients with chronic illness. The initial clinician–patient interactions often occur in an emergency room and inpatient setting, and are usually focused on pharmacological management and maintaining patient safety. During the initial episode first-episode patients typically experience a high level of confusion and psychological distress and may experience the first episode as a traumatic life event. As much as possible, clinical interactions should be reassuring, and directed at reducing the patient's acute distress. Forced treatment, restraint, and seclusion should be avoided whenever possible.

Contrary to the case in chronic schizophrenia, appropriate pharmacological treatment of the first episode of schizophrenia typically results in complete or near complete symptom remission,[23,24] thus traditional treatment settings, such as day treatment programs, clubhouses, or other psychosocial rehabilitation programs, may not be appropriate. Similarly, family members often report that their needs are not met in traditional family support groups where the focus is on severe and persistent mental illness.

The first episode of psychosis is a critical time where clinical interactions influence patients' attitudes and beliefs about their illness and treatment. An important treatment goal is for patients to develop attitudes and beliefs that will enhance treatment adherence, as remitted first-episode patients continue to be at high risk of relapse.[25] A psychotic relapse can be a dangerous and costly event, and is associated with risk of aggressive acts to others or to property, as well as suicide attempts in 5–25% and completed suicide in 5–10% in the first few years after a psychotic episode.[25–27] Patients also may lose recently regained psychosocial recovery, with disruption of school, work, friendships, and the ability to live independently. The health care costs of a relapse are often high, especially when hospitalization is necessary.[28] A recently recognized consequence of repeated psychotic relapses is the lengthening of time to respond to antipsychotic medications, and an increased risk of developing chronic, disabling, treatment-resistant symptoms.[29]

New treatment strategies are in development

to meet the special needs of first-episode patients.[30,31] We have developed ACE therapy (adherence-coping-education) with the goal of enhancing adherence and adaptive coping strategies in first-episode patients. ACE therapy is modified from cognitive and behaviorally oriented psychotherapeutic interventions which promote treatment adherence and self-esteem, lift mood, and mitigate self-stigma and severity of delusions in individuals with schizophrenia.[32,33] An educational component promotes the biopsychosocial explanation of illness, for example emphasizing that the illness is biologically based and vulnerable to stress, and that medications are protective against relapse. The protective role of medication to prevent relapse is emphasized, and patients are shown research indicating that up to 80% of individuals with first-episode psychosis who stop their antipsychotic medication experience symptom relapse.[2] It is also important to explore and identify barriers to treatment and help the patient develop strategies to adhere to treatment. For example, a patient who misses several appointments due to forgetfulness may benefit from such strategies as weekly phone contact the morning of the appointment as a reminder, or providing a calendar with prescheduled appointments written on it.

A second component of the therapy is designed to promote healthy adaptation to the illness. Cognitive-behavioral techniques are used to help patients accept and adapt to losses experienced during the first episode (for example, loss of academic term and friendships, stigma) and to accept the possibility of having a chronic vulnerability to future psychotic episodes. In addition, the diagnosis of a psychotic disorder may be an affront to the individual's beliefs about their efficacy, safety, identity, and ability to control their life. Therapy addresses the grieving process and the development of mastery over the psychotic experience, in order for the patient to regain and enhance self-efficacy and control. For example, a patient related a feeling of 'loss of control' over his life since the onset of his first episode. He stated a belief that the only way he could regain control was to stop taking medication, that this would return his life to the way it was before he became ill. He wanted to see if stopping medications would lead to his friends calling him again, his grades improving, and his enjoyment of and desire for usual activities returning. Here, the therapist acknowledged the patient's wish to regain the 'old self' and identified and explored feelings related to his loss (such as anger, guilt, shame, embarrassment, sadness). Alternative strategies to regain control were developed using reframing and normalizing techniques. For example, the therapist and patient developed ideas that 'control' is achieved by knowledge about the illness and the patient's actions as an active participant in treatment. The patient's decision to take medication was reframed as an active strategy that protected against relapse. Reasons for friends 'not calling' were explored and where feasible normalized (for example, the patient had not seen them for a long time), and then strategies to renew friendships developed.

In addition to individual work with patients, we have found group sessions to be very therapeutic. Group interactions reduce feelings of isolation, shame, guilt, and embarrassment commonly associated with recovery from a first psychotic episode. Furthermore, patients are sometimes more responsive to information and advice given by peers than by mental health professionals. For example, if a peer rather than a therapist confronts a patient on their substance use the patient may be less defensive or likely to minimize the issue. A group format can be another venue to address the issues of the meaning and experience of a first episode of psychosis, the impact of the illness on self-concept, and coping strategies to enhance recovery. Rather than leading the group's discussion, the therapist can maximize the supportive aspects of the group by encouraging group members to respond to one another. First-episode patients with good recovery will often assume an active role in the group. The therapist may model supportive behaviors such as engaging less active members, and being sensitive and respectful to others' views and feelings.

When possible, treatment for first-episode patients should include family involvement and education through individual and group sessions. During that first episode of a psychotic illness, family members are also struggling to understand the illness and meaning for their loved ones' future. They may feel a profound sense of loss when their relative is diagnosed, which may include loss of companionship and fulfillment of family roles and of occupational or life accomplishments.[34] Like patients, family members often experience anger, fear, embarrassment, and guilt. While there is a range of issues that may be addressed with families, it is important that the family members identify the critical therapeutic issues and acknowledge the strengths and the adaptive coping strategies that the families have utilized thus far. It is often unhelpful, and may be perceived as patronizing, if the therapist assumes that the family is lacking in skills or assigns the family treatment goals.

Individual work with families will often focus on education and fostering hopeful yet realistic expectations for the future. Common issues raised by family members include how to distinguish normal age-appropriate behaviors from behaviors associated with the illness, and then how to manage difficult behaviors at home. Families may need information and support in order to deal with delusion material. Also, families may need to learn how to monitor symptoms without becoming hypervigilant and infantalizing the ill family member.

Frequently families experience an overwhelming sense of isolation and loneliness, as well as victimization by the same societal stigmatization as patients themselves. Concern about negative misconceptions from others may limit the extent to which families will seek support from others, and when they do seek support, family members may find that their friends, family, clergy and co-workers have a negative rather than empathetic reaction. Offering groups for families is one way to minimize isolation and provide a supportive venue to discuss their family member's illness. The therapist's role will primarily be to provide information and to encourage members to share issues and concerns.

The first episode of psychosis is often a frightening and unanticipated event, but one that can be viewed with hope when identified and treated early. While research is needed to determine the best strategies for first-episode patients, our clinical observations indicate that comprehensive treatment, including pharmacological management and individual, family, and group interventions in the early stages, may enhance recovery. It has been professionally rewarding to work with this population and their families and to witness the marked symptomatic and functional recovery made by many first-episode patients.

Patient–clinician interactions in chronic schizophrenia

Chronic schizophrenia remains a debilitating disorder for many patients, despite the advances in pharmacological treatments. Most patients with chronic symptoms have experienced repeated relapses and have developed persistent residual symptoms resulting in personal and vocational skill deficits. Patients will often have a long history of recurrent episodes and multiple hospitalizations due to noncompliance with medication, treatment-refractory symptoms, and stressful life events.

Most treatment for patients with chronic illness occurs in outpatient and residential settings, with goals of symptom reduction and maximizing social and vocational function. Except for the most disabled patients, inpatient treatment is reserved for acute exacerbations. Inpatient treatment may afford an opportunity to provide education about the illness, and address risk factors for relapse, such as substance use, medication compliance, and stressful environments. Often, with short hospitalizations, there may be only time to identify critical treatment issues, with

most interventions occurring in the outpatient setting. Thus, communication between inpatient and outpatient treatment providers is often a critical component of treatment.

Patients with chronic, long-standing illness have well-developed beliefs and attitudes about their illness and treatment. Patients may bring into treatment 'baggage' from previous negative treatment experiences, such as medication side effects, involuntary commitment, forced medication, seclusion and restraint, and negative encounters with treatment providers in hospital or community settings that may interfere with developing a trusting therapeutic relationship. In contrast, if patients become overly dependent on treatment providers, autonomy may need to be encouraged. Examples range from the patient who skips appointments for months at a time, to the patient who will not make the simplest decision without first contacting his/her clinician.

A flexible therapeutic relationship and the development of common therapeutic goals are critical to establishing a therapeutic alliance. For example, when working with someone with poor insight, or who is resistant to medication, it may be helpful to find some area of need as a therapeutic goal, such as housing, setting up a bank account, or coordinating transportation. Helping the patient with their identified needs can lay the foundation for a therapeutic alliance. As trust and rapport are established, the therapist can then advance notions about the importance of medication and other treatment modalities. The focus on concrete or practical issues can be a tool to engage patients in maintenance treatment. For example, a patient was brought in by her mother for evaluation several weeks pregnant. She had broken off her medication and was demonstrating prodromal symptoms for relapse. She was living on the streets with her boyfriend, was malnourished and receiving no antenatal care. Being very invested in the pregnancy, we first engaged the patient around this issue. We assisted with coordinating and transporting for prenatal visits as well as working on accessing financial and housing resources. We also worked closely with the family to develop a support network for the patient with her pregnancy. Once a therapeutic alliance was established with the patient and her family, we could then further discuss starting a low dose of antipsychotic medication to which the patient agreed.

Psychotherapeutic interventions are targeted towards assisting patients to cope with persistent symptoms though case management, social skills training, cognitive remediation, cognitive-behavioral therapy, psychosocial rehabilitation, and psychopharmacologic maintenance. Treatments may target specific types of residual symptoms and adherence to treatment. In particular, chronic residual positive symptoms resistant to medication may respond to cognitive-behavioral (CBT) interventions.[35-39] As an adjunctive treatment, CBT is used to reduce the severity and functional impact of delusions and hallucinations by exploring the meaning and enhancing coping with the psychotic experiences. Patients will also often develop creative techniques to manage their symptoms (for example, distraction techniques such as listening to music, going for a walk). CBT expands the patient's repertoire of coping behaviors and helps the patient develop other specific techniques to deal with persistent positive symptoms. CBT may also be used to explore the patient's beliefs about medication and maximize treatment adherence.[32]

Cognitive remediation and vocational and social skills training are used primarily to address functional deficits, persistent negative symptoms, and cognitive deficits. Often these services are accessed through psychosocial rehabilitation programs and clubhouses, which may provide programs in vocational rehabilitation, occupational therapy, recreational therapy, and community reintegration. These programs may teach daily and community living skills (such as diet, personal hygiene, cooking, housekeeping, shopping, budgeting). Because patients with chronic symptoms may benefit from a range of services and supports, case management can be a valuable tool

to help access, coordinate, prompt, and monitor use of services. Collateral contacts may often include social services, social security, legal services, law enforcement, treatment providers, landlords, friends and family members.

Whether the therapeutic goals are improved symptom management or functional skills, it is frequently helpful to engage and collaborate with family members. As with the patient, family members have developed beliefs and attitudes about the illness as well as treatment providers. This is particularly true when there has been a long period of time without any education about the illness, hence resulting in the formation of a personalized lay view of it.[40] When patients have been ill for many years, families may have been blamed by health care providers for their loved one's illness. For example, Fromm-Reichman coined the term 'schizophrenogenic mother', theorizing that a mother who was domineering and overprotective induced schizophrenia in her child.[41] It was not until the 1970s that providing psychoeducation and involving families in the treatment process without blaming them was viewed as an effective component of comprehensive treatment for schizophrenia. The importance of family interventions increased with the understanding that high expressed emotion in families increases relapse risk in a member ill with schizophrenia. In addition, the burden placed on the family in providing care for their ill relative can be overwhelming to families and a focus of treatment.[42,43] For example, a series of family surveys indicated that families that provided care for their ill relatives had an increased risk of deterioration in their psychological and physical health; families frequently reported feeling confused, left out of treatment, and ignored by professionals.[44]

When engaging families as members of the 'treatment team', it is often helpful to determine their expectations about their role, and to understand and empathize with any previous negative experiences families may have had with health care providers. A frequent goal of family intervention is to validate family members' experience and view of the illness while providing education about the disorder and developing strategies to help families manage problem behaviors. Family members may have tried multiple strategies over many years to deal with disruptive behaviors, chronic symptoms, and recurrent relapses. Thus clinicians should respect and not judge any limits the family establishes around the care of their ill relative.

Advocacy work focusing on mental illness legislation, policies, and community education can be a means for families to channel their frustration with the system and society's stereotypical views of mental illness. Informing and referring families to organizations such as National Alliance for the Mentally Ill (NAMI) in the USA, and the National Schizophrenia Fellowship (NSF) in the UK as well as local mental health associations can provide access to advocacy opportunities and support services.

Benefits to multiple family groups for relatives of patients exhibiting a chronic course of illness include decreasing rates of relapse.[45–49] Regardless of whether psychoeducation is offered individually or in a group setting, it is important to keep in mind that families possess varying degrees of understanding of the symptomatology of the illness and that the clinician should not make assumptions about families' knowledge and coping skills. Finding opportunities to provide positive feedback for already existing adaptive coping skills (for example, sense of humor, low expressed emotion, direct communication) and strengths can enhance families' confidence and mastery in managing daily levels of stress resulting from caretaking responsibilities. The group therapist may need to emphasize the importance of self-care for family members, and encourage group members to support one another and give permission to engage in social and recreational activities apart from their ill relative. In addition to psychoeducation, families in our groups often benefit from discussions of practical issues such as financial planning (for instance, wills, social security benefits), legal issues (such as, guardianship, power of attorney, commitment laws), and housing (including group homes, family care homes, rest homes, supported apartments, shelters). The therapist should promote an atmosphere where families are acknowledged as 'experts' over their situation, and allow them to share their individual skills and knowledge with each other.

Patient with chronic schizophrenia and their relatives can benefit from a variety of services and supports focusing on alleviating the distress associated with residual symptoms. Comprehensive treatment should involve an individualized approach, selecting the appropriate intervention for each patient from the various services offered, such as individual cognitive-behavioral therapy, case management or psychosocial or vocational rehabilitation.

References

1. Lieberman JA, Pathophysiologic mechanisms in the pathogenesis and clinical course of schizophrenia, *J Clin Psychiatry* (1999) **60(Suppl 12):**9–12.
2. Robinson D, Woerner MG, Alvir JM et al, Predictors of relapse following response from a first episode of schizophrenia or schizoaffective disorder, *Arch Gen Pyschiatry* (1999) **56:**241–7.
3. Frank AD, Gunderson JG, The role of the therapeutic alliance in the treatment of schizophrenia. Relationship to course and outcome, *Arch Gen Psychiatry* (1990) **47:**228–36.
4. Perkins DO, Adherence to antipsychotic medications, *J Clin Psychiatry* (1999) **60(Suppl 21):**25–30.
5. Petrila JP, Sadoff RL, Confidentiality and the family as caregiver, *Hosp Community Psychiatry* (1992) **43:**136–9.
6. Wahl OF, Mental health consumers' experience of stigma, *Schizophr Bull* (1999) **25:**467–78.
7. Link BG, Phelan JC, Bresnahan M et al, Public conceptions of mental illness: labels, causes, dangerousness, and social distance, *Am J Public Health* (1999) **89:**1328–33.
8. Moldin SO, Gottesman II, At issue: genes, experience, and chance in schizophrenia – positioning for the 21st century, *Schizophr Bull* (1997) **23:**547–61.

9. Kendler KS, Diehl SR, The genetics of schizophrenia: a current, genetic-epidemiologic perspective, *Schizophr Bull* (1993) **19**:261–85.

10. Waddington JL, Lane A, Larkin C, O'Callaghan E, The neurodevelopmental basis of schizophrenia: clinical clues from cerebro-craniofacial dysmorphogenesis, and the roots of a lifetime trajectory of disease, *Biol Psychiatry* (1999) **46**:31–9.

11. Yung AR, McGorry PD, The initial prodrome in psychosis: descriptive and qualitative aspects, *Aus N Z J Psychiatry* (1996) **30**:587–99.

12. Yung AR, Phillips LJ, McGorry PD et al, Prediction of psychosis. A step towards indicated prevention of schizophrenia, *Br J Psychiatry Suppl* (1998) **172**:14–20.

13. Gross G, The onset of schizophrenia, *Schizophr Res* (1997) **28**:187–98.

14. Perkins DO, Nieri JM, Bell K, Lieberman J, Factors that contribute to delay in the initial treatment of psychosis. Presented at International Congress on Schizophrenia Research, Santa Fe, New Mexico, 1999 [abstract].

15. Huber G, Gross G, The concept of basic symptoms in schizophrenic and schizoaffective psychoses, *Recenti Prog Med* (1989) **80**:646–52.

16. Phillips LJ, McGorry P, Yung AR et al, The development of preventative interventions for early psychosis: interim findings and directions for the future. International Congress on Schizophrenia Research, Santa Fe, New Mexico, USA, 1999 [abstract].

17. Tanouye E, New weapons in the war on schizophrenia, *Wall Street Journal* (1900) B1–B8. 8–23.

18. Wyatt RJ, Neuroleptics and the natural course of schizophrenia, *Schizophr Bull* (1992) **17**:325–51.

19. McGlashan TH, Duration of untreated psychosis in first-episode schizophrenia: marker or determinant of course? *Biol Psychiatry* (1999) **46**:899–907.

20. Johannessen JO, Early intervention and prevention in schizophrenia – experiences from a study in Stavanger, Norway, *Seishin Shinkeigaku Zasshi* (1998) **100**:511–22.

21. McGorry PD, Edwards J, Mihalopoulos C et al, EPPIC: an evolving system of early detection and optimal management, *Schizophr Bull* (1996) **22**:305–26.

22. Larsen JK, Johannessen JO, Guldberg CA et al, Early intervention programs in first-episode psy-

23. chosis and reduction of duration of untreated psychosis, *Schizophr Res* (2000) **36**:344–5.

23. Lieberman JA, Koreen AR, Chakos M et al, Factors influencing treatment response and outcome of first-episode schizophrenia: implications for understanding the pathophysiology of schizophrenia, *J Clin Psychiatry* (1996) **57(Suppl 9)**:5–9.

24. Robinson DG, Woerner MG, Alvir JM et al, Predictors of treatment response from a first episode of schizophrenia or schizoaffective disorder. *Am J Psychiatry* (1999) **156**:544–9.

25. Wiersma D, Nienhuis FJ, Slooff CJ, Giel R, Natural course of schizophrenic disorders: a 15-year followup of a Dutch incidence cohort, *Schizophr Bull* (1998) **24**:75–85.

26. Robinson GL, Gilbertson AD, Litwack L, The effects of a psychiatric patient education to medication program on post-discharge compliance, *Psychiatr Q* (1986) **58**:113–18.

27. Torrey EF, Violent behavior by individuals with serious mental illness, *Hosp Community Psychiatry* (1994) **45**:653–62.

28. Weiden PJ, Olfson M, Cost of relapse in schizophrenia, *Schizophr Bull* (1995) **21**:419–29.

29. Lieberman JA, Sheitman B, Chakos M et al, The development of treatment resistance in patients with schizophrenia: a clinical and pathophysiologic perspective, *J Clin Psychopharmacol* (1998) **18**:20S–24S.

30. Jackson H, McGorry P, Edwards J et al, Cognitively-oriented psychotherapy for early psychosis (COPE). Preliminary results, *Br J Psychiatry Suppl* (1998) **172**:93–100.

31. Larsen TK, Johannessen JO, Opjordsmoen S, First-episode schizophrenia with long duration of untreated psychosis. Pathways to care, *Br J Pychiatry Suppl* (1998) **172**:45–52.

32. Kemo R, Kirov G, Everitt B et al, Randomised controlled trial of compliance therapy. 18-month follow-up, *Br J Psychiatry* (1998) **172**:413–19.

33. Norman RM, Townsend LA, Cognitive-behavioural therapy for psychosis: a status report, *Can J Psychiatry* (1999) **44**:245–52.

34. Solomon P, Draine J, Examination of grief among family members of individuals with serious and persistent mental illness, *Psychiatr Q* (1996) **67**:221–34.

35. Haddock G, Morrison AP, Hopkins R et al, Indi-

vidual cognitive-behavioural interventions in early psychosis, *Br J Psychiatry Suppl* (1998) **172:**101–6.

36. Tarrier N, Sharpe L, Beckett R et al, A trial of two cognitive behavioural methods of treating drug-resistant residual psychotic symptoms in schizophrenic patients. II. Treatment-specific changes in coping and problem-solving skills, *Soc Psychiatry Psychiatr Epidemiol* (1993) **28:**5–10.

37. Chadwick P, Birchwood M, The omnipotence of voices. A cognitive approach to auditory hallucinations, *Br J Psychiatry* (1994) **164:**190–201.

38. Kingdon D, Turkington D, John C, Cognitive behaviour therapy of schizophrenia. The amenability of delusions and hallucinations to reasoning [editorial] *Br J Psychiatry* (1994) **164:**581–7.

39. Freeman D, Garety P, Fowler D et al, The London–East Anglia randomized controlled trial of cognitive-behaviour therapy for psychosis. IV: Self-esteem and persecutory delusions, *Br J Clin Psychol* (1998) **37:**415–30.

40. Tarrier N, Barrowclough C, Providing information to relatives about schizophrenia: some comments, *Br J Psychiatry* (1986) **149:**458–63.

41. Fromm-Reichman F, Notes on the development of treatment of schizophrenics by psychoanalytic psychotherapy, *Psychiatry* (2000) **11:**263–73.

42. Penn DL, Mueser KT, Research update on the psychosocial treatment of schizophrenia, *Am J Psychiatry* (1996) **153:**607–17.

43. Steinglass P, Psychoeducational family therapy for schizophrenia: a review essay, *Psychiatry* (1987) **50:**14–23.

44. Hatfield AB, Consumer issues in mental illness, *New Dir Ment Health Serv* (1987) **34:**35–42.

45. Goldstein MJ, Psychoeducational and family therapy in relapse prevention, *Acta Psychiatr Scand Suppl* (1994) **382:**54–7.

46. Leff J, Berkowitz R, Shavit N et al, A trial of family therapy v. a relatives group for schizophrenia, *Br J Psychiatry* (1989) **164:**58–66.

47. Hogarty GE, Anderson CM, Medication, family psychoeducation, and social skills training: first year relapse results of a controlled study, *Psychopharmacol Bull* (1986) **22:**860–2.

48. Falloon IR, McGill CW, Boyd JL, Pederson J, Family management in the prevention of morbidity of schizophrenia: social outcome of a two-year longitudinal study, *Psychol Med* (1987) **17:**59–66.

49. McFarlane WR, Lukens E, Link B et al, Multiple-family groups and psychoeducation in the treatment of schizophrenia, *Arch Gen Psychiatry* (1995) **52:**679–87.

8

Case Management of Patients with Schizophrenia

Chiara Samele and Robin M Murray

Contents • Development of case management • Models of case management • Efficacy of case management • Factors influencing outcome • How long should case management go on for? • Methodological problems with case management evaluations • Financial cost of case management and ACT • Are case management and ACT worth implementing?

This chapter provides an overview of case management and assertive outreach treatment. It examines the development and implementation of case management, the models employed, its efficacy, the methodological problems involved in its assessment, and the benefits.

Development of case management

Case management arose, following the deinstitutionalization of the mentally ill and the shift towards community care, in response to the fragmentation of psychiatric care and the need to coordinate services.[1] Methods of bringing together the components of care were developed both in the United States, in federally funded initiatives such as the Community Support Program,[2] and in Britain. The latter mainly followed the House of Commons Social Services Committee's report[3] on community care, which encouraged the use of keyworkers, and a clear package of care for discharged patients.

Intagliata[4] identified some of the main components of case management, including assessment of needs, planning comprehensive services, arranging delivery of services, monitoring and assessing those services, and evaluation and follow-up; a chief aim was 'to enhance the continuity of care and its accessibility, accountability

and efficiency'. Despite this clarity of aim, the delivery of case management has varied enormously and this has led to confusion and contradictory approaches.[5]

Holloway[6] identified two main models of case management – service brokerage case management and clinical case management. In the brokerage model, the case manager, often an office-based administrator with no health or social service background, acts as an enabler, systems coordinator, and a broker of services. The brokerage model was seen as limited in value to patients with severe mental illness;[6] indeed, this was confirmed in controlled studies.[7,8] Clinical case management, on the other hand, took on all aspects of the patients' physical and social environment, including housing, psychiatric treatment, general health care, welfare entitlements, transportation, families and social networks.[9] This latter model has become the preferred approach in the United States where all states are required to show substantial progress towards the provision of case management services to all adults with severe mental illness.[10]

Models of case management

A number of clinical case management models have emerged. Assertive community treatment

(ACT), first developed by Stein and Test,[11] includes assertive outreach, teaching and assistance in daily living skills, 24-hour cover 7 days a week, assistance in finding work, and a focus on patients' strengths. The psychosocial rehabilitation model[12] comprises rehabilitation assessment and planning, coordinating and linking patients with community services, monitoring progress, and advocacy. The strengths model[13] focuses on patients' strengths and self determination, the case manager/patient relationship, and aggressive outreach. This model has been described as providing the support and skills needed to identify, and aim for, realistic personal goals rather than provide treatment for illness.[14] Thornicroft[15] lists 12 axes defining the precise characteristics of case management in terms of its practice: individual/team case management, direct care/brokerage, intensity of interventions, degree of budgetary control, health/social service function, status of case manager, specialization of case manager, staff:patient ratio, patient participation, point of contact, level of intervention, and target population. Case management teams are often interdisciplinary, usually headed by a consultant psychiatrist, consisting largely of psychiatric nurses, occupational therapists, a psychologist, and a psychiatric social worker, although this can vary.

Some degree of overlap exists between the different case management models. For example, ACT and case management share the same goals: (a) maintain contact with patients, (b) reduce the number and duration of hospital admissions, and (c) improve clinical and social outcome. The case manager's task is to: (a) assess the patients' needs, (b) develop a care plan, (c) arrange suitable care, (d) monitor the quality of care provided, and (e) maintain contact with the patient.[16] ACT goes a step further to: (f) provide rather than arrange care, (g) apply assertive outreach, (h) focus on medication compliance, and (i) offer emergency cover.

Efficacy of case management

Many studies on case management have been conducted in inner city settings. The majority of these have randomly allocated patients to one of two treatment groups, for example, intensive case management vs standard/generic care, or ACT vs standard/generic care. Evaluating the efficacy of case management has been measured using clinical outcome (that is, improvement in symptoms), and social outcome (quality of life). The most common outcome measure, however, is hospital utilization – both frequency and duration of stay. Several reviews of the outcome of case management practices have been published;[17–19] perhaps the most comprehensive is that by Marshall et al.[17] To qualify, studies had to be randomized control trials, have compared case management (or care management rather than ACT) to standard community care, and have included people with severe mental disorder between the ages of 18 and 65.

Impact on hospital utilization

Some studies using intensive case management have shown a significant reduction in hospital utilization.[8,20,21] However, in Marshall et al's review,[17] the numbers admitted to psychiatric hospital in the case management group approximately doubled (OR 1.84, 99%CI 1.33–2.57, $n = 1300$). The most impressive evidence for the reduction of hospital admissions and duration of stay is found with the ACT model when compared to standard care.[11,22,23] This is confirmed in Marshall et al's review,[17] where people allocated ACT were less likely to be admitted to hospital (OR 0.59, 99%CI 0.41–0.85) and spent less time in hospital.

Clinical and social outcome

Not all case management studies report clinical and social outcomes as part of their evaluation. Of the case management studies which included assessments of clinical symptoms, many found no differences between the case management group and controls.[24–26] Even with ACT, relatively few studies report a statistically significant decrease in symptomatology.[11,27] Similarly, very few studies, using case management or ACT, have shown an improvement in overall functioning and social performance.[28–30] Marshall et al[17] conclude that it appears unlikely that case management produces substantial improvement in clinical or social outcome, although ACT did show significant advantages over standard care in accommodation status and employment.

Quality of life and patient satisfaction

The majority of case management studies examining outcome in terms of quality of life report no significant difference between groups;[24,25,31] however some ACT studies report a significant improvement in quality of life.[11,32] Holloway and Carson's[25] study showed greater patient satisfaction with intensive case management compared to standard care. Marks et al's study[22] demonstrated similar significant differences in patient satisfaction for those who received ACT. It is difficult, however, to gain an overall idea of this patient satisfaction with intensive case management and ACT, since few studies have included this assessment.

Service engagement and compliance with medication

Case management appears to increase the number of people remaining in contact with services.[17] Approximately one extra person remained in contact with services for every 15 people receiving case management. Patients receiving ACT were also more likely to remain in contact with services compared to those receiving standard care. Holloway and Carson's study[25] also found a significant gain in service engagement among patients considered 'hard to treat' who received case management. Increased compliance with medication has been shown with patients receiving ACT,[11,20] although many studies do not report this.

Factors influencing outcome

Caseload size

For clinical case management to be effective, a small caseload appears to be necessary; one case manager per 10–15 patients is considered the optimal ratio.[33] Where caseloads are over 15 patients, the case manager becomes increasingly reactive (to crises) rather than proactive in the care of patients. Case managers with heavy loads are unable fully to assess patients' needs, and resort to doing things for the patient, in an effort to save time, rather than assisting them to become more independent.[34,35] Of the four main case management studies conducted in the United Kingdom[24,34,36,37] in which small caseload size was the central component, only one showed reduced hospital utilization.[36] A small caseload allowed the case manager to organize early discharge from hospital, thereby reducing costs.[36] Improved compliance with medication was also associated with small caseload in three of the studies.[34,36,37] Burns et al,[24] who carried out a large multi-center trial in the United Kingdom, failed to find any significant differences in clinical or social outcome variables, including days in hospital, even though caseload size for case managers was limited to between 10 and 15 patients.

Patients in case management studies

An overview by Clark and Fox[38] concluded that little is known about which patients benefit most from the different types of case management. There remains a need to identify which patients respond to intensive case management and those whose outcome is independent of it.[34] Recent studies have attempted to address this. For example, the UK700 trial yielded no significant benefit of intensive case management for patients of African-Caribbean origin.[24] However, in the same trial, Tyrer et al[39] examined the outcome of intensive case management of those patients who had psychotic disorder and borderline learning disability. Those comorbid patients who received intensive case management spent significantly fewer days in hospital than those receiving standard case management (mean 47.2 vs 104.8, $p = 0.003$) and had a reduced number of admissions (mean 0.55 vs 1.49, $p = 0.004$). Thus intensive case management may be especially useful for psychotic patients with learning disability (who may have particular difficulties in living in the community).

Holloway and Carson[25] found better engagement with services and greater patient satisfaction in patients considered 'hard to treat' who received intensive case management. Increasingly, specific groups of patients who suffer from severe comorbid mental illness and substance abuse,[40] or the homeless mentally ill,[41] have been targeted to receive ACT. However, the value of this is not yet clear.

Number of case manager contacts

The amount of contact with services differs enormously depending on the case management model applied. The minimum number of contacts can range from one or two times per week for some case management models[28] to daily for others.[42] Does the amount of case manager contact have any impact on outcome? This has been relatively underexplored in the case management literature. Dietzen and Bond[43] examined patterns of service use and outcome in seven programmes using the ACT model with frequently hospitalized patients. Four of the programmes with moderate to high levels of service intensity (an average of 11 contacts per patient per month) had a moderate or substantial impact in reducing days in hospital. The remaining three programmes with moderate to low service intensities (an average of 6.3 contacts per client per month) had minimal impact on hospital use. However, for the combined sample ($n = 155$ patients), there was no linear correlation between hospital use and the frequency of service either for the total contacts or for type of contact. In the UK700 trial, there was no significant impact on patients receiving intensive case management in terms of hospital use, or clinical and social outcome, despite the significantly greater number of contacts.[24]

Appropriate support services

In areas where resources are poor, the benefit of case managers linking patients to services is severely limited.[44] The case manager is more likely to be effective if local resources are available but poorly accessed.[10] In situations where local resources are easily accessed then case management may make a small contribution to improved outcome. Successful outcome has been associated with use of vocational services and day care facilities.

How long should case management go on for?

Where case management has been shown to be beneficial, this is not usually obvious until at least 1 year has passed.[35] Many case management and ACT studies have gone on for longer, often 2 years, and included follow-up assessments at various stages, either 6-monthly or yearly intervals, during the study period. Do the benefits of case management/ACT persist over time? One of the few longitudinal studies to address this question was by Borland et al,[21] who evaluated 5 years of continuous intensive case management in 72 patients with schizophrenia or bipolar disorder. Days in hospital were reduced by 75%, and the use of emergency services steadily decreased over the 5-year period. This, however, was offset by a 193% increase in days in structured residential care in the community. Patients' level of functioning remained the same over the 5-year period. Conversely, Marks et al[22] found significant improvements in terms of reduced days in hospital, improved symptomatology, and patients' and relatives' satisfaction at 20 months of ACT. At 30–45 months, these gains were lost and only patients' and relatives' greater satisfaction with ACT remained.[45] One of the main reasons given for the loss of gains was the attenuation of the quality of ACT and the low morale experienced by the ACT team in the latter phase of the study.

Methodological problems with case management evaluations

The most common methodological shortcoming suffered by studies of case management is small sample size; in some instances numbers within groups have been as low as 14.[20] Most case management studies have between 35 and 100 patients per group, resulting in low statistical power.[25,28,32]

Comparisons between studies have proved difficult given the definitional problems surrounding case management and the lack of description of the case management model employed.[46]

The various methodological problems contribute to the inconsistent findings of case management studies. Consequently, it is difficult to form any definitive conclusions concerning the potential benefits of case management on hospital utilization and clinical and social outcomes. Identifying the ingredients for a successful case management practice is not altogether clear either. Some suggestions point to: (a) a single point of accountability (that is, a keyworker), (b) the case manager/patient relationship and continuity of care, (c) compliance with medication, (d) good multidisciplinary team, (e) a psychiatrist integrated to the team, and (f) applying the ACT model.[44]

Financial cost of case management and ACT

There are also difficulties in drawing firm conclusions about the cost of case management and ACT. These relate to whether costs of inpatient care, health care costs or total costs are considered. In their economic evaluation of case management, Gray et al[47] found that costs were lower in the treatment group, but the difference was not significant. Some studies report increased cost, and others report a decrease in costs, but only when increased income through higher rates of employment is taken into account.[11]

Are case management and ACT worth implementing?

The evidence concerning the beneficial effects of case management is mixed. Some professionals favor the practice of case management as a well-structured approach to community care for people with severe mental illness. Certainly, there exists evidence that case management, and in particular ACT, encourages and enhances service engagement and compliance with medication. Factors such as continuity of care and better patient/health professional relationships are very important to achieve. Service interventions alone, however intensive, may not make any real impact in the long term.

The idea that case management or ACT should be introduced on the basis that it will be more cost effective or introduce savings is unwarranted. The costs may be higher, not just financially, but also in terms of staff hours in order to provide, for example, 24-hour cover, 7 days a week.

When implementing case management there are several factors to consider. The most important is the choice of case management model. How this decision is made depends on the service setting, the available resources, the structure of services, the motivation of staff, and the training and support that can be made available to them. It is important to consider the reasons for implementing a case management service (for example, whether the primary aim is to target special groups of patients) and the outcome to be achieved. Relying simply on reduced caseload for case managers, although this is a valuable first step, may not be enough to generate improvements. More may be required in terms of specific training and additional professional input, such as an out of hours service. In some cases this may not be feasible due to cost or the availability of other emergency services. However, if patients have to resort to emergency services outside the case management setup, this may be disruptive to their continuity of care.

References

1. Rössler W, Löffler W, Fätkenheuer B et al, Case management for schizophrenic patients at risk for rehospitalization: a case control study, *Eur Arch Psychiatry Clin Neurosci* (1995) **246**:29–36.

2. Tessler R, Goldman H, *The Chronic Mentally Ill: Assessing The Community Support Program* (Ballinger: Cambridge, MA, 1982).

3. House of Commons Social Services Committee, Second report. Session 1984–85. Community care (HMSO: London, 1985).

4. Intagliata J, Improving the quality of community care for the chronically mentally disabled: the role of case management, *Schizophr Bull* (1982) **8**:655–74.

5. Bachrach L, Case management: towards a shared definition, *Hosp Community Psychiatry* (1989) **40**:883–4.

6. Holloway F, Case management for the mentally ill: looking at the evidence, *Int J Soc Psychiatry* (1991) **37**:2–13.

7. Franklin JL, Solovitz B, Mason M et al, An evaluation of care management, *Am J Public Health* (1987) **77**:674–8.

8. Curtis JL, Millman EJ, Struening E et al, Effect of case management on rehospitalization and utilization of ambulatory care services, *Hosp Community Psychiatry* (1992) **43**:895–9.

9. Kanter J, Clinical case management: definition, principles, components, *Hosp Community Psychiatry* (1989) **40**:361–8.

10. Solomon P, The efficacy of case management services for severely mentally disabled clients, *Community Health J* (1992) **28**:163–80.

11. Stein LI, Test MA, Alternative to mental hospital treatment. I. Conceptual model, treatment program, and clinical evaluation, *Arch Gen Psychiatry* (1980) **37**:392–7.

12. Goering PN, Wasylenki DA, Farkas M et al, What difference does case management make? *Hosp Community Psychiatry* (1988) **39**:272–6.

13. Modrcin M, Rapp CA, Poertner J, The evaluation of case management services for the chronically mentally ill, *Evaluation and Programme Planning* (1988) **11**:307–14.

14. Rapp CA, Wintersteen R, The strengths model of case management: results from 12 demonstrations, *Psychosoc Rehabil J* (1989) **13**:23–32.

15. Thornicroft G, The concept of case management for long term mental illness, *Int Rev Psychiatry* (1991) **3**:125–32.

16. Holloway F, Home treatment as an alternative to acute psychiatric inpatient admission: a discussion. In: *Community Psychiatry in Action: Analysis and Prospects* (Cambridge University Press: Cambridge, 1995) 85–96.

17. Marshall M, Gray A, Lockwood A et al, Case management for people with severe mental disorders (Cochrane Review). In: *The Cochrane Library, Issue 3* (Update Software: Oxford, 1998).

18. Burns BL, Santos AB, Assertive community treatment: an update of randomized trials, *Psychiatr Serv* (1995) **46**:669–75.

19. Holloway F, Oliver N, Collins E et al, Case management: a critical review of the outcome literature, *European Psychiatry* (1995) **10**:113–28.

20. Bush CT, Lanford MW, Rosen P et al, Operation Outreach: intensive case management for severely psychiatrically disabled adults, *Hosp Community Psychiatry* (1990) **41**:647–9.

21. Borland A, McRae J, Lycan C, Outcomes of 5 years of continuous intensive case management, *Hosp Community Psychiatry* (1989) **40**:369–76.

22. Marks IM, Connolly J, Muijen M et al, Home-based versus hospital-based care for people with serious mental illness, *Br J Psychiatry* (1994) **165**:179–94.

23. Wright RG, Heiman JR, Shupe J *et al*, Defining and measuring stabilization of patients during 4 years of intensive community support, *Am J Psychiatry* (1989) **146**:1293–8.

24. Burns T, Creed F, Fahy T et al, Intensive versus standard case management for severe psychotic illness: a randomised trial, *Lancet* (1999) **353**:2185–9

25. Holloway F, Carson J, Intensive case management for the severely mentally ill. Controlled trial, *Br J Psychiatry* (1998) **172**:19–32.

26. McClary S, Lubin B, Evans C, Evaluation of a community treatment program for young adult schizophrenics, *J Clin Psychology* (1989) **45**:806–8.

27. Hoult J, Reynolds I, Charbonneay-Powis M et al, Psychiatric hospital *versus* community treatment: the results of a randomised trial, *Aust N Z J Psychiatry* (1983) **17**:160–7.

28. Issakidis C, Sanderson K, Teesson M et al, Intensive case management in Australia: a randomized

controlled trial, *Acta Psychiatr Scand* (1999) **99:**360–7.

29. Dincin J, Wasmer D, Witheridge TF et al, Impact of assertive community treatment on the use of State Hospital inpatient bed-days, *Hosp Community Psychiatry* (1993) **44:**833–8.

30. Arana JD, Hastings B, Herron E, Continuous care teams in intensive outpatient treatment of chronic mentally ill patients, *Hosp Community Psychiatry* (1991) **42:**503–7.

31. Bond GR, Miller LD, Krumweid RD et al, Assertive case management in three CMHCs: a controlled study, *Hosp Community Psychiatry* (1988) **39:**411–18.

32. Lafave HG, de Souza HR, Gerber GJ, Assertive community treatment of severe mental illness: a Canadian experience, *Psychiatr Serv* (1996) **47:**757–9.

33. Rubin A, Is case management effective for people with serious mental illness? A research review, *Health Soc Work* (1992) **17:**138–50.

34. Muijen M, Cooney M, Strathdee G et al, Community psychiatric nurse teams: intensive support versus generic care, *Br J Psychiatry* (1994) **165:**211–17.

35. Baker F, Intagliata J, Case management. In: Liberman RP, ed, *Handbook of Psychiatric Rehabilitation* (Macmillan: London, 1992).

36. Muijen M, Marks I, Connolly J et al, Home based care and standard hospital care for patients with severe mental illness, *BMJ* (1992) **304:**749–54.

37. Ryan P, Ford R, Clifford P, *Case Management and Community Care* (Sainsbury Centre for Mental Health: London, 1991).

38. Clark RE, Fox T, A framework for evaluating the economic impact of case management, *Hosp Community Psychiatry* (1993) **44:**469–73.

39. Tyrer P, Hassiotis A, Ukoumunne O et al, Intensive case management for psychotic patients with borderline intelligence, *Lancet* (1999) **354:**999–1000.

40. Wingerson D, Ries RK, Assertive community treatment for patients with chronic and severe mental illness who abuse drugs, *J Psychoactive Drugs* (1999) **31:**13–18.

41. Calsyn RJ, Morse GA, Klinkenberg WD et al, The impact of assertive community treatment on the social relationships of people who are homeless and mentally ill, *Community Ment Health J* (1998) **34:**579–93.

42. Thornicroft G, Breakey WR, The COSTAR Programme. 1: Improving social networks of the long-term mentally ill, *Br J Psychiatry* (1991) **159:**245–9.

43. Dietzen LL, Bond GR, Relationship between case manager contact and outcome for frequently hospitalized psychiatric clients, *Hosp Community Psychiatry* (1993) **44:**839–43.

44. UK700 Group, Comparison of intensive and standard case management for patients with psychosis. Rationale of the trial, *Br J Psychiatry* (1999) **174:**74–8.

45. Audini B, Marks IM, Lawrence RE et al, Home-based versus outpatient/in-patient care for people with serious mental illness. Phase II of a controlled study, *Br J Psychiatry* (1994) **165:**204–10.

46. Burns T, Case management, care management and care programming, *Br J Psychiatry* (1997) **170:**393–5.

47. Gray AM, Marshall M, Lockwood A et al, Problems in conducting economic evaluations alongside clinical trials. Lessons from a study of case management for people with mental disorders, *Br J Psychiatry* (1997) **170:**47–52.

9

Childhood- and Adolescent-onset Schizophrenia

Marianne Wudarsky, Marge Lenane and Judith L Rapoport

Contents • Introduction • Pharmacologic treatment of early-onset schizophrenia • Nondrug intervention

Introduction

Childhood onset schizophrenia (COS) is a rare, clinically severe form of schizophrenia.[1] Like other early-onset forms of multifactorial diseases (for example, juvenile onset diabetes mellitus, juvenile rheumatoid arthritis), childhood-onset schizophrenia is associated with greater disease severity than adult-onset schizophrenia[2] and may be more heritable.[3]

Recent work has shown that childhood onset schizophrenia is associated with disrupted cognitive, linguistic and social development well before the appearance of frank psychotic symptoms.[4] In addition, intellectual deterioration and brain morphologic changes may progress after psychosis onset.[5] This disruption of multiple developmental domains signals the important opportunity these patients present for examining genetic and neurodevelopmental hypotheses of schizophrenia.

Adolescent onset is considerably more common. Here too, however, as in childhood onset, there is less information about treatment than for adult-onset cases. This chapter summarizes the treatment of schizophrenia in childhood and adolescence. Because of the paucity of the data, some open trials and descriptive data have been included.

Pharmacologic treatment of early-onset schizophrenia

Typical antipsychotics

Since 1976, only three double-blind drug studies of antipsychotic medication efficacy for childhood/adolescent schizophrenia have been published.[6-9] The collective study populations number 120 for double-blind trials of typical and atypical agents combined. Table 9.1 summarizes controlled trials of typical antipsychotics.

The first placebo-controlled study involving schizophrenic adolescents was that of Pool et al in 1976.[6] This randomized, placebo-controlled, double-blind 4-week parallel trial compared haloperidol, loxapine and placebo treatments of 75 adolescent in-patients. The Brief Psychiatric Rating Score (BPRS) ratings showed improvement from baseline for all three groups at week 4, but treatment effects, if any, were weak. Haloperidol-treated subjects showed only a trend toward improved hallucinatory behavior over the placebo group. The loxapine group showed a significant difference for hallucinatory behavior over placebo only at week 4. Nevertheless, this study stands as a bellwether heralding the efficacy of antipsychotics for younger affected individuals and acknowledges the importance of separate studies for pediatric groups.

Table 9.1 Drug treatment studies of child and adolescent schizophrenia: typical antipsychotics.

Author/year	Number of pts and diagnosis	Age (mean and range)	Dose (mean mg/d; range)	Design	Outcome
Controlled trials					
Pool et al 1976[6]	75; schizophrenia continuous or episodic	15.65 13–18	Haloperidol 9.8 mg/d 2–16 mg/d Loxitane 87.5 mg/d 10–200 mg/d	Randomized, placebo-controlled, double-blind 4-week parallel group	No drug/placebo difference Extra Pyramidal Syndrome (EPS): 75%; sedation: 52%–80% in treatment group; most ill had greatest improvement
Realmuto 1984[6a]	21; schizophrenia	15.6 11.9–18.9	Thiothixene 16.2 mg 4.8–42.6 mg/d Thioridazine 178 mg 91–228 mg/d	Randomized, single-blind, 4- to 6-week parallel group; no placebo	Higher baseline BPRS than adults; mean BPRS decreased by 18; ~50% 'improved' by Clinical Global Impression (CGI); no treatment differences
Spencer et al 1992[7] and 1994[10] Spencer and Campbell, 1994[8]	24; schizophrenia	8.78 5.5–11.75	Haloperidol 1.80 mg/d 0.5–3.5 mg/d	Placebo-controlled, double-blind, cross-over; 4-week treatment and 4-week placebo	Significant BPRS-C and CGI change; (p = 0.003 and 0.001, respectively); 75% w/sedation; 25% w/EPS; 12.5% w/dystonia

Most intriguing is the dramatic benefit of haloperidol demonstrated by the New York University (NYU) studies compared with the Pool study. Spencer et al[7,10] and Spencer and Campbell[8] carried out a double-blind, 8-week, placebo-controlled, crossover trial of haloperidol. A series of reports describe a final study group of 24 schizophrenic children. The optimal haloperidol dose was low (mean: 1.80 mg/day). Haloperidol treatment was superior to placebo for Clinical Global Impression (CGI) Severity of Illness, CGI Global Improvement and four of eight Child Psychiatric Rating Scale (CPRS) items: ideas of reference, persecutory ideation, other thinking disorders and hallucinations. None receiving placebo improved. The best responders, as measured by the BPRS-C Total Pathology Score, were those older subjects who had a later onset of symptoms and higher IQ.[8,10] This is an important study as there will still be a need for haloperidol for pediatric cases, given the complication of weight gain experienced by some cases on atypical antipsychotics (see below). Moreover the efficacy of very low doses suggests that clinical practice may have utilized higher doses than needed.

Atypical antipsychotics
Open case series
More than 20 years after the European demonstration of clozapine's antipsychotic activity without extrapyramidal side effects,[11] the drug was shown to be a successful intervention in chronic neuroleptic resistant adults, with virtually no parkinsonian or dystonic side effects (see this volume, Chapter 4). Interest in its use for selected pediatric patients was natural. In spite of the risk for granulocytopenia (1.5–2.0%[12]) and agranulocytosis (0.8%[13]), and dose-dependent seizure incidence in adult patients (1–5%[14]), the option of real therapeutic benefit to a severely ill, treatment-refractory pediatric population or patients with high risk of tardive dyskinesia was compelling.

Following earlier chart review reports of adolescents who also benefited from clozapine,[15] a series of case reports[16–18] indicated promising results (see Table 9.2). As shown, EEG changes were prominent, but in general, side effects resembled those for adults.

Open trials
A systematic open trial of clozapine was reported for 11 treatment-refractory adolescents with childhood-onset schizophrenia,[19] comparing its therapeutic efficacy to prior haloperidol treatment. More than half of these patients improved on clozapine relative to haloperidol. The most pronounced side effect was weight gain (mean 15.4 pounds) during 6-week clozapine treatment. Three other systematic open trials and one retrospective review of clozapine treatment of children and adolescents numbering a total of 64 patients reported impressive treatment response.[18,20–22] Again, rates of EEG abnormalities in two studies are high.[18,22] Incidence of abnormal EEG changes in adults treated with clozapine have been reported to be between 64% and 83%.[23–25] Other major side effects were sedation and sialorrhea.

Because of clozapine's toxicity, studies of newer serotonin/dopamine antagonists are of particular importance for pediatric groups. To date, there have been two systematic open trials of risperidone, both in schizophrenic adolescents[26,27] most of whom had been on typical antipsychotics. Armenteros et al[27] reported that 67% of patients who completed the study showed at least a 20% reduction in total score Positive and Negative Syndrome Scale for Schizophrenia (PANSS) on a mean dose of 6.6 mg/day, with some response seen during the first week of treatment. This result parallels those of adult studies,[28,29] but additional trials are needed to verify possible unique response kinetics of risperidone in children.

In the Armenteros study,[27] 80% of adolescents experienced mild, transient somnolence. In total, 60% had either acute dystonia, Extra Pyramidal Syndrome (EPS) requiring continuous treatment with benztropine or orofacial dyskinesia on a mean dose of 6.6 mg/day. Additionally, 8 of 10

Table 9.2 Drug treatment studies of child and adolescent schizophrenia: atypical antipsychotics.

Author/year	Number of pts and diagnosis	Age (mean and range)	Dose (mean mg/d; range)	Design	Outcome
Open case series					
Seifen and Remschmidt 1986[15]	21; schizophrenia nonresponders	18.1 12–18	Clozapine 450 mg 225–800 mg	Retrospective chart review	52% 'marked improvement'; 33% EEG changes; 50% leukopenia; fatigue, dizziness, low BP, sialorrhea
Birmaher et al 1992[16]	3; schizophrenia nonresponders	17 17–18	Clozapine 333 mg 100–400 mg	Case studies	All improved in positive and negative symptoms; 2 with transient decrease in WBC
Blanz and Schmidt 1993[17]	53/57 schizophrenia nonresponders	16.8 10–21	Clozapine 285 mg 75–800 mg	Case studies	67% 'significantly improved'; 16% with tremor, akathisia, EPS; 51% with sedation; 35% – sialorrhea; 35% – low BP; 55% – EEG changes
Remschmidt et al 1994[18]	36; schizophrenia nonresponders	14–22	Clozapine 330 mg 50–800 mg	Retrospective chart review	75% improved; positive symptoms more responsive than negative; 44% with EEG changes; 5.5% discontinued due to leukopenia
Open trials					
Turetz et al 1997[22]	11; schizophrenia nonresponders	11.3 9–13	Clozapine 227 mg 193–262 mg	Open clozapine 16 weeks	>50% improvement in CGI, BPRS, PANSS; 90% with sialorrhea and sedation; 82% with EEG changes; 27% with agitation
Quintana and Keshivan 1995[26]	4; schizophrenia 3 nonresponders 1 treatment naïve	14.5 12–17	Risperidone 4.5 mg 4–5 mg	Open risperidone 6 months	3/4 had >40% decrease in BPRS; negative symptoms more responsive than positive; no Extra Pyramidal Syndrome (EPS) or Tardive Dyskinesia (TD)
Armenteros et al 1997[27]	10: schizophrenia 7 nonresponders and 3 medication naïve	15.1 12–18	Risperidone 6.6 mg 4–10 mg	Open risperidone 6 weeks	75% with at least a 20% decrease in PANSS; 50%: dystonia, EPS, dyskinesia

Table 9.2 *continued*

Author/year	Number of pts and diagnosis	Age (mean and range)	Dose (mean mg/d; range)	Design	Outcome
Kumra et al 1998[38]	23; schizophrenia nonresponders 8 treatment olanzapine 15 treatment clozapine	13.6 15.2	Olanzapine 17.5 mg 15–19 mg Clozapine 317 mg 117–464 mg	Open olanzapine – 8 weeks Open clozapine – 6 weeks	25% 'drug responsive' in olanzapine treatment group; 50% 'drug responsive' in clozapine treatment group
Frazier et al 1994[19]	11; schizophrenia nonresponders	14 12–17	Clozapine 370 mg 125–825 mg	Open trials of clozapine or haloperidol	30% improvement in BPRS in 56% on clozapine vs haloperidol; 82% on clozapine with BPRS >30% improved; side effects: sedation, sialorrhea, weight gain mean 15.4 lb in 6 weeks
Levkovitch et al 1994[20]	13; schizophrenia	16.6	Clozapine 240 mg	Open trials	77% improved significantly with a decline in BPRS by 50% after 2 mos of treatment; side effects: sedation, sialorrhea, low BP and fever
Kowatch et al 1995[21]	4/10 schizophrenia nonresponders 5/10 bipolar DO and 1/10 psychotic DO NOS	7.2 6–8	Clozapine 137.5 mg 75–225 mg	Open trials	75% with marked improvement on CGI; 25% with moderate improvement; 0% EPS; 75% sialorrhea; 100% with weight gain
Double-blind					
Kumra et al 1996[9]	21; schizophrenia nonresponders	14 12–16	Clozapine 240 mg 25–525 mg Halperidol 16 mg 7–27 mg	Randomized, double-blind 6-week parallel comparison	Clozapine treatment superior to halperidol re: Scale for the Assessment of Negative Symptoms (SANS) ($p < 0.01$), Scale for the Assessment of Positive Symptoms (SAPS) ($p < 0.01$) and BPRS ($p < 0.05$); 3/21 with seizures; 3/21 with EEG changes; 5/21 with Absolute Neutrophil Count (ANC) <1500 cc/mm^3

patients experienced weight gain with a substantial mean increase of 4.85 kg over 6 weeks. Nutritional counseling was instituted in the Armenteros study after the increase was observed but follow-up data concerning weight control were not reported.

There is some evidence that weight may be controllable. In a study of children with PTSD, weight gain on risperidone was held to 2.2 kg after a 16-week treatment trial.[30] A diet consisting of low-glycemic carbohydrates (to decrease insulin levels and glycogen synthesis) along with control of total caloric intake was instituted. The mechanism of the weight gain seen in children taking atypicals is unknown; clinically it appears to be an even more serious concern than for adults. The Kumra et al 1997[31] chart review reported hepatotoxicity in 2 of 13 patients treated with risperidone. Elevated liver transaminases and fatty infiltration of the liver were thought to be secondary to the onset of obesity in these patients. The authors emphasized the importance of obtaining baseline liver function tests and monitoring liver transaminases in those pediatric patients treated with risperidone. Kelly et al,[32] in the only known study comparing weight gain in adolescents taking conventional antipsychotics, risperidone and no medication, showed retrospectively that the risperidone-treated group gained significantly more body mass than did those taking conventional antipsychotics ($p = 0.001$).

The first double-blind clozapine study in treatment-resistant childhood-onset schizophrenic patients[9] showed clozapine to be superior to haloperidol for positive and negative symptoms. Adverse effects were a concern however. Five of twenty-one patients (24%) experienced significant neutropenia. This recurred on rechallenge for two of these patients, for whom clozapine was discontinued. Pediatric patients may be more susceptible than adults to this clozapine toxicity, perhaps secondary to higher concentrations of *N*-desmethylclozapine, the metabolite implicated in clozapine's hematopoietic toxicity.[33] It may be

that selected patients intolerant to clozapine can be successfully rechallenged some years later.[34]

In the Kumra et al 1996 study,[9] clozapine was also discontinued due to seizures in three patients who experienced continuing EEG abnormalities or seizure activity after the addition of anti-seizure medications. The increase of clozapine levels secondary to concurrent valproate[35] may account in part for the persistent EEG abnormalities along with individual variations in metabolism in the three patients ultimately discontinuing clozapine. Seizure incidence in this population may also be higher than in adults, as the 14% incidence of seizures in this small adolescent study group exceeds the 1.3–4% seizure incidence in adult and adolescent studies of much larger numbers.[36,37]

One of these patients, now 21 years old, is currently undergoing retreatment with clozapine at the National Institute of Mental Health (NIMH) after premedication with gabapentin at 1800 mg/day.[38] At the time of this writing, the patient is seizure free on the combination of 300 mg/day of clozapine and 2100 mg/day of gabapentin. This case supports careful rechallenge for 'failed' pediatric subjects as they increase in age.

There is a dearth of information on pediatric cases for olanzapine, a thienobenzodiazepine structurally related to clozapine but with a stronger binding affinity at dopamine D2 receptors. The only open published study of olanzapine in schizophrenic adolescents was by Kumra et al.[39] Two of eight treatment-refractory patients receiving olanzapine met criteria for response,[40] with decreases of at least 20% in BPRS total scores from baseline by treatment week 8. Although meager, the overall impression was that clozapine may be superior (with 8/15 responders) for this very ill, treatment-resistant group. As expected from adult studies, side effects of olanzapine included increased appetite, constipation, nausea/vomiting, headache, somnolence, insomnia, difficulty concentrating, tachycardia, transient transaminase elevations and agitation. The authors conclude

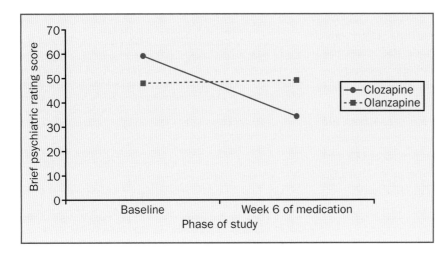

Figure 9.1 Comparisons between baseline and week 6 Brief Psychiatric Rating Scores for olanzapine ($n = 6$) and clozapine ($n = 7$) treatment. Ancova ($F = 7.3$; $p = 0.018$).

that olanzapine may be a good 'first-line' agent for the treatment of childhood-onset schizophrenia given its relative safety and therapeutic benefit for at least some patients. The small number of patients treated with olanzapine ($n = 8$) and comparison of data between double-blind and open-label trials limit these superficial findings. Since publication of these open-label/controlled trial comparisons, additional data continue to suggest a unique role for clozapine.

Observations from treatment week 6 BPRS scores for 13 COS patients who had open trials with either clozapine ($n = 7$) or olanzapine ($n = 6$), showed greater clozapine treatment effect (Ancova $F = 7.3$; $p = 0.018$; adjusted for baseline).

Of interest is that a subset of 4 patients who received clozapine in a double-blind clozapine/haloperidol trial and were treatment responsive at 6 weeks of treatment but who were intolerant of side effects (1 with neutropenia, 2 with seizures) were subsequently treated with open olanzapine. This group did less well with olanzapine. BPRS score differences (week 6 clozapine or week 6 olanzapine − baseline) for clozapine were greater ($t = 2.67$; $p < 0.04$).

Finally, of six treatment resistant COS patients randomized to either clozapine ($n = 4$) or olanza-

pine ($n = 2$), BPRS total score differences (week 8 − baseline) indicate the four receiving clozapine showed greater improvement (paired $t = 5.1$, $p = 0.015$) than olanzapine (paired $t = 4.4$, $p = 0.14$). At this juncture, it seems that clozapine remains the 'gold standard' for treatment of the severely ill, early onset cases in spite of the attendant risks.

Quetiapine, a more recently approved atypical antipsychotic agent, is structurally related to clozapine, though less active at dopamine D_1 and D_2 receptors. Because experimental canines with long-term exposure to quetiapine have shown lenticular changes, slit lamp examination before and 6 months into treatment is recommended. Daily doses up to 500–700 mg for effective control of psychosis in youths have been reported.[41] Szigethy et al[42] report a schizophrenic adolescent with onset of psychosis at age 8 who had a good response to quetiapine, 200 mg/day. His previous partial response to risperidone and olanzapine, and weight gain on both medications, spurred a quetiapine trial. After 2 months of treatment with quetiapine, BPRS score was 21 in comparison to a pretreatment score of 34. Newer atypicals such as quetiapine and ziprasidone await testing in adolescents.

There has been growing pressure from the public and NIMH to productively counter 'off-label' prescribing practices for pediatric patients with research knowledge concerning safety and efficacy of agents.[43] The reach of this maturing trend for appropriate pharmacologic research in childhood and adolescent psychiatric disorders is already manifested by the studies noted above and the creation by NIMH of a research consortium for such studies. In its most mature form, medical science will extend into the daily practices of child psychiatrists and to pediatric specialists battling against other illnesses with onset in childhood.

Nondrug intervention

In light of the extreme rarity of childhood-onset schizophrenia, and thus very limited research on this condition, it is understandable that there is little systematic research on family, residential or educational intervention. Because of this, we offer some brief descriptions reflecting our own work with families and community agencies.

Family coping and support strategies

The family can significantly and even dramatically influence their child's ability to lead a reasonably happy life. The family's acceptance of their child and his/her illness seems the most important nonpharmacological factor in maximizing the child's assets. Advocating for their child is one of the ways our most successful families have shown their acceptance, while simultaneously helping themselves.

Case studies

CASE 1.
Doug was 11 when he was admitted to the childhood-onset schizophrenia protocol. His symptoms included delusions, auditory and visual hallucinations and some autistic-like behaviors. Doug had good response to clozapine and has remained on it for the past 6 years.

Doug's father, a hard-driving businessman, always accepted Doug's limitations. An enthusiastic speaker, Mr Smith doesn't require much reciprocal conversation. He talks to Doug about a wide range of subjects, inviting Doug to see the world through his father's eyes. He often includes subtle encouragement in what he says to Doug: 'Doug, since you're so good at raking leaves, I know you'll want to hear about the earth warming and its impact on trees in North America.' 'You like to make pan-

cakes on Sundays so you'll know what it takes to make the kind of meal we had last week in New York. We had....'

Mr Smith's dogged pursuit of normalcy for his son has borne fruit. When Doug was 12, Mr. Smith approached the local Boy Scout Council, and he identified staff who would be receptive to Doug's becoming a Boy Scout. Mr Smith also met with the boys in Doug's future troop, stressing his son's assets, and ways Doug could contribute. He mentioned Doug's deficits almost as an aside. Over Doug's Boy Scout years, Mr. Smith contributed time to the troop, soliciting financial support for Doug's troop's projects, carpooling and giving staff feedback about how they were helping Doug. Doug is now only two badges from Eagle Scout!

Doug lived in a state where high schoolers must perform mandatory volunteer work in order to graduate. Mr Smith approached the local honor society and suggested that Doug be a 'volunteer opportunity' for the students. Mr Smith and school staff arranged for honor society students to perform their volunteer service by going with Doug to video stores, local ice cream parlors, music stores and the mall – all 'normal' activities for high schoolers and ways for Doug to increase his social skills. Doug made important connections with these students, some of whom still call Doug when they are home on college break or even stop by to go with him to a movie.

CASE 2.
The Lee family's financial situation was different, but Mrs Lee, a single mother and Pacific Rim immigrant with limited English, showed equal dedication to her daughter. Her advocacy allowed Kilani to have experiences and acquire skills she would never have attained. Mrs Lee persuaded reluctant church officials to give Kilani a chance at childcare during church services. Mrs Lee made herself personally available to childcare staff, supervising Kilani's work through the one-way mirror in the nursery until the staff were comfortable with Kilani's presence. Kilani's work has been wonderful and parents appreciate her gentle approach.

When it became obvious that Kilani would not rise to be a doctor, lawyer, or chief executive officer, this mother painfully gave up her former high aspirations and urged school personnel to provide job training for Kilani at their understaffed job training center. Now Kilani takes pride in the money she makes at a nearby college cafeteria, and enjoys depositing her paycheck in the account her mother helped her establish. Because Kilani so enjoyed the animal therapy program at NIMH, Mrs Lee and Kilani became co-volunteers at the local SPCA, spending 3 hours each week caring for abandoned animals. Thus Kilani is now a contributing member of her community, in a church nursery, college cafeteria and animal shelter.

Mrs Lee also educated the extended family. She has taught them not just to accept Kilani, but encouraged them to have the same expectations for appropriate behavior as they do from their unaffected children.

Because of Mrs Lee, Kilani has people around her who accept and love her. Nothing is curing her schizophrenia, but she feels good about herself and confident about her ability to be as independent as her illness permits.

Any clinician working with families should help them master such advocacy and support skills.

In a study of 21 schizophrenic children, Asarnow et al[44] found that confusing, unclear communication style or communication deviance (CD) on a Rorschach CD measure, similar to that reported in adults previously,[45,46] was a frequent attribute of parents of children with schizophrenia and schizophrenia spectrum disorders. It may prove helpful to expand parents' communication repertoire by training more direct ways for them to prevent the child from drifting off task or to positively redirect them when they offer disorganized or peculiar ideas. The efficacy of such an approach remains to be tested.

Parental expressed emotion (EE) was also examined by the Asarnow group[47] and was found to occur less commonly in parents of children with schizophrenia than in samples of parents of adult schizophrenics; in fact it did not differ from that of a normal comparison group. The authors question whether such a difference between the parent groups is associated with the different developmental stages during which the onset of the illness occurs and whether family coping styles differ with the child's age and developmental level. These findings underscore the importance of developing psychosocial and family interventions that are specifically responsive to the unique difficulties encountered by families disrupted by this much earlier and more severe form of the illness.

Studies of family interventions for adult-onset schizophrenia may be helpful for COS family treatment. Dixon and Lehman 1995 report[48] (and our own data suggest) that the positive effects of family interventions reach a wider spectrum of patients than just those from high-EE families. Combinations of engagement, support, psychoeducation and active problem solving appear more effective than brief psychoeducation alone in delaying relapse in adult patients. Multiple family groups rather than single family sessions may be more effective for patients with more positive symptoms who are Caucasian and whose families demonstrate high degrees of expressed emotion. Future studies are needed to identify the components of family interventions most important for COS.

Community resources

The availability of adequate community resources also influences clinical outcome. Here again, COS is too rare for systematic research but our clinical experience with its recruitment from widely differing geographic settings in the United States has been instructive. One of our patients, for example, came from a suburban college town in a midwestern state, which provided high-quality care to disabled residents. The hospital administrator and the child psychiatry unit head nurse called NIMH in advance of his discharge to obtain input for the next placement, given that he was too ill to return home (in spite of partial response to clozapine). They offered inpatient hospitalization, residential treatment facility and therapeutic foster care and eventually facilitated rehospitalization. In the 2 years since NIMH discharge, he has been in a hospital, a residential treatment center and at home. His residential treatment facility provided a family support group involving the family in all decisions. When their son seemed ready to live at home, transition was gradual, increasing the probability of success. When he is well enough to be home, the local mental health agency assists mother with an in-home worker to stay with him after school. Respite care also lets the parents have a few hours to themselves on weekends. When rehospitalization is needed, the staff handle it efficiently and compassionately, and this young boy is always in the most appropriate setting.

In contrast, another patient came from an urban community in a southwestern state with a penny-wise-pound-foolish program. This unfortunate youth has had multiple in-patient admissions. Referred to the NIMH study with diagnoses of psychotic disorder NOS and oppositional defiant disorder, he had a fairly good response to medication but still required a therapeutic setting and structured classroom to maintain behavioral improvements and academic progress. (He had made up a full grade during a 3-month inpatient NIMH stay.) His parents advocated for him, even contacting their state governor to get sustained, appropriate long-term outpatient care. The state education review board only authorized a 3-month admission to a highly structured, small-enrollment, state-funded school (which provided a multitude of services in a supportive setting), where he thrived and had friends for the first time. After 3 months the state education review board ignored his parents', psychiatrist's and NIMH requests for extension. His regular school had only resource-room access and within a couple of months he was hospitalized with suicidal ideation. The specialized school he had attended for 3 months cost $30,000 a year; rehospitalization for 3 months had a higher financial and emotional cost.

The efficacy of family, educators and mental health professional as advocates can be bolstered by the National Alliance for the Mentally Ill (NAMI), with its rich experience in working with systems of mental health care. NAMI's 'curriculum' for families is 'taught' by staff and family members and includes psychoeducation, 'tutorials' improving individuals' advocacy skills, and peer consultation directed at management of children with a prolonged dependency so that maturity and self-esteem can be bolstered nevertheless. Additionally, NAMI can help decrease the loneliness and isolation and stress of coping with a family member with chronic illness by its support system of peer families. NAMI's World Wide Web site offers local chapter addresses for easy access to NAMI's extensive network of chapter leaders. There is also a 'Youth' page that lists specific services for children and adolescents with brain disorders.

In summary, the growing research interest in childhood onset schizophrenia has increased awareness of these cases. A byproduct of this new interest will be better treatment guidelines.

References

1. Remschmidt HE, Schulz E, Martin M et al, Childhood-onset schizophrenia: history of the concept and recent studies, *Schizophr Bull* (1994) **20:** 727–45.

2. Gordon CT, Frazier J, McKenna K et al, Childhood-onset schizophrenia: an NIMH study in progress, *Schizophr Bull* (1994) **20:**697–712.

3. Childs B, Scriver CR, Age at onset and causes of disease, *Perspect Bio Med* (1986) **29:**437–60.

4. Alaghband-Rad J, McKenna K, Gordon CT et al, Childhood-onset schizophrenia: the severity of the premorbid course, *J Am Acad Child Adolesc Psychiatry* (1995) **34:**1273–83.

5. Rapoport JL, Giedd, J, Jacobsen LK et al, Childhood-onset schizophrenia; progressive ventricular enlargement during adolescence on MRI brain rescan, *Arch Gen Psychiatry* (1997) **54:**897–903.

6. Pool D, Bloom W, Mielke DH, et al, A controlled evaluation of loxitane in seventy-five adolescent schizophrenic patients, *Curr Ther Res* (1976) **19:** 99–104.

6a. Realmuto GM, Erickson WD, Yellin AM et al, Clinical comparison of thiothixene and thioridazine in schizophrenic adolescents, *Am J Psychiatry* (1984) **141:**440–2.

7. Spencer EK, Kafantaris V, Padron-Gayol MV et al, Haloperidol in schizophrenic children: early findings from a study in progress, *Psychopharmacol Bull* (1992) **28:**183–6.

8. Spencer EK Campbell M, Children with schizophrenia: diagnosis, phenomenology, and pharmacotherapy, *Schizophr Bull* (1994) **20:**713–25.

9. Kumra S, Frazier JA, Jacobsen LK et al, Childhood-onset schizophrenia: a double-blind clozapine-haloperidol comparison, *Arch Gen Psychiatry* (1996) **53:**1090–7.

10. Spencer EK, Alpert M, Pouget ER, Shell J, Baseline characteristics and side effect profile as predictors of haloperidol treatment outcome in schizophrenic children. Presented at the Thirty-fourth NCDEU/NIMH Annual Meeting, Marco Island, FL, 31 May–3 June 1994.

11. Hippius H, The history of clozapine, *Psychopharmacology* (1989) **99:**S3–S5.

12. Gerson SL, Clozapine: deciphering the risks, *N Engl J Med* (1993) **55:**94–7.

13. Alvir J, Lieberman JA, Safferman AZ et al, Clozapine-induced agranulocytosis, *N Eng J Med* (1993) **329:**162–7.

14. Safferman A, Lieberman JA, Kane JM et al, Update on the clinical efficacy and side effects of clozapine, *Schizophr Bull* (1991) **17:**247–61.

15. Seifen G, Remschmidt HG, Behandlungsergebnisse mit Clozapin bei schizophrenen jugendlichen, *Z Kinder Jugendpsychiat* (1986) **14:**245–57.

16. Birmaher B, Baker R, Kapur S et al, Clozapine for the treatment of adolescents with schizophrenia, *J Am Acad Child Adolesc Psychiatry* (1992) **31:**160 -4.

17. Blanz B, Schmidt MH, Clozapine for schizophrenia, *J Am Acad Child Adolesc Psychiatry* (1993) **32:**222–3.

18. Remschmidt H, Schulz E, Marti PD, An open trial of clozapine in thirty-six adolescents with schizophrenia, *J Child Adolesc Psychopharmacol* (1994) **4:** 31–41.

19. Frazier JA, Gordon CT, McKenna K et al, An open trial of clozapine in 11 adolescents with childhood-onset schizophrenia, *J Am Acad Child Adolesc Psychiatry* (1994) **33:**658–63.

20. Levkovitch Y, Kaysar N, Kronnenberg Y et al, Clozapine for schizophrenia, *J Am Acad Child Adolesc Psychiatry* (1994) **33:**431.

21. Kowatch RA, Suppes T, Gilfillan SK et al, Clozapine treatment of children and adolescents with bipolar disorder and schizophrenia: a clinical case series, *J Child Adolesc Psychopharmacol* (1995) **5:**241–53.

22. Turetz M, Mozes T, Toren P et al, An open trial of clozapine in neuroleptic-resistant childhood-onset schizophrenia, *Br J Psychiatry* (1997) **170:**507–10.

23. Treves IA, Neufeld MY, EEG abnormalities in clozapine-treated schizophrenia, *Eur Neuropsychopharmacol* (1996) **6:**93–4.

24. Tiihonen J, Nousiainen U, Hakola P, EEG abnormalities associated with clozapine treatment (letter), *J Clin Psychiatry* (1991) **148:**1406.

25. Olesen OV, Thomsen K, Jensen PN et al, Clozapine serum levels and side effects during steady state treatment of schizophrenic patients: a cross-sectional study, *Psychopharmacology (Berl)* (1994) **117:**371–8.

26. Quintana H, Keshivan M, Case study: risperidone in children and adolescents with schizophrenia, *J Am Acad Child Adolesc Psychiatry* (1995) **34:**1292–6.

27. Armenteros J, Whitaker AH, Welikson M et al, Risperidone in adolescents with schizophrenia: an open pilot study, *J Am Acad Child Adolesc Psychiatry* (1997) **36:**694–700.

28. Borison RL, Pathiraja AP, Diamond BI, Meibach RC, Risperidone: clinical safety and efficacy in schizophrenia, *Psychopharmacol Bull* (1992) **28:** 213–18.

29. Chouinard G, Jones B, Remington G et al, A Canadian multi-center placebo-controlled study of fixed doses of risperidone and haloperidol in the treatment of chronic schizophrenic patients, *J Clin Psychopharmacol* (1993) **13:**25–40.

30. Horrigan JP, Atypical neuroleptics and posttraumatic stress disorder in children. Talk presented at the Annual Meeting, American Academy of Child and Adolescent Psychiatry, Anaheim, CA, October 1998.

31. Kumra S, Herion D, Jacobsen LK et al, Case study: risperidone-induced hepatoxicity in pediatric patients, *J Am Acad Child Adolescent Psychiatry* (1997) **36:**701–5.

32. Kelly DL, Conely RR, Love RC et al, Weight gain in adolescents treated with risperidone and conventional antipsychotics, *J Child Adolesc Psychopharmacol* (1998) **8:**151–9.

33. Gerson SL, Arce C, Meltzer HY, N-desmethylclozapine: a clozapine metabolite that suppresses hemapoiesis, *Br J Haematol* (1994) **86:**555–61.

34. Usiskin SI, Nicolson R, Lenane M, Rapoport J, Retreatment with clozapine after erythromycin-induced neutropenia. *Am J Psychiatry* (2000), **157:**1021.

35. Centorrino F, Baldessarini RJ, Kando J et al, Serum concentrations of clozapine and its major metabolites: effects of cotreatment with fluoxetine or valproate, *Am J Psychiatry* (1994) **151:**123–5.

36. Devinsky O, Pacia S, Seizures during clozapine therapy, *J Clin Psychiatry* (1994) **55:**153–6.

37. Freedman J, Wirshing W, Russell A et al, Absence status seizures during successful long-term clozapine treatment of an adolescent with schizophrenia, *J Child Adolesc Psychopharmacol* (1994) **4:**53–62.

38. Usiskin SI, Nicolson R, Lenane M, Rapoport JL, Gabapentin prophylaxis of clozapine-induced seizures in a patient with childhood-onset schizophrenia (letter), *Am J Psychiatry* (2000) **157:**482–3.

39. Kumra S, Jacobsen LK, Lenane MC et al, Childhood-onset schizophrenia: an open-label study of

olanzapine in adolescents, *J Am Acad Child Adolesc Psychiatry* (1998) **37**:377–85.

40. Kane J, Honigfeld G, Singer, J, Meltzer H, Clozapine for the treatment-resistant schizophrenia: a double-blind comparison with chlorpromazine, *Arch Gen Psychiatry* (1988) **45**:789–96.

41. Sikich L, Atypical antipsychotics in the treatment of childhood and adolescent psychosis. Talk presented at the Annual Meeting of the American Academy of Child and Adolescent Psychiatry, Anaheim, CA, October 1998.

42. Szigethy E, Brent S, Findling RL, Quetiapine for refractory schizophrenia, *J Am Acad Child Adolesc Psychiatry* (1998) **37**:1127.

43. Vitiello B, Jensen PS, Psychopharmacology in children and adolescents: current problems, future prospects: summary notes on the 1995 NIMH–FDA conference, *J Child Adolesc Psychopharmacol* (1995) **5**:5–7.

44. Asarnow JR, Tompson MC, Goldstein MJ, Childhood-onset schizophrenia: a followup study, *Schizophr Bull* (1994) **20**:599–617.

45. Singer MT, Wynne LC, Thought disorder and family relations of schizophrenics: IV. Results and implications, *Arch Gen Psychiatry* (1965) **12**:201–9.

46. Jones JE, Patterns of transactional deviance in the TAT's of parents of schizophrenics, *Fam Process* (1977) **16**:327–37.

47. Asarnow JR, Tompson MC, Hamilton EB et al, Family-expressed emotion, childhood-onset depression, and childhood-onset schizophrenia spectrum disorders: is expressed emotion a non-specific correlate of child psychopathology or a specific risk factor for depression? *J Abnorm Child Psychol* (1994) **22**:129–46.

48. Dixon L, Lehman AF, Family interventions for schizophrenia, *Schizophr Bull* (1995) **21**:631–43.

10

The Detection and Optimal Management of Early Psychosis

Patrick D McGorry

Contents • Introduction • A framework for early intervention in schizophrenia and related psychoses • Preventive interventions in the real world • Conclusion

Introduction

The best progressive ideas are those that include a strong enough dose of provocation to make its supporters feel proud of being original, but at the same time attract so many adherents that the risk of being an isolated exception is immediately averted by the noisy approval of a triumphant crowd.

Milan Kundera[1]

In recent years there has been a growing sense of optimism about the prospects for better outcomes for schizophrenia and related psychoses, which has achieved the status of a 'progressive idea'. Some of this optimism has flowed from the development of a new generation of antipsychotic medications with greater efficacy and fewer toxic side-effects, but a second major factor has been the belated recognition that a special focus on the early phases of illness could result in a substantial reduction in morbidity and better quality of life for patients and their families. This is not a new idea, having been developed during the pre-neuroleptic era by Sullivan[2] in particular and others subsequently.[3,4] However, in the face of a number of severe obstacles, it remained dormant for decades, gradually re-emerging during the 1980s and especially the 1990s.

The Northwick Park study of Crow and colleagues in the United Kingdom[5] and the Hillside first-episode studies of Kane et al[6] and Lieberman et al[7,8] pioneered the first-episode focus as a research strategy with the potential to clarify a whole range of research questions which were difficult to explore in multiepisode and chronic patients. Importantly, the United Kingdom researchers were flexible enough to focus on first-episode psychosis rather than schizophrenia, a key issue to which I will return below. The obvious advantages of this approach led to a cohort of first-episode research studies which continues to this day; however, at first the clinical issues and the major preventive opportunities revealed by the first-episode strategy were not widely appreciated. However, when the clinical care of the first-episode and recent-onset patients was streamed separately from chronic patients in a research setting, something which is still difficult to achieve, it became obvious to clinician researchers that the patients had quite different clinical needs and that a preventive opportunity was staring them in the face.[9–11] The innovative work of Falloon[12] and the increasing devolution of mental health care into community settings provided further momentum, as did a genuine renaissance in biological and psychological treatments for psychosis. An exponential growth in interest in neuroscientific research in schizophrenia injected further optimism into the field with a new generation of clinician researchers coming to the fore. In Australia, a durable National Mental Health Strategy has catalysed and guided major reform and helped to generate a preventive mindset. Around the world a range of clinicians and researchers have established clinical programmes and research initiatives focusing on early psychosis and it now constitutes a growth point in clinical care as well as research. If this process, which is sociological as well as scientific, remains evidence-based, it has the potential to lead to a sea change in the way these illnesses are approached clinically.

For a variety of reasons, secondary prevention and early intervention are good intermediate options prior to the stage where primary prevention might become possible. To reduce the prevalence and impact of psychotic disorders in society as a whole would constitute a major achievement. Yet this has not occurred despite the development of highly effective treatments,[13] a result of failed implementation in the real world beyond the randomized controlled trial. Even with existing knowledge, substantial reductions in prevalence and improved quality of life are possible for patients provided societies are prepared to pay for it. Early intervention, with its promise of more efficient treatment through an enhanced focus on the early phases of illness, is an additional prevalence reduction strategy which is now available to be tested and, if cost-effective, to be widely implemented.

Evidence is critical if there is to be a real world shift in attitudes and clinical practice and if we are to avoid a further false dawn in the history of this field. However, for each element, we need to determine how much evidence is required before a change in practice is warranted. In deciding where the onus of proof should lie, we should also remember that the alternative to early and optimal intervention is delayed and substandard treatment with all its human consequences. Even

in developed countries, as consumers and carers will readily attest, the timing and quality of standard care is relatively poor, very much a case of 'too little, too late'. In developing countries, a significant proportion of cases never receives treatment.[14] While we do need evidence, there are obvious additional clinical and commonsense drivers for more timely and widespread treatment of better quality.

A framework for early intervention in schizophrenia and related psychoses

As well as evidence we need a conceptual framework which supports an early intervention strategy. While it is possible to discuss the preventive clinical management of early psychosis within the traditional framework of primary, secondary, and tertiary prevention, there is now an alternative. Building on the ideas of Gordon,[15] Mrazek and Haggerty[16] developed a more sophisticated framework for conceptualizing, implementing and evaluating preventive interventions within the full spectrum of interventions for mental disorders (Figure 10.1).

They classified preventive interventions as universal, selective and indicated. *Universal* preventive interventions are focused upon the whole population, for example, immunization and prevention of smoking, while *selective* preventive measures are aimed at asymptomatic subgroups of the population whose risk of becoming ill is above average, for example, annual mammograms for women with a positive family history of breast cancer. *Indicated* prevention is now defined as follows:

> Indicated preventive interventions for mental disorders are targeted to high-risk individuals who are identified as having minimal but detectable signs or symptoms foreshadowing mental disorder, or biological markers indicating predisposition for mental disorder, but who do not meet DSM-III-R diagnostic levels at the current time.

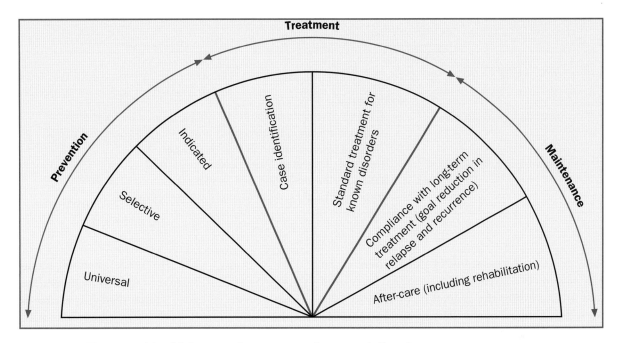

Figure 10.1 The mental health intervention spectrum for mental disorders.

This definition, a modification of Gordon's original concept, means that individuals with early and/or subthreshold features (and hence a degree of distress and disability) are now included within the focus of indicated prevention. This involves making subthreshold symptoms a risk factor in their own right in the context of a categorical model of illness, which has been widely accepted, at least in the epidemiological approach to mental disorders. This subthreshold phase is analogous to the increasingly important, but essentially retrospective, concept of prodrome. Some clinicians would regard this as early intervention or an early form of treatment; however, the situation with these individuals is not so clear-cut. While some of these cases will clearly have an early form of the disorder in question (when the subthreshold clinical features will then turn out to have been 'prodromal'), others will not, and will therefore constitute 'false positives' for the disorder in question. They might, however, have other less serious disorders, and many individuals, subthreshold for a potentially

serious disorder, may have nevertheless crossed a clinical threshold where they either require or request treatment. This will either be because they have reached the diagnostic threshold for other comorbid syndromes, or because the subthreshold symptoms of the putatively core disorder have become disabling or distressing. Clinicians working with such a range of comorbidity potentially have two objectives. Firstly, they may treat what is already present, and secondly they can try to reduce the risk of the existing syndromes worsening or evolving into a more serious syndrome, such as acute psychosis. In any event, as any clinician knows, help-seeking and treatment need in psychiatry are not perfectly correlated with diagnostic threshold; not surprisingly, patients do not always conform to the categories and thresholds found in diagnostic manuals.[17–19]

Beyond the subthreshold or prodromal phase, two additional secondary prevention foci can be discerned. Firstly, there is the issue of *timing* of treatment. Early case detection aimed at shortening delays in accessing treatment should reduce

Table 10.1 Two classification schemas.	
• Primary prevention	• Universal
	• Selective
	• Indicated
• Secondary prevention	• Early case identification (+ increased treated incidence)
	• Optimal/intensive treatment of first episode and critical period
	• Relapse prevention (after full remission)
• Tertiary prevention	• Relapse prevention (after partial remission)
	• Disability minimization and reduction
	• Improved quality of life (+ mental health promotion)

prevalence and morbidity provided there is an effective form of treatment available. The related task of increasing the treated incidence, particularly for high-incidence disorders, also aims to reduce prevalence and morbidity, and can be achieved through similar strategies (see below). Secondly, there is the *quality* of treatment. The notion that optimal treatment of the early phase of disorder could shorten the duration of illness and thus reduce the prevalence of the disorder, and further have a positive medium- to long-term effect on the course and outcome, is an attractive idea. The idea of a 'critical period' during which the disorder is more responsive to intervention has recently been developed for psychotic disorders and fits with the patterns of illness severity found in recent follow-up studies as well as the developmental stage of life in which these illnesses emerge.[11,20–24] If early detection provides one safety net to limit the psychosocial damage of these illnesses, then optimal and sustained treatment during this critical period when the vulnerability is at its peak can act as a second one, providing a degree of 'damage control'. Optimizing and intensifying early-phase treatment is therefore a third subtype of secondary prevention which could be implemented and evaluated within mental health services even at the present state of knowledge. Given the alternative for patients and families, we really should ask ourselves why not? Indicated prevention and early

case detection could also be explored as secondary preventive strategies by mental health professionals and services. These three foci can be collectively termed 'early intervention'. A fourth subtype of secondary prevention, relapse prevention in the context of full remission between episodes of disorder, genuinely falls within the scope and definition of secondary prevention. While there is substantial evidence supporting its widespread use and it should be a core part of the role of every mental health service, space considerations preclude its further consideration here. The remainder of the chapter will confine itself to early intervention as just defined (Table 10.1).

Preventive interventions in the real world

Prepsychotic intervention in schizophrenia and related psychoses

The best hope now for the prevention of schizophrenia lies with indicated preventive interventions targeted at individuals manifesting precursor signs and symptoms who have not yet met full criteria for diagnosis. The identification of individuals at this early stage, coupled with the introduction of pharmacological and psychosocial interventions, may prevent the development of the full-blown disorder.

Mrazek and Haggerty (p. 154)[16]

It is increasingly clear that deficits in social functioning are primarily established during the prepsychotic or prodromal phase. The level of social development achieved by the end of the prodromal phase, when the first psychotic symptom appears, determines the further social course of the disorder by setting a 'ceiling' for recovery.[25,26] This loss of function almost certainly develops in the majority of cases during an active period of illness proximal to attaining diagnostic threshold. In other words it is a 'prodromal' change not a 'premorbid' one, since during childhood most people with subsequent schizophrenia are only very subtly, if at all, different from their peers, and even less so from those who later develop an affective illness.[27,28] This means that in childhood the disorder is rarely clinically active, and it is far too early to make any accurate predictions regarding subsequent psychosis in adolescence or adulthood. While an early vulnerability may exist in a proportion of cases, other environmental risk factors[29] and putative problems with adolescent brain development processes (a second-stage process, termed neurodegenerative or neurotoxic by some)[30] clearly come into play during adolescence or later, though months or years prior to the emergence of the diagnostically defining features of psychotic disorder.[25]

Until recently it has not been possible systematically to identify those at incipient risk of transition to psychosis, that is people in the late prodromal phase of illness. However, a new approach termed the 'close-in' strategy,[31] has shown that it is possible to provide clinical access to the subgroup of young people who are at ultra high risk (UHR) of a first episode of psychosis, are already distressed and functioning poorly, and who are willing to accept professional help.[32-36] These studies have shown that even with good psychosocial care, 41% of operationally defined UHR patients make the transition to first-episode psychosis within a 12-month follow-up period. Several clinical features, such as depression and various negative and positive symptoms, enhance the capacity to predict transition to psychosis within this group even though a very diverse range of clinical features are present.[37-39] Prediction is better for those with a longer duration of symptoms in the late prodromal phase, but there is clearly a less specific early prodromal phase where prediction will be much less feasible. Nonspecific psychosocial interventions helpful in the reduction of risk for a range of disorders may find a place during this less differentiated phase. It is important to emphasize that these patients have experienced a recent change in subjective experience, have emerging and significant disability and are seeking help. They must be distinguished from a subgroup of the general population who report isolated psychotic symptoms in the apparent absence of disability or progressive change, and who do not desire assistance.[40]

A recent randomized controlled trial in this clinical population has shown a significant reduction in transition rate to psychosis for patients receiving specific treatment (ST) – very low dose risperidone (1–2 mg/day) and cognitive therapy – in comparison to non-specific treatment (NST) – supportive psychotherapy and symptomatic treatment.[41] A range of ethical and conceptual issues need to be considered in relation to this emerging field, but it is clear that these young people are a help-seeking clinical population and are both distressed and disabled by their symptoms, whatever their ultimate diagnosis. They also have a very substantial risk of developing a frank psychotic illness, usually, but not always, schizophrenia. Further research is urgently required to clarify the range of treatments which will alleviate their distress and disability and reduce their risk of subsequent psychosis.

In the interim there is a need for a clinical response from psychiatrists, community mental health services and primary care, since these young people are highly symptomatic and at increased risk of suicide, substance abuse and vocational failure. What should the clinician do when approached by a young person or by the family of a young person who appears to be at high risk? Firstly, if the symptoms are very non-specific, especially if they are of recent onset, and there is no family history of psychosis, then the approach should be a general and supportive one. This could include treating any specific features, such as depression, panic or obsessive-compulsive disorder, with a psychosocial approach initially, combined with the use of a selective serotonin reuptake inhibitor (SSRI), if symptoms are persistent or severe.

For those meeting the criteria for ultra high risk (UHR) as defined above, the offer, at least, of initial psychosocial treatment, including the emerging range of cognitive therapies, with or without syndrome-based drug treatments, aimed at the relief of such distress and disability in young people seems eminently justifiable as a component of youth-oriented mental health care. What the patient and family should be told about the level of risk of future psychosis has been debated; however, in our experience, an open approach of disclosure, guided by the curiosity of the patient and family, has worked well. If this offer is initially refused, as it may well be in this age group, this can usually be accepted, although some kind of assertive follow-up is also justifiable, combined with family contact because, in addition to the risk of psychosis, there is, as mentioned, a higher than expected rate of substance abuse, deliberate self-harm and suicide in this potentially prepsychotic population.[41]

Not uncommonly, the parents of the young person will be concerned about vocational failure and social withdrawal in their relative, but will be unable to persuade them to attend for assessment. This is partly because of problems relating to stigma and self-stigmatization. In this situation, rather than retreat behind the usual barriers erected by more traditional clinical approaches, it is more appropriate to ensure that a way is found for the young person to be assessed and offered help in a non-stigmatizing manner. This can be accomplished through home visits by the family doctor, by the school counsellor, or by mobile youth mental health teams linked to specialist youth health services or specialist mental health services. Early intervention teams can also be located in mainstream community facilities to facilitate such assessments and avoid stigma. Naturally, a good understanding of the range of normal psychology of adolescents and young adults, and of appropriate interviewing and engagement strategies, is invaluable. Engagement is more than half the battle in early intervention in psychosis and a youth mental health orientation is critical. It effectively deals with the false positive issue, which recedes when a broader focus on youth mental health with all of its comorbidity is embraced.

Even if psychosis does emerge and the symptoms cross the threshold for antipsychotic therapy, a key advantage of this focus on vulnerable, prepsychotic or potentially prodromal people is that a therapeutic relationship has been established when it is much more possible to do so. The young person has been less severely ill and more accessible to relationships generally. This means that recommendations re drug therapy are more likely to be accepted by patient and family when they are made and, in our experience, that hospitalization can be avoided in most cases, hence reducing the costs and trauma associated with treatment of the first psychotic episode. Furthermore, the duration of untreated psychosis (DUP) is reduced to an absolute minimum. Even if only a minority of first-episode cases can be engaged prior to psychosis and no transitions to psychosis can be prevented, the advantages are still potentially great. Treatment will be commenced 'on the right foot' in an atmosphere of trust rather than fear and disruption, and with fewer complications.

The final clinical issue in this phase of illness is whether there is a role for antipsychotic medications prior to reaching the threshold for diagnosis of a frank psychotic disorder. Despite the lower risks of disabling side-effects and better efficacy of the novel antipsychotic drugs, and the positive early research findings described above, caution is required here. If the indications for broadening the use of antipsychotic medications beyond frank and persistent psychosis as reflected in the DSM-IV[42] psychotic disorders are not very carefully defined and supported by high-quality research, then it is likely that much harm could be done. While we await such guidance from research, it seems reasonable for clinicians to proceed as follows.

The conservative engagement and monitoring strategies outlined above could be offered, and each syndrome, for example depression, as it manifests, could be specifically treated with pharmacological and psychosocial interventions within a youth mental health model. Antipsychotic medications should be withheld except in the following situations, when they could be considered. Patients who meet the UHR criteria as defined, and who are rapidly deteriorating (but have not become frankly psychotic in a persistent manner such that they meet criteria for schizophreniform disorder or another major DSM-IV[42] psychotic disorder) with increasing suicidality or risk of violence, or with increasingly disorganized, stigmatizing or embarrassing behaviours, could be offered a trial of low-dose antipsychotic medication which could be reviewed after say 6 weeks. If substantial improvement occurred then it would seem reasonable (as if the patient had had a first psychotic episode) to continue the treatment for 6–12 months and then, provided remission was maintained, to withdraw the medication cautiously and slowly at that point. If the first drug used were to have little beneficial effect, then the situation would be less clear-cut, though other antipsychotic treatment trials could be considered especially if the patient's condition continued to worsen. In the future a range of other strategies may prove to be worth trying, such as cognitive remediation, cognitive behaviour therapy, and putative neuroprotective agents, such as lithium and essential fatty acids. This proposed approach is clearly based on personal opinion and local experience with such patients and its validity needs to be thoroughly tested through further

clinical research. The value of such research cannot be overestimated given the critical nature of this phase of illness in relation to outcomes for patients.

Early case detection in first-episode psychosis

Once the currently accepted threshold for treatment with antipsychotic medication – the first clear and sustained emergence of psychotic features – is reached, there is a firmer foundation for early intervention. Despite this and the severity of these disorders, for a substantial proportion of people, such treatment is surprisingly delayed, often for very prolonged periods.[43,44] Hence for the typical case, the above description of the prepsychotic treatment strategy is a long way from present reality. Indeed for others, especially in the developing world,[14] treatment is *never* accessed. The duration of untreated psychosis (DUP), as a marker of delay in delivering effective specific treatment, is a potentially important variable in relation to efforts to improve outcome in first-episode schizophrenia, and more widely in first-episode psychosis.[45] Indeed, psychosis may be an easier and less conflicted target to detect than schizophrenia.[46,47] Schizophrenia, which requires a period of frank psychotic features for diagnosis, may take time to emerge as a stable diagnosis, and our primary treatment target is positive psychotic symptoms, for which we prescribe antipsychotic medications (notwithstanding their effects on other symptom domains). DUP is important because, unlike other prognostic variables such as genetic vulnerability, gender and age of onset, it is a potentially malleable variable which can become the focus of intervention strategies.

A strong and extensive literature supports a correlational link between DUP and both short- and long-term outcome,[43,48] although two recent studies have cast doubt on the link.[48,49] However, even if the link is as robust as it seems, there is one obvious and central question. Is the association causal, that is, is delay (prolonged DUP) in treatment a risk factor for worse outcome? Or is the link due to a common underlying factor, namely a more severe form of illness which has a more insidious onset with more negative symptoms, more paranoid ideation, less salience and awareness of change and less willingness to seek and accept treatment? Even if this is so, DUP may still be a key intervening variable through which these clinical features influence outcome, and hence reducing it may mitigate their effect. Space does not permit a detailed review of the evidence regarding this question and, though it is not yet clearly proven that reducing DUP improves outcome, there is a strong prima facie case, and as clinicians, we could agree with McGlashan[43] that delayed treatment is already a major public health problem and that '[prolonged] DUP, by itself, is reason enough for early intervention on a large and intensive scale' (p. 901).

What justifies such a statement is a clinical appreciation derived from patients and families directly of the destructive effects of delay and the rage of negative psychosocial outcomes which accumulate during the period of untreated psychosis.[48,51] These include vocational failure, self-harm, offending behaviour, family distress and dysfunction, aggression, substance abuse, and victimization by others.

Mental health services in partnership with local communities, primary care and individual clinicians could therefore embark upon a range of strategies to reduce delays in treatment onset. This is not a process which is seen as part of the mandate of clinicians or clinical services, indeed depending on the funding system, it is more common for the latter to regulate their workload by restricting access to new patients. There may be a reluctance to widen access because of a lack of resources, due to inadequate funding, to cope with a feared influx of referrals. This is a real issue since it is quite true that the effect of early detection strategies in community psychiatry settings (for example community education and mobile detection teams) will probably be twofold, as witnessed in recent Scandinavian studies.[43]

First, if intensive efforts are made to improve mental health literacy in the general community, recognition skills among general practitioners through training and consultation-liaison, and access to and engagement with specialist mental health services, then the duration of untreated psychosis for the average case should be substantially reduced, especially the relatively small subgroup with a very long DUP. This should make the work of the service easier and result in a reduced need for inpatient care and involuntary treatment. Secondly, there will be an increase in treated incidence of and hence workload due to psychosis of up to 40%, although this may largely involve milder and self-limited cases. Nevertheless, there would be a corresponding reduction in the prevalence of hidden psychiatric morbidity in the community. Clearly these effects will be complex to measure and monitor. To achieve them, an initial change in the culture of clinical practice will be required with reciprocal effects upon the complexion of the service. More resources will be required for services to become proactive in this way, to undertake the detection role and cope with the additional caseloads. Such a role should be built into part of the mandate of modern community-based mental health services and requires leadership from within psychiatry, but needs to be developed in partnership with communities and primary care. It also needs to be added to the existing budgets for health services on a regional basis rather than expecting direct service budgets to absorb such costs.

Optimal and intensive phase-specific intervention in first-episode psychosis and the 'critical period'

Since it does not require as much of a change in role as the previous two preventive foci, more intensive phase-specific treatment during the first episode of psychosis, and beyond into the critical period, is the most feasible proposition for most clinicians and researchers interested in secondary prevention. Several monographs have appeared on this subject recently.[24,52–54]

In general, there is some evidence that such

intensive treatment of young people at this phase of illness is effective;[24,48,54,55] and cost-effective[56] in real world settings at least in the short term, though more research is certainly required to examine the longer-term impact and to determine the most appropriate service models. Whether it is possible to reduce the intensity of treatment over a longer timeframe or not[21] is an important secondary research question.

First-episode psychosis

The key elements of management in first-episode psychosis are described in detail elsewhere.[27,52–54,,57] They can be summarized as follows.

ACCESS AND ENGAGEMENT. Most people, though not all, who develop psychotic disorders are young people with little or no experience of mental health services. They lack knowledge and carry the same fears and prejudices as the rest of the community regarding mental illness and will generally be reluctant to seek or accept help. This is not specific to first-episode psychosis but is a common problem in adolescent psychiatry, exaggerated by the sense of invulnerability which is part of normal adolescence. The presence of psychotic symptoms, particularly delusions, may further inhibit awareness and help-seeking. Access and engagement with services are processes that can be markedly enhanced by the way services are designed and operated. Mobile assessment available around the clock in a setting that suits the individual patient and family is a key advance in improving access to care. This should ideally be offered even prior to a crisis or high-risk situation having developed, so that a calm and careful process of assessment and initial management can be undertaken. Engagement with services is made more difficult if a traumatic crisis and involuntary treatment is the initial experience of the young patient and family. Many services still shield themselves behind concrete and self-serving interpretations of local mental health legislation requiring patients who are not actively seeking help on their own behalf or who

reject it, especially first-episode cases, to develop suicidal or violent behaviour before even direct assessment is offered. Although crises cannot always be avoided, the frequency can be reduced substantially if resources are devoted to a mobile early detection and assessment service.[58]

ASSESSMENT. The assessment process is of major importance at the point of first entry to specialist mental health care for obvious reasons. Ultimately, this should be comprehensive and include a developmental and family perspective. However, the goal of detailed assessment should not undermine the goals of engagement and initial management of the distressed young patient and their family, so it should be carried out in a stepwise fashion. The initial assessment should focus on the major diagnostic issues and levels of risk of harm to self or others. The rest can be pieced together over time. A key issue is to determine whether the patient is clearly psychotic, and if so whether there is also a major mood syndrome present. Substance abuse and dependence are frequently comorbid with positive psychotic symptoms, and it is important to identify the small proportion of cases where the psychosis represents a simple acute intoxication, rather than the more common scenario where each disorder acts as a risk factor for the other. As early detection strategies begin to bite, it is also likely that more sub-threshold cases, including those with isolated psychotic symptoms,[40] will be assessed. Some of these patients have psychotic symptoms that are not typical of the textbook or diagnostic manual and may confuse clinicians. Many of these patients do request and require treatment, sometimes with antipsychotics and often with other drug therapies as well; however, further research may be required to define carefully the range of appropriate treatment for such patients. Our existing treatment strategies are most clearly indicated when they are offered to severe acute cases or patients with prolonged untreated illness and significant disability, though the onset of clear-cut and sustained positive psychotic symptoms represents a watershed for any given patient. Although the novel antipsychotics have broader effects than those on positive symptoms alone, the clear emergence of frank and sustained (at least 1 week) positive symptoms is currently a necessary step to considering their use in clinical settings. Hence in detection and diagnosis *psychosis* is an appropriate target. Secondary targets then become mania, depression, and a range of other comorbid syndromes and syndromes, rather than DSM-IV or ICD-10[59] diagnoses per se, because they constitute a better guide to drug therapy.[45,60]

ACUTE TREATMENT. The initial decision is whether inpatient care is required. This will be influenced by patient factors, the degree of family and social support, and by the range of services available and local policies. Where this is possible, home-based acute care is preferred for a range of reasons and can be achieved in over 50% of cases with a highly structured intensive approach.[61,62] An antipsychotic-free period of at least 48 hours is usually advisable, during which benzodiazepines only are prescribed to alleviate the distressing symptoms of agitation, anxiety and insomnia. If sustained psychosis is confirmed then antipsychotic medication may be commenced. The second-generation or novel antipsychotics are indicated as first-, second- and even third-line therapy because of their greater efficacy and better tolerability. The starting dose should be very low (for example 0.5 mg risperidone or 2.5 mg olanzapine) and be increased to an initial 'step' and held there for the effect to be evaluated (for example, 2 mg risperidone or 7.5 mg olanzapine). Further increases should only occur in the setting of poor response and only then at intervals of approximately 3 weeks to allow the effect of the change in dose to become clear. The all-too-familiar weekly doubling of the dose at ward rounds should become a thing of the past. We now know that these dosages are sufficient to produce sufficient levels of D_2 blockade in the central nervous system to bring about a clinical response and that the threshold for clinical response is lower, albeit narrowly so, than the threshold at which neurological and other side-effects begin to be manifested. We are indebted to classic research conducted at the Karolinska Institute in Sweden and at the Clarke Institute in Canada for the demonstration of this narrow therapeutic window.[63,64] These low doses of antipsychotics are not intended or expected to deal with the behavioural disturbances and associated symptoms frequently seen in this acute phase. The latter should be managed if at all possible with benzodiazepines and psychosocial strategies during this period, since the use of parenteral or sedating oral typical neuroleptics will inevitably produce aversive neurological side-effects and undermine, perhaps terminally, an already fragile process of engagement and adherence to treatment.

Emergency situations requiring urgent sedation can be managed with intramuscular benzodiazepines such as midazolam or lorazepam in most cases. In occasional cases this will be ineffective and a short-acting sedating neuroleptic, droperidol 5 mg intramuscularly, is the next best option. Longer-acting depot preparations such as zuclopenthixol acetate seem superficially appealing because they purport to avoid the necessity for repeated injections during the acute phase, but their delayed onset of action and the almost inevitable production of distressing neurological side-effects mean that the risks outweigh the benefits for nearly all first-episode patients. Repeated injections are in any case very rarely required with good nursing care, a supportive milieu and liberal use of benzodiazepines in the acute phase. Naturally, intensive psychosocial support is essential for the patient and family during this highly stressful period, though services are often unable to provide this due to inadequate funding, low morale and poor skills, combined with an unfortunate lack of awareness or acknowledgement of its critical role. This is a deficiency in urgent need of reform. Home-based care is less stressful for the patient in particular and usually results in a reduced need for acute medication. The identification and treatment of the major affective syndromes, especially mania, is a key issue in the treatment of first-episode psychosis. A manic syndrome is present in up to 20% of cases of first-episode psychosis and should be rapidly treated with a mood stabilizer, ideally lithium carbonate, to promote full recovery while minimizing antipsychotic dosages. Depression, unless clearly dominating the clinical picture, commonly resolves in parallel with the positive psychotic symptoms; however, if it persists or worsens during the post-psychotic period, it should be actively treated with a combination of SSRI and psychological intervention. More detailed descriptions of the principles and practice of acute care can be found in Kulkarni and Power,[62] Aitchison et al[54] and the Australian Clinical Guidelines for Early Psychosis.[57]

THE RECOVERY PHASE. Up to 85–90% of first-episode patients will achieve a remission or partial remission of their positive psychotic symptoms within the 12 months following entry to treatment, though some potentially responsive patients will fail to engage with treatment or rapidly cease adherence to medication. A range of psychosocial strategies can augment and broaden the scope and depth of the recovery process, and these include psychological interventions,[65–67] family interventions[69] and group-based recovery programmes.[70] Some of these will increase the remission rate for positive symptoms and they all aim to improve negative symptoms, functioning and quality of life. Rapid discharge of responding patients following an acute first episode of psychosis to unsupported general practitioners is a poor practice. It represents a missed opportunity for maximizing and consolidating recovery and for secondary prevention. An integrated shared care model with the GP and other agencies is likely to prove more beneficial.

The critical period

This term can be regarded as covering the period following recovery from a first episode of psychosis and extending for up to 5 years subsequently. This is based on the notion[23] that this is the phase of maximum vulnerability. A number of recent research studies have focused on the treated course of early psychosis. These have shown that the early course of illness for both schizophrenia and affective psychosis is turbulent and relapse prone, with up to 80% of patients relapsing within a 5-year period. These findings suggest that drug therapy should be continued for most if not all patients for longer than 12 months after recovery from a first psychotic episode. However, it should be remembered that a subsample, at least 20%, never relapse, that some will not relapse for a prolonged period, and that relapse prevention is not the sole consideration in treatment but rather a means to an end. Adaptation to illness is a challenging, often overwhelming, task for these young people, and they usually need to be given time and special help to come to an acceptance of the need for maintenance treatment.[71]

A concerted effort should be made to maintain the engagement of most patients with clinical care during the early years after onset and to have in place a written relapse plan so that action can be taken if symptoms re-emerge, whether on or off medication. A good therapeutic and personal relationship with the patient and family is the key to success and should be nurtured, though continuity of care is at a premium in public psychiatry in developed countries. This deficiency is the Achilles' heel of the system, leaving patients who often have significant problems with trust and in forming social relationships with no safety net. Even with standard care, however, it has been shown that outcome at 13 years is much more positive than expected, supporting the notion of an early critical period, which may be turbulent but seems to abate after 2–5 years. With optimal care such outcomes could be substantially improved.

Conclusion

There is growing support for a more preventive stance in the treatment of schizophrenia and psychotic disorders. Primary prevention, specifically universal and selective preventive interventions, is beyond our capacities at the present stage of knowledge. However, indicated prevention for subthreshold symptoms has been endorsed as the frontier of prevention in schizophrenia,[16] and early detection and optimal early treatment are clearly within the mandate of clinicians and services, and can be justified despite predictable academic scepticism. This scepticism must be appropriately addressed through rigorous clinical research, but it may prove difficult to dissipate fully, and should not be allowed to snuff out precious therapeutic optimism which can improve morale within services as well as patient outcomes. Evidence will be a vital guide because a range of new clinical and ethical issues are being brought to light as the frontier advances, and it is important that changes in mental health care are based on solid foundations, not shifting sands, as so often in the past. Nevertheless, dispersing the mists of pessimism which have shrouded the clinical care of people with schizophrenia and encouraged stigma is an overdue and worthwhile endeavour. The treatment objectives and approaches described in this chapter characterize recent early steps in this direction, with the hope that further progress will rapidly occur.

References

1. Kundera M, *The Book of Laughter and Forgetting* (Faber & Faber: London, 1996) 273.

2. Sullivan HS, The onset of schizophrenia, *Am J Psychiatry* (1927) **151**:135–9. (1994: reprinted).

3. Cameron DE, Early schizophrenia, *Am J Psychiatry* (1938) **95**:567–78.

4. Meares A, The diagnosis of prepsychotic schizophrenia, *Lancet* (1959) **i**:55–9.

5. Crow T, Macmillan J, Johnson A, Johnstone E, A randomized controlled trial of prophylactic neuroleptic treatment, *Br J Psychiatry* (1986) **148**:120–7.

6. Kane JM, Oaks G, Rifkin A et al, Fluphenazine vs placebo in patients with remitted acute first-episode schizophrenia, *Arch Gen Psychiatry* (1982) **39**:70–3.

7. Lieberman JA, Matthews SM, Kirch DG, First-episode psychosis: Part II. Editors' introduction, *Schizophr Bull* (1992) **18**:349–50.

8. Lieberman JA, Jody D, Alvier JM et al, Brain morphology, dopamine, and eye-tracking abnormalities in first-episode schizophrenia. Prevalence and clinical correlates, *Arch Gen Psychiatry* (1993) **50**:357–68.

9. McGorry PD, The Aubrey Lewis Unit: the origins, development, and first year of operation of the clinical research unit at Royal Park Psychiatric Hospital. Dissertation submitted for Section 11 of MRANZCP examination, December 1985.

10. Copolov DL, McGorry PD, Singh BS et al, Origins and establishment of the Schizophrenia Research Programme at Royal Park Psychiatric Hospital, *Aust N Z J Psychiatry* (1989) **23**:443–51.

11. McGorry PD, The concept of recovery and secondary prevention in psychotic disorder, *Aust N Z J Psychiatry* (1992) **26**:3–17.

12. Falloon IRH, Early intervention for first episode of schizophrenia: a preliminary exploration, *Psychiatry* (1992) **55**:4–15.

13. Hegarty J, Baldessarini R, Tohen M et al, One hundred years of schizophrenia: a meta-analysis of the outcome literature, *Am J Psychiatry* (1994) **151**:1409–16.

14. Padmavathi R, Rajkumar S, Srinivasan T, Schizophrenic patients who were never treated – a study in an Indian urban community, *Psychol Med* (1998) **28**:1113–17.

15. Gordon R, An operational classification of disease prevention, *Public Health Rep* (1983) **98**:107–9.

16. Mrazek PJ, Haggerty RJ, eds, *Reducing Risks for Mental Disorders: Frontiers for Preventive Intervention Research* (National Academy Press: Washington, DC, 1994).

17. Regier DA, Kaelber CT, Rae DS et al, Limitations of diagnostic criteria and assessment instruments for mental disorders, *Arch Gen Psychiatry* (1998) **55**:109–15.

18. Spitzer RL, Diagnosis and need for treatment are not the same, *Arch Gen Psychiatry* (1998) **55**:120.

19. Frances A, Problems in defining clinical significance in epidemiological studies, *Arch Gen Psychiatry* (1998) **55**:119.

20. Birchwood M, MacMillian F, Early intervention in

schizophrenia, *Aust N Z J Psychiatry* (1993) **27:**374–8.

21. Birchwood M, Todd P, Jackson C, Early intervention in psychosis: the critical period hypothesis, *Br J Psychiatry* (1998) **172(Suppl 33):**53–9.

22. Loebel A, Lieberman JA, Alvir JM et al, Duration of psychosis and outcome in first-episode schizophrenia, *Am J Psychiatry* (1992) **149:**1183–8.

23. McGorry PD, Singh BS, Schizophrenia: risk and possibility. In: Raphael B, Burrows GD, eds, *Handbook of Studies on Preventive Psychiatry* (Elsevier Science Publishers: Amsterdam, 1995).

24. McGorry PD, Jackson HJ, eds, *The Recognition and Management of Early Psychosis: A Preventive Approach* (Cambridge University Press: Cambridge, 1999).

25. Häfner H, Nowotny B, Löffler W et al, When and how does schizophrenia produce social deficits? *Eur Arch Psychiatry Clin Neurosci* (1995) **246:**17–28.

26. Häfner H, Löffler W, Maurer K et al, Depression, negative symptoms, social stagnation and social decline in the early course of schizophrenia, *Acta Psychiatr Scand* (1999) **100:**105–18.

27. Jones P, Rodgers B, Murray R, Marmot M, Child development risk factors for adult schizophrenia in the British 1946 birth cohort, *Lancet* (1994) **344:**1398–402.

28. Van Os J, Jones P, Lewis G et al, Developmental precursors of affective illness in a general population birth cohort, *Arch Gen Psychiatry* (1997) **54:**625–31.

29. Mahy G, Mallett R, Leff J, Bhugra D, First-contact incidence rate of schizophrenia on Barbados, *Br J Psychiatry* (1999) **175:**28–33.

30. Rapoport J, Giedd J, Blumenthal J et al, Progressive cortical change during adolescence in childhood-onset schizophrenia, *Arch Gen Psychiatry* (1999) **56:**649–54.

31. Bell RQ, Multiple-risk cohorts and segmenting risk as solutions to the problem of false positives in risk for the major psychoses, *Psychiatry* (1992) **55:**370–81.

32. McGorry P, Phillips L, Yung A, Recognition and treatment of the pre-psychotic phase of psychotic disorders: frontier or fantasy? In: Mednick S, McGlashan T, Libiger J, Johannessen J, eds, *Early Intervention in Psychiatric Disorders* (Kluwer: Netherlands, in press).

33. McGorry PD, Yung AR, Phillips LJ, 'Closing in':

what features predict the onset of first episode psychosis within a high risk group? In: Zipursky RB, ed, *The Early Stages of Schizophrenia* (American Psychiatric Press: Washington, DC, in press).

34. Yung A, Phillips L, McGorry P et al, Prediction of psychosis, *Br J Psychiatry* (1998) **172(Suppl 33):**14–20.

35. Yung A, McGorry P, McFarlane C et al, Monitoring and care of young people at incipient risk of psychosis, *Schizophr Bull* (1996) **22:**283–303.

36. McGorry P, Jackson H, Edwards J et al, Preventively-oriented psychological interventions in early psychosis. In: *Psychological Treatments for Schizophrenia* (Institute of Psychiatry, University of Manchester: Oxford, 1999).

37. McGorry PD, Phillips LJ, Yung AR et al, The identification of predictors of psychosis in a high risk group, *Schizophr Res* (1999) **36:**49–50.

38. Schultze-Lütter F, Klosterkötter J, What tool should be used for generating predictive models? *Schizophr Res* (1999) **36:**10.

39. Phillips L, Yung A, Hearn N, McFarlane C et al, Preventive mental health care: accessing the target population, *Aust N Z J Psychiatry* (1999) **33:**912–17.

40. Van Os J, Bijl R, Ravelli A, Can the boundaries of psychosis be defined? *Schizophr Res* (2000) **41:**8.

41. Phillips L, McGorry P, Yung A et al, The development of preventive interventions for early psychosis: early findings and directions for the future, *Schizophr Res* (1999) **36:**331–2.

42. American Psychiatric Association: Diagnostic and Statistical Manual of Mental Disorders 4th ed (DSM-IV). American Psychiatric Association: Washington DC, 1994.

43. McGlashan T, Duration of untreated psychosis in first-episode schizophrenia: marker or determinant of course? *Biol Psychiatry* (1999) **46:**899–907.

44. Carbone S, Harrigan S, McGorry P et al, Duration of untreated psychosis and 12-month outcome in first-episode psychosis: the impact of treatment approach, *Acta Psychiatr Scand* (1999) **100:**96–104.

45. Harrigan SM, McGorry PD, Krstev H, Does treatment delay in first-episode psychosis really matter? *Schizophr Res* (2000) **41:**175.

46. McGorry P, A treatment-relevant classification of psychotic disorders, *Aust N Z J Psychiatry* (1995) **29:**555–8.

47. Driessen G, Gunther N, Bak M et al, Character-

istics of early- and late-diagnosed schizophrenia: implications for first-episode studies, *Schizophr Res* (1998) **33**:27–34.

48. McGorry P, Edwards J, Mihalopoulos C et al, EPPIC: An evolving system of early detection and optimal management, *Schizophr Bull* (1996) **22**:305–26.

49. Ho BC, Andreasen NC, Duration of initial untreated psychosis – methods and meanings. Paper presented at the Second International Conference on Early Psychosis 'Future Possible', 31 March and 1–2 April 2000, New York.

50. Craig TJ, Bromet EJ, Fennig S et al, Is there an association between duration of untreated psychosis and 24-month clinical outcome in a first-admission series? *Am J Psychiatry* (2000) **157**:60–6.

51. Lincoln C, Harrigan S, McGorry P, Understanding the topography of the early psychosis pathways, *Br J Psychiatry* (1998) **172(Suppl 33)**:21–5.

52. McGorry P, Edwards J, eds, *Early Psychosis Training Pack* (Gardiner-Caldwell Communications Ltd: Cheshire, 1997).

53. McGorry PD, ed, Preventive strategies in early psychosis: verging on reality, *Br J Psychiatry* (1998) **172(Suppl 33)**:1–136.

54. Aitchison K, Meehan K, Murrary R, *First Episode Psychosis* (Martin Dunitz: London, 1999).

55. Power P, Elkins K, Adlard S et al, Analysis of the initial treatment phase in first-episode psychosis, *Br J Psychiatry* (1998) **172(Suppl 33)**:71–6.

56. Mihalopoulos C, McGorry P, Carter R, Is phase-specific, community-oriented treatment of early psychosis an economically viable method of improving outcome? *Acta Psychiatr Scand* (1999) **100**:47–55.

57. National Early Psychosis Project Clinical Guidelines Working Party, Australian Clinical Guidelines for Early Psychosis. National Early Psychosis Project, University of Melbourne, Melbourne, 1998.

58. Yung AR, Jackson HJ, The onset of psychotic disorder: clinical and research aspects. In: McGorry PD, Jackson HJ, eds, *The Recognition and Management of Early Psychosis: A Preventive Approach* (Cambridge University Press: New York, 1999).

59. W.H.O. International Classification of Disease 10th Edition: ICD-10. Chapter V: Mental Behavioural and Developmental Disorders. WHO: Geneva, 1992.

60. Bermanzohn P, Hierarchical diagnosis in chronic schizophrenia: a clinical study of co-occurring syndromes, *Schizophr Res* (2000) **41**:43.

61. Fitzgerald P, Kulkarni J, Home-oriented management program for people with early psychosis, *Br J Psychiatry* (1998) **172(Suppl 33)**:39–44.

62. Kulkarni J, Power P, Initial management of first-episode psychosis. In: McGorry PD, Jackson HJ, eds, *Recognition and Management of Early Psychosis: A Preventive Approach* (Cambridge University Press: New York, 1999) 184–205.

63. Kapur S, Zipursky R, Jones C et al, Relationship between dopamine D_2 occupancy, clinical response, and side effects: a double-blind PET study of first-episode schizophrenia, *Am J Psychiatry* (2000) **157**:514–20.

64. Nyberg S, Farde L, Halldin C et al, D_2 dopamine receptor occupancy during low-dose treatment with haloperidol decanoate, *Am J Psychiatry* (1995) **152**:173–8.

65. Edwards J, Maude D, McGorry PD et al, Prolonged recovery in first-episode psychosis, *Br J Psychiatry* (1998) **172(Suppl 33)**:107–16.

66. Lewis SW, Tarrier N, Haddock G et al, The SOCRATES trial: a multicentre, randomised, controlled trial of cognitive-behaviour therapy in early schizophrenia, *Schizophr Res* (2000) **41**:9.

67. Power P, Bell R, Mills R et al, A randomised controlled trial of a suicide preventative cognitive oriented psychotherapy for suicidal young people with first episode psychosis, *Schizophr Res* (1999) **36**:332.

68. Edwards J, Cannabis and psychosis project: intervention and client group. Inaugural International Cannabis and Psychosis Conference, Melbourne, February 1999.

69. Gleeson J, Jackson HJ, Stavely H, Burnett P, Family intervention in early psychosis. In: McGorry PD, Jackson HJ, eds, *The Recognition and Management of Early Psychosis* (Cambridge University Press: New York, 1999) 376–406.

70. Albiston DJ, Francey SM, Harrigan SM, A group program for recovery from early psychosis, *Br J Psychiatry* (1998) **172(Suppl 33)**:117–21.

71. Jackson H, McGorry PD, Edwards J et al, Cognitively-oriented psychotherapy for early psychosis (COPE). Preliminary results, *Br J Psychiatry* (1998) **172(Suppl 33)**:93–100.

11

Chronic Schizophrenia

Peter J McKenna

Contents • Introduction • What is chronic schizophrenia? • The clinical picture of chronic schizophrenia • Course and fluctuations • Cognitive impairment as a symptom of chronic schizophrenia • Is there a dementia of dementia praecox? • Conclusion

Introduction

Much of schizophrenia is chronic schizophrenia. Much of what is at issue in schizophrenia, from the point of research, treatment, management, health economics and even government policy, also concerns chronic schizophrenia. Yet, as the author found some years ago in the course of researching a book, chronic schizophrenia is hardly ever discussed as a topic in its own right. Kraepelin[1] described it clinically. Bleuler[2] touched on its features at various points. Jaspers[3] deliberated about its essential nature to some extent. A few later authors have referred to it, usually in passing, or embedded in some theory-laden account, or as part of a research project. Beyond this essentially nothing has been written in the English language (and probably any other language).

While every psychiatrist would claim to be able to recognize chronic schizophrenia, its defining characteristics are uncertain and ambiguous. The condition was recently given a simple definition, of more than 2 years of illness, to which, however, no-one subscribes. Instead, the term continues to be used more-or-less interchangeably with a range of others, such as defect state, deficit syndrome, residual schizophrenia or burnt-out schizophrenia. To many, it also conjures up a mental picture

of the most severely ill, institutionalized, long-stay, 'back ward' patients. It is far from clear whether these stereotypes are valid or misleading, and to what extent, if any, chronic schizophrenia is a specific entity with a particular clinical presentation.

What is chronic schizophrenia?

Generally in medicine, the term 'chronic' is applied to diseases which are not self-limiting, and in which the symptoms are to some extent different from those of the initial, acute presentation. The term has additional connotations, of ongoing, insidious pathological process and incurability. As applied to schizophrenia, Jaspers[3] contrasted the essential features of acute psychoses – severe symptoms and signs in a state which is curable or at any rate capable of some improvement – with those of chronic psychosis – less conspicuous symptoms in a no longer curable state: 'Chronic states are sensible, oriented, quiet, orderly and relatively even ... we think of pathological states which develop slowly or remain as a residue of the stormy acute processes.' Rather differently from the rest of medicine, Jaspers did not consider the duration of the illness important; in some cases psychoses which had lasted for years could still reasonably be called acute.

Contemporary approaches have tended to

focus on one or another of the elements of the above definition. American psychiatry, in DSM-III and DSM-IIIR, initially opted for a simplistic approach, merely defining chronic schizophrenia as schizophrenia with a total duration of greater than 2 years. This and other course specifiers such as acute and subchronic were, however, dropped by DSM-IV. Neither DSM-IV nor ICD-10 include a classification for chronic schizophrenia, but the latter contains one for residual schizophrenia (with a synonym listed as chronic undifferentiated schizophrenia). This is defined as a chronic stage in the development of the disorder characterized by long-term negative symptoms. Florid symptoms have to be minimal or at least substantially reduced from the time of prior acute episodes. As will be seen below, this is quite misleading.

The clinical picture of chronic schizophrenia

While accepting that the end-states of schizophrenia could show an infinite number of gradations from recovery to severe disability, Kraepelin[1] and Bleuler[2] considered it convenient to distinguish mild and severe presentations. Kraepelin referred to the milder forms as 'weak-mindedness', Bleuler used the term 'cure with defect', and both authors' accounts were replete with terms such as 'dementia' and 'imbecility' in connection with some of the more severe end-states. In what follows, the less dated and prejudicial terms 'mild deterioration' and 'severe deterioration' are substituted throughout.

One mild (or more accurately not devastatingly severe) chronic state in Kraepelin's and Bleuler's classification was *simple deterioration* (simple weak-mindedness, simple dementia, cure with defect). The key features of this were deficits in emotion and volition, or negative symptoms in current terminology. Such patients appear superficially rational (their 'outward conduct ... is in general reasonable'), but they show obvious abnormalities – a stiff, constrained manner, odd behaviour,

minor peculiarities in speech, gait or movement, idiosyncratic dress or self-neglect. Mood may be predominantly cheerful, depressed, irritable, and so on, but the striking feature is the lack of any deep emotion. Allied to this is a pervasive indifference; the patients live 'a day at a time without endeavour, without wishes, without hope or fears'. Relationships with relatives become cool, sometimes hostile, and former interests are lost. The capacity for work is diminished: sometimes the patient can manage easier work than before, but many are unable to work. Thinking is affected: the circle of ideas is narrowed, and judgement becomes weak – the patients are no longer capable of taking a general view, of distinguishing the central from the side-issues, of planning anything for themselves, of foreseeing the consequences of their actions. Florid symptoms, however, are no longer much in evidence: delusions are denied, typically without much insight, or alternatively are just not spoken about any more. Hallucinations are no more than minor and occasional. An example of one of Kraepelin's[4] own such patients is described in Box 11.1 (this patient is also notable for the presence of apparent orofacial dyskinesia long before the introduction of neuroleptic drugs[5]).

The degree of deterioration can vary considerably. Some patients merely seem a little quieter than before, more self-willed, more capricious, more absent-minded; others do nothing, sit staring, etc. While many patients cannot work, or 'absolutely refuse to work', others remain steady, careful and precise workers in jobs which do not require much responsibility. The state also shows qualitative variations: some patients become taciturn, shy, withdrawn, or avoid people; others are docile; yet others may be self-willed, stubborn, overfamiliar, display signs of slight excitement, talk too much, engage in all kinds of impulsive actions, become promiscuous and so on – one of Kraepelin's patients, previously a respectable girl, gave birth to three illegitimate children in 5 years, one of which she smothered through carelessness.

In *paranoid* and *hallucinatory deterioration* the

Box 11.1 A case of simple deterioration (taken from Kraepelin 1905).[4]

The patient was a 21-year-old man who had become more and more solitary over the past few years. A year previously he failed university examinations and then became preoccupied with the belief that he was ugly, that he had a rupture and that he was suffering from wasting of the spinal cord, which he believed was the result of masturbation. He had stopped seeing friends because he believed that they knew about this and were making fun of him about it. Prior to admission he began crying a great deal, masturbated, ran about aimlessly, was occasionally excited and disturbed at night, played senseless tunes on the piano, and began to write obscure observations on life.

In hospital he was in a state of excitement for several days, during which he chattered in a confused way, made faces, ran about, wrote in disconnected scraps, which were crossed and recrossed with flourishes and meaningless combinations of letters. After this a tranquil state ensued. The patient would lie in bed for weeks or months, or sit around without feeling the slightest need to occupy himself, or at best turning over the pages of a book. He would stare ahead with expressionless features, over which a vacant smile would occasionally play. When he had visitors he would sit without showing any interest, would not ask about what was happening at home, hardly ever greeted his parents, and would go back indifferently to the ward. Occasionally he wrote letters expressing all kinds of distorted half-formed ideas, with a peculiar and silly play on words, in very fair style, but with little connection.

On examination, the patient was able to give an accurate account of his past experiences and displayed knowledge compatible with his education. He knew where he was and how long he had been in hospital, but was only imperfectly acquainted with the names of the people around him; he said that he had never asked about them. He could give only a meagre account of the events of the last year. He described his previous symptoms in an indifferent tone of voice, without looking up or troubling about his surroundings. Occasional wrinkling of the forehead or facial spasm was noted. Round the mouth and nose there was a fine, changing twitching. The patient made his statements slowly and in monosyllables and seemed to feel no desire to speak at all. He appeared to answer questions with whatever occurred to him without thinking, and with no visible effort of will. His expression betrayed no emotion; but he laughed for a moment now and then. All movements were languid, but made without difficulty. There was no sign of dejection, such as one would expect from the nature of his talk.

The patient returned to the care of his family unchanged.

---

above state is complicated by ongoing, persistent, obtrusive florid symptoms. In Bleuler's words, 'the delusions and hallucinations persist in a rather uniform, stable fashion, often with periodic aggravations, but they do not gain any further influence over the thought and actions'. Even though auditory hallucinations may continue to be as frequent and tormenting as in the acute phase, the attitude of the patient towards them appears changed; they no longer talk about or listen to their voices; they are no longer distressed, merely irritated by them. Delusions, especially of persecution, remain firmly held, and as time goes by they may become more fantastic and nonsensical, but they are recited in a monotonous way and without any substantial elaboration – peculiarly stoic or inconsequential attitudes to the imagined persecution are adopted.

The patients remain lucid on the whole, but when they touch on their delusions they may become incoherent. Mood tends to be depressed. There may be minor mannerisms, lip-smacking, stereotyped repetition of questions put to them, stilted speech, etc.

Both authors recognized one further form of mild end-state where deterioration of much the same order as above is accompanied by very marked incoherence of speech (confusional speech dementia, 'imbecility' with confusion of speech). Such patients tend to be accessible, mentally active and take a lively interest in their surroundings. Their behaviour is reasonable and they typically work diligently and to a surprisingly high standard. Delusions and hallucinations are usually present but only in the background and do not influence or preoccupy the patient. Speech, on the other hand, is rich, voluble and completely incoherent, interspersed with many neologisms.

More severe chronic states could take a multiplicity of presentations. Kraepelin recognized five main types: drivelling, dull, silly, manneristic and negativistic. Bleuler simplified these to paranoid, silly and apathetic forms. Their common denominator was very marked affective flattening and impairment of volition, coupled with a striking impoverishment of all mental life. Such patients show a complete emotional indifference, or alternatively a rigid inaccessibility, which is interrupted only by causeless, silly laughter, tearfulness, fits of anger, and so on. Many, if left to themselves, would do nothing or lie in bed all day. Others might be temporarily rousable to carry out some kind of simple work, but soon sink back into a state of apathy. Some are mute or nearly so. In Kraepelin's graphic description they 'live their lives dully and without taking any interest, do not trouble themselves about their relatives, do not reflect about their position, do not give utterance either to wishes or hopes or fears'. Catatonic phenomena, in the form of minor stereotypies, mannerisms, echophenomena, etc., or sometimes as a more pronounced feature, become common among all such patients, not just in those who originally had a catatonic presentation – Bleuler remarked that more than half of all institutionalized patients show catatonic symptoms temporarily or permanently.

Most, perhaps all such patients remain deluded and experience hallucinations to some extent. In *dull* or *apathetic* states delusions, hallucinations, and formal thought disorder are far in the background, and make only a minor contribution to a clinical picture dominated by severe apathy and self-neglect. In *paranoid* and *drivelling* states delusions and hallucinations, or formal thought disorder, respectively remain continuously present, often in a very florid form. Such patients express a wealth of often fantastic delusions 'without connection and without emphasis', hear voices (though often to a minor extent), are more hallucinated in other modalities, and may display an extraordinary degree of incoherence of speech. Sometimes catatonic symptoms dominate the picture as *manneristic* or *negativistic* deterioration. But, as always with schizophrenia, it is not a question of sharp delimitations; sometimes one symptom is to the forefront of the clinical picture and sometimes another, but all the forms merge into each other via innumerable transitions. A contemporary example of a severely deteriorated patient, in whom florid symptoms dominate the picture, is given in Box 11.2.

Finally, according to Kraepelin, there are some severely deteriorated patients in whom delusions and hallucinations are entirely lacking, and who, beyond a certain monotony and impoverishment of mental life, show little in the way of negative symptoms. Instead, their abnormalities lie in the realm of judgement and behaviour (*silly dementia*). Such patients are confident and cheerful, sometimes with passing moods of depression or anger, and keep themselves occupied. They are impulsive, easily led, lack judgement, and sometimes have a continual restless drive which results in reckless behaviour. They are thoughtless, show a striking lack of fine feeling, and 'chat casually about intimate matters'. When presented with tasks requiring planning or independent thought, they fail surprisingly badly.

Box 11.2 A case of severe deterioration.

The patient is a 51-year-old single man, who had worked briefly as a photographer's assistant before becoming ill. At the age of 17, over a few weeks he began alluding to delusions and auditory hallucinations. He went on to have a long series of acute admissions during which he was described as very thought-disordered, as well as floridly deluded and hallucinated. He has been continuously hospitalized since the age of 27.

Examined after some years in hospital, he was dishevelled, with a wrinkled and furrowed brow and a usually expressionless face sometimes breaking into a fatuous grin. He was observed to sometimes creep around the hospital, and could sometimes be seen in bizarre postures, e.g. staring motionless at a crack in a wall. At other times he would lie on his bed for long periods, or stride apparently purposefully around the hospital grounds. Mood was mostly one of complete indifference, but sometimes the patient would become angry and hostile; during these periods he was prone to beat his own chest with frightening force. Affect was grossly blunted and inappropriate. Speech would break down into severe incoherence under stress, or just if conversation continued for any length of time. Example: '[Medication] can kill the space area off if I died, space areas are normally after I died. Cubic space area and nature. That syrup does kill us off if we have it three or four times a day. It does kill us off, it does. Some of it is quite kind but some of it is duff bottles some of it. It deads me off. I can't awake all the time, day and night, to take medication all at once.' Delusions were produced continuously as he spoke, including but not limited to the following. Transmitters control his thoughts, tape recorders control his actions. The skin behind his eyes has broken away and there is nothing behind them. When he urinates, his nipples move up his chest and lodge on his forehead. His nipples control the traffic. His brain is upside down; there is a plastic bag in his brain; there is a man cycling in his brain. He built the hospital. When he first came into hospital it was because he had been found at the bottom of a river, together with pieces of other bodies in plastic bags. He has 500 bodies some or all of which are dead. He would usually acknowledge experiencing auditory hallucinations, but did not go into details, and these did not seem to be a major feature. He once reported seeing an army of caterpillars driving tanks up the hospital drive.

As mentioned in the introduction, next to nothing has been written about chronic schizophrenia clinically since Kraepelin and Bleuler. The European authors Kleist,[6] Leonhard[7] and Astrup,[8] whose names are closely associated with attempts to subclassify chronic schizophrenia, included very little clinical material in their accounts. The British psychiatrist Fish,[9] who wrote extensively on schizophrenia, is also disappointing. His writings on chronic schizophrenia are perhaps most notable for their revealing insights into the often grim realities of the lives of chronically hospitalized patients. For example, he noted the frequent discrepancy between delusions and behaviour; the self-styled Queen of Heaven is content to scrub the floors. A common pattern of abnormal behaviour seen in some patients is incessant letter-writing. The letters themselves could be well written or quite disjointed; they might cover the paper in a scrawl or be well laid out, but with additions made longitudinally in the margins. Collecting and hoarding form another common abnormal behaviour pattern. The pockets of male patients and the handbags of female patients are often found to be full of rubbish – pieces of stale food, wood, matchsticks, grass, stones, dead insects, pieces of string, pieces of toilet paper and scraps of soap. Hoarding may just be of old newspapers, etc., but can consist of more unpleasant things. One patient killed cats and other small animals, then wrapped them in cloth and stored them in her room; another caught and killed birds then carried the carcass around in her clothing. All sorts of unpleasant and antisocial behaviour can occur. Patients frequently steal food and cigarettes from their fellow patients, or are spiteful and play tricks: they may trip or push others over, spit on them, snatch their chairs away, and so on. Deteriorated patients often behave in very degraded ways. They may neglect themselves and become filthy. Some handle faeces, urine or nasal mucus, while others smear faeces on themselves, the fittings, or other patients. Fish was one of the very few authors to acknowledge that chronically hospitalized patients are not uncommonly incontinent.

A final subtle and subjective observation about chronic schizophrenia concerns the alleged persisting inner intactness of even severely ill patients. Although Kraepelin[1] stated bluntly that 'the essence of the personality is destroyed', Bleuler[2] and especially his son, M. Bleuler,[10,11] believed that trapped in even the most deteriorated schizophrenic was a full repertoire of emotions, intact but inaccessible most of the time. This latter author described instances of normal and touching emotion, real joy and compassion in schizophrenic patients considered to be burnt-out, petrified, without human feelings. While it is debatable whether this applies to all schizophrenic patients, it is certainly true that many quite severely deteriorated and/or psychotic patients have surprising reserves of human warmth (and other emotions) – one of the present author's predecessors, who lived in the hospital grounds as medical superintendent, was perfectly happy to let an extremely deluded chronically hospitalized woman regularly babysit his children!

Many of the above clinical impressions are borne out in what appears to be the only formal clinical survey of chronic schizophrenia. Owens and Johnstone[12,13] assessed 510 patients meeting Feighner criteria for schizophrenia who had been continuously hospitalized in a large mental hospital for more than a year (mean 26 ± 13 years). One-third of the patients were found to show no positive symptoms (delusions, hallucinations and formal thought disorder). Of the majority who did have these, a picture of ongoing very florid symptoms was not uncommon – just under 20% of the whole population scored maximally on the delusions and hallucination items of the rating scale, and similar levels of incoherence of speech were present in 7%. Another third of the patients did not show any very marked negative symptoms (however, as the authors noted, these were rated conservatively). Impairment and disorganization of behaviour was very common, and a sizeable minority of patients were 'only able to conform to the rudiments of acceptable behaviour'. A final surprising finding was that, despite requiring chronic hospitalization, 7% of the patients surveyed were free from all positive symptoms and exhibited no definite negative symptoms. An example of this kind of patient is described in Box 11.3.

Course and fluctuations

It is a fond belief of some psychiatrists, and seemingly most planners of mental health services, that chronic schizophrenia is a static, stable condition; the patients are 'burnt out', their needs do not change, and they have something more akin to disability than illness. The reality has always been rather different. Kraepelin[1] cautioned that one must always be prepared for acute exacerbations. Bleuler[2] stated that advances, halts, exacerbations and remissions could be seen at all stages, and that even severe schizophrenics almost never show complete cessation of the process. Several subsequent studies have attested to the clinical changes that can take place many years after the onset of illness.[14,15]

The definitive findings on this issue were provided by M. Bleuler,[10,11] who carried out a personal 20-year follow-up study of 208

Box 11.3 A chronically hospitalized patient without positive or negative symptoms.

This 55-year-old man first became ill at the age of 32, when he developed persecutory and referential delusions revolving around spying and heard voices telling him to commit suicide. He improved on treatment and returned to work as a driver. He remained well for the next 13 years, but then had a series of relapses where he showed delusions and mild formal thought disorder. He had a further hospitalization after an incident where he rammed his car into the doorway of a police station; his explanation was that he wanted to write it off for insurance purposes. Shortly afterwards he jumped off a bridge into a river, having taken a decision to 'bow out peacefully' in the face of (groundless) fears about losing his social security. There were no psychotic symptoms and no evidence of sustained depressed mood. Attempts at discharge failed, partly because of further suicide attempts, and the patient became chronically hospitalized.

The patient has shown much the same mental state for 10 years. He is well kempt and usually well dressed, although this is variable. His behaviour appears entirely normal during interview. His mood varies from affable to moody and unco-operative, but most of the time is neutral and quite friendly. Affect is mildly flattened – once the patient recounted a visit from his ex-wife, in which she broke down crying, with detached amusement. Talk is normal in quantity and the patient is quite a good conversationalist, much given to telling crude jokes; however, he has a tendency to tell the same stories over and over again. He has shown mild poverty of content of speech in the past, but this has faded over the years. Delusions and hallucinations cannot be elicited.

The main feature of the patient's presentation has been his impulsive and reckless behaviour. Once he jumped from a first-floor window and was seriously injured. There was no evidence of depression or psychotic symptoms immediately before or after the incident, and the only explanation he gave was that he had become depressed at the thought of being in hospital for a long time. For some time afterwards he referred to himself as 'the man they couldn't kill'. Later he persuaded a fellow patient (who could not drive) to buy a car, took it and drove it, some of the time on the wrong side of the road, and running into several other cars, apparently using this as an alternative to braking. His only explanation for this incident was that he was bored and wanted to get out of hospital for a time. On one occasion he left hospital and lived in a disused car for a few days. On another, he was found to have cans of petrol in his room and set off the fire alarm in the course of trying to burn the flex off some copper wire he was hoping to sell. He is constantly being discovered writing to various bodies claiming money and developing other ill-thought-out money-making schemes. When he did receive some money, he bought an almost unroadworthy used car, despite the fact he is banned from driving.

well-diagnosed schizophrenic patients admitted to one hospital. He emphasized 'the very long course that schizophrenia runs for many years and decades after its onset'. Even during the last 5 years of the follow-up period nearly 25% of the patients were still experiencing quite severe worsening and improvements. The remainder had reached a position where their clinical state had persisted relatively unchanged for at least 5 years. But even these patients were not completely stable; minor fluctuations still took place and there could also be longer-term trends, often in the direction of improvement.

M. Bleuler's wider conclusion was that schizophrenia is not strictly a progressive disorder. Rather, it follows a complex course. Initially it evolves clinically over a period of on average 5 years, but with wide individual variations. After this no further permanent deterioration takes place, and, if anything, there is a tendency towards improvement. Exacerbations and improvements still take place but are on the whole less marked than early in the course of the illness. Ultimately, a certain stability is reached by many but not all patients.

Cognitive impairment as a symptom of chronic schizophrenia

Although Kraepelin[1] considered that dementia praecox exhibited many features in common with other forms of dementia, he felt that the injury predominated in the emotional and volitional spheres and that memory and orientation were comparatively little affected; 'patients are able, when they like, to give a correct detailed account of their past life, and often know accurately to a day how long they have been in the institution'. One of Bleuler's[2] reasons for renaming dementia praecox as schizophrenia was that he believed the connotation of intellectual decline to be misleading. He argued that what he variously referred to as schizophrenic dementia, schizophrenic intellectual deterioration and the schizophrenic disorder of intelligence was fundamentally different from 'dementia, in the sense of the organic psychoses'.

Notwithstanding this equivocation, if not ambivalence, it soon became orthodoxy that the deficits of chronic schizophrenia did not extend into the realm of intellectual function. Nevertheless, as psychological studies began to be carried out over the first half of the century, schizophrenic patients, as a group, were reliably found to have lower IQs than the rest of the population,[16] and to perform more poorly than normals on just about any cognitive task they were given.[17] Invariably, chronic schizophrenic patients – by which was usually meant chronically hospitalized patients – were found to show the greatest deficits. The studies of this era culminated in the publication of three reviews in 1978[18–20] which all came to the conclusion that it was impossible to distinguish chronic schizophrenic patients from patients with organic brain disease on the basis of their performance on a variety of neurophysical tests.

Following this, and with the publication of many more recent, well-controlled, diagnostically scrupulous and neuropsychologically sophisticated studies,[21,22] cognitive impairment is now widely accepted in schizophrenia. Performance has been found to be affected across all domains of neuropsychological function, but it is widely believed that deficits in memory and executive ('frontal') function are particularly marked.[22,23] A typical contemporary study is that of Saykin et al:[24] these authors administered a comprehensive battery of tests to 37 patients with first-episode schizophrenia, 65 with chronic schizophrenia and 131 normal controls. All three groups were similar in terms of age and education and any minor differences were controlled for in the analysis. The findings are shown in Figure 11.1, where the patients' performance is expressed as z-scores, that is in terms of standard deviations below the mean for the control group, which by definition is represented by the upper zero line. Both groups of patients performed significantly worse than the normal controls, and the chronic patients also performed significantly more poorly than the first-episode patients.

It should be noted that cognitive impairment in chronic schizophrenia is not trivial. In the above study, the average level of performance of the chronic patients fell most of the time between two and three standard deviations below that of the controls, a level that would be expected to be found in less than 5% of the normal population. Two recent studies have also compared the range and extent of memory impairment[25] and executive impairment[26] found in chronic schizophrenic patients to that of patients with moderate or severe head injury. Both studies used measures which were designed to pick up the kind of memory and executive difficulties encountered in

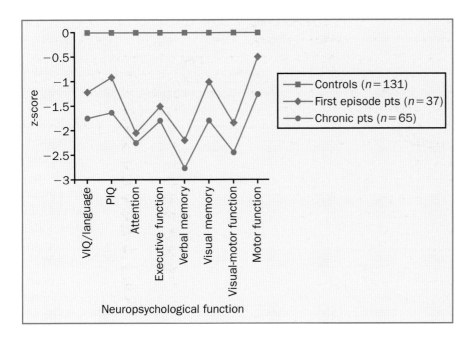

Figure 11.1 Profile of cognitive impairment in first-episode and chronic schizophrenic patients. (Reproduced with permission from Saykin et al 1994.)[24]

daily living. The findings are shown in Figure 11.2. Despite the fact that the chronic schizophrenic patients in both studies encompassed all grades of severity (they were not just chronically hospitalized patients), just as in an earlier generation of studies, their cumulative percentage curves appear indistinguishable from those of brain-injured patients.

The fact that the chronic patients in the study of Saykin et al[24] were drug-free (and the first-episode patients had never been treated) makes it unlikely that cognitive impairment in schizophrenia could be due to neuroleptic drug treatment. The unanimous conclusion of many studies has also been that drug treatment had little effect on most aspects of cognitive function in both normal individuals and schizophrenic patients.[27–29] Another attempt to explain away schizophrenic cognitive impairment has been to attribute it to the effects of symptoms, either lack of motivation and persistence due to negative symptoms, or generally poor co-operation, or distraction

because of hallucinations, anxiety, thought disorder, etc. In fact, studies which have rated patients' motivation, attention and co-operation have found little to suggest that these variables are relevant to performance.[25,30,31] The argument that schizophrenic symptoms are distracting and so impair cognitive performance has suffered a loss of credibility as a result of the development of drugs which can produce symptomatic improvement even in chronic, treatment-resistant patients. Thus Goldberg et al[32] rated symptoms and a range of cognitive functions in 15 chronic schizophrenic patients before and after treatment with the atypical neuroleptic clozapine. The symptom ratings showed decreases of about 40%; however, there was no change in any of the cognitive test scores. Similarly, two patients who became entirely free of both positive (and negative) symptoms on clozapine and appeared normal in every respect continued to show a typical pattern of memory, executive and other deficits after recovery.[33]

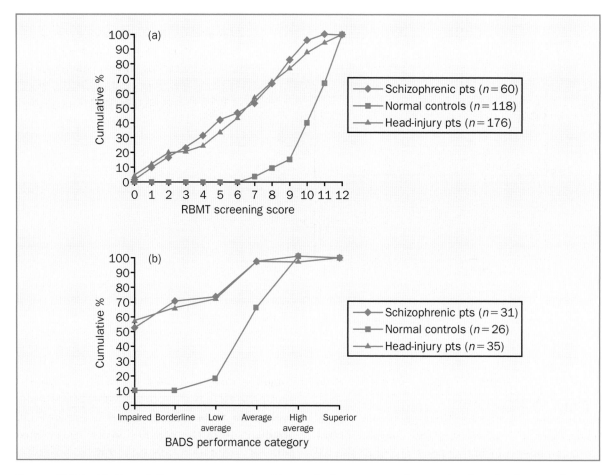

Figure 11.2 (a, b) Cumulative scores on tests of 'everyday' memory and executive function in chronic schizophrenic patients, patients with head injury and normal controls. RBMT, Rivermead Behavioural Memory Test; BADS, Behavioural Assessment of the Dysexecutive Syndrome. (From McKenna et al 1990, Evans et al 1997.)[25,26]

Is there a dementia of dementia praecox?

In Owens and Johnstone's[12] survey of chronically hospitalized patients, poor performance was found on a simple test covering orientation, recall, general knowledge, etc., in around 40% of the sample. Marked cognitive impairment has been found in other similar studies.[34-36] Between 16% (meeting diagnostic criteria) and 25% (clinically diagnosed) of chronically hospitalized schizophrenic patients also show the phenomenon of age disorientation, being unable to give their age correctly, typically underestimating it by a margin of 5 years or more.[37,38] This has been shown not to be a function of coexisting learning disability, prior physical treatments or institutionalization, and it forms part of a wider pattern of cognitive impairment.[38,39] Both general intellectual impairment and age disorientation increase in prevalence with advancing age in these populations of schizophrenic patients. Figure 11.3 shows a progressive lowering of mean scores on a widely used clinical dementia scale, the Mini-Mental State

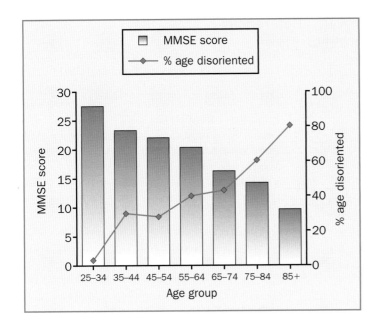

Figure 11.3 Mini-Mental State Examination (MMSE) scores and age disorientation among chronically hospitalized schizophrenic patients in different age groups. (From Davidson et al 1995, Harvey et al 1995.)[35,36]

Examination (MMSE),[40] which is paralleled by steadily increasing numbers of patients showing age disorientation. Over the age of 65, around two-thirds of institutionalized schizophrenic patients have MMSE scores in the demented range.[35,41]

The obvious interpretation of these findings is that something essentially indistinguishable from dementia supervenes in a minority of patients with schizophrenia. However, while accepted by some,[42,43] such a view is controversial. Since there is evidence of lifelong IQ disadvantage of the order of 5–10 points in future schizophrenic patients,[44] and because neuropsychological deficits can be demonstrated at the time of first presentation,[24] many researchers believe that cognitive impairment in schizophrenia is a 'neuro-developmental' phenomenon.[45] While this does not in any way preclude further postmorbid decline, all studies which have retested first-episode schizophrenic patients after up to 2 years have failed to find evidence for any progression of neuropsychological deficits.[46] One recent study also failed to document intellectual decline in the

longer term: Russell et al[47] traced 34 patients who had presented to child psychiatry services in late childhood or adolescence, had undergone IQ testing, and then went on to become schizophrenic (or were already psychotic at the time of initial evaluation in a few cases). Repeat IQ testing of these patients, some of whom were chronically hospitalized, was carried on average 19 years later. The mean IQ at initial testing was found to be 84.2, and that at follow-up was 82.0, a non-significant difference.

Conclusion

It is perhaps not surprising that chronic schizophrenia has proved difficult to define. There is no doubt that the disorder may be characterized only by negative symptoms varying in severity from a minor degree of lack of volition and flattening of affect to very marked apathy, emotional impoverishment, and impaired self-care. However, it may equally be characterized just by positive symptoms: even among chronically hospitalized patients the presentation may consist of florid schizophrenic symptoms which are present against a background of only the most subtle negative symptoms. Despite this apparent dissociation between positive and negative symptoms, when chronic schizophrenic patients show both sets of symptoms, as they perhaps most typically do, there often seems to be a relationship between them, so that it is the patients with the worst degrees of deterioration who are prone to show the most fantastic delusions, the most tormenting hallucinations, and the most incoherence of speech. And finally there are a few patients who show no clear symptoms, but are nevertheless still severely handicapped by the effects of chronic schizophrenia on behaviour and judgement.

Just what makes schizophrenia chronic may remain elusive, but it is possible to correct some common misapprehensions about the disorder. One of these is that it is a static, unchanging end-state. There is a certain amount of truth to this, in that fluctuations are certainly less marked in long-established schizophrenia than in the acute phase. But, as Owens et al[13] put it, 'the idea of "burned out" schizophrenia is no longer acceptable, referring as it does more to the clinician's interest than to the realities of the established disorder'. Also no longer acceptable is the time-honoured view that schizophrenia does not compromise intellectual function. While the degree of cognitive impairment is often minor and demonstrable only on detailed testing in acutely ill patients, there can be no doubt that in chronic schizophrenia it is as genuine and substantial as in any neurological disorder. In general rarely, but quite commonly in elderly chronically hospitalized patients, schizophrenic cognitive impairment appears to warrant a designation of dementia, in its clinical features, if not in its development.

References

1. Kraepelin E, *Dementia Praecox and Paraphrenia*, RM Barclay, 1919 (Livingstone: Edinburgh, 1913).

2. Bleuler E, *Dementia Praecox or the Group of Schizophrenias*, J Zinkin, 1950 (International Universities Press: New York, 1911).

3. Jaspers K, *General Psychopathology*, J Hoenig, MW Hamilton, 1963 (Manchester University Press: Manchester, 1959).

4. Kraepelin E, *Lectures on Clinical Psychiatry*, 3rd English edn, T Johnstone, 1917 (W Wood: New York, 1905).

5. Owens DGC, *A Guide to the Extrapyramidal Side-effects of Antipsychotic Drugs* (Cambridge University Press: Cambridge, 1999).

6. Fish FJ, The classification of schizophrenia: the views of Kleist and his co-workers, *J Ment Sci* (1957) **103**:443–63.

7. Leonhard K, *The Classification of Endogenous Psychoses*, R Berman (Irvington: New York, 1959).

8. Astrup C, *The Chronic Schizophrenias* (Universitetsforlaget: Oslo, 1979).

9. Hamilton M, *Fish's Schizophrenia*, 3rd edn (Wright: Bristol, 1984).

10. Bleuler M, The long-term course of the schizophrenic psychoses, *Psychol Med* (1974) **4**:244–54.

11. Bleuler M, *The Schizophrenic Disorders: Long-Term Patient and Family Studies*, SM Clemens (Yale University Press: New Haven, 1978).

12. Owens DGC, Johnstone EC, The disabilities of chronic schizophrenia – their nature and the factors contributing to their development, *Br J Psychiatry* (1980) **136**:384–93.

13. Owens DGC, Johnstone EC, Frith CD, Chronic schizophrenia and the defect state – a case of terminological inexactitude. In: Schiff AA, Roth M, Freeman HL, eds, *Schizophrenia: New Pharmacological and Clinical Developments*, Royal Society of Medicine Services International Congress and Symposium Series, 94 (Royal Society of Medicine Services Ltd: London, 1985).

14. Ciompi L, The natural history of schizophrenia in the long term, *Br J Psychiatry* (1980) **136**:413–20.

15. Harding C, Course types in schizophrenia: an analysis of European and American studies, *Schizophr Bull* (1988) **14**:633–44.

16. Payne RW, Cognitive abnormalities. In: Eysenck

HJ, ed, *Handbook of Abnormal Psychology* (Pitman: London, 1973).

17. Chapman LJ, Chapman JP, *Disordered Thought in Schizophrenia* (Appleton-Century-Crofts: New York, 1973).

18. Goldstein G, Cognitive and perceptual differences between schizophrenics and organics, *Schizophr Bull* (1978) **4:**160–85.

19. Heaton RK, Baade LE, Johnson KL, Neuropsychological test results associated with psychiatric disorders in adults, *Psychol Bull* (1978) **85:**141–62.

20. Malec J, Neuropsychological assessment of schizophrenia versus brain damage: a review, *J Nerv Ment Dis* (1978) **166:**507–16.

21. Elliott R, Sahakian BJ, The neuropsychology of schizophrenia: relations with clinical and neurobiological dimensions, *Psychol Med* (1995) **25:**581–94.

22. Goldberg TE, Gold JM, Neurocognitive deficits in schizophrenia. In: Hirsch SR, Weinberger DR, eds, *Schizophrenia* (Blackwell: Oxford, 1995).

23. McKenna PJ, *Schizophrenia and Related Syndromes* (Oxford University Press: Oxford, 1994).

24. Saykin AJ, Shtasel DL, Gur RE et al, Neuropsychological deficits in neuroleptic naive patients with first-episode schizophrenia, *Arch Gen Psychiatry* (1994) **51:**124–31.

25. McKenna PJ, Tamlyn D, Lund CE et al, Amnesic syndrome in schizophrenia, *Psychol Med* (1990) **20:**967–72.

26. Evans J, Chua SE, McKenna PJ, Wilson BA, Assessing the dysexecutive syndrome in schizophrenia, *Psychol Med* (1997) **27:**625–46.

27. King DJ, The effect of neuroleptics on cognitive and psychomotor function, *Br J Psychiatry* (1990) **157:**799–811.

28. Goldberg TE, Weinberger DR, Effects of neuroleptics on the cognition of patients with schizophrenia: a review of recent studies, *J Clin Psychiatry* (1996) **57**(supplement 9):62–5.

29. Mortimer AM, Cognitive function in schizophrenia: do neuroleptics make a difference? *Pharmacol Biochem Behav* (1997) **56:**789–95.

30. Goldberg TE, Weinberger DR, Berman KF et al, Further evidence for dementia of prefrontal type in schizophrenia? A controlled study of teaching the Wisconsin Card Sorting Test, *Arch Gen Psychiatry* (1987) **44:**1008–14.

31. Duffy L, O'Carroll R, Memory impairment in schiz-

ophrenia – a comparison with that observed in the alcoholic Korsakoff syndrome, *Psychol Med* (1994) **24:**155–66.

32. Goldberg TE, Greenberg R, Griffin S, The impact of clozapine on cognition and psychiatric symptoms in patients with schizophrenia, *Br J Psychiatry* (1993) **162:**43–8.

33. Laws K, McKenna PJ, Psychotic symptoms and cognitive deficits: what relationship? *Neurocase* (1997) **3:**41–50.

34. Waddington JL, Youssef HA, Dolphin C, Kinsella A, Cognitive dysfunction, negative symptoms and tardive dyskinesia in schizophrenia, *Arch Gen Psychiatry* (1987) **44:**907–12.

35. Davidson M, Harvey PD, Powchik P et al, Severity of symptoms in chronically hospitalised geriatric schizophrenic patients, *Am J Psychiatry* (1995) **152:**197–207.

36. Harvey PD, Lombardi J, Kincaid MM et al, Cognitive functioning in chronically hospitalized schizophrenic patients: age-related changes and age disorientation as a predictor of impairment, *Schizophr Res* (1995) **17:**14–24.

37. Stevens M, Crow TJ, Bowman MJ, Coles EC, Age disorientation in schizophrenia: a constant prevalence of 25 per cent in a chronic mental hospital population? *Br J Psychiatry* (1978) **133:**130–6.

38. Liddle PF, Crow TJ, Age disorientation in chronic schizophrenia is associated with global intellectual impairment, *Br J Psychiatry* (1984) **144:**193–9.

39. Buhrich N, Crow TJ, Johnstone EC, Owens DGC, Age disorientation in chronic schizophrenia is not associated with pre-morbid intellectual impairment or past physical treatments, *Br J Psychiatry* (1988) **152:**466–9.

40. Folstein MF, Folstein SE, McHugh PR, 'Mini-Mental State': a practical method for grading the cognitive state of patients for the clinician, *J Psychiatr Res* (1975) **12:**189–98.

41. Arnold SE, Gur RE, Shapiro RM et al, Prospective clinicopathological studies of schizophrenia: accrual and assessment, *Am J Psychiatry* (1995) **152:**731–7.

42. Johnstone EC, Crow TJ, Frith CD et al, The dementia of dementia praecox, *Acta Psychiatr Scand* (1978) **57:**305–24.

43. Harrison P, On the neuropathology of schizophrenia and its dementia: neurodevelopmental,

neurodegenerative or both? *Neurodegeneration* (1995) **4:**1–12.

44. Jones P, Done DJ, From birth to onset: a developmental perspective of schizophrenia in two national birth cohorts. In: Keshevan MS, Murray RM, eds, *Neurodevelopment and Adult Psychopathology* (Cambridge University Press: Cambridge, 1997).

45. Keshevan MS, Murray RM, eds, *Neurodevelopmental and Adult Psychopathology* (Cambridge University Press: Cambridge, 1997).

46. Rund BR, A review of longitudinal studies of cognitive functions in schizophrenia, *Schizophr Bull* (1998) **24:**425–36.

47. Russell AJ, Munro JC, Jones PB et al, Schizophrenia and the myth of intellectual decline, *Am J Psychiatry* (1997) **154:**635–9.

12

Treatment-resistant Schizophrenia

Herbert Y Meltzer and A Elif Kostakoglu

Contents • Introduction • The role of clozapine in the evolution of the concept of treatment resistance • The concept of treatment-resistant schizophrenia • Treatment resistance at the time of the United States clozapine efficacy and safety trial • Prevalence of treatment-resistant schizophrenia by United States clozapine multicenter criteria • Revised criteria for treatment resistance • Response of neuroleptic-resistant patients to atypical antipsychotic drugs • Determination of the presence of treatment resistance • Characteristics of treatment-resistant schizophrenia • Development of treatment resistance: first-episode vs later development during the course of treatment • Course of treatment resistance • Biological basis of treatment resistance • Treatment of treatment-resistant schizophrenia with atypical antipsychotic drugs • Cost-effectiveness of clozapine in treatment-resistant schizophrenia • Adjunctive treatments • Conclusion

Introduction

Treatment-resistant schizophrenia is a concept which is best understood in the context of the criteria for the diagnosis of schizophrenia, the definitions of treatment response and resistance, and the effectiveness of current treatments relative to those criteria, since the criteria for the diagnosis of schizophrenia and the standards for treatment response are themselves shaped by the effectiveness of available treatments. Thus, treatment-resistant schizophrenia is a moving target. However, for the purpose of this chapter, the definition to be used will focus heavily on lack of response of positive symptoms, that is, delusions and hallucinations, to the typical neuroleptic drugs for reasons which will be discussed subsequently. The mutability of the definition of treatment-resistant schizophrenia can be illustrated by recalling that what Bleuler considered schizophrenia at the time he identified it as a syndrome in 1906 is not the same as what is con-

sidered schizophrenia under DSM-IV[1] criteria. The current criteria rely more heavily on specific symptoms, particularly positive symptoms, the duration of those symptoms, and the absence of independent mood disturbances that meet the criteria for bipolar disorder than did the Bleulerian concept.

The concept of treatment-resistant schizophrenia is more important today than ever before, because (1) it provides a guide to treatment choice in an era where the options to treat schizophrenia, at least from a pharmacologic perspective, have never been more abundant; and (2) the nature of the similarities and differences among treatments has made it particularly difficult for clinicians to choose among them. In addition, the concept of treatment-resistant schizophrenia is important because it provides the impetus to develop more effective treatments for those aspects of schizophrenia, for example, negative symptoms and cognitive function, which current treatments fail to address adequately for some or all patients. The belief that overall treatment response is 'adequate' for a given patient or for schizophrenics as a class contributes to the complacency which denies many patients the opportunity to receive treatments that may be more effective but are also more expensive, even if the cost-effectiveness is greater. In addition, the idea that treatment response is adequate does not provide governments or industry with optimal incentive to develop more effective and safer treatments. Finally, treatment-resistant schizophrenia is important because it can be the basis for identification within the group of patients diagnosed as having schizophrenia of a subgroup who have a unique etiology, possibly on a genetic basis or that of some gene–environment interaction. This can not only lead to the development of effective treatments for these individuals but also, by reducing heterogeneity, enhance the ability to study the etiology of schizophrenia in those who do respond adequately to current treatments.

The role of clozapine in the evolution of the concept of treatment resistance

Current interest in treatment-resistant schizophrenia is intertwined with the development of clozapine, the prototypical atypical antipsychotic agent, its history, and its profile of efficacy and side effects relative to the typical neuroleptic drugs, that is haloperidol, chlorpromazine, etc. As will be discussed, the severity of some of the side effects of clozapine made it necessary to establish a set of criteria for response to the typical neuroleptic drugs which would justify, in 1986, the increased risk of testing and potentially approving clozapine as a treatment of schizophrenia, or a subgroup of those patients, compared to the efficacy, tolerability, and safety of the typical neuroleptic drugs. Regulatory authorities in the United States considered that persistent positive symptoms, despite at least three trials of typical neuroleptic drugs adequate in dosage (high) and

duration (≥ 6 weeks), would justify the risk of clozapine, that is agranulocytosis, occurring in approximately 1% of patients. Other outcome criteria to justify a clozapine trial could have been proposed, for example, persistent negative symptoms, cognitive dysfunction, poor quality of life, and tardive dyskinesia at a particular level of severity. The original concept of treatment resistance remains important because of the continuing need to identify the population of patients who should be treated with clozapine rather than other available pharmacologic treatments and because of the importance of understanding the basis of failure of positive symptoms to respond to typical neuroleptic drugs. Furthermore, the concept is important because it provides a framework for discussion of the criteria for response to neuroleptic treatment.

The concept of treatment-resistant schizophrenia

Chlorpromazine was discovered in 1954 and was quickly recognized to be the first effective treatment of schizophrenia on the basis of its ability to treat the positive symptoms of schizophrenia. Subsequently, other antipsychotic drugs of the same chemical class, trifluoperazine, perphenazine, and thioridazine, as well as other drugs of different chemical classes, such as haloperidol, molindone, thiothixene, and pimozide, were identified on the basis of their ability to block a specific group of dopamine receptors which are now labeled as D_2 receptors. These receptors are abundant in the striatum, mesolimbic system, and pituitary gland and are responsible for the motor side effects, antipsychotic action, and prolactin-stimulating effect of the typical neuroleptic drugs, respectively. These drugs were designated to be neuroleptics because of their ability to cause catalepsy in animals, due to their deleterious effect on the function of the extrapyramidal motor system. Large-scale controlled clinical trials in the last decade after their introduction demonstrated that approximately 70% of people with schizophrenia responded to these agents with complete or nearly complete remission of positive symptoms, whereas 30% had persistent moderate to severe delusions or hallucinations despite an adequate trial of one or more typical neuroleptic drugs.[2] The latter group was considered to be treatment resistant. The fact that these agents did not improve the negative or mood symptoms of schizophrenia, or cognitive dysfunction, was noted but for various reasons, which may seem hard to understand at the current time, was not considered worthy of contributing to the categorization of individuals as neuroleptic responsive or resistant. Perhaps the basis for this was that few patients with schizophrenia, if any, could be shown to have a clearly definable improvement in either negative symptoms, for example, volition, affect, capacity for pleasure, and energy level, or cognition, for example, working memory, reference memory, attention, or executive function, to these agents, so that response to these features of schizophrenia could not be used for categorization. Thus, they were, for some of the purposes noted above, such as impetus to develop new treatments, more or less ignored.

Treatment resistance at the time of the United States clozapine efficacy and safety trial

Prior to the development of typical neuroleptics, treatment-resistant schizophrenic patients were likely to comprise those patients who required more or less permanent institutionalization. The number of such patients decreased greatly following the development of neuroleptics and community mental health centers. The ability of antipsychotic drugs to produce a greater effect on psychosis than placebo, along with safety considerations, were the only criteria for approval of an antipsychotic drug before the issue of the approval of clozapine in the United States became a possibility. Clozapine had been approved in some European countries between 1970 and 1975 and was undergoing testing in the

United States when the deaths of eight patients in Finland who were taking clozapine, along with other drugs, were attributed to clozapine-induced agranulocytosis. Although careful inquiry by epidemiologists never conclusively linked their deaths to clozapine because of other agents the patients were receiving and the peculiar localization of the deaths to a small area of Finland and specific hospitals, clozapine was withdrawn from use around the world.[3] However, four factors provided a strong rationale for further study of the drug's risks and benefits. First, many patients who had been receiving clozapine prior to its withdrawal relapsed, despite being transferred to other antipsychotic drugs. Their physicians successfully petitioned the manufacturer, Sandoz (now Novartis), and regulatory agencies to have it remain available on a strictly regulated compassionate need basis with weekly blood monitoring to detect granulocytopenia or agranulocytosis, so that treatment could be stopped prior to the development of infection. Secondly, although no formal trials were carried out, clinicians and investigators using clozapine developed the impression that it was more effective for the treatment of positive symptoms in some patients than the typical neuroleptics. Thirdly, clozapine was definitively shown to be more benign with regard to extrapyramidal side effects (EPS) than any other antipsychotic. Finally, in the 5 years of use before 1975 and during the subsequent decade of compassionate use, clozapine was never reported to produce tardive dyskinesia, whereas the incidence with typical neuroleptic drugs is about 25% in younger adults receiving drugs for 5–10 years or longer. For these reasons, Sandoz submitted a New Drug application to the United States Food and Drug Administration (FDA) to have clozapine approved for use in schizophrenia, focusing on its advantages for tardive dyskinesia rather than superior efficacy. This application was rejected by the FDA, which requested a double-blind efficacy trial to show that it was superior with regard to psychopathology reduction in patients who did not have an adequate response to typical neuroleptics. The criteria which were developed for that purpose for the pivotal United States study are given in Box 12.1. They include: persistent positive symptoms and poor global function as measured by the Clinical Global Impression Scale (CGI)[4] and poor work and social function, despite evidence from medical records of adequate trials of at least three different neuroleptics from two different classes of these agents, together with prospective demonstration that an adequate trial of haloperidol was ineffective. These criteria were the benchmark for the definition of treatment resistance. Three hundred patients were recruited for this double-blind, 6-week trial which did, in fact, demonstrate superior efficacy for clozapine with regard to both positive and negative symptoms as well as EPS. Thirty percent of the patients who were randomized to clozapine responded by the predetermined criterion of having at least a 20% decrease in the Brief Psychiatric Rating Scale (BPRS)[5] score and a total score less than 36, rating each of the 18 items on a scale of 1 to 7. Ultimately, clozapine was approved on the basis of this trial for use in neuroleptic-resistant and neuroleptic-intolerant patients.

Prevalence of treatment-resistant schizophrenia by United States clozapine multicenter criteria

Before discussing whether this is the optimal definition for treatment-resistant schizophrenia, some commentary on the proportion of patients who meet these criteria is in order. There have been no systematic studies of first-episode patients with prolonged follow-up periods to determine what proportion of them would meet these criteria. As will be discussed, some patients who are treatment resistant by these criteria are so from first contact with health care providers. Others do not meet these criteria until many years later. Therefore, only very prolonged follow-up, with nearly complete data on the entire cohort, could lead to reliable estimates of the proportion of patients with schizophrenia who are treatment resistant. These data are not available.

Studies of the proportion of treatment-resistant patients in specific groups, such as those who are treated at a community mental health center or hospital, will be biased by the method of ascertainment. In a survey of patients hospitalized chronically in Connecticut,[6] 60% of 803 patients with schizophrenia or schizoaffective disorder were judged to be eligible for clozapine by the criteria of Kane and colleagues.[7] Studies of very large catchment areas are superior but even they can be biased because of the likelihood that treatment-resistant patients may be more highly represented in populations that represent the poorer parts of inner cities. Using the same criteria, a clozapine eligibility rate of 30% was found[8] in a stabilized, random cluster sample of 293 schizophrenic patients in a Californian mental health catchment area. However, using

---

Box 12.1 Criteria for treatment resistance in the United States multicenter trial.

1. Current presence of very high levels of psychopathology according to the Brief Psychiatric Rating Scale and Clinical Global Impressions Scale, including persistent positive psychotic symptoms.
2. No period of good social or occupational functioning within the preceding 5 years.
3. Drug refractory condition defined by failure to improve despite at least three periods of treatment with at least two different classes of typical neuroleptics at doses ⩾1000 mg/day chlorpromazine equivalents for 6 weeks or more, and following a prospective trial of haloperidol at 10–60 mg/day.

less stringent criteria, namely two trials of neuroleptics (≤ 600 mg/day chlorpromazine) for at least 4 weeks, the presence of tardive dyskinesia and an evaluation of Global Assessment of Functioning,[9,10] 42.9% of the patients were eligible.[8] These latter criteria would seem more realistic and reflect the broader view of treatment resistance advocated in this review.

The estimate of 30% treatment-resistant patients which emerged from the early studies of typical neuroleptics is likely to be too low. In a review of twentieth-century outcomes, a total of 320 primary reports, involving 51 800 patients from 368 cohorts between 1895 and 1991, Hegarty and colleagues[11] judged patients to be 'improved' if they had no more than mild psychotic symptoms and, importantly, attainment of substantial levels of functioning. This latter criterion included without significant deficit, socially recovered, or working or living independently. To compare across these decades, which encompassed studies prior to and after the introduction of neuroleptics, only cohorts with ≤ 10 years of follow-up were included. The average number of cohorts per decade meeting the criteria of presumptive schizophrenia was 38.7 (SD = 27.1) with an average duration of follow-up of 5.6 years (SD = 6.5). Somatic treatment predominantly involved electroconvulsive therapy (ECT) during the 1940s and 1950s, whereas neuroleptic drugs were the main somatic treatment subsequently. The mean proportion of patients with good outcome over the entire century was 40.2%. Prior to the introduction of neuroleptic drugs, it was 34.9%. After the introduction of neuroleptics, it increased to 48.5%, but fell back to 36.4% in the last decade of the twentieth century. Thus, the majority of patients treated with neuroleptic drugs did not have a good outcome because of persistent psychotic symptoms, poor social function, or both. This apparent decline in outcome after 1986 may reflect changes in diagnostic practices, with more severe, treatment-resistant cases and fewer misdiagnosed bipolar or schizotypal patients in study populations, or changes in

health care delivery systems that have led to a decline in treatment effectiveness.

As an example of one outcome study, Helgason[12] investigated an epidemiological sample of 107 schizophrenic patients who sought psychiatric care in Iceland for the first time between 1966 and 1967. No more than 31% of the patients had a good outcome in terms of symptom response and social function. It should be borne in mind that this sample was from a country with a progressive mental health system available to all on an equal basis, relatively little poverty, and well-trained psychiatrists.

These results, which are consistent with those of Hegarty and colleagues,[11] reinforce the view that only 35–45% of patients with schizophrenia achieve good outcome with classical neuroleptic drugs. Furthermore, Hegarty and colleagues[11] did not include consideration of the level of cognitive function, quality of life assessment, or mortality and morbidity, including that due to EPS and tardive dyskinesia. Had these important criteria been included, the percentage of good responders is likely to have been even lower. Thus, poor outcome is the norm rather than the exception in schizophrenia, at least when outcome criteria other than temporary control of positive symptoms are considered.

Revised criteria for treatment resistance

The criteria for neuroleptic resistance utilized in the United States multicenter clozapine trial have been criticized as too narrow, imprecise, and vague.[13–16] For example, poor functioning for 5 years was a criterion for entry into the clozapine trial. However, patients may fail to respond to three neuroleptic trials of adequate duration within the first 4–6 months of treatment with these agents. There is no evidence that more prolonged treatment with these agents will lead to improvement. Secondly, the clozapine multicenter trial criteria emphasized persistent positive symptoms, ignoring the disabling effects of cognitive dysfunction and negative symptoms. While they did include poor function, this was not defined adequately. It is also unclear that three trials with typical neuroleptic drugs are required, since current evidence suggests that no more than one trial with a typical neuroleptic, providing it is of adequate duration, 4–12 weeks at most, and at adequate dosage, should be able to define neuroleptic resistance. The issue of adequate dosage is a difficult one. In the United States multi-center trial, very high dosage of neuroleptics was required, based on the prevailing view that higher dosage might lead to better response with typical neuroleptic drugs in some of the patients who did not respond to usual doses. Subsequent research, involving both clinical trials and understanding the relationship between clinical response and occupancy of D_2 receptors, has indicated that much lower doses of neuroleptic may be optimal with regard to the balance between efficacy, EPS and other dose-related side effects. It has been suggested that an adequate trial of a typical neuroleptic drug might be as low as 2 mg/day in haloperidol equivalents and should rarely exceed 10–15 mg/day. In any event, there is no longer any reason to believe that trials with doses as high as 1000 mg/day chlorpromazine equivalents (approximately 40 mg/day haloperidol) are necessary for an adequate trial and that higher doses might, in fact, diminish response in some patients. There is little question that higher doses reduce tolerability. Thus, shortly after the criteria

listed in Box 12.1 were published, numerous criticisms were raised, and alternatives suggested. Box 12.2 provides a broader conceptualization of treatment resistance based upon a multidimensional model.

Adjunctive treatments such as antidepressants, mood stabilizers and anxiolytics to improve response in mood, aggression, impulsivity, and anxiety are sometimes helpful and may be used to increase the proportion of neuroleptic responders. However, there is no reliable evidence that these agents affect positive symptoms and cognition in patients receiving typical neuroleptic drugs. If patients have minimal psychotic, negative, and mood symptoms, but have persistent problems with regard to work and social function, a more prolonged trial might be indicated before considering them neuroleptic resistant. However, it is likely that this failure to recover function is related to cognitive impairment, which does not respond to typical neuroleptic drugs regardless of duration of treatment, but does respond to clozapine or other atypical antipsychotics as discussed in detail elsewhere in this volume.

An international study group to define treatment resistance in schizophrenia has proposed a multidimensional approach, including psychopathology (positive and negative symptoms), functional disability, and behavior.[15] They incorporate the dimensions included in Box 12.2 and provide a useful rating scale to measure treatment responsiveness on a continuum.

Box 12.2 Pathological dimensions of treatment resistance.

1. Persistent moderate, severe positive, negative, or disorganization symptoms.
2. Cognitive dysfunction in multiple spheres which interfere with work and social function.
3. Recurrent mood disturbances and suicidality.
4. Poor work and social function.
5. Poor (subjective) quality of life.
6. Bizarre behavior.
7. One adequate trial of a typical neuroleptic which is tolerable to the patient at doses of 2–20 mg/day of haloperidol or equivalent for a duration of 6–12 weeks.

The importance of recognition of treatment resistance early in the course of this continuum is becoming apparent. Newly diagnosed schizophrenic patients who remain symptomatic and dysfunctional at the end of a first or second course of treatment with typical neuroleptic drugs are more likely to return to work or school if more effective medication, together with adequate psychosocial treatment, is given as early as possible. Evidence is also accumulating that prolonged periods of psychosis in the early stages of illness due to inadequate antipsychotic treatment have an adverse effect on outcome, and increase the likelihood of hospitalization and social disability.[17–19]

Regardless of whether a uni- or multidimensional approach is used to evaluate treatment response in schizophrenia, there will be differences in what is considered good, intermediate, or poor global response or outcome. For example, the opinions of patients, families, mental health workers, health care administrators, and fiscal personnel on this matter may vary greatly. Patients who lack insight into their illness and its influence on their quality of life may feel satisfied with their treatment, despite persistent positive or negative symptoms or poor work function. Patients with little overt psychopathology while taking neuroleptic drugs may consider their treatment response unacceptable because of moderate-to-severe parkinsonian side effects or tardive dyskinesia. Other patients may feel demoralized, depressed, and even suicidal because of their inability to resume intellectual, social or work activities at the level achieved prior to the psychosis. Similarly, parents, siblings, and children of schizophrenic patients, especially early in the course of illness, may regard any outcome rather than a return to the premorbid level of functioning as unsatisfactory. Later in the course of illness, the same individuals may be grateful for even small improvements.

Most mental health clinicians focus their evaluation of treatment response on the severity of psychotic (positive symptoms, disorganization) and negative symptoms, aggressiveness, and the extent to which daily behavior is consistent with societal expectations. Nevertheless, the financially pressed custodians of mental health resources may consider treatment response to be satisfactory if hospitalization and costly emergency room visits are avoided, with less importance attached to quality of life or persistent psychopathology.

Response of neuroleptic-resistant patients to atypical antipsychotic drugs

Numerous studies have suggested that there is no benefit to be obtained from trying two or more typical neuroleptic drugs before deciding that a patient is neuroleptic resistant. All of these agents act as D_2 receptor blockers. Other pharmacologic features such as alpha-2 adrenergic receptor blockade might add to efficacy but there are no data to support this as yet. Therefore, it is desirable that patients who fail to respond to a typical neuroleptic drug of any type should be treated with an atypical antipsychotic. Atypical antipsychotic drugs are defined as those drugs which produce fewer EPS at clinically effective doses.[20] As discussed elsewhere in this volume, there are now atypical antipsychotic drugs other than clozapine, for example, risperidone, olanzapine, and quetiapine, and these agents may be superior to haloperidol and other typical neuroleptics with regard to some of the dimensions of outcome listed in Box 12.2, including control of positive symptoms, negative symptoms, mood disturbances and cognition. Iloperidone and ziprasidone are two more atypical antipsychotic drugs in late stages of development. These five atypical antipsychotic drugs share some pharmacologic properties as discussed elsewhere in this volume. These drugs are considered by most but not all authorities to be superior to the typical neuroleptic drugs with regard to extrapyramidal function at equivalent doses. A few investigators argue that were patients treated with doses of haloperidol as low as 2–5 mg/day, there would be no difference in efficacy or EPS between any of these drugs, including clozapine, and haloperidol. However, the data to support this assertion are meager. If they have any validity, it is with regard to first-episode patients. Thus, after patients fail to respond to an adequate trial of a typical neuroleptic, they are then likely to be given an atypical agent. Many clinicians use an atypical other than clozapine as first-line treatment. Some may choose clozapine as a first-line treatment because of its demonstrated superior efficacy, freedom from risk of tardive dyskinesia, and usefulness as mood stabilizer and antidepressant.

Determination of the presence of treatment resistance

Before concluding that a schizophrenic patient is treatment resistant, factors which may account for limited response to typical neuroleptic drugs should be considered.

Compliance

First, compliance with medication should be assured, for example by using depot neuroleptic drugs or by measuring plasma neuroleptic levels, or those of a biological marker such as prolactin (all classical neuroleptics increase prolactin levels due to blockade of anterior pituitary dopamine (D_2) receptors). However, some male patients treated with low doses of neuroleptic drugs for long periods may have plasma prolactin levels within normal limits. Compliance with risperidone may also be monitored via prolactin determinations. Compliance with other atypical antipsychotic drugs may require determination of plasma levels.

Dosage

Secondly, the dose of medication should be carefully chosen. As mentioned above, there is evidence that lower doses of neuroleptic drugs are at least as effective as higher doses in the majority of patients. Lower doses are associated with fewer EPS which would be expected to translate into

better compliance (the use of antiparkinsonian drugs will also reduce EPS). While an adequate neuroleptic dose may be as little as 5–10 mg/day of haloperidol or its equivalent, some patients may require more (up to 20 and possibly even 40 mg haloperidol/day or its equivalent).

Choice of drug

A third issue is choice of drug and the number of trials with different drugs. There is little evidence for superiority of one classical neuroleptic drug over another with regard to the remission of positive symptoms. Thus, a second trial with a classical neuroleptic drug of a different class (for example, butyrophenone followed by a phenothiazine) is rarely effective. The explanation for the rare exceptions is obscure and may be related to total duration of treatment rather than a unique mechanism of action.

Other factors

In addition, a clinical judgement about psychosocial stressors and concomitant substance abuse, especially stimulant drugs, should be made. In some instances, 'expressed emotion' (the influence of the family or other care givers) on the psychopathology of patients through excessive critical comments and intrusiveness into the patient's daily life may be a significant stressor. While such an influence appears to be greater in the absence of neuroleptic drug treatment, there is still a measurable deleterious effect on behavior and psychopathology during neuroleptic treatment.

Substance abuse may cause relapse and non-compliance but there is usually limited ability to influence such behavior when it is present. However, participation in mutual support organizations, frequent urine testing and withholding of rewards (such as privileges or money) if abuse is detected are sometimes helpful.

Augmentation of classical neuroleptics with other psychotropic drugs (for example, benzodiazepines for anxiety, antidepressants for depression) may be attempted. Lithium carbonate, carbamazepine and sodium valproate may be useful to diminish hypomania and mood instability in schizoaffective patients. Carbamazepine may also be helpful in decreasing aggression. However, overall, these strategies are of limited value in the majority of patients.[21]

Characteristics of treatment-resistant schizophrenia

More males than females are likely to be treatment resistant but the proportions are not markedly different. Neuroleptic-resistant schizophrenia differs from non-neuroleptic-resistant schizophrenia in having an earlier age at onset (approximately 2 years earlier on average)[22] with an absence of gender difference from that usually found in neuroleptic-responsive patients (approximately 2 years earlier in males).[23–25] Family history of schizophrenia is not more common in patients with schizophrenia who are neuroleptic resistant. There is some evidence that monozygotic twins are usually concordant with regard to neuroleptic response.[26] Perinatal complications, which are more frequent in patients with schizophrenia than the general population, have been reported more frequently in neuroleptic-resistant than responsive patients.[27]

Premorbid function
In a study comparing premorbid function in neuroleptic-resistant and responsive schizophrenic patients,[28] greater impairment in late adolescent psychosexual, but not childhood, functioning was found to be a predictor of poor response to neuroleptic treatment. Utilizing the Premorbid Asocial Adjustment Scale[29] to assess premorbid psychosocial and psychosexual functioning in 411 schizophrenic or schizoaffective patients, 204 of whom were treatment resistant, patterns of asociality were found to be different in the two groups. Premorbid asociality during the pre-adult years was not consistently worse in patients with poor response to treatment.

Development of treatment resistance: first-episode vs later development during the course of treatment

Treatment resistance may be present from the first episode of psychosis. Although most patients at the onset of the psychotic phase of schizophrenia respond well to neuroleptics in terms of delusions and hallucinations, and remain responsive except for occasional relapses, 5–20% of first-episode patients have persistent positive symptoms during the initial episode.

These studies indicate that patients who are resistant to neuroleptic drugs from the beginning of treatment will generally have persistent positive symptoms in addition to negative symptoms, cognitive dysfunction, and poor work and social function. They will lack insight into their illness and are at greater risk of suicide or self-harm than in the later stages of illness. For the families of such patients, the burden will be great.

In a recent study,[30] comparisons among 223 patients with poor responses to typical neuroleptics were made between primary and delayed-onset treatment resistance. No significant differences between the two groups were found in terms of gender, family history of schizophrenia, and premorbid indices. Age of onset, the duration of the prodrome, the age at which antipsychotic treatment was started, the time period between the appearance of first symptoms and the initiation of treatment, and the duration period of the first hospitalization period also did not show significant differences. However, the number of hospitalizations for the primary onset group was greater and the compliance with treatment was worse. In addition, the duration of treatment after initial psychotic symptoms was shorter and the number of suicide attempts higher in the primary onset group.

Identifying a patient as a primary or late-onset treatment-resistant patient raises the matter of choosing appropriate treatment. Initiation of treatment with an atypical antipsychotic in the delayed treatment-resistant patients could alter the evolution of illness in this group; identification of the primary onset treatment-resistant patients at an early stage and intervening with clozapine or another atypical antipsychotic could also affect the outcome in this group in a more favorable manner.

There is also an iatrogenic form of treatment resistance[31] which can develop following withdrawal of clozapine treatment from patients who have previously responded to typical antipsychotic agents, as shown in the study of Gerlach and colleagues.[32] This may serve to indicate that the capacity for antipsychotic responsiveness can actually be lost in patients with schizophrenia.[31]

Course of treatment resistance

Once present, neuroleptic resistance is usually permanent. True neuroleptic resistance should be distinguished from a transient relapse despite being compliant with therapy. Relapse may occur because of increased stress, but it may indicate diminished effectiveness of neuroleptics to control psychosis as the disease progresses. Environmental stressors if present must be identified and reduced when possible. In cases of transient relapse, positive symptoms will eventually respond to neuroleptic drug administration. A temporary increase in neuroleptic dose or augmentation with valproic acid or carbamazepine may be helpful.

Biological basis of treatment resistance

Neuroleptic drugs are effective in treating positive symptoms and disorganization in about 70% of patients with schizophrenia. This is due to their ability to block the D_2 receptors in the mesolimbic system; these receptors are negatively coupled to a second messenger system – the enzyme adenylate cyclase. There is a strong correlation between the binding of classical neuroleptic drugs to D_2 receptors and their average clinical dose. There is no evidence that patients who are resistant to clas-

sical neuroleptic drugs fail to absorb these agents from the gastrointestinal tract. As the natural tendency of clinicians is to increase the dose of a neuroleptic when patients fail to have an adequate response, the dose and plasma levels of poor responders are often significantly higher than those of good responders. Paradoxically, this may diminish response because of increased side effects and noncompliance. Positron emission tomography (PET) studies and single photon emission computerized tomography studies have demonstrated that occupancy of D_2 receptor sites in the striatum is not significantly different between treatment-responsive patients and treatment-resistant patients. Thus, treatment resistance may be due to: (1) failure to translate receptor occupancy into inhibition of adenylate cyclase; (2) a defect in a subsequent biological cascade of intracellular events; or (3) the possibility that excessive dopaminergic activity is not the basis for positive symptoms or disorganization. Excessive activation of D_2 receptors may contribute to some positive symptoms and explain partial response to classical neuroleptic drugs in a few patients. There is recent evidence from PET studies that neuroleptic-responsive patients have a higher dopamine turnover in the striatum than neuroleptic-resistant patients. Toward this end it has been hypothesized that a process of neurochemical sensitization may develop over sustained or repeated periods of psychosis (and associated DA dysregulation).[33]

The mechanism responsible for treatment resistance at the onset of psychosis and that acquired during the course of illness may differ. It has been suggested that two forms of pathology may lead to treatment resistance that can manifest at different stages of the illness.[34,35] Genetically determined factors which preclude response to neuroleptics may be present in those who do not respond during the first episode. Neurodegenerative changes which develop during the course of illness in patients who had been neuroleptic responsive may contribute to diminished response to neuroleptic drugs. Abrupt onset resistance might also reflect developmental neuro-chemical changes or neurostructural deficits that preclude the suppression of psychosis by anti-dopaminergic drugs. A similar process could also develop in later stages of the illness. This process may involve change in the capacity for modulation of dopaminergic activity by mechanisms such as altered response to 5-HT$_{1A}$, 5-HT$_{2A}$ or 5-HT$_{2C}$ receptor stimulation, all of which play a role in the response to clozapine but less so for typical neuroleptics.

There is minimal evidence to suggest a structural basis for neuroleptic resistance. In a meta-analysis covering 18 studies until 1990, Friedman and colleagues[36] concluded that structural brain abnormalities did not predict antipsychotic response. However, they also pointed out that structural brain abnormalities in early-onset patients had a greater impact on treatment response than in late-onset patients. In two other meta-analysis studies,[37,38] the ventricular brain ratios in schizophrenics and patients with mood disorders were very similar, suggesting that structural changes at that level of analysis were nonspecific.

Treatment of treatment-resistant schizophrenia with atypical antipsychotic drugs

The pharmacologic treatment of schizophrenia is covered in detail elsewhere in this volume. This section will briefly review some of the issues concerning the use of atypical antipsychotic drugs in neuroleptic-resistant schizophrenia. The following tables (Tables 12.1 and 12.2) summarize some studies, the details of which will be discussed in following sections, conducted on treatment-resistant patients meeting the Kane et al criteria[7] with the three major atypical antipsychotics (clozapine, olanzapine, and risperidone) currently on the market. There have only been two case reports indicating improvement in some treatment-refractory schizophrenic patients with quetiapine.

Clozapine

The most consistent results regarding efficacy in this group of patients have been observed with clozapine (Table 12.1). The data from both open and controlled studies show superior effects of clozapine on positive and negative symptoms, compared to prior treatment with typical neuroleptics.[16,39–42] It has been found that up to 60% of neuroleptic-resistant patients treated with clozapine respond to it. Half of these respond within 6 weeks of treatment, while the other half respond within 6 months of treatment. Response to clozapine has been shown to be related to polymorphisms of the 5-HT$_{2A}$ receptor.[43] The average dose of clozapine in neuroleptic-resistant patients is 400–500 mg/day but some respond to doses as low as 100–200 mg/day and others receive maximal benefit from doses as high as 900 mg/day. Additional information about the use of clozapine is provided elsewhere in this volume. Some investigators believe clozapine is also able to treat primary negative symptoms.[44–46] However, Carpenter and colleagues have presented evidence that it is not effective in the treatment of negative symptoms in so-called deficit state schizophrenia.[47,48]

Clozapine has been found effective to treat the cognitive deficit in schizophrenia.[49,50] It is most effective in improving semantic memory and reference memory but has no effect on most measures of executive function and working memory.[49] Clozapine does not increase serum prolactin levels in man.[51] Sexual function is much less affected than with typical neuroleptic drugs. Clozapine has been reported to be effective to reduce suicidality and depression in schizophrenia[52] and also improve quality of life in treatment-resistant patients.[53] As mentioned previously, it does not produce tardive dyskinesia and produces fewer EPS than any other antipsychotic drug. Its main drawbacks are a 1% incidence of agranulocytosis, major motor seizures, weight gain, sedation, hypersalivation, hypotension, and tachycardia.

When side effects or nonresponse require the termination of clozapine, abrupt discontinuation can produce withdrawal symptoms. Therefore treatment with the replacement agent may need to be started immediately or even prior to cessation of clozapine to prevent withdrawal effects.[54]

Table 12.1 Summary of clozapine studies in treatment-resistant patients.

Clozapine (CLZ) studies	Features	Sample size	Duration of treatment	Results
Kane et al 1988[7]	Open, nonblinded, prospective, schizophrenic patients	268	6 weeks	CLZ produces significantly greater improvement in BPRS (negative and positive symptoms) and CGI
Meltzer et al 1989[55]	Open, nonblinded, prospective, schizophrenic patients	51	10.3 ± 8.1 months, median 7.6 months, up to 78 weeks	Higher BPRS total and BPRS paranoid disturbance determine good response
Meltzer 1991[44]	Open, nonblinded, prospective, schizophrenic patients	85	12 months	Patients with high positive vs low negative symptoms show greater improvement in positive symptoms; reverse found in patients with high negative vs low positive symptoms
Pickar et al 1992[39]	Crossover, placebo-controlled, double-blind, prospective, schizophrenic and schizoaffective patients	21	On fluphenazine 13–76 days, on placebo 17–55 days, then CLZ	CLZ significantly reduces total as well as positive and negative symptoms compared to placebo and fluphenazine
Tandon et al 1993[56]	Open, nonblinded, prospective, schizophrenic patients	40	8 weeks	Both negative and positive symptoms show significant improvement
Miller et al 1994[45]	Open, nonblinded, prospective, schizophrenic patients	34	6 weeks	Significant improvement in negative, psychotic, disorganization and EPS symptoms
Lindenmayer et al 1994[57]	Open, nonblinded, prospective, schizophrenic patients	15	26 weeks	Significant improvement in positive, negative, cognitive, excitement and depression subscales after 12 weeks, but no further significant improvement between 12 and 26 weeks
Lieberman et al 1994[41]	Open, nonblinded, prospective, schizophrenic patients	66 resistant and 18 intolerant (total 84)	52 weeks	52-week response rate for the total group is 57%. In addition, clozapine exhibits therapeutic effects on negative symptoms, but these are not independent from improvement in positive and EPS symptoms
Rosenheck et al 1999[42]	Double blind (CLZ vs haloperidol – HAL), prospective, schizophrenic patients	205 on CLZ, 217 on HAL	12 months	CLZ's effect on positive and negative symptoms is a single, undifferentiated effect; significantly superior on positive symptoms at all times and negative symptoms at 3 months; CLZ has no independent effect on negative symptoms at any time, after controlling for positive symptoms

BPRS, Brief Psychiatric Rating Scale; CGI, Clinical Global Impressions

Table 12.2 Summary of olanzapine studies in treatment-resistant patients.

Olanzapine (OLZ) studies	Features	Sample size	Duration of treatment	Results
Martin et al 1997[58]	Open, nonblinded, prospective, schizophrenic patients, OLZ: 15–25 mg/day	25	6 weeks, optional extension up to 26 weeks	Significant improvement in positive and negative symptoms by the end of 6 weeks; further improvement in patients completing the extension phase
Conley et al 1998[59]	Double-blind (OLZ vs CPZ), prospective, schizophrenic patients, OLZ: 25 mg/day	84 who failed a 6-week HAL trial	8 weeks	No difference in the efficacy of the 2 drugs, total amount of improvement with either drug modest
Sanders and Mossman 1999[60]	Open, nonblinded, prospective, schizophrenic and schizoaffective patients, OLZ: 10–20 mg/day	16	12 week	OLZ not effective in chronic, severe, treatment-resistant psychosis
Dursun et al 1999[61]	Open, nonblinded, prospective, schizophrenic patients, OLZ: 5–40 mg/day	16	16 weeks	OLZ at moderate to high doses effective for a significant proportion of the treatment-resistant patients
Breier and Hamilton 1999[62]	Double-blind (OLZ vs HAL), prospective, schizophrenic, schizoaffective and schizophreniform patients, 2:1 assignment (OLZ:HAL), OLZ: 5–20 mg/day	526 treatment resistant (352 on OLZ, 174 on HAL) and 1420 treatment nonresistant	6 weeks	OLZ superior to HAL regarding improvement in total, positive, negative, depressive and EPS symptoms in treatment-resistant patients; greater response rate in treatment-nonresistant patients

CPZ, chlorpromazine; HAL, haloperidol

Cost-effectiveness of clozapine in treatment-resistant schizophrenia

Treatment-resistant schizophrenia is a particularly costly form of schizophrenia because of the frequent hospitalization and crisis care required. A more effective but expensive antipsychotic which reduces hospitalization can lower overall costs, as shown with clozapine.[63–65] Despite the higher cost for clozapine relative to other drugs, and the cost of weekly monitoring, the total cost of treatment with clozapine may be lower than that of other drugs if all the direct costs associated with treating schizophrenia are considered. Indeed, Meltzer and colleagues[64] found that clozapine reduced

the direct costs associated with treatment-resistant schizophrenia by nearly 50% per year. To the extent that clozapine facilitates return to gainful employment and decreases the interference with the ability of family members to continue working, clozapine may also reduce the indirect costs of schizophrenia.

Clozapine and electroconvulsive therapy

There is some evidence that ECT can augment the response to clozapine. A recent review[66] of 36 published cases of clozapine treatment combined with ECT reports that 67% of patients benefited from the combination. The indications for combination treatment in these cases were resistance or intolerance to typical neuroleptics, or resistance to clozapine or ECT alone. The number of ECT sessions was 12 ± 6; the clozapine dose during ECT was 385 ± 172 mg/day. The procedure was reported to be safe and well tolerated. Adverse reactions occurred in 16.6% of the patients, including ECT-induced seizures (one case), supraventricular (one case) and sinus tachycardia, and elevation of blood pressure. Kales and colleagues[67] have also reviewed prior reports of combined clozapine and ECT and added their own results obtained by a retrospective review of five patients, four treatment resistant and one intolerant. They also found the combination to be safe and effective in most cases. However, the longest duration of follow-up was 2 and 3.5 months. Among the other reports of the combination, only Benatov and colleagues[68] presented data on treatment-resistant schizophrenic patients only, reporting the combination to be safe for all three patients and effective (> 40% improvement on BPRS) in two. The follow-up period in this report was also comparably longer, indicating 6–24 months of improvement in three and transient improvement in one case. Kales and colleagues[67] reported that patients with marked symptomatic improvement did not sustain improvement beyond 10 weeks. Maintenance ECT was not effective in the only patient in whom it was attempted. They proposed that the initial positive response to the combination was due to a synergistic action which was halted with the discontinuation of ECT. Kupchik et al[66] suggested that the efficacy of the combination treatment was based on mechanisms such as clozapine-induced lowering of the seizure threshold or ECT compromising the blood–brain barrier so that greater amounts of clozapine penetrate to the brain. Maintenance ECT strategies with combination treatment, especially studies with durations of follow-up $\geqslant 6$ months, are needed.

Other atypical antipsychotics

Double-blind studies comparing typical neuroleptics to olanzapine have shown conflicting results ranging from 7%[59] to 35% response.[62] In a double-blind study comparing risperidone to typical neuroleptics,[69] the response rate was 32%. In double-blind studies comparing risperidone to clozapine, the response rates have been found to be even higher, ranging from 53–63% depending upon the dose of risperidone[70] to as high as 67%.[71] These discrepancies appear to be due to differences in the degree and severity of neuroleptic resistance as well as dosage of neuroleptic drugs. Doses of the other atypical agents that have been found to be effective in neuroleptic-responsive schizophrenic patients may be insufficient for neuroleptic-resistant schizophrenia. However, doses of olanzapine between 20 and 30 mg/day or risperidone between 6 and 12 mg/day have rarely been effective in treatment-resistant schizophrenia in the authors' experience. Risperidone perhaps losing its optimal efficacy at higher doses has recently been an important issue of consideration.[72,73] Even higher doses of olanzapine are being studied but it is unlikely that higher doses of risperidone would be tried because of high EPS. The availability and extent of utilization of these agents in different countries is markedly different at the time of writing. The general consensus is that these agents are useful in some neuroleptic-resistant patients but that the proportion is less than that of clozapine. More head-to-head trials with careful determination of neuroleptic resistance by various criteria are needed to clarify this issue. It is likely that factors such as age, duration of illness, gender, dose of antipsychotic, duration of trial, and concomitant psychosocial treatments will influence the outcome. Since the atypical antipsychotic agents other than clozapine have definite advantages over the typical neuroleptic drugs as first-line agents, for example fewer EPS and possibly advantages for negative and positive symptoms as well as some elements of cognitive function, it is certainly justified to include one or more of these agents in the first two trials of antipsychotic drugs in schizophrenia. Should they not have been, it is a matter of patient preference and clinical judgement as to whether to try one or more of these agents before beginning a trial with clozapine in a neuroleptic-resistant patient.

Olanzapine

There are several open studies of olanzapine in treatment-resistant schizophrenia (Table 12.2).[58,60,61] The first two of these studies were positive, the third was not. Higher doses (25–40 mg/day) were used in the successful studies. There have been case reports of higher doses of olanzapine improving social functioning but not psychopathology,[74] as well as improving psychopathology.[75] The efficacy of olanzapine at higher doses in treatment-resistant schizophrenic patients requires further evaluation in controlled trials.

The results of controlled trials (Table 12.2)[59,62] of olanzapine's efficacy for treatment-resistant patients are inconsistent. Breier and Hamilton[62] reported that a significantly greater proportion of treatment-resistant patients responded to olanzapine (47.4%) than haloperidol (34.9%). They noted greater improvement in positive, negative, and depressive symptoms in the olanzapine-treated group compared to the control group. However, Conley et al[59] found no difference in efficacy between the patients treated with olanzapine or chlorpromazine. The response rate in both groups was quite low, 7% for the olanzapine and 0% for the chlorpromazine group. The Conley study included patients who had been previously treated with risperidone and clozapine (only patients intolerant to clozapine included) as well as typical neuroleptics. The patients in the Breier and Hamilton study were not as severely ill, consisting of both in- and outpatients who had to fail at least one neuroleptic trial over a period of at least 8 weeks during the previous 2 years. These two studies indicate the importance of defining treatment-resistant schizophrenia in a consistent manner. However, the similarities between the Kane et al[7] and Conley studies point to the fact that olanzapine may not be as effective in this sub-population of schizophrenics as clozapine is, at

least with the relatively low doses (25 mg/day in the Conley study) utilized in treating nonresistant schizophrenics. No direct comparison studies of olanzapine and clozapine have yet been undertaken to clarify this issue.

Risperidone

Some early open and nonblinded studies conducted on treatment-resistant schizophrenic patients with risperidone[76,77] indicated its effectiveness on positive but not negative symptoms. A recent double-blind study,[69] using the same criteria as Kane et al,[7] reported significantly higher improvement in BPRS total score during a fixed-dose phase comparing risperidone with haloperidol (Table 12.3). Direct comparison of risperidone to clozapine in treatment-resistant schizophrenia has also been made in multiple studies (Table 12.4). An open, nonblinded, prospective study conducted by Flynn and colleagues[78] found clozapine to be superior to risperidone as determined by CGI, Positive and Negative Syndrome Scale (PANSS[79]) total score, positive subscale, and factors of psychomotor retardation, psychosocial withdrawal, and excitement. Forty-four percent of the clozapine group and 28% of the risperidone group responded. The open nature of the study and the small sample size (57 in the clozapine group, 29 in the risperidone group) might have affected the outcome. However, their patients did not meet stringent treatment resistance criteria. Another open and nonblinded study conducted by Lindenmayer and colleagues[80] found that clozapine showed superior efficacy on all outcome measures, but the differences did not reach statistical significance, suggesting that the study was underpowered.

The double-blind study of Bondolfi et al[71] found clozapine and risperidone equally effective to reduce psychotic symptoms. At end point in the Bondolfi study, 67% of the risperidone group and 65% of the clozapine group responded as determined by 20% reduction in the PANSS score. This study has been criticized on multiple

Table 12.3 Summary of risperidone studies conducted on treatment-resistant patients.

Risperidone (RISP) studies	Features	Sample size	Duration of treatment	Results
Smith et al 1996[76]	Open, nonblinded, prospective, schizophrenic and schizoaffective patients, RISP: 6–16 mg/day	25	6 months	RISP reduces positive but not negative symptoms in a subgroup of treatment-resistant patients (significantly decreases in BPRS total and BPRS psychosis factor); high baseline negative symptom scores correlated with poorer response to RISP
Jeste et al 1997[77]	Open, nonblinded, prospective, schizophrenic patients (27.6% of 910 patients treatment resistant) RISP: 4–12 mg/day	945	10 weeks (fixed dose in the last 4 weeks)	Both treatment-resistant and nonresistant patients show significant improvement in positive, negative, and affective symptoms and improvement in psychosocial functioning; at weeks 2 and 6, treatment-nonresistant patients have significantly better response
Wirshing et al 1999[69]	Double blind (RISP vs HAL), prospective, schizophrenic and schizoaffective patients, fixed dose of RISP: 6 mg/day, flexible dose of RISP: 3–15 mg/day	67	8 weeks (4 weeks of fixed dosing, 4 weeks of flexible dosing)	RISP superior to HAL in efficacy at the end of first 4 weeks, but not after additional 4 weeks; predictors of robust response: more severe positive symptoms, conceptual disorganization, less depression, akathisia and tardive dyskinesia

grounds and does not constitute evidence for the equivalence of these drugs.[81,82] A 6-month study of only treatment-resistant patients with schizophrenia confirmed with a final run-in trial with typical neuroleptic drugs, a slower titration of clozapine, and multiple fixed doses of risperidone or clozapine is needed to confirm that risperidone is as effective as clozapine in treatment-resistant patients.

Another double-blind study[70] comparing risperidone with clozapine in a 4-week prospective trial found both treatments reduced psychotic symptoms without significant differences; however, this study was conducted on chronic schizophrenic patients, who were not necessarily defined as treatment resistant.

In conclusion, although there is some evidence that risperidone is effective in at least some treatment-resistant patients, it has not been shown to have efficacy equal to that of clozapine in treatment-resistant patients.

Quetiapine

Although there are no reported studies conducted in treatment-resistant schizophrenics to assess the efficacy of quetiapine, there are case reports which suggest that some patients in this subpopulation respond to quetiapine.[83,84]

Combination antipsychotic therapy

Although there is no basis from controlled studies demonstrating the added benefit of combining antipsychotic drugs, it is a widespread practice used in the treatment of chronic and refractory patients. However, there is a possibility that patients who are partial responders to clozapine

Table 12.4 Summary of risperidone vs clozapine studies in treatment-resistant patients.

RISP vs CLZ studies	Features	Sample size	Duration of treatment	Results
Bondolfi et al 1998[71]	Double-blind (RISP vs CLZ), prospective, schizophrenic patients, RISP dose fixed: 6 mg/day, CLZ dose fixed: 300 mg/day for 1 week, then adjusted	86	8 weeks	Both treatments significantly reduced severity of psychotic symptoms; no significant differences between groups
Lindenmayer et al 1998[80]	Open, nonblinded, prospective, schizophrenic patients	35	12 weeks	Both medications significantly effective on overall psychopathology; CLZ numerically superior to RISP on PANSS total, positive, negative, excitement, and cognitive factors
Flynn et al 1998[78]	Open, nonblinded, prospective, schizophrenic and schizoaffective patients	57 on CLZ, 29 on RISP	At least 4 weeks	CLZ has better efficacy compared to RISP; RISP shows better response rates than previously reported for typical antipsychotics

or a long-acting depot medication may benefit from the addition of an agent from a different class.[85,86] Clozapine-responsive patients who have limited tolerance to its side effects have been successfully augmented with sulpiride in a double-blind trial.[87] When a patient has failed sequential trials of all atypical antipsychotics and refuses clozapine, combination therapy may also be a reasonable strategy.

Adjunctive treatments

Adding another class of psychiatric medication may be attempted to enhance therapeutic efficacy when there has only been a partial response to an antipsychotic or to treat residual or other nonpsychotic symptoms. However, most of these agents have been found to have limited benefit and require further study.

Benzodiazepines

Benzodiazepines have also commonly been used as adjunctive therapy in schizophrenia. As adjunctive treatment, benzodiazepines have been found to be most effective for anxiety and psychotic agitation and are commonly used in the initial stages of treatment.[88] Patients with motor disturbances including akathisia and catatonia benefit from benzodiazepines. Other indications for the addition of a benzodiazepine to antipsychotic medication include general augmentation, treatment of anxiety, and short-term treatment of psychotic agitation or insomnia.[89] Although there is no clear difference in efficacy between benzodiazepines, lorazepam, diazepam, and clonazepam have been used most frequently. Most likely these benzodiazepines are favored for availability in parenteral form and increased potency. Wassef et al[90] have extensively reviewed the role of GABA-ergic drugs, including benzodiazepines and valproic acid, in the treatment of schizophrenia.[89]

Lithium

Several studies using lithium as an adjunct in treatment-resistant patients suggest that it may enhance the efficacy of antipsychotic medication.[87] Additionally, it may be beneficial for affective symptoms, impulsivity, or violent behavior.[84,87] Usually, lithium is added to the ongoing antipsychotic treatment regimen and titrated to a dose that produces a therapeutic serum level (0.8–1.2 mEq/L). Treatment-emergent problems associated with lithium include worsening of pre-existing EPS, additive cognitive side effects, and possibly increased risk of neurotoxicity, in addition to lithium's usual side effect profile.[91]

Anticonvulsants

Anticonvulsants have been found to augment the efficacy of antipsychotic medications in some studies,[92] and may be most useful for specific subgroups of patients.[93] Manic, impulsive, or violent behavior may respond well to the addition of carbamazepine or valproic acid.[88,94,95] Patients with concurrent seizure disorder or who have had a clozapine-related seizure may also benefit from the addition of an anticonvulsant.[96] Valproic acid is usually preferred over carbamazepine due to the greater metabolic interactions and blood dyscrasias associated with the latter agent. Titration to a dose range that produces therapeutic serum levels is recommended.

Antidepressants

Depression is common in schizophrenia. Addition of an antidepressant is indicated when symptoms of depression are present. Both selective serotonin reuptake inhibitors (SSRIs) and tricyclic antidepressants (TCAs) have been used to treat depression in schizophrenic populations.[88,97,98] Residual negative symptoms, obsessive-compulsive symptoms, and other anxiety symptoms may also respond to SSRIs.[99]

Drug–drug interactions can occur when either SSRIs or TCAs are administered concurrently with antipsychotic medications. Increased plasma levels of either the antidepressant or antipsychotic medication may result from pharmacokinetic interactions.[100] In particular, fluvoxamine, which is metabolized via the CYP1A2 system, can substantially increase clozapine levels.[100,101]

Beta-blockers

High-dose propranolol (in doses up to 1200 mg/day) has been shown to augment antipsychotic efficacy in treatment-refractory schizophrenia.[93] Propranolol may produce its beneficial effect through its ability to treat EPS (akathisia), by increasing antipsychotic serum levels, decreasing anxiety symptoms, or through potential anticonvulsant effects.[93]

Glycine and D-cycloserine

Recently, much interest has surrounded the use of glycine and partial agonists (such as D-cycloserine) acting through the glycine site on N-methyl-D-aspartate (NMDA) receptors in the treatment of negative symptoms in schizophrenia. Early trials with low-dose glycine produced mixed results. More recent studies with higher doses of glycine (30–60 mg/day) have shown improvement in negative symptoms when added to antipsychotic medication.[102,103] Trials with D-cycloserine have also demonstrated improvement in negative symptoms when added to ongoing typical antipsychotic treatment.[104,105] Although these agents warrant further study, the current consensus is that adjunctive glycine or glycine agonists provide some benefit as adjunctive treatment for negative symptoms.

Conclusion

Treatment-resistant schizophrenia may be a genuine subtype of schizophrenia. It most likely has various biological characteristics which diminish response to classical neuroleptic drugs from the onset of illness or at later stages of its evolution. While the most evident features of treatment-resistant schizophrenia may be psychopathological, for example, persistent moderate to severe positive, negative, or disorganization symptoms, other features should also be appreciated as important signs of treatment resistance, such as impaired work and social function, cognitive dysfunction, suicidality, repeated hospitalizations (not due to noncompliance), and severe aggression. All of these factors contribute to a poor quality of life for the schizophrenic.

An adequate response to classical neuroleptics or the newer antipsychotic drugs should include good social function as well as remission of psychopathology. On this basis, fewer than 40% of patients with schizophrenia are adequate responders. Treatment resistance can be present from the very first administration of neuroleptic drugs during the initial period of administration of these agents. Switching from one class of classical neuroleptic to another or using higher than normal doses is rarely efficacious. Also, auxiliary treatment with other classes of psychotropic drugs is rarely successful.

Clozapine is effective in 30% of treatment-resistant patients within 6 weeks and in 50–60% of treatment-resistant patients after 3–6 months of treatment, as judged by a number of outcome measures including psychopathology, cognitive function, social and work function, suicidality, and quality of life. The efficacy of the other atypical antipsychotics in the treatment-resistant subpopulation and comparative efficacy with clozapine are still under investigation. There is clear evidence, however, that these agents are effective for at least some treatment-resistant patients.

References

1. American Psychiatric Association, *Diagnostic and Statistical Manual of Mental Disorders*, 4th edn (American Psychiatric Association: Washington, DC, 1994).
2. Davis JM, Casper R, Antipsychotic drugs: clinical pharmacology and therapeutic use, *Drugs* (1977) **14:**260–82.
3. Amsler HA, Teerenhovi L, Barth E et al, Agranulocytosis in patients treated with clozapine. A study of the Finnish epidemic, *Acta Psychiatr Scand* (1977) **56:**241–8.
4. Guy W, ed, Early Clinical Drug Evaluation Unit (ECDEU) *Assessment Manual for Psychopharmacology*, Department of Health, Education and Welfare (DHEW) Publication No. (ADM) 76-338, National Institute of Mental Health, Rockville, MD.
5. Overall JE, Gorham DR, Brief Psychiatric Rating Scale, *Psychol Rep* (1962) **10:**149–65.
6. Essock SM, Hargreaves WA, Dohm F-A et al, Clozapine eligibility among state hospital patients, *Schizophr Bull* (1996) **22:**15–25.
7. Kane J, Honigfeld G, Singer J, Meltzer H and the Clozaril Collaborative Study Group, Clozapine for the treatment-resistant schizophrenic: a double blind comparison with chlorpromazine, *Arch Gen Psychiatry* (1988) **45:** 789–96.
8. Juarez-Reyes MG, Shumway M, Battle C et al, Restricting clozapine use: the impact of stringent eligibility criteria, *Psychiatr Serv* (1995) **46:**801–6.
9. Endicott J, Spitzer RL, Fleiss JL, Cohen J, The Global Assessment Scale: a procedure for measuring overall severity of psychiatric disturbance, *Arch Gen Psychiatry* (1976) **33:**766–71.
10. Shaffer D, Gould MS, Brasic J et al, A Children's Global Assessment Scale (CGAS), *Arch Gen Psychiatry* (1983) **40:**1228–31.
11. Hegarty JD, Baldessarini RJ, Tohen M et al, One hundred years of schizophrenia: a metaanalysis of the outcome literature, *Am J Psychiatry* (1994) **151:**1409–16.
12. Helgason L, Twenty years' followup of first psychiatric presentation for schizophrenia: what could have been prevented? *Acta Psyciatr Scand* (1990) **81:**231–5.
13. Meltzer HY, Commentary: defining treatment refractoriness in schizophrenia, *Schizophr Bull* (1990) **16:**563–5.
14. Marder SR, Defining and characterising treatment-resistant schizophrenia, *Eur Psychiatry* (1995) **10(Suppl 1):**7S–10S.
15. Brenner HD, Merlo MCG, Definition of therapy-resistant schizophrenia and its assessment, *Eur Psychiatry* (1995) **10(Suppl 1):**11S–17S.
16. Meltzer HY, Treatment-resistant schizophrenia – the role of clozapine, *Curr Med Res Opin* (1997) **14:**1–20.

17. May PR, Tuma AH, Yale C et al, Schizophrenia – a follow-up study of results of treatment. II: Hospital stay over two to five years, *Arch Gen Psychiatry* (1976) **33:**481–6.

18. Loebel AD, Lieberman JA, Alvin J Jr et al, Duration of psychosis and outcome in first-episode schizophrenia, *Am J Psychiatry* (1992) **149:**1183–8.

19. Wyatt RJ, Neuroleptics and the natural course of schizophrenia, *Schizophr Bull* (1991) **17:**325–51.

20. Meltzer HY, Yamamoto BK, Lowy MT, Stockmeier CA, The mechanism of action of atypical antipsychotic drugs: an update. In: Watson SJ, ed., *Biology of Schizophrenia and Affective Disease-ARNMD Series* (American Psychiatric Press: Washington, DC, 1996) 451–92.

21. Meltzer HY, Treatment of the neuroleptic-nonresponsive schizophrenic patients, *Schizophr Bull* (1992) **18:**515–42.

22. Meltzer HY, Rabinowitz J, Lee MA et al, Age of onset and gender of schizophrenic patients in relation to neuroleptic resistance, *Am J Psychiatry* (1997) **154:**475–82.

23. Seeman MV, Gender differences in schizophrenia, *Can J Psychiatry* (1982) **27:**108–11.

24. Seeman MV, Current outcome in schizophrenia: women vs. men, *Acta Psychiatr Scand* (1986) **73:** 609–17.

25. Szymanski S, Lieberman J, Pollack S et al, Gender differences in neuroleptic nonresponsive clozapine-treated schizophrenics, *Biol Psychiatry* (1996) **39:**249–54.

26. Torrey EF, Bowler AE, Taylor EH, Gottesman II, *Schizophrenia and Manic-Depressive Disorder* (Basic Books: New York, 1994) 157.

27. Robinson DG, Woerner MG, Alvir JM et al, Predictors of treatment response from a first episode of schizophrenia or schizoaffective disorder, *Am J Psychiatry* (1999) **156:**544–9.

28. Findling RL, Jayathilake K, Meltzer HY, Premorbid asociality in neuroleptic-resistant and neuroleptic-responsive schizophrenia, *Psychol Med* (1996) **26:**1033–41.

29. Gittleman-Klein R, Klein DF, Premorbid asocial adjustment and prognosis in schizophrenia, *J Psychiatr Res* (1969) **7:**35–53.

30. Meltzer HY, Lee MA, Cola P, The evolution of treatment resistance: biologic implications, *J Clin Psychopharmacol* (1998) **18(Suppl 1):**5S–11S.

31. Meltzer HY, Lee MA, Ranjan R et al, Relapse following clozapine withdrawal: effect of cyproheptadine plus neuroleptic, *Psychopharmacology* (1996) **124:**176–87.

32. Gerlach J, Koppelhus P, Helweg E, Monrad A, Clozapine and haloperidol in a single-blind crossover trial: therapeutic and biochemical aspects in the treatment of schizophrenia, *Acta Psychiatr Scand* (1974) **50:**410–24.

33. Lieberman JA, Sheitman B, Kinon BJ, Neurochemical sensitization in the pathophysiology of schizophrenia: deficits and dysfunction in neuronal regulation and plasticity, *Neuropsychopharmacology* (1997) **17:**205–29.

34. Lieberman JA, Sheitman B, Chakos M et al, The development of treatment resistance in patients with schizophrenia: a clinical and pathophysiological perspective, *J Clin Psychopharmacol* (1998) **18:** 20S–24S.

35. Lieberman JA, Is schizophrenia a neurodegenerative disorder? A clinical and neurobiological perspective, *Biol Psychiatry* (1999) **46:**729–39.

36. Friedman L, Lys C, Schulz SC, The relationship of structural brain imaging parameters to antipsychotic treatment response: a review, *J Psychiatr Neurosci* (1992) **17:**42–54.

37. Van Horn JD, McManus IC, Ventricular enlargement in schizophrenia. A meta-analysis of studies of the ventricle:brain ratio (VBR), *Br J Psychiatry* (1992) **160:**687–97.

38. Elkis H, Friedman L, Wise A, Meltzer HY, Meta-analyses of studies of ventricular enlargement and sulcal prominence in mood disorders: comparisons with controls or patients with schizophrenia, *Arch Gen Psychiatry* (1995) **52:**735–46.

39. Pickar D, Owen R, Litman RE et al, Clinical and biologic response to clozapine in patients with schizophrenia. Crossover comparison with fluphenazine, *Arch Gen Psychiatry* (1992) **49:** 345–53.

40. Breier A, Buchanan RW, Kirkpatrick B et al, Effects of clozapine on positive and negative symptoms in outpatients with schizophrenia, *Am J Psychiatry* (1994) **151:**20–6.

41. Lieberman JA, Safferman AZ, Pollack S et al, Clinical effects of clozapine in chronic schizophrenia: response to treatment and predictors of outcome, *Am J Psychiatry* (1994) **151:**1744–52.

42. Rosenheck R, Dunn L, Peszke M et al and the Department of Veterans Affairs Cooperative Study Group on Clozapine in Refractory Schizophrenia, Impact of clozapine on negative symptoms and on the deficit syndrome in refractory schizophrenia, *Am J Psychiatry* (1999) **156:**88–93.

43. Masellis M, Basile V, Meltzer HY et al, Serotonin subtype 2 receptor genes and clinical response to clozapine in schizophrenia patients, *Neuropsychopharmacology* (1998) **19:**123–32.

44. Meltzer HY, The effect of clozapine and other atypical antipsychotic drugs on negative symptoms. In: Marneros A, Andreasen NC, Tsuang MT, eds, *Negative Versus Positive Schizophrenia* (Springer-Verlag: Heidelberg, 1991) 365–75.

45. Miller DD, Perry PJ, Cadoret RJ, Andreasen NC, Clozapine's effect on negative symptoms in treatment-refractory schizophrenics, *Compr Psychiatry* (1994) **35:**8–15.

46. Meltzer HY, Is another view valid? *Am J Psychiatry* (1995) **152:**821–5.

47. Carpenter WT Jr, Conley RR, Buchanan RW et al, Patient response and resource management: another view of clozapine treatment of schizophrenia, *Am J Psychiatry* (1995) **152:**827–32.

48. Buchanan RW, Breier A, Kirkpatrick B et al, Positive and negative symptom response to clozapine in schizophrenic patients with and without the deficit syndrome, *Am J Psychiatry* (1998) **155:**751–60.

49. Hagger C, Buckley P, Kenny JT et al, Improvement in cognitive functions and psychiatric symptoms in treatment refractory schizophrenic patients receiving clozapine, *Biol Psychiatry* (1993) **34:**702–12.

50. Meltzer HY, McGurk SR, The effects of clozapine, risperidone, and olanzapine on cognitive function in schizophrenia, *Schizophr Bull* (1999) **25:**233–55.

51. Meltzer HY, Fang VS, Effect of clozapine on human serum prolactin levels, *Am J Psychiatry* (1979) **136:**1550–5.

52. Meltzer HY, Okayli G, Reduction of suicidality during clozapine treatment in neuroleptic-resistant schizophrenia: impact on risk–benefit assessment, *Am J Psychiatry* (1995) **152:**183–90.

53. Meltzer HY, Burnett S, Bastani B, Ramirez LF, Effects of six months of clozapine treatment on the quality of life of chronic schizophrenic patients, *Hosp Comm Psychiatry* (1990) **41:**892–7.

54. Tollefson GD, Dellva MA, Mattler CA et al, Controlled, double-blind investigation of the clozapine discontinuation symptoms with conversion to either olanzapine or placebo. The collaborative Crossover Study Group, *J Clin Psychopharmacol* (1999) **19:**435–53

55. Meltzer HY, Bastani B, Kwon KY et al, A prospective study of clozapine in treatment-resistant schizophrenic patients. I. Preliminary report, *Psychopharmacology* (1989) **99(Suppl):**68S–72S.

56. Tandon R, Goldman R, DeQuardo JR et al, Positive and negative symptoms covary during clozapine treatment in schizophrenia, *J Psychiatr Res* (1993) **27:**341–7.

57. Lindenmayer JP, Grochowski S, Mabugat L, Clozapine effects on positive and negative symptoms: a six month trial in treatment refractory schizophrenics, *J Clin Psychopharmacol* (1994) **14:**201–4.

58. Martin J, Gomez JC, Garcia-Bernardo E et al, Olanzapine in treatment-refractory schizophrenia: results of an open label study. The Spanish group for the study of olanzapine in treatment-refractory schizophrenia, *J Clin Psychiatry* (1997) **58:**479–83.

59. Conley RR, Tamminga CA, Bartko JJ et al, Olanzapine compared with chlorpromazine in treatment-resistant schizophrenia, *Am J Psychiatry* (1998) **155:**914–20.

60. Sanders RD, Mossman D, An open trial of olanzapine in patients with treatment-refractory psychoses, *J Clin Psychopharmacol* (1999) **19:**62–6.

61. Dursun SM, Gardner DM, Bird DC, Flinn J, Olanzapine for patients with treatment-resistant schizophrenia: a naturalistic case-series outcome study, *Can J Psychiatry* (1999) **44:**701–4.

62. Breier A, Hamilton SH, Comparative efficacy of olanzapine and haloperidol for patients with treatment-resistant schizophrenia, *Biol Psychiatry* (1999) **45:**403–11.

63. Revicki DA, Luce BR, Wechsler JM et al, Cost-effectiveness of clozapine for treatment-resistant schizophrenic patients, *Hosp Comm Psychiatry* (1990) **41:**850–4.

64. Meltzer HY, Cola P, Way L et al, Cost effectiveness of clozapine in neuroleptic-resistant schizophrenia, *Am J Psychiatry* (1993) **150:**1630–8.

65. Reid WH, Mason M, Toprac M, Savings in hospital bed-days related to treatment with clozapine, *Hosp Comm Psychiatry* (1994) **45:**261–4.

66. Kupchik M, Spivak B, Mester R et al, Combined electroconvulsive-clozapine therapy, *Clin Neuropharmacol* (2000) **23:**14–16.

67. Kales HC, Dequardo JR, Tandon R, Combined electroconvulsive therapy and clozapine in treatment-resistant schizophrenia, *Prog Neuropsychopharmacol Biol Psychiatry* (1999) **23:**547–56.

68. Benatov R, Sirota P, Megged S, Neuroleptic-resistant schizophrenia treated with clozapine and ECT, *Convuls Ther* (1996) **12:**117–21.

69. Wirshing DA, Marshall BD, Green MF et al, Risperidone in treatment-refractory schizophrenia, *Am J Psychiatry* (1999) **156:**1374–9.

70. Klieser E, Lehmann E, Kinzler E et al, Randomised, double-blind controlled trial of risperidone versus clozapine in patient schizophrenia, *J Clin Psychopharmacol* (1995) **15(Suppl 1):**45S–51S.

71. Bondolfi G, Dufour H, Patris M et al, Risperidone versus clozapine in treatment-resistant chronic schizophrenia: a randomized double-blind study, *Am J Psychiatry* (1998) **155:**499–504.

72. Collaborative Working Group on Clinical Trial Evaluations, Clinical development of atypical antipsychotics: research design and evaluation, *J Clin Psychiatry* (1998) **59(Suppl 12):**10S–16S.

73. Lane HY, Chang WH, Clozapine versus risperidone in treatment-refractory schizophrenia: possible impact of dosing strategies, *J Clin Psychiatry* (1999) **60:**487–8.

74. Sheitman BB, Lindgren JC, Early J, Sved M, High dose olanzapine for treatment-refractory schizophrenia, *Am J Psychiatry* (1997) **154:**1626.

75. Mountjoy C, Baldacchina A, Stubbs J, British experience with high-dose olanzapine for treatment-refractory schizophrenia, *Am J Psychiatry* (1999) **156:**158–9.

76. Smith RC, Chua JW, Lipetsker B, Bhattacharyya A, Efficacy of risperidone in reducing positive and negative symptoms in medication-refractory schizophrenia: an open prospective study, *J Clin Psychiatry* (1996) **57:**460–6.

77. Jeste DV, Klausner M, Brecher M et al, A clinical evaluation of risperidone in the treatment of schizophrenia: a 10-week, open-label, multicenter trial. ARCS Study Group. Assessment of Risperdal in a clinical setting, *Psychopharmacology* (1997) **131:**239–47.

78. Flynn SW, MacEwan GW, Altman S et al, An open

79. comparison of clozapine and risperidone in treatment-resistant schizophrenia, *Pharmacopsychiatry* (1998) **31:**25–9.

79. Kay SR, Fiszbein A, Opler LA, The positive and negative syndrome scale (PANSS) for schizophrenia, *Schizophr Bull* (1987) **13:**261–76.

80. Lindenmayer JP, Iskander A, Park M et al, Clinical and neurocognitive effects of clozapine and risperidone in treatment-refractory schizophrenic patients: a prospective study, *J Clin Psychiatry* (1998) **59:**521–7.

81. Meltzer HY, Risperidone and clozapine for treatment-resistant schizophrenia, *Am J Psychiatry* (1999) **156:**1126–7.

82. Rubin E, Risperidone and clozapine for treatment-resistant schizophrenia, *Am J Psychiatry* (1999) **156:**1127.

83. Szigethy E, Brent S, Findling R, Quetiapine for refractory schizophrenia, *J Am Acad Child Adolesc Psychiatry* (1998) **37:**1127–8.

84. Reznik I, Benatov R, Sirota P, Seroquel in a resistant schizophrenic with negative and positive symptoms, *Harefuah* (1996) **130:**675–7.

85. Marder SR, Management strategies for the treatment of schizophrenia, *J Clin Psychiatry* (1996) **57(Suppl 11):**26–30.

86. Naber D, Optimizing clozapine treatment, *J Clin Psychiatry* (1999) **60(Suppl 12):**35–8.

87. Shiloh R, Zemishlany Z, Aizenberg D et al, Sulpiride augmentation in people with schizophrenia partially responsive to clozapine: a double-blind, placebo-controlled study, *Br J Psychiatry* (1998) **171:**569–73.

88. American Psychiatric Association, *Practice Guidelines for the Treatment of Schizophrenia* (American Psychiatric Association: Washington, DC, 1997).

89. Wolkowitz OM, Pickar D, Benzodiazepines in the treatment of schizophrenia: a review and reappraisal, *Am J Psychiatry* (1991) **148:**714–26.

90. Wassef AA, Dott SG, Harris A et al, Critical review of GABA-ergic drugs in the treatment of schizophrenia, *J Clin Psychopharmacol* (1999) **19:**222–32.

91. Freeman M, Stoll A, Mood stabilizer combinations: a review of safety and efficacy, *Am J Psychiatry* (1998) **155:**12–21.

92. Fein S, Treatment of drug refractory schizophrenia, *Psychiatr Annals* (1998) **28:**215–19.

93. Johns C, Thompson J, Adjunctive treatments in

schizophrenia: pharmacotherapies and electroconvulsive therapy, *Schizophr Bull* (1995) **21:**607–19.

94. Okuma T, Yamashitu I, Tahaharhi R et al, A double-blind study of adjunctive carbamazepine versus placebo on excited states of schizophrenia and schizoaffective disorders, *Acta Psychiatr Scand* (1989) **80:**250–9.

95. Luchin DJ, Carbamazepine in violent nonepileptic schizophrenia, *Psychopharmacol Bull* (1984) **20:** 571–96.

96. Kane JM, Lieberman JA, eds, *Adverse Effects of Psychotropic Drugs* (Guilford Press: New York, 1992).

97. Siris SG, Depression in schizophrenia. In: Hirsch SR, Weinberger DR, eds, *Schizophrenia* (Blackwell Science: Oxford, 1995) 128–45.

98. Goff DC, Kamal KM, Sarid-Segal O et al, A placebo-controlled trial of fluoxetine added to neuroleptics in patients with schizophrenia, *Psychopharmacology* (1995) **117:**417–23.

99. Sussman N, Augmentation of antipsychotic drugs with selective serotonin reuptake inhibitors, *Primary Psychiatry* (1997) **4:**24–31.

100. Ereshefsky L, Drug interactions: update for new antipsychotics, *J Clin Psychiatry* (1996) **57(Suppl 11):**12–25.

101. Hiemke C, Weigmann H, Hartter S et al, Elevated serum levels of clozapine after addition of fluvoxamine, *J Clin Psychopharmacol* (1994) **14:**279–81.

102. Heresco-Levy U, Javitt DC, Ermilov M et al, Efficacy of high-dose glycine in treatment of enduring negative symptoms of schizophrenia, *Arch Gen Psychiatry* (1999) **56:**29–36.

103. Farber NB, Newcomer JW, Olney W, Glycine agonists: what can they teach us about schizophrenia? *Arch Gen Psychiatry* (1999) **56:**13–17.

104. Goff DC, Guochuan T, Levitt J et al, A placebo-controlled trial of D-cycloserine added to conventional neuroleptics in patients with schizophrenia, *Arch Gen Psychiatry* (1999) **56:**13–17.

13

Affective Symptoms in Schizophrenia

Sukhwinder S Shergill and Robin M Murray

Since Kraepelin[1] distinguished dementia praecox from manic-depressive psychosis, there has been continuing controversy about the precise nature of the relationship between schizophrenia and affective disorder. One of the driving forces behind this debate has been the evidence that depression is a common feature of schizophrenia. Thus, Johnson et al[2] found that 19% of schizophrenic patients had depressive symptoms while Leff et al[3] reported such symptoms in 45% of schizophrenic patients. In a review of studies, Siris[4] concluded that the modal rate is around 25%.

It is not surprising that many people with schizophrenia are depressed, since they suffer from a chronic illness which greatly disrupts their life. However, depression often occurs in the first schizophrenic breakdown. Thus, Koreen et al[5] noted that 33 out of 64 patients suffering their first episode of schizophrenia had a Hamilton Depression Scale (HAM-D) score greater or equal to 15. Similarly, 38% of the 1379 patients with first-onset schizophrenia studied by Jablensky et al[6] appeared sad, mournful or hopeless. Furthermore, those who have examined the prodroma of relapse into psychosis report that symptoms such

as anxiety and depression are particularly common.[7,8] It is difficult to dismiss depressive symptoms at first onset, or early relapse, of psychosis as a reaction to chronic illness.

Much less is known about the frequency of manic symptoms in schizophrenia. This is partly because, for somewhat arbitrary reasons, patients with both manic and schizophrenic symptoms are most often classified as having schizoaffective disorder, or bipolar disorder with psychotic symptoms.

In this chapter, we will initially consider how best to conceptualize the relationship between schizophrenia and affective disorder and then describe the treatment options. However, before addressing these questions, we will first briefly review the current diagnostic categories to which patients with both schizophrenic and affective symptoms may be assigned.

Categorical diagnosis

The development of operational definitions has meant that both schizophrenia and affective disorder can now be diagnosed with reasonable reliability. Unfortunately, different nosological systems categorize a widely varying proportion of

Table 13.1 Diagnostic criteria for schizoaffective disorder and postpsychotic depression.

DSM-IV Schizoaffective disorder

An uninterrupted period of illness during which there is either a major depressive episode, a manic episode or a mixed episode concurrent with symptoms that meet criterion A for schizophrenia.

During the period of illness there have been delusions or hallucinations for at least 2 weeks in the absence of prominent mood symptoms.

Symptoms that meet criteria for a mood disorder are present for a substantial portion of the total duration of the active and residual periods of the illness.

Exclusion of direct physiological cause secondary to substance misuse or general medical condition.

Note: Subtype bipolar or depressive type.

ICD-10 Schizoaffective disorder

Subtyped into manic and depressive type.

MANIC TYPE

Prominent elevation of mood, or elevation of mood with increased excitement or irritability; within the same episode, at least one or preferably two typical schizophrenic symptoms, as specified for ICD-10 schizophrenia (diagnostic guidelines a–d should be present).

DEPRESSIVE TYPE

Prominent depression with a minimum of two characteristic depressive symptoms, as listed for ICD-10 depressive episode; within the same episode, at least one and preferably two typical schizophrenic symptoms, as specified for ICD-10 schizophrenia (diagnostic guidelines a–d should be present).

DSM-IV Post-psychotic depressive disorder of schizophrenia

Criteria are met for a major depressive episode.

The major depressive episode is superimposed on and occurs only during the residual phase of schizophrenia.

The major depressive episode is not due to the direct physiological effects of a substance or a general medical condition.

ICD-10 Post-schizophrenic depression

Presence of a schizophrenic illness within the previous 12 months.

Some schizophrenic symptoms still present.

Depressive symptoms are prominent and distressing, fulfilling criteria for a depressive episode and present for a minimum of 2 weeks.

patients as having the conditions. For example, Castle et al[9] demonstrated that the total number of cases of schizophrenia who presented to south London psychiatrists over a 20-year period varied from 135 to 470, according to which diagnostic criteria for schizophrenia were used. The avail-ability of a similar variety of criteria for diagnosing affective disorder has a predictable consequence; for example, the frequency of depression in schizophrenic patients ranges widely in different studies, depending largely on the criterion used for diagnosing depression.[4]

Which of the numerous operational definitions of schizophrenia and affective disorder should be used? In an ideal world, psychiatric diagnostic categories would be based on knowledge of their underlying aetiology. In the absence of such knowledge, it is sensible to stick to the two nosological systems in most widespread use: (a) the tenth revision of the *International Classification of Diseases and Related Health Problems* (ICD-10),[10] and (b) the fourth edition of the *Diagnostic and Statistical Manual of Mental Disorders* (DSM-IV).[11]

Patients with both schizophrenic and affective symptoms

Kendell and Brockington[12] specifically tried to find a clear differentiation between the symptoms of schizophrenia and affective psychosis, but failed because many patients have symptoms of both disorders. How is the clinician to diagnose such patients?.

Schizoaffective disorder

The ICD-10 and DSM-IV systems suggest that the diagnosis of schizophrenia should only be made if the schizophrenic symptoms antedate affective symptoms; if they occur together contemporaneously, or within a few days of each other, then these two systems suggest that diagnosis of schizoaffective disorder, depressive or manic type, should be made. Although the nosological position of schizoaffective disorders with respect to schizophrenia and affective illness is unclear, in both the ICD-10 and DSM-IV they are placed in the group of schizophrenia/psychotic disorders (see Table 13.1). Both classificatory systems indicate that the presence of mood incongruent delusions and hallucinations in affective disorder, in themselves, is not grounds for justifying a diagnosis of schizoaffective disorder. The DSM-IV criteria specify 2 weeks of psychotic symptoms in the absence of significant mood disturbance in an attempt to distinguish this diagnostic category from psychotic depression, but this is not stipulated in ICD-10.

Post-psychotic depression

A closely related category is that described as postschizophrenic depression in ICD-10, or postpsychotic depressive disorder of schizophrenia in DSM-IV (see Table 13.1). These diagnoses are reserved for a depressive episode occurring in the aftermath of a schizophrenic illness. Both sets of criteria characterize a depressive illness sufficient to fulfil criteria for at least a mild depressive episode (present for at least 2 weeks), occurring within 1 year of onset of a schizophrenic episode and with the continued presence of some schizophrenic symptoms.

Psychotic depression

Some symptoms can occur in both schizophrenia and depression; for example, although delusions and hallucinations typically occur in schizophrenia, they can also occur in psychotic depression. The presence of such psychotic features in a depressive illness indicates severe disorder and this is reflected in both the ICD-10 and DSM-IV, where only the severe depressive illness category includes the option of the presence of psychotic features. The delusions or hallucinations can be subclassified as either mood-congruent or mood-incongruent. In the past, there was a tendency to describe patients with mood-incongruent psychotic features as schizoaffective while those with mood-congruent psychotic features were classified as psychotic depression. However, both DSM-IV and ICD-10 suggest that both should be included within the psychotic mood disorder category.

Negative and depressive symptoms

Thus, the conventional diagnostic systems distinguish categorically between schizophrenia and depression, and have ways of coping, however inadequately, with patients who have symptoms of both disorders. Nevertheless, it can be very difficult to distinguish some characteristics of schizophrenia and depression; a particular problem is the similarity of the negative symptoms of schizophrenia to depression. Many of the supposedly characteristic negative symptoms can simulate aspects of depression, and some features (such as anhedonia, anergia, blunted affect and social withdrawal) are common to both states. Therefore, before diagnosing depression in schizophrenia, one must first exclude the possibility that apparent depressive symptoms are in fact negative symptoms. Patients tend to be less distressed by negative symptoms than by depressive symptoms[13] and the latter are generally accompanied by depressive mood and/or depressive cognitions.[14] In the longer term, a valuable pointer may come from the relapsing and remitting nature of depressive symptoms when compared to the more persistent course of negative features. However, the fact that negative symptoms are often divided into primary and secondary complicates the situation; the latter may be attributed to medication, an understimulating environment, or indeed depressive illness.

Sax et al[15] examined the relationship between negative, positive and depressive symptoms in acutely ill first-onset unmedicated patients with schizophrenia and psychotic depression. Depressive symptoms were correlated with negative symptoms, specifically anhedonia/asociality and avolition/apathy, across both diagnostic groups. However, in the schizophrenia group, only positive symptoms were associated with depressive symptoms suggesting that depressive symptoms may be secondary to the severity of positive symptoms (or vice versa). The idea that negative symptoms and depression are closely aligned receives support from a study that Dolan et al[16] carried out using positron emission tomography in (a) schizophrenic patients with psychomotor poverty and (b) depressive patients with retardation. They concluded that the physiological state underlying psychomotor poverty and retardation was similar across the diagnoses.

Is the outcome of schizophrenia and depression different?

If schizophrenia and depression are quite separate conditions then their course and outcome ought to be different. It is true that, on average, the outcome for schizophrenia is worse than for depression, but considerable overlap exists, with many schizophrenic patients showing good outcome and many depressed patients having poor outcome.[17] The intermediary forms of illness, the schizoaffective disorders, have an illness course which is also intermediate; that is, more benign than in schizophrenia, but worse than in affective disorders.[18] Within the category of schizophrenia, the presence of affective symptoms is generally regarded as having an ameliorating effect.[19] However, one must remember that approximately 10% of schizophrenic patients kill themselves,[20] and that this is a particular risk for those with a history of depressive episodes, more especially those with prominent hopelessness.[21] The proportion of schizophrenic patients who attempt suicide is, of course, higher than the proportion who succeed – perhaps 20%; patients who make such attempts are more likely to meet criteria for major depression than those who do not.[22] The reader is referred to Chapter 3 for a more detailed discussion.

A continuous psychopathological spectrum

It is clear from the literature on (a) genetic liability to psychotic illness,[23–30] (b) obstetric complications,[30–32] (c) childhood function[33,34] and (d) life events[35–40] that there is little support for the idea that there are qualitative differences in phenomenology between schizophrenia and affective psychosis. Phenomeno- logical distinctions between schizophrenia and depression, and particularly between the various overlapping categories in which symptoms of both disorders occur, can only be made with difficulty, and comorbidity is very common. Furthermore, some patients present such different clinical pictures at different periods that they receive a schizophrenic diagnosis at one point and an affective diagnosis at another.[41,42] In other words, there appears to be a psychopathological continuum rather than discrete disease entities, and consequently patients may change their position on the continuum.

This spectrum of psychotic psychopathology appears to be under the influence of two major aetiological effects.[43,44] The first is 'neurodevelopmental impairment', the effect of which operates across psychosis but is maximal in chronic cases with an early onset and poor outcome. Such cases tend to have a history of a family member with a schizophrenia-like illness or of obstetric complications; they are more likely to have shown poor premorbid function. On the other hand, many patients develop schizophrenia, particularly of the relapsing remitting type, without any evidence of developmental attenuation; such sufferers often have a personal or family history of affective symptoms, and tend to become ill after some precipitating event. Thus, 'social adversity' acts on genetic predisposition to affective psychosis to produce an acute psychosis. The effect of this factor is maximal at the acute onset–good outcome pole of psychosis; such cases tend to show little in the way of structural brain abnormality on magnetic resonance imaging (MRI) scan. For example, Kohler et al[45] used structural MRI to compare schizophrenic patients with high scores on the Hamilton depression scale and those with low scores, and showed that the patients with depression were more likely to have normal temporal lobe volumes than non-depressed patients, who had smaller volumes.

These two main effects, neurodevelopmental and affective, may operate separately at the extreme poles of the spectrum of psychotic illness; however, in many cases the two appear to coexist and indeed interact. These issues are discussed in detail in Chapter 3.

Treating dimensions rather than categories

Factor-analytical studies show that symptomatology in psychosis can be broken down into dimensions. Initially, factor analysis by Liddle[46] and others of symptoms present in chronic schizophrenic patients produced three main syndromes: *psychomotor poverty*, including poverty of speech, decreased spontaneity, decreased facial expression and gestures, lack of affective responsiveness, slowness, social withdrawal, and self neglect: *disorganization*, including inappropriate affect, incoherent speech, distractibility, bizarre reasoning, and loose associations; and *reality distortion*, including delusions and hallucinations.

Subsequently, Maziade et al[47] reported that such factors could be derived not only in schizophrenic patients but also in those with bipolar disorder. Similarly, Toomey et al[48] reported common symptom factors in schizophrenia and mood disorders in their comparison of the factor structure of the symptomatology in schizophrenia, major depression and bipolar disorder patients. Van Os et al[49] pointed out that the above analyses deliberately excluded affective symptoms which are, as we have noted, common in schizophrenia, and their studies have added two affective factors which are present not only in affective psychoses but also in schizophrenia; *a manic syndrome* (excitement, poor impulse control, hostility and tension), and a *depression component* (anxiety, guilt, depression and somatic concerns). A similar result was found in a factor analysis of 509 unselected first-episode psychosis patients, where mania and depression formed two distinct factors, with positive symptoms and a mixture of negative and disorganization symptoms comprising the other two factors, in a four-factor solution.[50]

Several studies have investigated the predictors of these various symptom dimensions. Thus, results of a factor analysis of PSE symptoms in 189 psychotic patients which we have carried out at the Institute of Psychiatry in London demonstrated that delusions and hallucinations, and negative symptoms, were both predicted by family history of schizophrenia and by developmental delay; delusions and hallucination were also associated with schizotypal symptoms in relatives. However, disorganization, generally regarded as the third core dimension of schizophrenic psychopathology, was predicted by the combination of a family history of bipolar disorder and low premorbid IQ.

Thus, symptoms in psychosis can be grouped into dimensions that occur across the existing diagnostic categories. Although these are not specific to individual diagnoses, the positive and negative dimensions tend to be more prominent at the neurodevelopmental end of the spectrum and mania and depression towards the life events/genetic predisposition end; disorganization appears to occupy an intermediate position. Since the predictive validity of symptom dimensions is greater than that of diagnostic categories,[49] the obvious implication is that it is more important to treat the specific symptoms of psychosis that an individual patient presents rather than the diagnosis he or she is accorded. Thus, an individual who has both positive and depressive symptoms requires treatment for both of these.

The remainder of this chapter will be concerned with pharmacological treatment for the affective dimensions, but we wish to emphasize that drug treatment cannot be seen outside the context of a good therapeutic relationship and shared understanding of the illness. Furthermore, a therapeutic alliance between doctor and patient not only facilitates compliance, but also enables the doctor to provide a thorough explanation of likely adverse effects of any drug treatment given, the anticipated time taken to respond to treatment, as well as the relevance and likely duration of drug treatment within an overall treatment plan. We will not discuss the important role of psychological management of affective symptoms further in this chapter. Since cognitive behaviour therapy (CBT) for schizophrenia is aimed not only at psychotic symptoms but also at coexistent depression, the reader is particularly referred to Chapter 4. Here we will simply cover the use of antidepressant medication, antipsychotic medication – both conventional and atypical – and of mood stabilizers.

Depressive symptoms

Antidepressant medication

Studies using a variety of older antidepressants in schizophrenia, prior to the introduction of the selective serotonin reuptake inhibitors (SSRIs), suggested that antidepressants on their own were ineffective in treating depressive symptoms when compared to placebo.[51] However, the use of antidepressant medication in schizophrenic patients, as an adjunct to antipsychotics, has been examined in placebo-controlled studies and has been generally demonstrated to improve depressive symptoms[52–55] despite at least one negative study.[56] More recent studies using the SSRIs fluoxetine (20 mg/day)[54] and sertraline (50 mg/day) respectively as adjuncts to conventional antipsychotic drugs also report significant reductions in depressive symptoms.[55] A note of caution is necessary concerning the use of amitriptyline, which has been associated with exacerbation of psychotic symptoms despite improving depressive symptoms.[53,56]

There are few data on the length of time that adjunctive treatment with antidepressants should be continued. However, one study suggests that the antidepressant treatment should be sustained for at least 9 weeks and that discontinuation of pharmacotherapy, even after a year of treatment, risks relapse with both depressive and psychotic symptoms.[57]

Conventional antipsychotics

Despite methodological inadequacies in individual studies, the weight of evidence suggests that depressive symptoms in schizophrenia can be reduced by treatment with conventional antipsychotics, such as chlorpromazine, haloperidol, sulpiride, and thioridazine.[58–61] This is despite the reports, from uncontrolled studies, that depressive symptoms can emerge after commencement of treatment with these antipsychotic agents.[62,63] More rigorous placebo-controlled studies suggest that chlorpromazine does not differ from placebo in its ability to cause depressive symptoms,[64] and long-term depot antipsychotic treatment is protective against depressive symptoms.[65] There are still concerns that some adverse side effects of conventional antipsychotic drugs may mimic depressive symptoms,[66] and that other sequelae such as akathisia may mimic agitation. Therefore, it is important to avoid excessive doses of these drugs. Overall, there is little to suggest that any particular conventional antipsychotic is better than another for depressive symptoms in schizophrenia.

Atypical antipsychotics

It has been suggested that atypical antipsychotics may have intrinsic antidepressant effects. At present, the evidence is mostly based on case reports or industry-sponsored studies. Although we report the available information, we should point out that systematic data on the efficacy of atypical antipsychotics in treatment of mood disorders in schizophrenia are very limited.

The impetus for the study of the antidepressant effect of atypical antipsychotics was provided by reports that clozapine was effective in the treatment of affective symptoms in both schizophrenia and schizoaffective disorder.[67–71] These studies have methodological constraints, including use of adjunct medication and lack of appropriate controlled design, but do suggest that clozapine may be beneficial in the treatment of patients with coexisting psychotic and affective symptoms.

Several case reports have suggested that risperidone has beneficial effects on depressive as well as psychotic symptoms,[72,73] However, the results of two controlled studies are not so encouraging. One study reported an advantage of risperidone over the combined administration of haloperidol and amitriptyline in psychotic depression,[74] with both regimes producing similar improvements in patients with schizophrenia or schizoaffective disorder. The other found haloperidol to be superior to risperidone in improving anxiety and depression ratings, although both drugs showed similar antipsychotic efficacy.[75]

The antidepressant efficacy of olanzapine in schizophrenia, schizoaffective and schizophreniform disorder has been compared to that of risperidone and haloperidol in controlled studies sponsored by its makers.[76–78] These studies suggest that olanzapine may lead to greater reduction in depressive symptoms. A similar advantage in antidepressant efficacy in schizophrenia has also been claimed for quetiapine when compared to either risperidone[79] or haloperidol and placebo,[80] although only the second study followed a randomized control design. Finally, there is some preliminary evidence that ziprasidone may also have beneficial effects, compared to placebo, on the depressive symptoms of schizophrenia and schizoaffective disorder.[81]

Mood stabilizers

There is very limited information on the use of mood stabilizers in the treatment of schizophrenic patients with depression. Lithium augmentation has been suggested to be beneficial in the treatment of depressive symptoms unresponsive to antipsychotics alone.[82,83] Carbamazepine as a sole agent in the treatment of schizophrenia has been shown to be effective in reducing depressive symptoms in at least one study,[84] and in improving affective and psychotic symptoms in patients with affective disorder with schizophrenic symptoms.[85] Valproic acid augmentation has been used to reduce both psychotic[86] and depressive symptoms[87] in both schizophrenic and schizoaffective patients unresponsive to neuroleptic treatment.

Summary

The use of antidepressant medication may be summarized as follows.

- Conventional antipsychotics in appropriate doses do not appear to precipitate depression in schizophrenic patients.
- Conventional antipsychotics are beneficial in relieving depressive symptoms associated with psychotic symptoms.
- Atypical antipsychotics may be more effective in relieving depressive symptoms in schizophrenia than conventional antipsychotics.
- Antidepressants when combined with antipsychotics produce clear reduction in depressive symptoms.
- Resistant depressive symptoms may benefit from the addition of a mood stabilizer to antipsychotic treatment.

Manic symptoms

The short-term treatment of manic symptoms in a patient who has received a diagnosis of schizophrenia is similar to that of an individual with severe manic symptoms without psychosis. Thus, it usually involves the use of sedative medication in the form of conventional antipsychotics such as haloperidol or of relatively short-acting benzodiazepines such as lorazepam or clonazepam. In the longer term, the options are to use mood stabilizers as adjuncts to antipsychotic medication or solely antipsychotic medication. Wherever possible, the therapeutic options discussed below are based on data from studies of patients presenting with psychosis and manic features; however, because of the shortage of such data, some studies discussed concerned patients with only mania.

Conventional antipsychotic drugs

Conventional antipsychotics have comparable efficacy to lithium in acute mania.[88] During the maintenance phase, lithium was shown to have superior efficacy in a meta-analysis of four controlled studies.[89] The difference may be more significant for the prevention of depressive episodes; depot antipsychotics on their own seem effective in reducing recurrent manic but not depressive symptoms.[90,91] For the latter, their combined administration with lithium or carbamazepine appears more advantageous.[82,84]

Atypical antipsychotic drugs

Clozapine may be helpful in the treatment of treatment-refractory mania when other more conventional choices have not been effective;[92] indeed, some studies, albeit retrospective, have reported that patients with schizoaffective and bipolar disorder with psychotic features had higher response rates (74%) compared to those with typical schizophrenia (52%).[68,71] It has also been suggested that, in addition to its antimanic effect, clozapine may also act as a mood stabilizer (review by McElroy et al[88]).

Both olanzapine and risperidone have been shown to result in a significant improvement in the symptoms of acute mania when compared to placebo,[88,93] although there are also concerns that risperidone may precipitate manic episodes, especially in the absence of concomitant mood stabilizing medication.[94,95] Olanzapine has shown some promise in the treatment of the acute phase of bipolar type schizoaffective disorder, but with the most prominent effects on depressive symptoms.[96]

Mood stabilizers
Acute treatment

Both lithium and carbamazepine can be used in the treatment of acute manic episodes, prophylaxis of both manic and depressive episodes, and treatment of depressive episodes. They are effective against mania,[90,91] as discussed earlier, and probably more effective than antipsychotic medication in mood stabilization, providing protection against depressive episodes as well. Carbamazepine is similar in structure to the tricyclic antidepressant imipramine. Sodium valproate was used originally as an antiepileptic in France and was then used for the treatment of bipolar affective disorder (BAD) where lithium and carbamazepine were contraindicated or had failed.[97] However, it is increasingly being used in preference to these drugs, and this is the authors' practice since it appears effective in acute mania,[98] especially mixed affective states, and in patients with schizomania (together with an antipsychotic). The benzodiazepine clonazepam is also useful in treatment of acute mania with or without psychotic symptoms.[99]

Lamotrigine is an anticonvulsant drug licensed for monotherapy of certain types of epilepsy. It acts by inhibiting the release of the excitatory neurotransmitters glutamate and aspartate by blocking sodium channels and stabilizing presynaptic neuronal membranes. There are case reports and open studies suggesting that it has a beneficial effect in the treatment of mania, usually in treatment-refractory patients, and as an adjunct to more conventional pharmacological approaches.[100] It should be used with caution, particularly in combination with valproate (which elevates lamotrigine levels), because of the possibility of severe side effects such as skin rashes and fever, which can necessitate discontinuation of therapy.[101] The recommended strategy to reduce the risk of adverse side effects is to build up the dose of the lamotrigine slowly, and the manufacturers have provided a starting kit with this in mind. The authors have only used it in a few patients with resistant schizomanic disorder but have not been impressed with the results.

Maintenance treatment

The decision to commence prophylactic or maintenance treatment in a patient who has both psychosis and manic symptoms is based on the assessment of several factors: the severity of previous episodes of illness, the risk of adverse effects from treatment, the likelihood of a recurrence in the near future and patients' willingness to commit themselves to treatment. Once the acute manic episode has resolved, maintenance treatment with lithium has been demonstrated to decrease the relapse rate of BAD from approximately 80% (with placebo) to 35%.[102,103] There is evidence that maintenance lithium should be continued for at least 2 years from relapse, as subsequent relapses may occur when lithium is discontinued and treatment with lithium may not be as effective in subsequent episodes. It is suggested that, if a further relapse occurs during lithium maintenance, the lithium should not be discontinued but augmented with carbamazepine or valproate.

In a randomized multicentre study, the prophylactic efficacy of lithium and carbamazepine was compared in schizoaffective disorder. A total of 90 ICD-9 schizoaffective patients were included in the maintenance phase (2.5 years). They were also diagnosed according to Research Diagnostic Criteria (RDC) and DSM-III-R and classified into subgroups. Lithium and carbamazepine seem to be equipotent alternatives in the maintenance treatment of broadly defined schizoaffective disor-

ders. However, in subgroups with depressive or schizophrenia-like features and regarding its long-term tolerability, carbamazepine seems to be superior.[104]

General consensus suggests that lithium treatment should be maintained for at least 2 years, and ideally for 5 years, before an attempt (always slow) to discontinue treatment should be considered. Rapid-cycling illness, where there have been more than four episodes in the year, is less responsive to lithium treatment, and in such patients carbamazepine is probably more effective.[105] However, the results of a meta-analysis of selected studies highlighted the paucity of high-quality controlled studies and contended that there were insufficient data to support this view.[106] A more recent review has supported the continued use of carbamazepine.[107] Similar arguments can be marshalled for the use of sodium valproate in the prophylactic treatment of BAD. Here, too, there are a number of clinical studies suggesting efficacy, but also a lack of good-quality controlled studies.[108] Valproate has been shown to benefit some patients with inadequate response to lithium and carbamazepine when used alone, as an adjunct to lithium or with both lithium and carbamazepine as triple therapy.[109] This latter study reported the following response rates from their prospective randomized study: 33% with lithium, 43% with carbamazepine, 50% with carbamazepine and lithium, 60% with valproate and lithium and 62% with all three.

The vast majority of the data concerning prophylaxis of manic and depressed episodes come from studies of patients who have received a categorical diagnosis of BAD rather than schizophrenia with mania or schizoaffective disorder. However, the authors' view, as outlined earlier, is that one should treat the symptoms a patient presents rather than the categorical diagnosis he/she receives.

Summary

The acute and prophylactic treatment of mania may be summarized as follows.

- Mood stabilizers are effective as acute and maintenance treatment in patients with recurrent manic episodes.
- Conventional, and some atypical, antipsychotics are effective in acute mania.
- Conventional antipsychotics show superior efficacy in preventing manic but not depressive relapses.
- Clozapine may have antimanic and mood stabilizing properties. The role of other atypical antipsychotics remains unclear though there are encouraging reports concerning olanzapine.
- In poor responders, treatment with combined mood stabilizers may be more effective than using a single agent.
- The comparative efficacy of combined prophylactic treatment with mood stabilizers and antipsychotics over treatment with mood stabilizers alone is to be determined; however, such combinations may be more beneficial for patients with prominent psychotic symptoms.

References

1. Kraepelin E, *Psychiatrie, ein Lehrbuch fur Studierende und Artze*, 5th edn (Barth: Leipzig, 1896).
2. Johnson DAW, Pasterski G, Ludlow JM et al, The discontinuance of maintenance neuroleptic therapy in chronic schizophrenic patients: drug and social consequences, *Acta Psychiatr Scand* (1983) **67:**339–52.
3. Leff J, Tress K, Edwards B, The clinical course of depressive symptoms in schizophrenia, *Schizophr Res* (1988) **1:**25–30.
4. Siris SG, Diagnosis of secondary depression in schizophrenia: implications for DSMIV, *Schizophr Bull* (1991) **17:**75–98.
5. Koreen AR, Siris SG, Chakos M et al, Depression in first-episode schizophrenia, *Am J Psychiatry* (1993) **150:**1643–8.
6. Jablensky A, Sartorius N, Ernberg G et al, Schizophrenia: manifestations, incidence and course in different culture. A World Health Organization ten-country study, *Psychol Med Monogr Suppl* (1992) **20:**1–97.
7. Herz M, Melville C, Relapse in schizophrenia, *Am J Psychiatry* (1980) **137:**801–5.
8. Hirsch SR, Jolley AG, Barnes TRE et al, Dysphoric and depressive symptoms in chronic schizophrenia, *Schizophr Res* (1989) **2:**259–64.
9. Castle D, Wessely S, Murray R, Sex and schizophrenia: effects of diagnostic stringency, and associations with premorbid variables, *Br J Psychiatry* (1993) **162:**658–64.
10. World Health Organization, *The ICD-10 Classification of Mental and Behavioural Disorders. Clinical Descriptions and Diagnostic Guidelines* (World Health Organization 21: Geneva, 1992).
11. American Psychiatric Association, *Diagnostic and Statistical Manual of Mental Disorders* (American Psychiatric Association: Washington, DC, 1994).
12. Kendell RE, Brockington IF, The identification of disease entities and the relationship between schizophrenic and affective psychoses, *Br J Psychiatry* (1980) **137:**324–31.
13. Selten JP, Gernaat HB, Nolen WA et al, Experience of negative symptoms: comparison of schizophrenic patients to patients with a depressive disorder and to normal subjects, *Am J Psychiatry* (1998) **155:**350–4.
14. Kibel DA, Laffont I, Liddle PF, The composition of the negative syndrome of chronic schizophrenia, *Br J Psychiatry* (1993) **162:**744–50.
15. Sax K, Strakowski S, Keck P et al, Relationships between negative, positive and depressive symptoms in schizophrenia and psychotic depression, *Br J Psychiatry* (1996) **168:**68–71.
16. Dolan RJ, Bench CJ, Liddle PF et al, Dorsolateral prefrontal cortex dysfunction in the major psychoses; symptom or disease specificity? *J Neurol Neurosurg Psychiatry* (1993) **56:**1290–4.
17. Lee A, Murray R, The long term outcome of Maudsley depressives, *Br J Psychiatry* (1988) **153:**741–51.
18. Samson J, Simpson J, Tsuang M, Outcome studies of schizoaffective disorders, *Schizophr Bull* (1988) **14:**543–54.
19. McGlashan T, Carpenter WT, An investigation of the postpsychotic depressive syndrome. *Am J Psychiatry* (1976) **133:**4–19.
20. Caldwell CB, Gottesman II, Schizophrenics kill themselves to: a review of risk factors for suicide. *Schizophr Bull* (1990) **16:**571–89.

21. Drake RE, Cotton PG, Depression hopelessness and suicide in chronic schizophrenia. *Br J Psychiatry* (1986) **148**:554–9.

22. Jones P, Rodgers B, Murray R, Marmot M, Child developmental risk factors for adult schizophrenia in the British 1946 birth cohort. *Lancet* (1994) **344**:1398–402.

23. Taylor M, Are schizophrenia and affective disorder related? A selective literature review, *Am J Psychiatry* (1992) **149**:22–32.

24. Cardno AG, Marshall EJ, Coid B et al, Heritability estimates for psychotic disorders: the Maudsley twin psychosis series, *Arch Gen Psychiatry* (1999) **56**:162–8.

25. Kendler KS, Karkowski LM, Walsh D, The structure of psychosis: latent class analysis of probands from the Roscommon Family Study, *Arch Gen Psychiatry* (1998) **55**:492–9.

26. Kendler KS, McGuire M, Gruenberg AM et al, The Roscommon Family Study. I. Methods, diagnosis of probands, and risk of schizophrenia in relatives, *Arch Gen Psychiatry* (1993) **50**:527–40.

27. Maier W, Lichtermann D, Minges J et al, Continuity and discontinuity of affective disorders and schizophrenia. Results of a controlled family study, *Arch Gen Psychiatry* (1993) **50**:871–83.

28. Kendler KD, Hays P. Schizophrenia subdivided by the family history of affective disorder: a comparison of symptomatology and cause of illness, *Arch Gen Psychiatry* (1983) **40**:951–5.

29. Subotnik KL, Nuechterlein K Asarnow R et al, Depressive symptoms in the early course of schizophrenia: relationship to family psychiatric illness, *Am J Psychiatry* (1997) **154**:1551–6.

30. Maj M, Starace F, Pirozzi R, A family study of DSMIIIR schizoaffective disorder, depressive type, compared with schizophrenia and psychotic and nonpsychotic major depression, *Am J Psychiatry* (1991) **148**:612–16.

31. Cannon T, On the nature and mechanisms of obstetric influences in schizophrenia: a review and synthesis of epidemiologic studies, *Int Rev Psychiatry* (1997) **9**:387–93.

32. Verdoux H, Geddes JR, Takei N et al, Obstetric complications and age at onset in schizophrenia: an international collaborative meta-analysis of individual patient data, *Am J Psychiatry* (1997) **154**:1220–7.

33. Hultman CM, Ohman A, Cnattingiuus S et al, Prenatal and neonatal risk factors for schizophrenia, *Br J Psychiatry* (1997) **170**:128–33.

34. Davies N, Russell A, Jones P, Murray RM, Which characteristics of schizophrenia predate psychosis? *J Psychiatr Res* (1998) **32**:121–31.

35. Done J, Sacker A, Crow TJ, Childhood antecedents of schizophrenia and affective illness: intellectual performance at ages 7 and 11, *Schizophr Res* (1994) **11**:96–7.

36. Kuipers L, Bebbington P, Expressed emotion research in schizophrenia: theoretical and clinical implications, *Psychol Med* (1988) **18**:893–909.

37. Malla A, Cortese L, Shaw TS, Ginsberg B, Life events and relapse in schizophrenia: a one year prospective study, *Soc Psychiatry Psychiatr Epidemiol* (1990) **25**:221–4.

38. Brown GW, Harris TO, Peto J, Life events and psychiatric disorders. Part 2: Nature of causal link, *Psychol Med* (1973) **3**:159–76.

39. Dohrenwend BP, Shrout PE, Link BG et al, Life events and other possible psychosocial risk factors for episodes of schizophrenia and major depression: a case-control study. In: Mazure CM, ed, *Does Stress Cause Psychiatric Illness?* (American Psychiatric Press: Washington, DC, 1995).

40. Van Os J, Fahy T, Bebbington P, The influence of life events on the subsequent course of psychotic illness, *Psychol Med* (1994) **24**:503–13.

41. Chen YR, Swann AC, Johnson BA, Stability of diagnosis in bipolar disorder, *J Nerv Ment Dis* (1998) **186**:17–23.

42. Sheldrick C, Jablensky A, Sartorius N et al, Schizophrenia succeeded by affective illness: catamnestic study and statistical enquiry, *Psychol Med* (1977) **7**:619–24.

43. Murray RM, Van Os J, Predictors of outcome in schizophrenia, *J Clin Psychopharmacol* (1998) **18(Suppl 1)**:2S–4S.

44. Van Os J, Jones P, Sham P et al, Risk factors for onset and persistence of psychosis, *Soc Psychiatry Psychiatr Epidemiol* (1998) **33**:596–605.

45. Kohler C, Swanson C, Gur R et al, Depression in schizophrenia: MRI and PET findings, *Biol Psychiatry* (1998) **43**:173–80.

46. Liddle PF, The symptoms of chronic schizophrenia. A re-examination of the positive-negative dichotomy, *Br J Psychiatry* (1987) **151**:145–51.

47. Maziade M, Roy MA, Martinez M et al, Negative, psychoticism and disorganized dimensions in patients with familial schizophrenia or bipolar disorder: continuity and discontinuity between the major psychoses, *Am J Psychiatry* (1995) **152:**1458–63.

48. Toomey R, Faraone S, Simpson J et al, Negative, positive and disorganised symptom dimensions in schizophrenia, major depression and bipolar disorder, *J Nerv Men Dis* (1998) **186:**470–6.

49. Van Os J, Gilvarry C, Bale R et al, A comparison of the utility of dimensional and categorical representations of psychosis. UK700 Group, *Psychol Med* (1999) **29:**595–606.

50. McGorry PD, Bell RC, Dudgeon PL, Jackson HJ, The dimensional structure of first episode psychosis: an exploratory factor analysis, *Psychol Med* (1998) **28:**935–47.

51. Siris SG, van Kammen DP, Docherty JP, Use of antidepressant drugs in schizophrenia, *Arch Gen Psychiatry* (1978) **35:**1368–77.

52. Siris SG, Morgan V, Fagerstrom R et al, Adjunctive imipramine in the treatment of postpsychotic depression. A controlled trial, *Arch Gen Psychiatry* (1987) **44:**533–9.

53. Prusoff BA, Williams DH, Weissman MM et al, Treatment of secondary depression in schizophrenia. A double blind placebo controlled trial of amitryptiline added to perphenazine, *Arch Gen Psych* (1979) **36:**569–75.

54. Goff DC, Brotman AW, Waites M et al, Trial of fluoxetine added to neuroleptics for treatment resistant schizophrenic patients, *Am J Psychiatry* (1990) **147:**492–4.

55. Kirli S, Caliskan M, A comparative study of sertraline versus imipramine in postpsychotic depressive disorder of schizophrenia, *Schizophren Res* (1998) **33:**103–11.

56. Kramer MS, Vogel WH, DiJohnson C et al, Antidepressants in depressed schizophrenic inpatients. A controlled trial, *Arch Gen Psychiatry* (1989) **46:**922–8.

57. Siris SG, Adan F, Strahan A et al, Comparison of 6 with 9 week trials of adjunctive imipramine in postpsychotic depression, *Compr Psychiatry* (1989) **30:**483–8.

58. Dufresne RL, Valentino D Kass DJ, Thioridazine improves affective symptoms in schizophrenic patients, *Psychopharmacol Bull* (1993) **29:**249–55.

59. Krakowski M, Czobor P, Volavka J, Effect of neuroleptic treatment on depressive symptoms in acute schizophrenic episodes, *Psychiatry Res* (1997) **71:**19–26.

60. Abuzzahab FS Sr, Zimmerman RL, Psychopharmacological correlates of postpsychotic depression: a double-blind investigation of haloperidol versus thiothixene in outpatient schizophrenia, *J Clin Psychol* (1982) **43:**105–10.

61. Alfredsson G, Harnryd C, Weisel FA, Effects of sulpiride and chlorpromazine on depressive symptoms in schizophrenic patients – relationship to drug concentrations, *Psychopharmacology* (1984) **84:**237–41.

62. Harrow M, Yonan CA, Sands JR et al, Depression in schizophrenia: are neuroleptics, akinesia, or anhedonia involved? *Schizophr Bull* (1994) **20:**327–38.

63. Knights A, Okasha MS, Salih MA et al, Depressive and extrapyramidal symptoms and clinical effects: a trial of fluphenazine versus flupenthixol in maintenance of schizophrenic outpatients, *Br J Psychiatry* (1979) **135:**515–23.

64. Hogarty GE, Munetz MR, Pharmacogenic depression among outpatient schizophrenic patients: a failure to substantiate, *J Clin Psychopharmacol* (1984) **4:**17–24.

65. Wisted B, Palmstierna T, Depressive symptoms in chronic schizophrenic patients after withdrawal of long-acting neuroleptics, *J Clin Psychiatry* (1983) **44:**369–71.

66. Siris SG, Akinesia and postpsychotic depression: a difficult differential diagnosis, *J Clin Psychiatry* (1987) **48:**240–3.

67. McElroy SL, Dessain EC, Pope HG Jr et al, Clozapine in the treatment of psychotic mood disorders, schizoaffective disorder, and schizophrenia, *J Clin Psychiatry* (1991) **52:**411–14.

68. Banov MD, Zarate CA, Tohen M et al, Clozapine therapy in refractory affective disorders. Polarity predicts response in long term follow-up, *J Clin Psychiatry* (1994) **55:**295–300.

69. Calabrese JR, Kimmel SE, Woyshville MJ et al, Clozapine for treatment refractory mania, *Am J Psychiatry* (1996) **153:**759–64.

70. Zarate CA Jr, Tohen M, Baldessarini RJ, Clozapine in severe mood disorders, *J Clin Psychiatry* (1995) **56:**411–17.

71. Naber D, Hippius H, The European experience

with the use of clozapine, *Hosp Community Psychiatry* (1990) **41**:886–90.

72. Hillert A, Maier W, Wetzel H et al, Risperidone in the treatment of disorders with a combined psychotic and depressive syndrome – a functional approach, *Pharmacopsychiatry* (1992) **25**:213–17.

73. Keck PE Jr, Wilson DR, Strakowski SM et al, Clinical predictors of acute risperidone responses in schizophrenia, schizoaffective disorder and psychotic mood disorders, *J Clin Psychiatry* (1995) **56**:466–70.

74. Muller-Seicheneder F, Muller MJ, Hillert A et al, Risperidone versus haloperidol and amitriptyline in the treatment of patients with a combined psychotic and depressive syndrome, *J Clin Psychopharmacol* (1998) **18**:111–20.

75. Ceskova E, Svestka J, Double-blind comparison of risperidone and haloperidol in schizophrenic and schizoaffective psychoses, *Pharmacopsychiatry* (1993) **26**:121–4.

76. Tran PV, Hamilton SH, Kuntz AJ et al, Double-blind comparison of olanzapine versus risperidone in the treatment of schizophrenia and other psychotic disorders, *J Clin Psychopharmacol* (1997) **17**:407–18.

77. Tollefson GD, Sanger TM, Lu Y et al, Depressive signs and symptoms in schizophrenia: a prospective blinded trial of olanzapine and haloperidol, *Arch Gen Psychiatry* (1998) **55**:250–8.

78. Tollefson GD, Beasley CM Jr, Tran PV et al, Olanzapine versus haloperidol in the treatment of schizophrenia and schizoaffective disorder and schizophreniform disorder: results of the international collaborative trial, *Am J Psychiatry* (1997) **154**:457–65.

79. Mullen J, Reinstein M, Bari M et al, Quetiapine and risperidone in outpatients with psychotic disorder: results of the quest trial, *Schizophr Res* (1999) **36**:290.

80. Arvanitis LA, Miller BG, Kowalcyk BB et al, Efficacy of Seroquel in affective symptoms of schizophrenia. In: Abstracts of the Thirty-sixth Annual Meeting of the American College of Neuropsychopharmacology, Honolulu, 1997.

81. Keck PE Jr, Harrigan EP, Reeves KR, The efficacy of Ziprasadone in schizophrenia and schizoaffective disorder: an update, *Biol Psychiatry* (1997) **42(Suppl)**:42s.

82. Lerner Y, Mintzer Y, Schestatzky M, Lithium combined with haloperidol in schizophrenic patients, *Br J Psychiatry* (1988) **153**:359–62.

83. Terao T, Oga T, Nozaki S et al. Lithium addition to neuroleptic treatment in chronic schizophrenia: a randomised double-blind placebo-controlled crossover study, *Acta Psychiatr Scand* (1995) **92**:220–4.

84. Sramek J, Herrera J, Costa J et al, A carbamazepine trial in chronic treatment refractory schizophrenia, *Am J Psychiatry* (1988) **145**:748–50.

85. Placidi GF, Lenzi A, Lazzerini F et al, The comparative efficacy and safety of carbamazepine versus lithium: a randomized double blind 3 year trial in 83 patients, *J Clin Psychiatry* (1986) **47**:490–4.

86. Schaff MR, Fawcett J, Zajecka JM, Divalproex sodium in the treatment of refractory affective disorders, *J Clin Psychiatry* (1993) **54**:380–4.

87. Hayes SG, Long-term use of valproate in primary psychiatric disorders, *J Clin Psychiatry* (1989) **50**:35–9.

88. McElroy SL, Keck PE, Strakowski SM, Mania, psychosis and antipsychotics, *J Clin Psychiatry* (1996) **57(Suppl 3)**:14–26.

89. Janicak PG, Newman RH, Davis JM, Advances in the treatment of manic and related disorders, *Psychiatr Annals* (1992) **22**:92–103.

90. White E, Cheung P, Silverstone T, Depot antipsychotics in bipolar affective disorder, *Int Clin Psychopharmacol* (1993) **8**:119–22.

91. Ahlfors UG, Baastrup PC, Dencker SJ et al, Flupenthixol decanoate in recurrent manic-depressive illness: a comparison with lithium, *Acta Psychiatr Scand* (1981) **64**:226–37.

92. Calabrese JR, Kimmel SE, Woyshville MJ et al, Clozapine for treatment-refractory mania, *Am J Psychiatry* (1996) **153**:759–64.

93. Sanger T, Tohen M, Tollefson G et al, Olanzapine vs placebo in the treatment of acute mania, *Schizophr Res* (1998) **29**:152.

94. Dwight MM, Keck PE Jr, Stanton SP et al, Antidepressant activity and mania associated with risperidone treatment of schizoaffective disorder, *Lancet* (1994) **344**:554–5.

95. Sajatovic M, DiGiovanni SK, Bastani B et al, Risperidone therapy in the treatment of refractory acute bipolar and schizoaffective mania, *Psychopharmacol Bull* (1996) **32**:55–61.

96. Tran PV, Tollefson GD, Sanger TM et al, Olanzapine versus haloperidol in the treatment of schizoaffective disorder. Acute and long-term therapy. *Br J Psychiatry* (1999) **174:**15–22.

97. Goodwin FK, Jamison KR, *Manic-depressive Illness* (Oxford University Press: New York, 1990).

98. Bowden CL, Brugger AM, Swann AC et al, Efficacy of divalproex vs lithium and placebo in the treatment of mania, *JAMA* (1994) **271:**918–24.

99. Chouinard G, Young SN, Annable L, Antimanic effects of clonazepam, *Biol Psychiatry* (1983) **18:**451–66.

100. Berk M, Lamotrigine and the treatment of mania in bipolar disorder, *Eur Neuropsychopharmacol* (1999) **9(Suppl 4):**S119–23.

101. Matsuo F, Lamotrigine, *Epilepsia* (1999) **40(Suppl 5):**S30–6.

102. Pien RF, Maintenance treatment. In: Paykel ES, ed, *Handbook of Affective Disorders* (Churchill Livingstone: Edinburgh, 1992) 419–35.

103. Guidelines for the treatment of bipolar affective disorder, *J Clin Psychiatry* (1996) **57(Suppl 12A):**7–42.

104. Greil W, Ludwig-Mayerhofer W, Erazo N et al, Lithium vs carbamazepine in the maintenance treatment of schizoaffective disorder: a randomised study, *Eur Arch Psychiatry Clin Neurosci* (1997) **247:**42–50.

105. Post RM, Uhde TW, Roy-Byrne W et al, Correlates of antimanic response to carbamazepine, *Psychiatry Res* (1987) **21:**71–83.

106. Dardennes R, Even C, Bange F et al, Comparison of carbamazepine and lithium in the prophylaxis of bipolar disorders. A meta-analysis, *Br J Psychiatry* (1995) **166:**378–81.

107. Post RM, Denicoff KD, Frye MA et al, Re-evaluating carbamazepine prophylaxis in bipolar disorder, *Br J Psychiatry* (1997) **170:**202–4.

108. McElroy SL, Keck PE, Pope HG et al, Valproate in the treatment of bipolar disorder: literature review and clinical guidelines, *J Clin Psychopharmacol* (1992) **12(Suppl 1):**425–525.

109. Denicoff KD, Earlian E, Smith-Jackson RN et al, Valproate prophylaxis in a prospective clinical trial of refractory bipolar disorder, *Am J Psychiatry* (1997) **154:**1456–8.

14

Suicidal Behaviour in Schizophrenia

Povl Munk-Jørgensen

Contents • Introduction • Suicide risk • Suicide attempts • Suicidal ideation • Psychopathology • Suicide prevention

Introduction

Schizophrenia is a severe disease with a mortality comparable with those in other long-term diseases, suicide being the main cause of death. The standard mortality ratio by suicide for a number of mental disorders, including schizophrenia, is shown in Table 14.1.

As shown, the standardized suicide ratio among schizophrenics is calculated as 9.0, approximately an average measure of the examples presented.[1] One of the most urgent questions regarding the excessive mortality is whether it has changed, and especially whether the mortality by suicide has changed.

The reorganization of psychiatry during the last third of the twentieth century ought to have improved the situation of psychiatric patients such as schizophrenics, and this ought to be measurable by, for instance, a decreasing mortality by suicide. In the first part of the twentieth century, the asylum period, the mortality among schizophrenics was high, mainly owing to tuberculosis and other infectious diseases, and malnutrition. Suicide was a common cause of death, but proportionally this only formed a limited part of the excessive mortality. In the middle of the century, bizarre treatment modes contributed to mortality

to a worrying degree: cardiazol convulsions, insulin coma and leucotomy.[2]

After the first period of increased mortality due to the somatic consequences of asylum life, and the later addition of iatrogenic excessive mortality, psychiatry in the 1960s looked forward to conditions improved by the introduction of neuroleptics and antidepressants in the 1950s. Unfortunately, this did not happen. Schizophrenics are still at excessive risk of death, mainly by suicide.

Suicide risk

The lifetime risk of suicide in schizophrenia is approximately 10–13%, with most reports giving figures closer to 10% than to 13%.[3,4] Suicides among schizophrenic patients constitute a substantial proportion of total suicides. In a Finnish study, 7% of all who committed suicide in Finland in the period April 1987 to March 1988 could be identified as schizophrenics.[5] In an Australian study of self-inflicted burns, it was found that 16% were schizophrenics.[6] These prevalence figures, 7% and 16%, must be read against a background of a schizophrenia prevalence in the general population of about 0.5–0.7%.

The figures 10–13% for suicide risk originate from studies performed mainly during the late asylum period, when potent antipsychotic drug

Table 14.1 Death by suicide: standardized suicide ratio for selected disorders and treatment settings (both genders).[1]

Risk factors	SMR	95% CI
Alcohol dependence and abuse	5.5	10.7–15.9
Mixed drug abuse	13.1	10.7–15.9
Schizophrenia	9.0	8.4– 9.6
Major depression	21.2	17.9–15.0
Bipolar disorders	11.7	6.1–20.6
Dysthymia	11.9	11.3–12.6
Panic disorder	7.5	2.8–16.3
Neurosis	2.5	1.8– 3.4
Psychiatric inpatients	11.2	9.9–12.5
Psychiatric outpatients	23.0	13.4–36.8
Psychiatric community care patients	14.4	10.3–19.6

SMR, standard mortality ratio; CI, confidence interval.

therapy was available. At that time most schizophrenics were institutionalized in hospitals or in nursing homes with the opportunity for more intensive observation. Both factors should have lowered the suicide risk.

During the past two to three decades the organization of the treatment system has radically changed. Even in countries where decentralization has progressed more conservatively, the number of schizophrenia bed days in hospital settings is now only one-third of the figures from 25 years ago. This means that patients representing two-thirds of all schizophrenia bed days are now under a lower degree of supervision and observation than formerly. This, alongside an unchanged relapse rate despite availability of improved antipsychotic medical treatment, must be interpreted as continuous problems with treatment compliance. The logical hypothesis would be that lifetime suicide risk would increase.

Studies from Denmark (Figure 14.1) show that the standard mortality ratio for suicide among first-admitted non-organic psychosis during 4-year

follow-up doubled between the beginning of the 1970s and the end of the 1980s.[7]

The interpretation of these results is complicated by the fact that the number of suicides in the general population has decreased, as has the number of first-admitted schizophrenics. But irrespective of interpretations it can be concluded

Box 14.1 Risk factors for suicide in the general population.

- Male sex
- Former suicide attempt
- Substance use disorder
- Living alone
- Old age
- Mental disorder
- Severe physical illness
- Living from social security benefit
- Loss of close relative

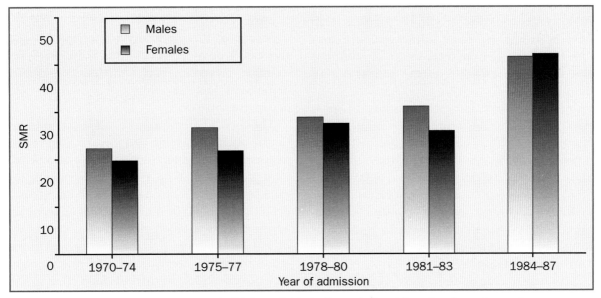

Figure 14.1 Standard mortality ratio (SMR) for suicide in first-admitted functional psychoses.[7]

that it has not been possible to derive any advantage for schizophrenic patients from the decreasing risk of suicide seen in the general population.

The strongest risk factors for suicide in the general population are presented in Box 14.1. Suicides in the general population are characterized by a higher occurrence among males than among females as opposed to the situation among suicide attempters. The same conditions are evident among schizophrenics, though not with as marked differences as in the general population. Fewer schizophrenics than other mentally disordered individuals give warnings before suicide; consequently, these suicides are more unpredictable than those among other mentally ill patients. As quoted above, the standardized mortality ratio is 9.0. Calculated for specific high-risk groups the risk ratio (RR) increases dramatically, for example in a Danish study it was found that for young males <30 years, during the first year after classification as schizophrenic for the first time, the RR was found to be higher than 160, and for an equally defined female group higher than 320 (the gender differences are due to the male suicide rate in the general population being twice the female rate).[8]

In clinical practice, these general risk factors must always be considered when treating and caring for schizophrenic patients. In addition to this, risk factors specifically identified among schizophrenics are shown in Box 14.2.

> **Box 14.2 Specific risk factors for suicide in schizophrenia.**
>
> • Revolving door admissions
> • Depressive symptoms, past and present
> • Previous admission to general hospital
> • First onset of schizophrenia at early age
> • Early phase of illness
> • Psychotic exacerbation
> • Recently discharged from psychiatric in-patient treatment

Inpatient suicide

A specially tragic subgroup of schizophrenia suicides is the inpatient suicide, because not only the victim and the relatives are involved but also the staff responsible for the patient during hospitalization.

Inpatient suicide by a schizophrenic is not a rare event. The literature demonstrates that approximately 5% of all suicides are psychiatric inpatient suicides. A Canadian study assessing more than 3000 suicides found that almost 3.4% of all suicides occurred among inpatients, and of these schizophrenic patients constituted one-third.[9] Suicidal behaviour is frequent during the first days of hospitalization, although it is seen during the whole period.

Inpatient suicide is defined as suicide under inpatient treatment even if the patient is temporarily away from the hospital on leave, trial discharge, etc. Consequently, the suicide need not be committed in the hospital to be defined as inpatient suicide. More than half of all inpatient suicides happen while the patient is away from the hospital during permitted absences for various purposes or after leaving the hospital without approval from the treating psychiatrists. Inpatient suicides have been shown to be correlated to several risk factors, which are listed in Box 14.3. General risk factors such as male sex, living alone, and substance abuse have not been listed, although they are also valid as risk factors in inpatients.

Several of the predictors are self-evident and can hardly be of any use in preventive work; for example, prescriptions of neuroleptics and antidepressants indicate nothing but psychotic and depressive patients.

The correlation to previous self-harm, previous suicide attempts, suicide ideation and an unstable treatment organization such as higher number of ward transfers may be helpful information; for example, observation of patients harbouring suicidal thoughts could be intensified and unnecessary ward transfers avoided. In practice, great care should be shown in permitting leave and extramural training in activities of daily living among patients presenting suicidal ideation. Due to the comprehensive psychiatric treatment performed in the outpatient services, including various forms of community psychiatric and social psychiatric treatments it might be necessary to introduce a new measure: 'under treatment suicide'.

Suicide attempts

In a recent study from the UK700 group a 2-year prevalence of parasuicide of almost 20% in chronic psychoses was demonstrated by Walsh and her colleagues.[10]

The schizophrenic's lifetime risk of suicide attempt is 20–40%. Thus, in a long-term follow-up (average 19 years) of schizophrenia spectrum disorders from Chestnut Lodge in the United States, it was found that 23% of schizophrenic and schizoaffective patients had attempted suicide and 6.7% had committed suicide; consequently, in total 30% had behaved in a suicidal manner.[11]

One must be aware that the same predictors pertain for suicide attempts as for accomplished suicides, with some minor differences. Warnings are fewer, and depressive symptoms less common (although these occur in half of the cases). Socially, fewer attempters are living alone than are completers.

Box 14.3 Risk factors for suicide among in-patients.

- Diagnosis of schizophrenia
- More frequent prescription of neuroleptics and antidpressants
- Previous self-harm/suicide attempts
- Suicidal ideation at the time of admission
- Suicidal ideation during hospitalization
- Higher number of ward transfers

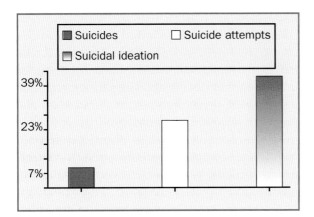

Figure 14.2 Suicide, suicide attempts and suicidal ideation in an average 19-year follow-up.[11]

Suicidal ideation

Suicidal ideation among schizophrenic patients is often hidden: that is the patient does not present these thoughts spontaneously. On the other hand, when the patient is questioned about it, it is very frequent. From the previously mentioned long-term follow-up study from Chestnut Lodge by Fenton and colleagues,[11] it can be concluded that 39.3% of the schizophrenic and schizoaffective patients had experienced suicidal thoughts during the average follow-up period of 19 years (Figure 14.2).

The 6.7% who committed suicide during the period must also have had suicidal thoughts, which brings the total up to 46%.

Among first episode schizophrenics, approximately 10% will have suicidal ideation within the first year of conspicuous illness. Frequently, postpsychotic suicides happen in the group of higher-educated patients who may be supposed to be well informed about their own situation. Furthermore, in a cohort of schizophrenic outpatients, those with recurrent suicidal thoughts or behaviour paid more attention to their own symptoms, negative as well as positive, than patients without suicidal behaviour.[12]

Psychopathology

Depression and depressive symptoms

Suicide has often been described in the residual phase following a psychotic episode. The occurrence of depressive symptoms has been found to be increased among first-episode schizophrenics both during the psychotic episode and in the months following.[13]

In the Finnish psychological autopsy study, 64% of the schizophrenics who had committed suicide were found to have presented depressive symptoms prior to the suicide.[5] Subsyndromal depression is described in between 20% and 25% of first-episode schizophrenics.

Among unselected schizophrenic patients, 5% with major depression should be expected if the occurrence of depression is the same as in the general population. However, it does not make sense to state prevalence values for schizophrenic patients in the same way as for the general population, that is in average values, as the occurrence fluctuates during different periods of the course of illness. The literature shows a higher occurrence than that expected in the general population. A rate of 5–10% of major depression in schizophrenic patients in stable treatment seems not to be an overestimate. On the other hand, dysphoria is seen in up to 50% of schizophrenics.

Other symptoms

Aggression is often described in suicidal schizophrenic patients. In a 2-year follow up of first-episode schizophrenic patients, it was found that three-quarters of the males and half of the females showed aggressive behaviour.[14] There seems to be a correlation between suicidal behaviour and both positive and negative symptoms but the findings are inconclusive. However, command hallucinations seem to be correlated with suicidal behaviour.

Substance abuse has dramatically increased among schizophrenic patients during recent decades. Consequently, even in general psychiatric wards in provincial towns that are not

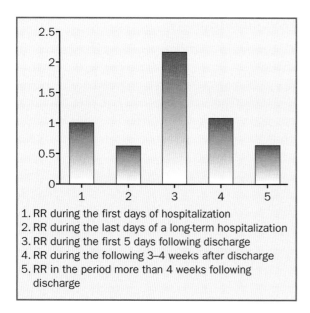

1. RR during the first days of hospitalization
2. RR during the last days of a long-term hospitalization
3. RR during the first 5 days following discharge
4. RR during the following 3–4 weeks after discharge
5. RR in the period more than 4 weeks following discharge

Figure 14.3 Relative suicide risk (RR) in schizophrenia at various times in relation to hospitalization.[8,17] Suicide risk at time of admission = 1.

over-burdened as those in socially depressed areas in cities, it can be expected that up to 50–60% of the patients will be substance abusers, taking a mixture of drugs, legal and illegal, and alcohol.[15] Having in mind that substance abuse is a general risk factor of suicide, the figures are alarming.

Hopelessness, ruminative thinking, social withdrawal and lack of activity are key symptoms in the suicidal schizophrenic patient.

Suicide prevention

None of the predictors previously mentioned has a predictive value that makes it directly useful in the preventive treatment of the specific patient because suicide in the schizophrenic patient, however, is a relatively rare event. The actions to be taken must be of such a general nature that these, besides being directed specifically towards suicide/suicidal attempts, must have a general, positive value for all patients, not only the potentially suicidal patients. As the most

important factor, sufficient and long-term neuroleptic treatment is emphasized. The antipsychotic treatment of schizophrenic patients who have committed suicide has been found to be inadequate. In the Finnish study of schizophrenics' suicides, more than half of the patients had received insufficient neuroleptic treatment or were non-compliant, while about one-quarter comprised compliant non-responders. Three-quarters of these patients received insufficient medical treatment, therefore.[16]

No matter how the cause/effect relations are in correlation with insufficient neuroleptic treatment and suicide, a general decrease of the relapse frequency should be expected among schizophrenic patients by intensified efforts in drug treatment.

Included in sufficient neuroleptic treatment is also the effort of avoiding dropout; from drug treatment in particular and from treatment contact in general.

Schizophrenic patients frequently drop out of treatment and therefore require a maximum effort to maintain contact and ensure continuous neuroleptic treatment. The use of novel antipsychotics with their lower adverse effects may facilitate the latter. Psychoeducative treatment might be expected to increase compliance in the shape of both more contact with the health service system and improved drug compliance. However, in this connection one must be aware of the increased risk of suicide found among patients who have more insight into their own disease.

One must assume that decentralized community-based organization of the psychiatric treatment services is a risk factor in itself. As postpsychotic depression is a distinct risk factor, the tendency towards short-term admissions only may prove fatal to some schizophrenic patients. The benefit achieved by a fast return home for the majority might be a risk factor imposed on the few who are in danger of committing suicide. The greatest risk of suicide in a course of illness is in the first week following discharge, most clearly shown by Mortensen's group from Denmark. This risk is markedly increased for up to 6 months after discharge.[8,17]

In a recent study of suicides after discharge from psychiatric inpatient care (also including schizophrenia) in Manchester, the Danish findings were replicated.[18] Furthermore, the suicide victims had experienced a significant care reduction compared with non-suicide mental disorder controls (odds ratio: 3.7, 95% CI: 1.8–7.6). But the risk caused by a decentralized community model might be neutralized by attention to the psychopathological predictors, especially depressive symptoms, suicidal thoughts, and to a lesser degree psychotic symptoms. This calls for the use of structured interviews at regular intervals. It is known that a general non-structured interview with a patient overlooks more than half of the symptomatology present compared with what is uncovered by use of a structured interview technique. This practice is especially recommended where depressive symptoms are involved, since less attention is often paid to these than to the psychotic symptoms.

The psychiatrist must be ready to take the consequences of the findings and never discharge a schizophrenic patient who has postpsychotic depressive symptoms or a patient whose psychotic symptoms are not adequately treated, no matter what the local political ideology dictates. Do not ever discharge a schizophrenic patient on a Friday when all decentralized services are closed, but wait until Monday morning. Never ask the discharged patient to contact the decentralized community service, but let the staff from the service follow up the patient so that continuity is guaranteed.

Social efforts can be used, as these will benefit all, including the patients who are potential suicides. Social and other demographic predictors alone are useless in the prophylactic treatment of suicide. Living alone and unemployment are predictors for suicide but are of no use in clinical prophylactic efforts towards the individual schizophrenic patient, as the great majority of all schizophrenic patients are unemployed and live alone, and as only a minority will attempt suicide/commit suicide.

The same can be said about substance use disorders. There has been a dramatic increase in the occurrence of these disorders among schizophrenic patients. A general effort to control abuse among schizophrenic patients might benefit the group generally and probably also the few potential suicides.

All schizophrenic patients are at all times in the course of illness at risk of committing suicide. Therefore, there must be a generally increased attention to, and initiatives towards, a maximal effort aiming at sufficient treatment with high compliance.

Finally, a profile of the maximum high-risk patient: he is a young male with recent onset of schizophrenia. He has formerly shown suicidal behaviour. He is unemployed, and lives alone under unfavourable conditions. He is in the postpsychotic phase, and has continuous depressive symptoms. He tries to avoid drug treatment, and prefers to return to his substance abuse. He is intelligent and has, when not psychotic, a clear insight into his own disease. He has just been discharged on a Friday afternoon to his own apartment, where he must be alone during the weekend, and has been told to go to the nearby community mental health centre on Monday.

References

1. Harris EC, Barraclough B, Excess mortality of mental disorder, *Br J Psychiatry* (1998) **173**:11–53.
2. Brown S, Excess mortality of schizophrenia, *Br J Psychiatry* (1997) **171**:502–8.
3. Harkavy-Friedman JM, Nelson E, Assessment and intervention for the suicidal patient with schizophrenia, *Psychiatr Q* (1997) **68**:361–75.
4. Harkavy-Friedman JM, Nelson E, Management of the suicidal patient with schizophrenia, *Psychiatr Clin North Am* (1997); **20**:625–40.
5. Heilä H, Isometsä ET, Henriksson MM et al,

Suicide and schizophrenia: a nationwide psychological autopsy study on age- and sex-specific clinical characteristics of 92 suicide victims with schizophrenia, *Am J Psychiatry* (1997) **154:**1235–42.

6. Cameron DR, Pegg ST, Muller M, Self-inflicted burns, *Burns* (1997) **23:**519–21.

7. Ministry of Health's Life Expectancy Committee, Development in suicide mortality in Denmark 1955–1991 (in Danish), Ministry of Health (1994).

8. Mortensen PB, Suicide among schizophrenic patients: occurrence and risk factors, *Clin Neuropharmacol* (1995) **18:**51–8

9. Proulx F, Lesage AD, Grunberg F, One hundred in-patient suicides. *Br J Psychiatry* (1997) **171:**247–50.

10. Walsh E, Harvey K, White I et al, Prevalence and predictors of parasuicide in chronic psychosis, *Acta Psychiatr Scand* (1999) **100:**375–82.

11. Fenton WS, McGlashan TH, Victor BJ, Blyler CR, Symptoms, sub type, and suicidality in patients with schizophrenia spectrum disorders, *Am J Psychiatry* (1997) **154:**199–204.

12. Amador XF, Friedman JH, Kasapis C et al, Suicidal behavior in schizophrenia and its relationship to awareness of illness, *Am J Psychiatry* (1996) **153:**1185–8.

13. Addington D, Addington J, Patten S, Depression in people with first-episode schizophrenia, *Br J Psychiatry* (1998) **172(Suppl 33):**90–2.

14. Steinert T, Wiebe C, Gebhardt RP, Aggressive behavior against self and others among first-admission patients with schizophrenia, *Psychiatr Serv* (1999) **50:**85–90.

15. Hansen SS, Munk-Jørgensen P, Guldbæk B et al, Psychoactive substance use diagnoses among psychiatric inpatients, *Acta Psychiatr Scand* (2000), in press.

16. Heilä H, Isometsä ET, Henriksson MM et al, Suicide victims with schizophrenia in different treatment phases and adequacy of antipsychotic medication, *J Clin Psychiatry* (1999) **60:**200–8.

17. Rossau CD, Mortensen PB, Risk factors for suicide in patients with schizophrenia: nested case-control study, *Br J Psychiatry* (1997) **171:**355–9.

18. Appleby L, Dennehy JA, Thomas CS et al, Aftercare and clinical characteristics of people with mental illness who commit suicide: a case-control study, *Lancet* (1999) **353:**1397–400.

15(i)

Violent Patients: Managing Acute Disturbance

Ceri L Evans and Lyn S Pilowsky

The management of psychiatric patients who are either actively violent or appear to be on the threshold of violence constitutes a psychiatric emergency. The risk of significant physical and psychological harm to the patient, staff or other patients as a result of violent behaviour means that there is a demand for early and safe containment of potentially dangerous situations. However, despite the obvious need for effective and consistent approaches to the management of acute disturbance, the development of clinical guidelines has been hampered by the relative shortage of relevant empirical evidence to support particular clinical interventions. Nevertheless, most modern psychiatric units dealing with potentially violent patients have constructed guidelines for rapid tranquillization (RT), albeit with widely varying protocols. This chapter is mainly concerned with summarizing the empirical evidence concerning pharmacological interventions in the acute management of violent behaviour in mental health care settings. In an attempt to put the use of RT within a realistic clinical context, principles relating to various non-drug aspects of management of acute disturbance are also presented within a practical sequential

framework, although it is not intended that this material should constitute a comprehensive treatment algorithm.

Clinical priorities

There are three overriding priorities to keep in mind when managing violent behaviour in psychiatric settings. The first objective, the rapid establishment of a safe environment for both staff and patients, is paramount; protection of property is rightly regarded as having a lower priority. Second, attempts should be made to relieve the acute distress of the patient who is either involved with or who is threatening violent behaviour. Third, good management should also enable adequate diagnostic and risk formulation to take place, with a view to effective future risk management.

Gaining control

The achievement of containment and control is, in a broad sense, the initial objective in the management of violent behaviour. On arriving at the scene of a violent incident, medical staff will often find that nursing staff have already established a level of physical control over the situation, and the violent activity will typically have concluded. Many patients will require 'control and restraint' (C and R) procedures to terminate their violent actions. Although the meaning of restraint varies between countries, with several European countries and American states employing belts, cuffs or straightjacket-type apparatus to restrict patients' movements, it is taken here to mean a co-ordinated and safe physical immobilization of a patient. No strong empirically based statements can be made concerning the methods of control and restraint, but it is obviously appropriate for staff to be in adequate numbers, to have been adequately trained, and to be appropriately led in a clinical sense, before C and R is performed. Once immobilization of the patient has been achieved, the immediate physical environment can be made safe, other patients can be moved to appropriate areas of the ward if this has not already been accomplished, the help of additional staff for restraining the patient or for supervision of other patients can be enlisted, and time can be created for rational decision-making.

On some occasions a violent act will not yet have occurred but will be deemed imminent, and the patient may need to be interviewed. There are well-accepted guidelines for safe interviewing techniques involving potentially violent patients, including the removal from the interviewing location of potential weapons, the careful positioning of staff nearest to exits or escape routes and emergency alarms, and use of appropriate staff numbers.[1] On other occasions, the high level of violence or situational factors, such as use of a weapon, will make it inappropriate for staff to attempt C and R procedures, and the help of additional professional services such as the police may be required. Once the senior members of the managing team who have the authority for overseeing the incident are identified, a safe environment has been established, and a level of control attained, attention can be turned to the careful selection, sequencing and implementation of various non-pharmacological and pharmacological options, on the basis of the clinical situation.

Differential diagnosis

There are two distinct but related tasks with respect to clinical formulation of the violent or near-violent incident, with the pressure to make decisions relatively quickly often contributing to an anxiety-provoking situation. The first task is to arrive at a provisional diagnosis for the patient, although this may already be established. It is often adequate to decide in general terms whether the patient has an organic presentation with an acute confusional state, an acute psychosis, or an acute stress reaction with a vulnerable premorbid personality, that is, non-organic and non-psychotic. Although less specific, this kind of categorization can assist decision-making about the likely usefulness of a pharmacological intervention, and the degree of urgency attached to medical examination and investigation. A broad range of diagnoses is associated with acutely disturbed and violent behaviour, including psychotic disorders, personality disorders, substance abuse, neurotic conditions, and a wide list of organic pathologies.[2]

The second task is to formulate the clinical situation from a forensic, risk assessment perspective, of which diagnosis only forms a part. Making a diagnosis alone is inadequate as a risk assessment. Basic risk assessment requires consideration of various elements concerning 'the patient, the circumstances, and the victim' (the 'triad') as a minimum analysis of violent behaviour.[3] Situational factors are likely to be crucial in any adequate assessment, as it has been demonstrated that a range of ward-environment factors either precede or are associated with violent behaviour, including overcrowding, certain times of the day such as medication time, substance misuse, provocation by other patients or visitors, the turning down of requests, and the availability of weapons.[4] Restricting the assessment solely to diagnostic issues is likely to undermine effective interventions and later risk management.

Non-pharmacological interventions

The two general strategies that can be utilized are either attempting to 'de-escalate' the situation using psychological approaches such as distraction or 'talking down', or the use of seclusion. Psychological approaches are based on giving the patient concerned real options (if they are available) within clear boundaries, so that he or she has the opportunity to 'save face' and can avoid the perception that a 'back down' is necessary. This requires a style of interviewing that is non-confrontational but firm, with the measured use of an empathic attitude with non-threatening non-verbal cues.[5] The use of seclusion can often be avoided with the astute use of restraint and other clinical measures. Although temporarily removing staff and other patients from potentially violent behaviour, seclusion has not been shown to influence the course of the illness, to improve compliance with oral medication or to reduce future violent behaviour,[6] although it can have a positive effect on staff morale. The establishment and maintenance of a quiet, calm atmosphere makes a major contribution to successful outcomes in situations requiring RT.

Pharmacological interventions

There is a range of important methodological factors which undermine the degree of confidence it is appropriate to have concerning the use of medications in RT. The lack of consistency between studies in terms of the use of defining terminology, for instance 'disturbed' vs 'violent', and in the assessment measures utilized, means that it is not possible to make strong statements concerning between-study comparisons. Furthermore, the contribution of mental state and diagnostic issues, and situational variables, have not generally been considered in enough depth to make it possible to consider how these factors interact with medication in emergency situations. The evidence-base is, therefore, largely reliant upon 'open' or poorly controlled studies across all drug groups, and, as a result, there are significant variations in medication regimens employed for RT in practice. In particular, there is no convincing consensus in the literature for appropriate emergency dosages for any of the classes of drugs to be discussed here. This is mainly due to pharmacokinetic factors contributing to interindividual variation in response to psychotropic drugs, and to their sedative effect in particular. Effect varies with patient size, severity of illness, responsiveness of tissues and concentration of drug at the site of action. It has been suggested that dosage should be guided by the level of clinical improvement, with an emphasis on avoidance of oversedation before diagnostic issues are resolved.[7]

Antipsychotics

The therapeutic effect looked for with the use of antipsychotics in RT is rapid sedation (with a time scale of minutes to hours); rapid 'neuroleptization' has been discredited as a realistic and safe option in these circumstances, and it is accepted that the true 'antipsychotic' effect has an irreducible time scale of several days to weeks.[8] The antipsychotic drugs which have been the most fully investigated and therefore favoured for use in RT have been the high potency neuroleptics haloperidol and droperidol.[7,9–11] Other antipsychotics, including loxapine, thioridazine and molindone, do not show increased efficacy over haloperidol.[12] Newer drugs including the atypical antipsychotics such as clozapine have yet to be assessed in emergency settings. The acetate form of the zuclopenthixol depot injection is a valuable introduction because of its intermediate action, with sedative properties apparent up to 3 days, thus avoiding the need for repeated antipsychotic injections,[13] although this medium-term injectable antipsychotic is contraindicated in antipsychotic naïve or struggling patients.

A major factor influencing drug selection is safety, including the presence or absence of side effects. Chlorpromazine, despite retaining widespread popularity as a drug of first choice in RT,[14] is not advised for parenteral use because it is painful when given by the intramuscular route, and has been associated with profound hypotension secondary to its alpha-adrenergic blocking properties, and even sudden death.[15] Haloperidol and droperidol are both reported to have a low incidence of side effects,[7] and their cardiorespiratory safety is well established even in cardiac intensive care settings,[16] although there are some reports of serious adverse side effects, including cardiac arrest, and death;[17] these adverse reactions may be related to direct exposure of high concentrations of drug to cardiac tissue and prolongation of the Q–Tc interval.[18] The use of intravenous haloperidol is considered controversial[2] even though it is in common practice.[19] Supporters of the intravenous route point to its safety and its rapidity of onset, although droperidol has been shown to be almost as rapid in action when given intramuscularly (5–20 minutes) as when given intravenously. The risk of extrapyramidal side effects is greatest with high potency antipsychotics such as haloperidol and droperidol, and preventative use of anticholinergic medication has been advocated for high-risk groups including young males, the elderly, patients with Parkinson's disease and patients with a history of extrapyramidal reactions.[12]

Few surveys have examined dosages used in actual practice. The mean dose of haloperidol given to 136 casualty patients for RT was 8 mg,[11] compared to a general psychiatric hospital survey which found the mean dose of haloperidol used in RT to be 22 mg (range 10–60 mg), for droperidol 14 mg (range 10–20 mg) and for chlorpromazine 162 mg (range 50–400 mg).[13]

Benzodiazepines

Even though they have no antipsychotic activity, the sedative and anxiolytic effects of benzodiazepines are often utilized in psychiatric emergencies because of the low toxicity of this class of drugs. They can reduce the antipsychotic requirement and can be used in patients for whom antipsychotics are relatively contraindicated, for example if patients are prone to seizures or if they have previously had idiosyncratic reactions to neuroleptics. Benzodiazepines have been used effectively in drug-induced agitation, early psychotic relapse, and combined with lithium in mania.[20,21]

The benzodiazepines most commonly used in psychiatric emergencies are diazepam and lorazepam. Diazepam is suitable for use as an intravenous preparation, where the dose can be titrated against patient response, as opposed to erratic and slowly absorbed intramuscular injections which should be avoided. Diazepam has been shown to be as effective as haloperidol.[21] Lorazepam is also effective and well tolerated, although there are important pharmacokinetic differences between diazepam and lorazepam. Diazepam is a long-acting drug with a long elimination half-life, is prone to accumulation, has active metabolites and is therefore susceptible to causing residual effects, particularly with repeated dosing. Lorazepam is a short-acting medication with a short elimination half-life and minimal accumulation, and has no active metabolites.[22] In addition, lorazepam is not eliminated by hepatic oxidation (as is diazepam), and therefore it is useful in patients with liver disease or when drug interactions are potentially important. Other benzodiazepines which have been shown to be useful in RT include clonazepam[23] and midazolam.[24]

The main safety risk with benzodiazepines is respiratory depression through oversedation, although the therapeutic index is wide and flumazenil, a specific antagonist, can rapidly reverse this side effect. They cannot be considered as entirely safe as they have also been implicated in the sudden death of patients prescribed other medication.[15] Clonazepam has been linked with aggressive reactions, although the evidence is inconclusive.[25]

The mean dose of diazepam administered to patients subjected to RT in a general psychiatric hospital was 27 mg (range 10–80 mg).[26] To minimize the danger of overdose in emergencies, it is sensible to titrate dose against clinical response, with diazepam requiring a slow rate of intravenous injection, that is a *maximum* rate of 5 mg/minute.[27] Suggested regimens for RT are published, for example in the *British National Formulary* (BNF),[27] although these may be inadequate when dealing with highly disturbed psychiatrically ill patients.[2]

Combined antipsychotics and benzodiazepines

The use of combined antipsychotic and benzodiazepine medications is common in RT.[19,20] It has been argued that this combination can act synergistically, reducing the amount of each drug required, and therefore leading to reduced incidence of side effects.[7] A survey of RT practices in a general psychiatric hospital reported that the level of aggression declined more rapidly if the combination of drugs was used as opposed to single classes of drugs, staff expressed greater satisfaction with the outcome of the violent patient episode, and patients were less likely to require the administration of second doses of medication.[26] Other reports of the successful use of an antipsychotic/benzodiazepine combination include combined haloperidol/lorazepam in patients seriously ill with cancer,[28] and in managing disruptive patients on an open general ward.[29] The main argument against using drug combinations of this kind is that they can lead to accidental overdosage of medication; in the survey described above,[26] serious adverse effects were rare, although one patient suffered a cardiorespiratory collapse directly attributable to overdosage (60 mg diazepam and 80 mg haloperidol as a single dose over 10 minutes).

Other medications

Antipsychotics and benzodiazepines are used in most RT procedures, but other classes of drug are included in treatment algorithms as drugs of last resort, although they require extreme caution. Sodium amylobarbitone, a barbituate, is sedative but is cautioned against because of potentially lethal respiratory depression, hypotensive reactions and hazardous drug reactions. Paraldehyde is similarly cautioned against because of respiratory depression and a propensity to cause sterile abscesses and nerve damage when given intramuscularly; it should never be given intravenously. Anticonvulsant medications such as carbamazepine and sodium valproate are effective in acute mania, but the therapeutic effect is typically delayed for several days and they cannot therefore be considered RT agents. Nadolol, a betablocker with mainly peripheral actions, has been demonstrated to be an effective adjunct in the treatment of acutely aggressive schizophrenic patients, although it is not used within an RT framework.[30]

Aftercare

Management of the patient does not end with RT as there are several important clinical issues to address. Patients subjected to RT require close nursing supervision for a minimum of 1 hour, including the regular measurement of vital signs (including pulse oximetry if available). This allows the clinical staff to detect signs of respiratory depression and idiosyncratic drug reactions, or alternatively to recognize the sedative drug effect wearing off and thus detect early further dangerous behaviour, so that appropriate interventions can be instigated. Patients with medical illness will require thorough examination, investigation and treatment. Careful documentation of both the violent incident and RT procedure and response must occur to facilitate liaison between the emergency and clinical teams (if they differ), to assist with clinical formulation of both diagnosis and future risk assessment, for medicolegal reasons and to assist with clinical audit. Decisions will have to be made regarding whether the patient is appropriately cared for in his or her current location or whether placement is required elsewhere, whether the medication regimen needs to be changed, whether seclusion of the patient is needed, and whether there are issues regarding the legal status of the patient. Notification of a senior colleague may be indicated. It may be necessary or appropriate for the ward to hold various group sessions for support, transfer of information or for review of the management strategy for the patient. The effects of the violent incident on other patients in the ward setting will need to be considered.

New directions

Although the management of violent disturbance has not been systematically researched and therefore several possible research strategies remain unexplored, two particular opportunities suggest themselves as potentially fruitful lines of investigation. There is a need for well-designed studies comparing candidate medications for RT, that is, randomized, controlled, double-blind trials with good power (large patient groups), and reliable and valid assessment and outcome measures. A range of studies partially fulfils these require-

ments, but very few are methodologically sound, and even fewer attempt to address the relationship between the role of medication and non-pharmacological interventions. There is also developing interest in the role of atypical antipsychotics in the treatment of violent disturbance, notwithstanding that they are not considered 'emergency' treatments. There is growing evidence that the use of atypical neuroleptics such as clozapine and olanzapine in psychiatric settings where aggression is problematic is beneficial in reducing violent behaviour.[31–33]

Summary

Violence or imminent violence in the mental health setting constitutes a psychiatric emergency, although there is wide variation in the clinical management of these situations. Clinical priorities are safety, reducing the distress of the patient, and formulation focusing on both diagnostic and risk management issues. After establishing control of the situation, planned non-pharmacological

---

Box 15(i).1 Pharmacological management of behavioural emergencies. Taken from Pilowsky and Kerwin 1997.[34]

1. Use benzodiazepine alone (lorazepam/diazepam) or in combination with a high-potency neuroleptic (haloperidol/droperidol).
2. Give dose benzodiazepine (lorazepam i.m. or i.v. 1–3 mg or diazepam *only* i.v. up to 20 mg) and/or (if benzodiazepine contraindicated).
3. Give haloperidol/droperidol i.m. or i.v. up to 20 mg.
   Advantage of i.v. route: greater flexibility, more control over dose levels, rapid onset (seconds to minutes).
   Advantage of i.m. route: no problem with access, slower onset (5–30 minutes).
4. When giving i.v. medication, deliver at 1 mg/minute for up to 5 mg, then wait 5–15 minutes to assess effect on target behaviours (for example, degree of struggle against physical restraint).
5. Do not use i.v. sedation outside a hospital setting unless resuscitation back-up available.
6. If sedation not obtained by the above, may need further medication or other strategies (behavioural, electroconvulsive therapy); therefore urgent consultation with senior specialist colleagues will be necessary before proceeding.
7. In patients well known to treating team, with good tolerance to antipsychotic medication, in whom long-term treatment must be initiated, zuclopenthixol acetate (a medium-term injectable antipsychotic) may be used. This is not a first-line treatment for a behavioural emergency.

interventions can be considered; although RT may be indicated, it should not be considered an automatic response to violent behaviour. Use and selection of medication for RT should take into account the nature of the patient's illness, their current medication regimen, their physical status, and the side effect and adverse effect profile of the drugs under consideration. In general, the use of benzodiazepines or high-potency antipsychotic drugs individually is considered safe and effective if dose is titrated against response (see Box 15(i).1), with the use of combined antipsychotic and benzodiazepine medications possibly conferring synergistic benefits. Responsible aftercare of the patient is indicated.

References

1. Coid J, Interviewing the aggressive client. In: Kidd B, Stark C, eds, *Management of Violence and Aggression in Health Care*, (Gaskell: London, 1995) 27–48.

2. Kerr I, Taylor D, Acute disturbed or violent behaviour: principles of treatment, *J Psychopharmacol* (1997) **11:**271–7.

3. Scott P, Assessing dangerousness in criminals, *Br J Psych* (1977) **131:**127–42.

4. Powell G, Caan W, Crowe M, What events precede violent incident in psychiatric hospitals? *Br J Psych* (1994) **165:**107–12.

5. Brown TM, Scott AIF, *Handbook of Emergency Psychiatry* (Churchill Livingstone: London, 1990).

6. Angold A, Seclusion, *Br J Psych* (1989) **154:**437–44.

7. Dubin WR, Rapid tranquillization: antipsychotics or benzodiazepines? *J Clin Psych* (1988) **49(Suppl):**5–12.

8. King DJ, Neuroleptics and the treatment of schizophrenia. In: King DJ, ed, *Seminars in Clinical Psychopharmacology* (Gaskell: London, 1995) 259–327.

9. Ayd FJ, Intravenous haloperidol therapy, *Int Drug Ther Newsletter* (1978) **13**.

10. Ayd FJ, Parenteral (IM/IV) droperidol for acutely disturbed behaviour in psychotic and nonpsychotic individuals, *Int Drug Ther Newsletter* (1980) **15**.

11. Clinton JE, Sterner S, Stelmachers Z, Ruiz E, Haloperidol for sedation of disruptive emergency patients, *Ann Emerg Med* (1987) **16:**319–22.

12. Goldberg RJ, Dubin WR, Fogel BS, Review: behavioural emergencies; assessment and psychopharmacologic management, *Clin Neuropharmacol* (1989) **12:**233–48.

13. Chakravarti SK, Muthu A, Muthu PK et al, Zuclopenthixol acetate (5% in Viscoloe): single-dose treatment for acutely disturbed psychotic patients, *Curr Med Res Opin* (1990) **12:**58–65.

14. Cunnane JG, Drug management of disturbed behaviour by psychiatrists, *Psychiat Bull* (1994) **18:**138–9.

15. Jusic N, Lader M, Post-mortem antipsychotic drug concentrations and unexplained deaths, *Br J Psych* (1994) **165:**787–91.

16. Tesar GE, Murray GB, Cassem NH, Use of high dose intravenous haloperidol in the treatment of agitated cardiac patients, *J Clin Psychopharmacol* (1985) **5:**344–7.

17. Goldney R, Bowes J, Spence N et al, The psychiatric intensive care unit, *Br J Psych* (1985) **146:**50–4.

18. Metzger E, Friedman R, Cardiac effects of haloperidol and carbamazepine treatment, *Am J Psych* (1996) **153:**135.

19. Nielssen O, Buhrich N, Finlay-Jones R, Intravenous sedation of involuntary psychiatric patients in New South Wales, *Aust N Z J Psychiatry* (1997) **31:**273–8.

20. Modell JG, Lonox RH, Weiner S, Inpatient clinical trial of lorazepam for the treatment of manic agitation, *J Clin Psychopharmacol* (1985) **5:**109–13.

21. Lerner Y, Lwow E, Levitnin A, Belmaker R, Acute high dose parenteral haloperidol treatment of psychosis, *Am J Psychiatry* (1979) **36:**1061–5.

22. Cooper SJ, Anxiolytics, sedatives and hypnotics. In: King DJ, ed, *Seminars in Clinical Psychopharmacology* (Gaskell: London, 1995) 103–37.

23. Chouinard G, Annable L, Turlier L et al, A double-blind randomised clinical trial of rapid tranquillization with IM clonazepam and IM haloperidol in agitated psychotic patients with manic symptoms, *Can J Psychiatry* (1993) **38(Suppl 4):**S114–S120.

24. Mendoza R, Djenderedjian AH, Adams J, Anath J, Madazolam in acute psychotic patients with hyperarousal, *J Clin Psychiatry* (1987) **48:**291–2.

25. Dietch JT, Jennings RK, Aggressive dyscontrol in patients treated with benzodiazepines, *J Clin Psychiatry* (1988) **49:**1262–6.

26. Pilowsky LS, Ring H, Shine P et al, Rapid tranquillisation – a survey of emergency prescribing in a

general psychiatric hospital, *Br J Psychiatry* (1992) **160:**831–5.

27. *British National Formulary*, no. 36 (The British Medical Association and The Pharmaceutical Press: London, 1998).

28. Adams F, Emergency intravenous sedation of the delirious medically ill patient, *J Clin Psych* (1988) **49(Suppl):**22–7.

29. Chakrabarti GN, Rapid relief of psychotic states by intravenous administration of haloperidol followed by intravenous diazepam, *Proc V11th Congress Psychiatr Vienna* (1983) 573.

30. Allan ER, Alpert M, Sison CE, Citrome L et al, Adjunctive nadolol in the treatment of acutely aggressive schizophrenic patients, *J Clin Psych* (1996) **57:**455–9.

31. Hector RI, The use of clozapine in the treatment of aggressive schizophrenia, *Can J Psychiatry* (1998) **43:**466–72.

32. Glazer WM, Dickson RA, Clozapine reduces violence and persistent aggression in schizophrenia, *J Clin Psychiatry* (1998) **59(Suppl 3):**8–14.

33. Evans C, Millet B, Olie JP, Pilowsky LS, Prescribing in psychiatric intensive care (PICU) – a place for atypical antipsychotic drugs? *Schizophr Res* (2000) **41:**B99.

34. Pilowsky LS, Kerwin RW, Biological treatments in psychiatry. In: Murray R, Hill P, McGuffin P, eds, *The Essentials of Postgraduate Psychiatry*, 3rd edn (Cambridge University Press: Cambridge, 1997) 605–35.

15(ii)

The Long-term Treatment of Violent Patients

Jan Volavka

Most schizophrenic patients do not exhibit violent behavior. However, violence in a small proportion of such patients has become an important factor that limits continuity of care and increases family burden. Mothers living with adult children who have schizophrenia and comorbid substance use disorders are particularly at risk for victimization.[1] Among patients with lower level of functioning, more frequent contact with family and friends is linked to a higher probability of violent events. However, among higher-functioning patients, frequent social contact is associated with lower risk of violence and greater satisfaction with relationships.[2]

In most patients who do exhibit violent behavior, it usually subsides within several weeks after they start antipsychotic treatment and – if applicable – stop using alcohol and drugs. In these *transiently violent* patients, ensuring continued adherence to antipsychotic treatment and abstinence from substance use will constitute a long-term prevention of violent behavior.[3] However, there is a subgroup of schizophrenic patients who continue to be violent in spite of antipsychotic treatment and lack of access to alcohol and drugs. Such patients contribute disproportionate numbers of violent incidents recorded in psychiatric hospitals: in one survey, 5% of the inpatients were responsible for 53% of violent incidents.[4] These *persistently violent* patients present a major challenge to long-term management.

Transiently violent schizophrenic patients

In these patients, the *adherence to antipsychotic treatment* when they are in the community is very important. In some patients, extrapyramidal side effects are the reason for non-adherence. Switching such patients to an atypical antipsychotic that causes fewer side effects and using the minimal effective dose levels may solve the problem. Other patients stop their medicine because they have difficulty remembering to take it or to keep their appointments. These patients may be managed using an intramuscular depot form of haloperidol or fluphenazine. For various reasons, including poor insight into their illness, some violent schizophrenic patients resist, overtly or covertly, taking any form of medication. As long as they are in the hospital, this resistance can usually be overcome by clinical and legal methods that vary across hospitals and jurisdictions. However, the situation is more difficult when these patients are residing in the community. There are patients who become violent in the community after they stop their medication, the violence leads to a hospital admission, they respond well to medication in the hospital and are discharged, then stop taking the medicine, become violent, and the cycle starts again. The combination of nonadherence to treatment and the abuse of drugs and alcohol is particularly likely to result in violent behavior.

In order to break this cycle of violence, some states in the United States and several other countries have adopted or are experimenting with outpatient commitment programs intended largely for psychotic patients with records of repeated violent behavior and poor cooperation with treatment. Under this system, a court orders the patient to follow a course of treatment (usually including antipsychotic medication) while living in the community. The patient is supervised; if he or she fails to comply, the police can be called and the patient is involuntarily hospitalized. Proponents of this system suggest that the outpatient commitment programs improve adherence to treatment, reduce violent behavior by patients in the community, reduce the need for hospitalization, and may result in shorter hospital stays for the involuntarily hospitalized patients committed through these programs. While civil libertarians complain that the outpatient commitment violates patients' rights, proponents argue that these programs are needed to help the schizophrenic patients who have no insight into their illness, and to protect their potential victims. However, the effectiveness of outpatient commitment has not yet been formally demonstrated.

It appears that much of the violent behavior by patients in the community is associated with inadequate services available to the patients rather than with their refusal to accept treatment. Egregious violent acts are typically committed by patients who had repeatedly and unsuccessfully attempted to obtain psychiatric care.[5] Such patients are then provided with long-term care in forensic facilities or in prisons.

Persistently violent schizophrenic patients

These patients are best managed at specialized secure units with highly trained staff. Their illness (and its neurobiological underpinning) is apparently different from the more typical schizophrenia seen in the transiently violent and the nonviolent patients. Some of these persistently violent patients exhibit comorbid psychopathy[6] or neurological impairments.[7,8] The implications of these comorbid problems for the management of such patients are not yet clear.

Various behavioral management approaches are used to treat persistently violent patients;[9,10] some of these methods are explicitly based on social learning.[11] The evidence for long-term effectiveness of such behavioral and learning programs is not robust; in fact, some programs intended to reduce dangerousness may actually increase it.[12] If the hospitalized or incarcerated patients respond to long-term care, their discharge may be considered, depending on their legal status. Patients with a history of persistent or serious criminal violence may be released into the community only after a risk assessment; scientific bases for such assessment can be found elsewhere.[13]

Pharmacological treatment of persistently violent patients
Antipsychotics

These patients do not respond to typical antipsychotics; nevertheless, they are sometimes treated with high doses of these agents.[14] The antiaggressive effects of atypical antipsychotics are under intensive investigation. The specificity of such antiaggressive effects is an important consideration. It can be understood in two ways: first, in order to be specific, the antiaggressive effect should not be mediated by sedation; the independence of antiaggressive and sedative effects of clozapine has been demonstrated.[15] Second, the specific antiaggressive effect should be relatively independent of general antipsychotic effects; this independence has also been demonstrated for clozapine.[16] This type of specificity is important for the consideration of an agent as a potential antiaggressive treatment in persons who are not psychotic.

Many reports support a long-term, perhaps

Table 15(ii).1 Effects of clozapine on aggressive and hostile behavior in schizophrenia and schizoaffective disorder

Author, year	n	Trial duration	Measure of effect
Maier 1992[17]	25	6–15 months	Security Level, discharge
Volavka et al 1993[16]	223	1 year	BPRS Hostility item
Ebrahim et al 1994[19]	27	6 months	Seclusion and restraint, BPRS, Level of Privileges
Chiles et al 1994[15]	139	3 months	Seclusion and restraint, NOSIE
Buckley et al 1995[20]	30	6 months	Seclusion and restraint, BPRS
Rabinowitz et al 1996[21]	75	6 months	Incidents of physical or verbal aggression, BPRS Hostility item

BPRS, Brief Psychiatric Rating Scale; NOSIE, Nurses' Observation Scale for Inpatient Evaluation.

specific antiaggressive efficacy of clozapine in schizophrenic and schizoaffective patients. This evidence, however, is based on open, uncontrolled studies in which patients were assigned to clozapine treatment on a clinical basis (rather than being randomized) and the data were collected in a retrospective record review;[15–21] some of these studies are summarized in Table 15(ii).1. A typical study is exemplified in Figure 15(ii).1: after the introduction of clozapine, the number of incidents of physical and verbal aggression decreased. However, the lack of controls for the placebo effect, time effect, baseline effect, etc. makes this study difficult to interpret. In spite of the methodological weaknesses of individual studies, the cumulative evidence for the antiaggressive effects of clozapine appears to be relatively strong. The antiaggressive effects of clozapine are not limited to patients with the diagnoses of schizophrenia or schizoaffective disorder.[22]

Other atypical antipsychotics may also have antiaggressive effects that may be similar to those of clozapine, but not many data are yet available.

There is some evidence that risperidone may reduce hostility[23] and aggression[24] in schizophrenic patients. Analogous data for olanzapine are currently being analysed. In general, the literature on antiaggressive effects of antipsychotics is plagued by serious methodological problems that are reviewed and analysed elsewhere.[22]

Adjunctive treatments

Many schizophrenic patients who are persistently violent are treated with a combination of an antipsychotic and an adjunctive medication.

CARBAMAZEPINE

The antiaggressive effects of carbamazepine as an adjunctive treatment in schizophrenic and schizoaffective patients were suggested by two placebo-controlled studies.[25,26] The first was small and included patients with other diagnoses. The second study[26] involved 162 schizophrenic or schizoaffective patients receiving various antipsychotics (open-label) who were randomized to one of two adjunctive treatments: carbamazepine or placebo (double-blind). The study demonstrated

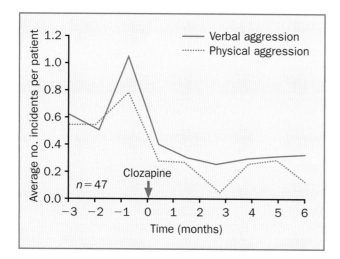

Figure 15(ii).1 A study of clozapine effects on overt aggression.[21]

a significantly better effect of carbamazepine on agitation and aggression; unfortunately, these two behaviors were commingled in data analysis. Thus, the report does not permit an assessment of antiaggressive effects *per se*. In addition to these placebo-controlled studies, other observations suggest antiaggressive effects of carbamazepine in schizophrenic and schizoaffective patients.[27-29] Thus, adjunctive carbamazepine may indeed possess antiaggressive effects in such patients. However, definitive studies demonstrating such effects are lacking.

VALPROATE

In a survey of 12 444 inpatients in New York State psychiatric hospitals, 28% of all patients diagnosed with schizophrenia received valproate (valproic acid and divalproex sodium),[30] and that proportion is increasing.[31] A previous survey of a smaller subset of the same inpatient population suggested that the intended effects of this treatment are improvements of impulse control and reduction of aggressive behavior.[32]

Valproate may have antiaggressive effects, but the evidence for its efficacy is based largely on uncontrolled studies and case reports describing mostly patients with dementia, mental retardation, and brain injuries. Very little is known about the antiaggressive efficacy of valproate in patients with schizophrenia.[33] A small controlled study suggested that adjunctive valproate may have antipsychotic effects in schizophrenia,[34] but this finding was not confirmed in another small study.[35] Thus, the widespread use of valproate that is intended to control aggressive behavior in schizophrenic patients does not appear to be based on robust evidence of effectiveness. This is troubling, particularly in view of its potential for hepatotoxicity.

SELECTIVE SEROTONIN REUPTAKE INHIBITORS (SSRIs)

Since reduced central serotonin turnover is associated with impulsive aggression,[13] SSRIs would be expected to inhibit aggression. Indeed, in a double-blind crossover study, citalopram showed convincing antiaggressive effects as adjunctive treatment in forensic patients diagnosed with schizophrenia.[36]

BENZODIAZEPINES

For a long time, benzodiazepines as needed (p.r.n.) have been commonly used in the short-term management of aggression. More recently, however, these compounds are increasingly used on a continuous basis (i.e., not merely p.r.n.) for the long-term management of persistently violent patients. Thus, for many months, some of these patients are receiving regular daily doses of benzodiazepines intended to control aggressive behavior. The effectiveness of such long-term treatment has not been demonstrated; indeed, one might expect the development of tolerance (and attendant loss of efficacy) after several weeks of continued administration of benzodiazepines.

In some psychiatric facilities, clonazepam is prescribed routinely to control aggression in schizophrenic patients. There are several case reports suggesting antiaggressive effects of clonazepam in various disorders other than schizophrenia. However, in a double-blind, placebo controlled trial, adjunctive clonazepam had no beneficial effect in schizophrenic patients, and some of the patients showed an *increase* of violent behavior after clonazepam.[37] Thus, continuous benzodiazepine treatment of persistent aggressive behavior in schizophrenia does not appear to be based on evidence of effectiveness. The use of clonazepam to control aggression in schizophrenic patients who do not have concomitant seizure disorder seems particularly questionable.

BETA-ADRENERGIC BLOCKING AGENTS

These compounds have been used to treat persistent aggressive behavior in a variety of conditions (see Volavka,[13] 279–83). Isolated cases of successful treatment of aggression with propranolol in particularly assaultive schizophrenic patients have been reported.[38,39] A retrospective chart review demonstrated antiaggressive effects of nadolol in 6 patients with chronic schizophrenia.[38] A double-blind, placebo-controlled parallel-group trial of nadolol in aggressive, mostly schizophrenic patients ($n = 41$) has demonstrated the superiority of nadolol in reducing incidents of overt aggression.[40] Unfortunately, there appeared to be a considerable difference in the level of aggression between the two treatment groups at the baseline; it is not clear whether this difference affected the outcome.

Interestingly, nadolol is a relatively lipophobic compound that is accordingly believed not to cross the blood–brain barrier to any great extent (although this belief is not universal; see Whitman et al[39]). Thus, these encouraging results with a lipophobic drug suggest that at least some of the antiaggressive action of beta-blocking agents may have a peripheral mechanism of action. Peripheral components of akathisia, tension, or anxiety might be improved by nadolol, and the antiaggressive effect may be mediated by these improvements. Thus, although rigorously designed studies have not yet been done, adjunctive beta-adrenergic blocking agents may have antiaggressive effects in persistently violent schizophrenic patients. The mechanism of this effect is unclear.

References

1. Estroff SE, Swanson JW, Lachicotte WS et al, Risk reconsidered: targets of violence in the social networks of people with serious psychiatric disorders, *Soc Psychiatry Psychiatr Epidemiol* (1998) **33(Suppl 1):**S95–101.

2. Swanson J, Swartz M, Estroff S et al, Psychiatric impairment, social contact, and violent behavior: evidence from a study of outpatient-committed persons with severe mental disorder, *Soc Psychiatry Psychiatr Epidemiol* (1998) **33(Suppl 1):**S86–94.

3. Swartz MS, Swanson JW, Hiday VA et al, Violence and severe mental illness: the effects of substance abuse and nonadherence to medication, *Am J Psychiatry* (1998) **155:**226–31.

4. Convit A, Isay D, Otis D, Volavka J, Characteristics of repeatedly assaultive psychiatric inpatients, *Hosp Community Psychiatry* (1990) **41:**1112–15.

5. Winerip M, Bedlam on the street, *The New York Times*, 23 May 1999, Magazine, pp 42–70.

6. Nolan KA, Volavka J, Mohr P, Czobor P, Psychopathy and violent behavior among patients with schizophrenia or schizoaffective disorder, *Psychiatr Serv* (1999) **50:**787–92.

7. Krakowski M, Czobor P, Violence in psychiatric patients: the role of psychosis, frontal lobe impairment, and ward turmoil, *Compr Psychiatry* (1997) **38:**230–6.

8. Krakowski MI, Czobor P, Clinical symptoms, neurological impairment, and prediction of violence in psychiatric inpatients, *Hosp Community Psychiatry* (1994) **45:**700–5.

9. Rice ME, Harris GT, Varney GW, Quinsey VL, *Violence in Institutions: Understanding, Prevention, and Control*, (Hogrefe & Huber Publishers: Toronto, 1989).

10. Ball GG, Modifying the behavior of the violent patient, *Psychiatr Q* (1993) **64:**359–69.

11. Bellus SB, Vergo JG, Kost PP et al, Behavioral rehabilitation and the reduction of aggressive and self-injurious behaviors with cognitively impaired, chronic psychiatric inpatients, *Psychiatr Q* (1999) **70:**27–37.

12. Rice ME, Violent offender research and implications for the criminal justice system, *Am Psychol* (1997) **52:**414–23.

13. Volavka J, *Neurobiology of Violence* (American Psychiatric Press: Washington, DC, 1995).

14. Krakowski MI, Kunz M, Czobor P, Volavka J, Long-term high-dose neuroleptic treatment: who gets it and why? *Hosp Community Psychiatry* (1993) **44:**640–4.

15. Chiles JA, Davidson P, McBride D, Effects of clozapine on use of seclusion and restraint at a state hospital, *Hosp Community Psychiatry* (1994) **45:**269–71.

16. Volavka J, Zito JM, Vitrai J, Czobor P, Clozapine effects on hostility and aggression in schizophrenia, *J Clin Psychopharmacol* (1993) **13:**287–9.

17. Maier GJ, The impact of clozapine on 25 forensic patients, *Bull Am Acad Psychiatry Law* (1992) **20:**297–307.

18. Ratey JJ, Leveroni C, Kilmer D et al, The effects of clozapine on severely aggressive psychiatric inpatients in a state hospital, *J Clin Psychiatry* (1993) **54:**219–23.

19. Ebrahim GM, Gibler B, Gacono CB, Hayes G, Patient response to clozapine in a forensic psychiatric hospital, *Hosp Community Psychiatry* (1994) **45:**271–3.

20. Buckley P, Bartell J, Donenwirth K et al, Violence and schizophrenia: clozapine as a specific antiaggressive agent, *Bull Am Acad Psychiatry Law* (1995) **23:**607–11.

21. Rabinowitz J, Avnon M, Rosenberg V, Effect of clozapine on physical and verbal aggression, *Schizophr Res* (1996) **22:**249–55.

22. Volavka J, Citrome L, Atypical antipsychotics in the treatment of the persistently aggressive psychotic patient: methodological concerns, *Schizophr Res* (1999) **35:**S23–33.

23. Czobor P, Volavka J, Meibach RC, Effect of risperidone on hostility in schizophrenia, *J Clin Psychopharmacol* (1995) **15:**243–9.

24. Buckley PF, Ibrahim ZY, Singer B et al, Aggression and schizophrenia: efficacy of risperidone, *J Am Psychiatry Law* (1997) **25:**173–81.

25. Neppe VM, Carbamazepine as adjunctive treatment in nonepileptic chronic inpatients with EEG temporal lobe abnormalities, *J Clin Psychiatry* (1983) **44:**326–31.

26. Okuma T, Yamashita I, Takahashi R et al, A double-blind study of adjunctive carbamazepine versus placebo on excited states of schizophrenic and schizoaffective disorders, *Acta Psychiatr Scand* (1989) **80:**250–9.

27. Hakola HP, Laulumaa VA, Carbamazepine in treatment of violent schizophrenics [letter], *Lancet* (1982) **i:**1358.

28. Yassa R, Dupont D, Carbamazepine in the treatment of aggressive behavior in schizophrenic patients: a case report, *Can J Psychiatry* (1983) **28:**566–8.

29. Luchins DJ, Carbamazepine in violent non-epileptic schizophrenics, *Psychopharmacol Bull* (1984) **20:**569–71.

30. Citrome L, Levine J, Allingham B, Utilization of valproate: extent of inpatient use in the New York State Office of Mental Health, *Psychiatr Q* (1998) **69:**283–300.

31. Citrome L, Levine J, Allingham B, Valproate use in schizophrenia: 1994–1998, Poster presentation NR 307, American Psychiatric Association Annual Meeting, Washington, DC, 1999. [Abstract].

32. Citrome L, Use of lithium, carbamazepine, and valproic acid in a state-operated psychiatric hospital, *J Pharm Technol* (1995) **11:**55–9.

33. Wassef AA, Dott SG, Harris A et al, Critical review of GABA-ergic drugs in the treatment of schizophrenia, *J Clin Psychopharmacol* (1999) **19:**222–32.

34. Wassef AA, Dott SG, Harris A et al, Randomized, placebo-controlled pilot study of divalproex sodium in the treatment of acute exacerbations of chronic schizophrenia, *J Clin Psychopharmacol* (2000) **20:**357–61.

35. Hesslinger B, Normann C, Langosch JM et al, Effects of carbamazepine and valproate on haloperidol plasma levels and on psychopathologic outcome in schizophrenic patients, *J Clin Psychopharmacol* (1999) **19:**310–15.

36. Vartiainen H, Tiihonen J, Putkonen A et al, Citalopram, a selective serotonin reuptake inhibitor, in the treatment of aggression in schizophrenia, *Acta Psychiatr Scand* (1995) **91:**348–51.

37. Karson CN, Weinberger DR, Bigelow L, Wyatt RJ, Clonazepam treatment of chronic schizophrenia: negative results in a double-blind, placebo-controlled trial, *Am J Psychiatry* (1982) **139:**1627–8.

38. Sorgi PJ, Ratey JJ, Polakoff S, Beta-adrenergic blockers for the control of aggressive behaviors in patients with chronic schizophrenia, *Am J Psychiatry* (1986) **143:**775–6.

39. Whitman JR, Maier GJ, Eichelman B, Beta-adrenergic blockers for aggressive behavior in schizophrenia [letter], *Am J Psychiatry* (1987) **144:**538–9.

40. Ratey JJ, Sorgi P, O'Driscoll GA et al, Nadolol to treat aggression and psychiatric symptomatology in chronic psychiatric inpatients: a double-blind, placebo-controlled study, *J Clin Psychiatry* (1992) **53:**41–6.

16

Substance Abuse Comorbidity

Robert E Drake and Kim T Mueser

Contents • Introduction • Epidemiology, phenomenology, and correlates • Service issues
• Assessment • Treatment • Conclusions

Introduction

Over the past two decades there has been a growing awareness of the problem of co-occurring substance use disorder (SUD) in persons with schizophrenia. In this article, the terms 'dual diagnosis', 'dual disorders', and 'SUD comorbidity' are used interchangeably to denote the problem of co-occurring SUD and schizophrenia. Following a brief overview of the epidemiology, phenomenology, and correlates of dual diagnosis, we review current approaches to service organization, assessment, and treatment.

Epidemiology, phenomenology and correlates

Persons with schizophrenia are at increased risk for comorbid SUD.[1] For example, in the Epidemiologic Catchment Area study, the rate of lifetime SUD in the general United States population was 17%, compared to 48% for persons with schizophrenia.[2] In addition to the high rate of lifetime SUD in persons with schizophrenia, rates of recent alcohol and drug disorders are also high. Most studies suggest that between 25% and 35% of persons with schizophrenia manifest SUD over the past 6 months. While much of the early research on the high comorbidity of SUD in schizophrenia was reported in the United States,

numerous studies from other countries have replicated these findings.[3–8] Dual diagnosis tends to be more common in those patients who are young, male, single, and less educated; in those with histories of conduct disorder; and in those with family histories of SUD.[1,6] Those who are homeless, in jail, or who present to an emergency room or hospital setting are also more likely to have SUD than other patients.

For people with schizophrenia, alcohol is the most common substance of abuse, followed by cannabis and cocaine.[9] Their SUD tends to be a social behavior and is associated with problems of disinhibition, aggression, and psychosocial instability.[10–13] Patients with schizophrenia report reasons for use that tend to be very similar to the reasons cited by others with SUD.[14,15] In other words, they report using alcohol and other substances to combat loneliness, social anxiety, boredom, and insomnia rather than specific symptoms of schizophrenia or side effects of medications. Finally, as with SUD in the general population, SUD in persons with schizophrenia tends to be a chronic, relapsing disorder with persistence over many years.[16,17]

People with schizophrenia have heightened sensitivity to the effects of psychoactive substances, with the result that they incur negative consequences with remarkably low amounts of use and rarely sustain nonsymptomatic, or non-problematic, usage.[18] Not only are they more sensitive to the effects of psychoactive substances, but they are also more likely to encounter such substances. As a result of deinstitutionalization and other risk factors, such as poverty, poor education, poor social skills, lack of vocational skills and opportunities, and residence in drug-infested neighborhoods, they experience a high rate of regular exposure to psychoactive substances and of social pressures to use them.

Individuals with schizophrenia predictably suffer adverse consequences that are somewhat different from those encountered by others in the general population.[19] Dual diagnosis is associated with higher rates of specific negative outcomes: severe financial problems due to poor money management; unstable housing and homelessness; medication noncompliance, relapse, and rehospitalization; violence, legal problems, and incarceration; depression and suicide; family burden; and high rates of sexually transmitted diseases. Many common problems related to SUD in the general population, such as marital and vocational difficulties, are less frequent in persons with schizophrenia. One important consequence of the clinical and social effects of SUD in this population is that dually diagnosed patients tend to utilize more psychiatric services than singly diagnosed patients, especially costly services such as emergency room visits and inpatient hospitalizations.[20,21]

Because of the high prevalence and chronicity of SUD in persons with schizophrenia, the serious negative effects of dual diagnosis on the course of illness and on social problems, and the high cost of treatment, the development of more effective interventions for dual diagnosis has been a high priority since the mid-1980s. Current approaches to the care of persons with dual disorders involve substantive changes in traditional methods of service organization and clinical intervention.

Service issues

Early reviews of dual diagnosis services[22] identified two fundamental problems. First, most patients with dual diagnosis received no SUD treatment, largely because of difficulties in accessing services. Second, when they did receive SUD treatment, it was not tailored to the needs of persons with a comorbid mental illness. Poor access and inadequate treatment were in part attributed to the historical split between mental health and substance abuse treatment services.

In the United States and many other countries, mental health and substance abuse treatment services have been separated for years. Different organizations provide mental health and substance abuse services; financing mechanisms are separate and often compete for scarce public health funds; education, training, and procedures for establishing professional credentials differ between the two systems; and eligibility criteria for receipt of services differ as well. As a consequence of these factors, two general approaches to the treatment of patients with dual diagnosis predominated until recently. In the sequential treatment approach, patients were directed to obtain definitive treatment in one system before entering treatment in the other system. For example, a person with schizophrenia might have been told that his or her SUD should be completely in remission before mental health treatment would be appropriate. In the parallel treatment approach, patients were directed to pursue independent treatments in each of the two systems. In other words, a patient in treatment in one system might be referred for an evaluation at a separate agency in the other treatment system. Both approaches placed the burden of integrating services entirely on patients rather than on providers, and ignored the need to modify mental health and SUD services for persons with comorbid disorders.[23]

In practice, most patients with schizophrenia were quickly excluded from substance abuse treatment programs if they sought services. On the other hand, they experienced poor outcomes in the mental health system because their SUD was undetected or untreated. Even worse, patients with dual diagnosis were sometimes excluded from both systems because of having comorbid disorders. For example, the dually diagnosed individual could be determined ineligible for mental health hospitalization or housing because of SUD and simultaneously ineligible for SUD hospitalization or housing because of psychosis. Thus, sequential and parallel approaches defended providers' professional and financing boundaries but did not serve patients well.[24]

By the end of the 1980s, clinicians, advocates, and researchers called for the formation of integrated programs that combined mental health and substance abuse services.[22] Consequently, new models with a primary aim of integrating services have rapidly developed and evolved since the mid-1980s.[25–30]

Integrated treatment

The essence of integration is that the same clinicians or teams of clinicians, working in one setting, provide both mental health and substance abuse interventions in a coordinated fashion. Clinicians take responsibility for combining the interventions so that they are tailored for the presence of comorbidity. Integration is often accomplished through the use of multidisciplinary teams that include both mental health and substance abuse specialists who share responsibility for treatment and cross-training. Integration must be supported and sustained by a common administrative structure and confluence of funding streams.[31] For the dually diagnosed individual, the services appear seamless, with a consistent approach, philosophy, and set of recommendations; the need to negotiate with separate systems, providers, or payers disappears.

Integration involves modifications of traditional approaches to both mental health and substance abuse treatment.[32] For example, skills training focuses on the need to develop meaningful relationships and the need to deal with social situations involving substance use. Pharmacotherapy takes into account not only the need to control symptoms but also the potential of some medications for abuse. SUD interventions are modified in accordance with the vulnerability of patients with schizophrenia to confrontational interventions, their need for support, and their typical lack of motivation to pursue abstinence.

Although the models for providing integrated treatment vary, programs that have demonstrated positive outcomes have several common service features.[33] First, they are almost always developed within outpatient mental health programs, primarily because adding substance abuse treatment to the existing array of community support services already available for persons with schizophrenia is more feasible than reproducing all of these services within a substance abuse treatment context.

Second, awareness of SUD is insinuated into all aspects of the existing mental health program rather than isolated as a discrete substance abuse treatment intervention. As described below, components such as case management, assessment, individual counseling, group interventions, family psychoeducation, medication management, money management, housing, and vocational rehabilitation incorporate special features that reflect awareness of dual diagnosis.

Third, successful programs address the difficulty that dually diagnosed patients have in linking with services and maintaining treatment adherence by providing continuous outreach and close monitoring techniques, which are described below. These approaches enable patients to access services and to maintain needed relationships with a consistent program over months and years. Without such efforts, noncompliance and dropouts are high.

Fourth, integrated programs recognize that recovery tends to occur over months or years in the community. People with severe mental illness and SUD do not develop stable remission quickly, even in intensive treatment programs. Rather, they tend to develop stable remission over longer periods, with a cumulative rate of approximately

10–15% attaining stable remissions per year, in conjunction with a consistent dual diagnosis program. Successful programs therefore take a long-term, outpatient perspective.

Fifth, most dual diagnosis programs recognize that the majority of psychiatric patients have little readiness for abstinence-oriented SUD treatments. Rather than just treating the highly motivated patients, they therefore incorporate motivational interventions that are designed to help patients who either do not recognize their SUD or do not desire substance abuse treatment become ready for more definitive interventions that are aimed at abstinence. Motivational interventions involve helping the individual to identify his or her own goals and then to recognize that using psychoactive substances interferes with attaining those goals.[34]

Integrated programs are consistently able to engage dually diagnosed patients in services and to help them to reduce SUD behaviors and attain stable remission.[33] Other outcomes related to hospital use, psychiatric symptoms, and quality of life are positive but less consistent. However, despite the encouraging findings regarding integrated treatment programs and the widespread acceptance that integrated treatment is superior to non-integrated treatment for this population, implementation continues to be slow because of problems related to organizing and financing dual diagnosis programs. Organizational guidelines have been developed for dual diagnosis programs,[31] but few large systems have successfully integrated services.

Assessment

Several interlocking steps comprise the standard approach to assessment of SUD: detection, classification, specialized (or functional) assessment, and treatment planning.[35] Each of these requires some modification for patients with schizophrenia.

Detection
Screening is critical because SUD tends to be covert and treatment depends on detection. SUD frequently goes undetected in psychiatric care settings.[36] The single most important reason is that many mental health programs do not screen at all. Even when screening is attempted, however, schizophrenic patients are prone to poor self-reporting, in part due to the inadequacy of standard substance abuse screening instruments for this population.

Several helpful approaches to the problem of detection are recommended. First, clinicians in mental health settings should ask all clients about their substance use and related problems. Perhaps the most efficient method is with a new screening instrument, the Dartmouth Assessment of Lifestyle Instrument, which has been developed specifically for persons with severe mental illness.[37]

Second, clinicians should maintain a high index of suspicion for SUD, even in the face of denial, particularly among young male patients with other characteristics that suggest SUD. Denial of SUD in situations of symptomatic or psychosocial instability should lead to multimodal assessment, such as urine drug screens, interviews with collaterals, and longitudinal observations in the community. Laboratory tests may yield false negatives and are ineffective when there are delays between drug use and testing, but they often detect current use that is denied by patients.[38,39] Collateral reports from trained case managers are also an effective way of identifying SUD in psychiatric patients.[40] Case managers have the opportunity to synthesize medical information from various assessment contacts, direct observations of the patient in the community, collateral reports from relatives, and self-reports over multiple occasions, leading to higher sensitivity to SUD.

Finally, all patients who have a past history of SUD or a current self-report of any regular use of alcohol or other substances should be followed up carefully. SUD tends to be a chronic, relapsing disorder so that currently nonabusing patients with a history of SUD are highly vulnerable.

Classification

The classification of SUD is relatively straightforward. If a person repeatedly uses a psychoactive substance that results in medical, emotional, social, or vocational impairments or physical danger, a diagnosis of SUD should be made.[41,42] Substance abuse (or harmful use), as opposed to substance dependence, is common in persons with severe mental illness, and the distinction may have important treatment implications.[43] Furthermore, we also recommend using the classification of 'use without impairment' as a marker for potential problems.[40]

Although diagnosing SUD is relatively straightforward, comorbid psychiatric symptoms, syndromes, and diagnoses are often difficult to sort out because psychiatric symptoms of all kinds can occur as a result of SUD.[44] Criteria from the Diagnostic and Statistical Manual of Mental Disorders, Fourth Edition (DSM-IV)[41] specify making a diagnosis only after observing the patient for 1 month without substance use and without medications. The International Classification of Diseases, Tenth Revision,[42] on the other hand is less specific, stating that psychiatric syndromes such as schizophrenia should not be diagnosed during acute substance intoxication or withdrawal. Although standardized and simple, the DSM-IV recommendation has little empirical basis and is unrealistic for patients who have psychotic symptoms because they usually require immediate medications and are often not abstinent for sufficient time to observe them. Rather than the simple DSM rule, Weiss et al[45] recommend using more specific abstinence criteria based on the known effects of particular substances of abuse in relation to the disorders being classified. They also recognize that longitudinal evaluation, corroborating data from collaterals, and multiple data sources are often necessary to make accurate diagnoses.

Attempts to classify individuals with SUD and co-occurring psychotic symptoms have been fraught with difficulties such that many patients fall into an uncertain category.[46] In practice, clinicians often treat these patients with uncertain diagnoses as though they have schizophrenia, withdraw medications when feasible, and reassess the diagnosis if and when they attain stable abstinence.

Specialized assessment

A specialized, or functional, assessment of substance use behavior is the cornerstone upon which dual diagnosis treatment planning is based.[47] Specialized assessment entails a detailed evaluation of the patient's SUD, including motives for use, expectancies related to specific substances, and motivation for change; of how the patient's SUD interacts with adjustment in different domains of functioning, including housing, relationships, illness management, and work; and of the patient's personal goals. All of these factors help the clinician to develop an individualized treatment plan, consistent with the patient's personal strengths and goals, that identifies specific targets and intervention approaches.

This type of behavioral analysis assumes that motivating factors sustain continued substance use and that addressing these factors will facilitate substance use reduction and abstinence. For example, dual diagnosis patients often report that substance use enhances social opportunities, helps them deal with boredom, anxiety, and dysphoria, and is an important source of recreation. Substance abuse treatment addresses specific, individual issues of this type.

While the details of specialized assessment are beyond the scope of this chapter, it should be clear that the assessment covers areas such as social relationships with family and friends, leisure and recreational activities, work and education, financial matters, legal involvement, and spirituality. One goal is to evaluate the patient's strengths and potential resources. For example, if the patient expresses a desire to work, treatment can focus on securing competitive work and developing strategies for reducing the impact of substance use on getting or maintaining employment.

Another goal is to assess the patient's awareness of negative consequences associated with substance use, insight into having a substance abuse problem, motivation for change, and preferences for treatment. Many patients need interventions specifically designed to help them develop motivation. Moreover, other interventions are keyed to the patient's stage of treatment participation.[32,48] The concept of stage of treatment is based on the four-stage model developed by Osher and Kofoed:[26] engagement (no regular contact with dual diagnosis clinician), persuasion (contact with clinician but no reduction in substance abuse), active treatment (significant reduction in substance abuse), and relapse prevention (no problems with substance abuse in past 6 months). Treatment goals are determined partly by the patient's stage of treatment. In the *engagement* stage, patients have no working relationship with a clinician and are not motivated to change their substance use behavior, and therefore treatment goals primarily focus on establishing regular contact and helping patients get their basic needs met. At the *persuasion* stage, patients have regular contact with their clinicians, but are minimally invested in changing their substance use behavior. In this stage of treatment, realistic goals are to learn more and talk about their substance use behavior, and to work on other rehabilitation goals that are personally relevant. In *active treatment* patients have begun to reduce their substance use, and goals emphasize further reduction or abstinence. In *relapse prevention* patients have not recently had problems related to substance use. Typical goals are to keep the substance abuse in remission and to work on other areas of personal growth.

Treatment planning

The final step in assessment, treatment planning, involves combining and integrating information obtained during the first three steps of assessment into a coherent set of activities. Treatment plans may involve interventions that either directly address SUD (for example, developing motivation

to reduce or cease substance use) or other areas that impact on SUD (for example, helping the patient find competitive work in order to decrease opportunities for using substances and improve self-esteem).

The treatment plan must, of course, address pressing needs, such as a grave risk to the patient or others, problems with housing, untreated medical conditions, and lack of psychiatric stabilization. More important, however, is the long-term plan to target behaviors for change based on the specialized assessment. Long-term goals might include, for example, changing the patient's social network, finding a job, and learning behavioral techniques to handle social anxiety. A wide variety of treatment strategies is available for achieving changes in target behaviors.[32]

Treatment

As described above, effective dual diagnosis services require the integration of mental health and substance abuse services, which involves organizing and financing programs. Within the integrated treatment paradigm, however, a variety of specific components have been developed and are currently being refined. Individual components have different targets and are therefore often designed to be used in combination. For example, within a dual diagnosis program, case management and close monitoring are used to link dually diagnosed individuals with treatment, substance abuse treatments to address substance use and high-risk behaviors, family psychoeducation and housing supports to ensure that the environment supports stability and abstinence, rehabilitation to promote functioning in meaningful roles, and medications to target symptoms of mental illness and to inhibit SUD behaviors.

Before discussing individual components, we reiterate that dual diagnosis treatment occurs primarily in the outpatient setting. Inpatient care is reserved for stabilization, assessment, and linkage with the outpatient program.[49] We have described the process of clinical care in greater detail elsewhere.[32] Specific components of dual diagnosis services have received minimal research attention, and we have reviewed the current research base for these interventions elsewhere as well.[50] Here we will briefly describe the common components of integrated treatment.

Case management

The most common approach to integrating mental health and substance abuse treatments and to linking dual diagnosis patients with outpatient services is through the use of multidisciplinary case management teams.[51] To integrate services, mental health and substance abuse specialists on the same team blend their respective skills into common procedures by sharing training experiences, responsibility for care, and the onus of developing a melded philosophy. Clinicians on these teams often provide interventions to address trauma sequelae as well as the symptoms of mental illness and SUD.

To link dually diagnosed patients with services and maintain treatment relationships, teams rely heavily on outreach, practical assistance, and sharing decision-making with the patient. Multidisciplinary teams typically require several months of training and working together to mature. Specific criteria for assessing the quality of dual diagnosis treatment can be used to guide and monitor implementation,[52] and the quality of dual diagnosis services predicts substance abuse treatment outcomes.[53]

Close monitoring

In addition to outreach and direct substance abuse treatment, dual diagnosis teams often provide a variety of interventions that can be described by the rubric 'close monitoring'.[54] Close monitoring techniques include medication supervision, protective payeeships, guardianships for medications, urine drug screens, housing supports, probation, parole, and outpatient commitments. Many of these approaches rely on the patient's cooperation, while others assume some degree of coerciveness based on the patient's incapacity to manage his or her own affairs or on the need to protect the patient and others from dangerousness.

Substance abuse treatment

Once patients are engaged in outpatient services, all dual diagnosis programs provide some form of substance abuse treatment. Because the patients are often unmotivated to pursue abstinence, most programs focus initially on education, harm reduction, and increasing motivation rather than on abstinence.[29,30,54,55] As described above, motivational approaches are designed to help the patient to recognize that SUD is interfering with his or her own goals and thereby to nurture the patient's desire to reduce and then eliminate SUD. The other common approach to substance abuse treatment involves some form of cognitive-behavioral counseling. The two approaches are often combined or offered in stages so that skills for achieving and maintaining abstinence are taught after motivation is developed.[56]

Substance abuse interventions can be provided in individual, group, or family formats. Clinicians on multidisciplinary teams often use all of these approaches based on the patient's preference and a shared decision-making model.[32] In practice, most dual diagnosis programs assume that the peer-orientated group is a powerful vehicle and address substance-abusing behaviors in one or more type of professionally led group. The groups vary in orientation from 12-step to education-supportive to social skills training to stage-wise. Because high rates of serious infectious diseases, such as HIV and hepatitis, are associated with SUD, these sessions also address risk behaviors.

An adjunctive approach to substance abuse treatment is linkage with self-help groups such as Alcoholics Anonymous in the community or with self-help groups that are specifically for dual diagnosis patients. Clinical experience suggests that these linkages require some preparation and debriefing by mental health staff and that they are more effective once patients are actively pursuing abstinence.

Rehabilitation

Recovery from SUD extends into a longitudinal process because it typically involves building a new life rather than just avoiding substances.[57] Stable abstinence usually requires major alterations in how one handles internal and external stress, social networks, habits, self-perceptions, and vocational activities. Since most dual diagnosis patients have become entangled in the social scene of substance abuse over years, their recovery from SUD also takes years.[16] Many dual diagnosis programs attempt to substitute day treatment, rehabilitation groups, or sheltered work for previous activities and relationships. The weakness of these approaches is that mental health activities are difficult to sustain over time, and more important, patients do not value them and often find them demeaning.[58] Supported education or supported employment, which help patients to succeed in normal roles in the community, offer greater promise. For example, standard approaches to supported employment can support the patient's movement toward abstinence.

Housing

Since dual diagnosis patients commonly have difficulties maintaining housing and since living in drug-infested housing settings often sustains their SUD, housing has been a specific focus of dual diagnosis interventions, particularly for the homeless.[59] Patients, even those who are homeless, tend to prefer independent housing. Some have argued on ideological grounds that independent housing is preferable, while others have argued that the special vulnerabilities of dual diagnosis can only be addressed in structured living situations that include close monitoring by professional staff. One well-known program has created a housing continuum that allows dual diagnosis patients to enter housing while they are still actively abusing substances but also provides a range of staffed and supported housing arrangements for those who are in varying stages of recovery.[60]

Pharmacology

Medication nonadherence correlates with comorbid SUD,[61] perhaps in part because dually diagnosed individuals are often told that using alcohol or street drugs in addition to their prescribed medications poses a grave health risk. On the other hand, clinical experience suggests that medication adherence and symptom control are often prerequisites to successful SUD treatment. Most programs therefore adopt efforts to improve compliance by providing education, medication management skills, medication supervision, use of depot forms of antipsychotic medications, and coercive means such as outpatient commitment and guardianship.

For patients with schizophrenia, antipsychotic medications are the mainstay of pharmacological treatment. Typical antipsychotic medications, per se, probably do not decrease SUD behaviors and may actually precipitate or worsen SUD.[62] There is emerging evidence, however, that the atypical antipsychotic drug clozapine may reduce SUD in dual diagnosis patients.[63] Mood stabilizers are also a mainstay of treatment of severe mental illness and are frequently prescribed for dually disordered patients. Another critical issue in dual diagnosis treatment concerns the effectiveness of antianxiety medications and their potential for abuse. Clinical discussions of pharmacology for dual diagnosis inevitably produce strong but mixed opinions about whether long-acting benzodiazepines are helpful or harmful. There is also concern about the potential for abuse of antiparkinsonian medications.

Finally, many psychiatrists prescribe antidipsomanic medications to help dual diagnosis patients achieve stable remission. Kofoed et al[64] reported the usefulness of adjunctive disulfiram in an open clinical trial, and naltrexone is often used as well.

Conclusions

Comorbid SUD is a common complication of severe mental illness and is associated with several adverse consequences. Over the past two decades the health care field has recognized the ineffectiveness of providing care to dually diagnosed individuals in two separate service systems and has rapidly developed service models that integrate mental health and substance abuse treatments. Recent evidence regarding the general integrated treatment approach is consistent and positive, but much work remains to be done on organizing and financing of integrated programs. Furthermore, the basic components of integrated treatment – case management, close monitoring, substance abuse treatment, family psychoeducation, rehabilitation, housing, and medications – are still being developed and refined.

References

1. Mueser KT, Bennett M, Kushner MG, Epidemiology of substance use disorders among persons with chronic mental illnesses. In: Lehman AF, Dixon L, eds, *Double Jeopardy: Chronic Mental Illness and Substance Abuse* (Harwood Academic: New York, 1995) 9–25.

2. Regier DA, Farmer ME, Rae DS et al, Comorbidity of mental disorders with alcohol and other drug abuse, *JAMA* (1990) **264:**2511–18.

3. Cantwell R, Brewin J, Glazebrook C et al, Prevalence of substance misuse in first-episode psychosis, *Br J Psychiatry* (1999) **174:**150–3.

4. Duke PJ, Pantelis C, Barnes TRE, South Westminster Schizophrenia Survey: alcohol use and its relationship to symptoms, tardive dyskinesia and illness onset, *Br J Psychiatry* (1994) **164:**630–6.

5. Fowler IL, Carr VJ, Carter NT, Lewin TJ, Patterns of current and lifetime substance use in schizophrenia, *Schizophr Bull* (1998) **24:**443–55.

6. Menzes PR, Johnson S, Thornicroft G et al, Drug and alcohol problems among individuals with severe mental illnesses in South London, *Br J Psychiatry* (1996) **168:**612–19.

7. Scott J, Homelessness and mental illness, *Br J Psychiatry* (1993) **162:**314–24.

8. Soyka M, Albus M, Kathmann N et al, Prevalence of alcohol and drug abuse in schizophrenic inpatients, *Eur Arch Psychiatry Clin Neurosci* (1993) **242:**362–72.

9. Lehman AF, Myers CP, Dixon LB, Johnson JL, Detection of substance use disorders among psychiatric inpatients, *J Nerv Ment Dis* (1996) **184:** 228–33.

10. Dixon L, Haas G, Weiden P et al, Acute effects of drug abuse in schizophrenic patients: clinical observations and patients' self-reports, *Schizophr Bull* (1990) **16:**69–79.

11. Rasanen P, Tiihonen J, Isohanni M et al, Schizophrenia, alcohol abuse, and violent behavior: a 26-year follow-up study of an unselected birth cohort, *Schizophr Bull* (1998) **24:**437–41.

12. Scott H, Johnson S, Menezes P et al, Substance misuse and risk of aggression and offending among the severely mentally ill, *Br J Psychiatry* (1998) **172:**345–50.

13. Smith J, Hucker S, Schizophrenia and substance abuse, *Br J Psychiatry* (1994) **165:**13–21.

14. Addington J, Duchak V, Reasons for substance use in schizophrenia, *Acta Psychiatr Scan* (1997) **96:** 329–33.

15. Mueser KT, Nishith P, Tracy JI, Expectations and motives for substance use in schizophrenia, *Schizophr Bull* (1995) **21:**367–78.

16. Drake RE, Mueser KT, Clark RE, Wallach MA, The course, treatment, and outcome of substance disorder in persons with severe mental illness, *Am J Orthopsychiatry* (1996) **66:**42–51.

17. Kozaric-Kovacic D, Folnegovic-Smalc V, Folnegovic Z, Marusic A, Influence of alcoholism on the prognosis of schizophrenic patients, *J Stud Alcohol* (1995) **56:**622–7.

18. Mueser KT, Drake RE, Wallach MA, Dual diagnosis: a review of etiological theories, *Addict Behav* (1998) **23:**717–34.

19. Drake RE, Brunette MF, Complications of severe mental illness related to alcohol and other drug use disorders. In: Galanter M, ed, *Recent Developments in Alcoholism, vol 14. Consequences of Alcoholism* (Plenum: New York, 1998) 285–99.

20. Dickey B, Azeni H, Persons with dual diagnosis of substance abuse and major mental illness: their excess costs of psychiatric care, *Am J Public Health* (1996) **86:**973–7.

21. Maslin J, Graham H, Birchwood M, COMPASS Programme Service Development Group. The prevalence of co-morbid severe mental illness/psychotic symptoms and problematic substance use in the mental health and addiction services within

NBMHT, Northern Birmingham Mental health Trust (NBMHT), Birmingham, England, 1999.

22. Ridgely MS, Osher FC, Goldman HH, Talbott JA, *Executive Summary: Chronic Mentally Ill Young Adults with Substance Abuse Problems: A Review of Research, Treatment, and Training Issues* (Mental Health Services Research Center, University of Maryland School of Medicine: Baltimore, MD, 1987).

23. Kavanagh DJ, Greenaway L, Jenner L et al, and members of the Dual Diagnosis Consortium, Contrasting views and experiences of health professionals on the management of comorbid substance abuse and mental disorders, *Aust NZ J Psychiatry* (2000) **34:**279–89.

24. Rorstad P, Checinski K, *Dual Diagnosis: Facing the Challenge* (Wynne Howard Publishing: Kenley, 1996).

25. Minkoff K, An integrated treatment model for dual diagnosis of psychosis and addiction, *Hosp Community Psychiatry* (1989) **40:**1031–6.

26. Osher FC, Kofoed LL, Treatment of patients with psychiatric and psychoactive substance abuse disorders, *Hosp Community Psychiatry* (1989) **40:**1025–30.

27. Dailey DC, Moss HB, Campbell F, *Dual Disorders: Counseling Clients with Chemical Dependency & Mental Illness* (Hazelden: Center City, MN, 1993).

28. Ziedonis DM, Fisher W, Assessment and treatment of comorbid substance abuse in individuals with schizophrenia, *Psychiatr Annals* (1994) **24:**477–83.

29. Carey KB, Substance use reduction in the context of outpatient psychiatric treatment: a collaborative, motivational, harm reduction approach, *Community Ment Health J* (1996) **32:**291–306.

30. Mercer-McFadden C, Drake RE, Brown NB, Fox RS. The Community Support Program demonstrations of services for young adults with severe mental illness and substance use disorders, *Psychiatric Rehab J* (1997) **20:**13–24.

31. Mercer CC, Mueser KT, Drake RE, Organizational guidelines for dual disorders programs, *Psychiatr Q* (1998) **69:**145–68.

32. Mueser KT, Drake RE, Noordsy DL, Integrated mental health and substance abuse treatment for severe psychiatric disorders, *J Pract Psychiatry Behav Health* (1998) **4:**129–39.

33. Drake RE, Mercer-McFadden C, Mueser KT et al, Treatment of substance abuse in patients with severe mental illness: a review of recent research, *Schizophr Bull* (1998) **24:**589–608.

34. White A, Kavanagh DJ, Wallis G et al, *Start Over and Survive (SOS) Treatment Manual: Brief Intervention for Substance Abuse in Early Psychosis* (University of Queensland: Brisbane, Australia 1999).

35. Drake RE, Rosenberg SD, Mueser KT, Assessing substance use disorder in persons with severe mental illness. In: Drake RE, Mueser, KT, eds, *Dual Diagnosis of Major Mental Illness and Substance Abuse, vol 2. Recent Research and Clinical Implications* (Jossey-Bass: San Francisco, 1996) 3–17.

36. Ananth J, Vanderwater S, Kamal M et al, Missed diagnosis of substance abuse in psychiatric patients, *Hosp Community Psychiatry* (1989) **4:**297–9.

37. Rosenberg SD, Drake RE, Wolford GL et al, The Dartmouth Assessment of Lifestyle Instrument (DALI): a substance use disorder screen for people with severe mental illness, *Am J Psychiatry* (1998) **155:**232–8.

38. McPhillips MA, Kelly FJ, Barnes TRE et al, Comorbid substance abuse among people with schizophrenia in the community: a study comparing self-report with analysis of hair and urine, *Schizophr Res* (1997) **25:**141–8.

39. Shaner A, Khaka E, Roberts L et al, Unrecognized cocaine use among schizophrenic patients, *Am J Psychiatry* (1993) **150:**777–83.

40. Drake RE, Osher FC, Noordsy D et al, Diagnosis of alcohol use disorders in schizophrenia, *Schizophr Bull* (1990) **16:**57–67.

41. American Psychiatric Association, *Diagnostic and Statistical Manual of Mental Disorders*, 4th edn. (American Psychiatric Association: Washington, DC, 1994).

42. World Health Organization, *The ICD-10 Classification of Mental and Behavioral Disorders: Clinical Descriptions and Diagnostic Guidelines* (World Health Organization: Geneva, 1992).

43. Minkoff K, Substance abuse versus substance dependence, *Psychiatr Serv* (1997) **48:**867.

44. Rounsaville BJ, Clinical assessment of drug abusers. In: Kleber HD, ed, *Treatment of Drug Abusers (Non-Alcohol), A Task Force Report of the American Psychiatric Association* (American Psychiatric Association Press: Washington, DC, 1989) 1183–91.

45. Weiss RD, Mirin SM, Griffin ML, Methodological considerations in the diagnosis of coexisting psychiatric disorders in substance abusers, *Br J Addict* (1992) **87:** 179–87.

46. Shaner A, Roberts LJ, Eckman TA et al, Sources of diagnostic uncertainty for chronically psychotic cocaine abusers, *Psychiatr Serv* (1998) **49:**684–90.

47. Carey KB, Correia CJ, Severe mental illness and addictions: assessment considerations, *Addict Behav* (1998) **23:**735–48.

48. McHugo GJ, Drake RE, Burton HL, Ackerson TH, A scale for assessing the stage of substance abuse treatment in persons with severe mental illness, *J Nerv Ment Dis* (1995) **183:**762–7.

49. Drake RE, Noordsy DL, The role of inpatient care for patients with co-occurring severe mental disorder and substance use disorder, *Community Ment Health J* (1995) **31:** 279–82.

50. Drake RE, Mueser KT, Psychosocial approaches to dual diagnosis, *Schizophr Bull* (2000) **26:**105–18.

51. Fariello D, Scheidt S, Clinical case management of the dually diagnosed patient, *Hosp Community Psychiatry* (1989) **40:**1065–7.

52. Teague GB, Bond GR, Drake RE, Program fidelity in assertive community treatment, *Am J Orthopsychiatry* (1998) **68:**216–32.

53. McHugo GJ, Drake RE, Teague GB et al, The relationship between model fidelity and client outcomes in the New Hampshire Dual Disorders Study, *Psychiatr Serv* (1999) **50:**818–24.

54. Drake RE, Bartels SB, Teague GB et al, Treatment of substance use disorders in severely mentally ill patients, *J Nerve Ment Dis* (1993) **181:**606–11.

55. Kavanagh DJ, An intervention for substance abuse in schizophrenia, *Behaviour Change* (1995) **12:**20–30.

56. Bellack AS, DiClemente CC, Treating substance abuse among patients with schizophrenia, *Psychiatr Serv* (1999) **50:**75–80.

57. Vaillant GE, *The Natural History of Alcoholism Revisited* (Harvard University Press: Cambridge, MA, 1995).

58. Estroff S, *Making It Crazy* (University of California Press: Berkeley, 1981).

59. Osher FC, Dixon LB, Housing for persons with co-occurring mental and addictive disorders. In: Drake RE, Mueser KT, eds, *Dual Diagnosis of Major Mental Illness and Substance Abuse, vol 2. Recent Research and Clinical Implications* (Jossey-Bass: San Francisco, 1996) 53–64.

60. Bebout RR, The Community Connections housing program: preventing homelessness by integrating housing and supports, *Alcohol Treatment Q* (1999) **17:**93–112.

61. Swartz MS, Swanson JW, Hiday VA et al, Violence and severe mental illness: the effects of substance abuse and nonadherence to medication, *Am J Psychiatry* (1998) **155:**226–31.

62. Voruganti LNP, Heslegrave RJ, Awad AG, Neuroleptic dysphoria may be the missing link between schizophrenia and substance abuse, *J Nerv Ment Dis* (1997) **185:**463–5.

63. Buckley PF, Substance abuse in schizophrenia: a review, *J Clin Psychiatry* (1998) **59(Suppl 3):**26–30.

64. Kofoed L, Kania J, Walsh T, Atkinson RM, Outpatient treatment of patients with substance abuse and coexisting psychiatric disorders, *Am J Psychiatry* (1986) **143:**867–72.

17

Issues Affecting Women with Schizophrenia

Ruth A Dickson and William M Glazer

Introduction

Gender issues have long been of interest to both schizophrenia researchers and clinicians given the differences in the neurobiology, epidemiology, treatment responses, and social context of this illness in women versus men. The literature supports superior premorbid functioning, a later onset of illness, fewer hospitalizations, better response to treatment, and better outcomes in women compared to men. Symptom patterns differ, with women having more positive and fewer negative symptoms of schizophrenia, the latter especially in women with late-onset schizophrenia, and more mood symptoms.[1-5] Differences, or lack thereof, between the sexes have also been described in neuroimaging studies and neuropsychological functions.[6,7] Estrogen's effects are often cited as a possible biological modulator influencing the time of onset, course, and response to treatment in women with schizophrenia. There are several reviews on these aspects of gender and schizophrenia.[8-11]

Despite the acknowledged importance of the sex of the person in understanding schizophrenia, there has been only limited progress made in developing a gender-based therapeutic approach to patients that could, hypothetically, improve treatment for both men and women. The few model treatment programs designed for women with schizophrenia include a spectrum of integrated psychosocial services that are necessary to provide comprehensive care throughout the life cycle.[12] The goal of this chapter is to discuss treatment of women with schizophrenia, focusing on: (a) the use of antipsychotic drugs, in particular the second generation of drugs; and (b) sexual and reproductive health issues unique to women.

Women and antipsychotic drug therapy

There is an expanding literature on psychopharmacology and sex-based differences,[13] but this area continues to be underresearched in patients with schizophrenia. Some 60% of all antipsychotics are prescribed to women, and approximately 30% to women aged 20–50 years (IMS).[14] Clinical trials of these drugs are conducted in patients with schizophrenia, but once marketed, these compounds are used 'off label' extensively in patients with other diagnoses including mood disorders, organic brain syndromes, and some personality disorders.

Thus, understanding gender aspects of antipsychotic treatment has relevance beyond treating patients with schizophrenia.

During the past decade, new drugs for the treatment of schizophrenia have been introduced. The first generation of neuroleptic drugs, or 'typical' antipsychotics, includes all the compounds with the exceptions of clozapine, risperidone, olanzapine, quetiapine and other drugs such as ziprasidone, in development but not yet released, which are collectively termed 'atypicals,' 'novel' compounds or second-generation drugs.

Recent changes in legislation and attitudes encourage the recruitment of women to clinical trials of new drugs, but historically, women of childbearing potential have been excluded and/or recruited in much lower numbers than have males.[15] In addition, many programs for seriously mentally ill individuals treat more males than females, therefore making recruitment of females more difficult for investigators even with the shifts in ethical and scientific perspectives that promote inclusion of women in drug testing. For the most part, the samples enrolled in clinical trials of the second generation of antipsychotic drugs reflect this male bias.[16,17] Thus, at the time of marketing of new medications and to this date, there is limited information on the efficacy and tolerability of these drugs in premenopausal women and during times of life unique to women, such as pregnancy and the postpartum period.

Efficacy

The introduction of the second generation of antipsychotics raised questions about differential efficacy of these new compounds in the sexes. In women with treatment-resistant schizophrenia, one study found that response to clozapine was not as robust in women as in men[18] but this was a small select sample of women. Analysis of the Canadian Clozaril Support and Assistance Network database does not support that women drop out of clozapine treatment at a higher rate than do men, a finding that would be expected if

the drug were less efficacious and/or less tolerated in women than in men (RAD, personal communication, Novartis Canada, 1999). Study of differences in response to olanzapine vs haloperidol found that women and men on olanzapine respond equally well.[19] Comparable studies by gender are not available for risperidone and quetiapine.

Dose of antipsychotic medication

In general, lower doses of conventional antipsychotic drugs are used in premenopausal women than in men and postmenopausal women. The neuromodulating effects of estrogen and the more rapid decline of dopamine receptors with age in men than in women may explain this observation.[9,20] Whether higher doses of medications are required in individual menopausal women as estrogen levels decline is controversial.

Of the new generation of antipsychotics, clozapine is the most studied. A study of clozapine levels in a Chinese population found that female patients had 35% higher clozapine level than did men. Aging is another variable that raises plasma levels of clozapine and its two major metabolites.[21] This study confirmed earlier findings[22] that women require lower doses of clozapine than do men to achieve comparable clozapine plasma levels. Dosage studies by sex are not available for the other new antipsychotics but it is likely that, as with the traditional drugs and clozapine, premenopausal women require lower doses than men. Recommended doses of antipsychotic drugs are for the most part based on clinical trial experience with male patients. Therefore, the clinician should be cautious in prescribing these medications at the 'standard' doses to women and consider starting at lower doses.

The dose of the drug should be titrated to the minimal effective level not only as is commonly accepted to increase the tolerability and to reduce the chance of developing extrapyramidal side effects (EPS), but to avoid menstrual disruptions.[23] Any potential protective effect of estrogen in a premenopausal woman is lost if, during antipsychotic therapy, an anovulatory state develops. Relative 'overdosing' of women with antipsychotic drugs may have a negative impact on response of symptoms of schizophrenia to treatment.[11]

Side effects of antipsychotic drugs

Sex differences also influence risk for side effects of antipsychotic drugs. For example, older women may be at higher risk of clozapine-induced granulocytopenia,[24] but the risk with current blood monitoring systems is low relative to risks from the illness itself. Two areas of particular interest with the new antipsychotics, movement disorders and neuroleptic-induced hyperprolactinemia (NIHP), are discussed below.

Gender and drug-induced movement disorders

Neurological movement disorders are the most researched side effects of antipsychotic drug treatment and the side effects that have been most reduced with the widespread use of the second generation of drugs. The sex of the patient has not been shown to be a consistent risk factor for either acute EPS (parkinsonism, dystonias, or akathisia) or tardive movement disorders (TD) secondary to treatment with first-generation antipsychotic medications. Numerous studies have identified possible demographic risk factors for the development of TD.[25] While early research identified an increased frequency of TD in older females, over time, the etiologic role of gender has been less clear.[26] Methodological problems, in particular selection biases and temporal ambiguities (of cause and effect) in evaluating risk factors in prevalence studies have contributed to conflicting results and perpetuated the clinical lore that female sex is a causative factor for TD. Two incidence studies have found an effect of gender, with males at higher risk, in older men[27] and in males with a deteriorating course of illness.[28]

There are no reviews focused specifically on gender as a risk factor utilizing the new antipsychotic drugs. From the literature on traditional drugs, one would expect women and men to benefit equally from drugs that reduce these distressing side effects. It is, in part, the reduced liability of the new antipsychotics to induce movement disorders that has allowed for and facilitated a shift to investigating other side effects of drug treatment.

Neuroleptic-induced hyperprolactinemia

Neuroleptic-induced hyperprolactinemia has recently been the focus of renewed interest given the variable propensities of the new antipsychotics to induce prolactin elevations and the heightened awareness of sex-specific treatment issues. This section focuses on neuroendocrine side effects of antipsychotic drugs, specifically those secondary to hyperprolactinemia that have an impact on reproductive functioning. More extensive reviews of NIHP, including sexuality, behavior, and potential long-term side effects in both men and women, are given by Dickson and Glazer[16,17] (Box 17.1).

Prolactin is an anterior pituitary polypeptide hormone that in mammals has a major role in lactogenesis. The neurotransmitter dopamine released by the hypothalamus into the portal circulation plays a primary role in regulation, acting as the principal prolactin inhibitory factor. Control of prolactin release is complex, with many physiologic and neuroendocrine stimulatory and inhibitory factors interacting, affecting the amount of prolactin secreted by the pituitary lactotrophs.[29]

Clozapine,[30] olanzapine,[31] and quetiapine[32] cause limited or mild prolactin elevation and collectively are termed 'prolactin-sparing' antipsychotics (Figure 17.1).[16] Ziprasidone, a new antipsychotic in development, also has minimal and transient effects on serum prolactin levels. Risperidone is comparable to haloperidol in its propensity to raise serum prolactin levels with 4–6 mg reported to be equivalent to approximately 20 mg haloperidol.[33] In small samples of

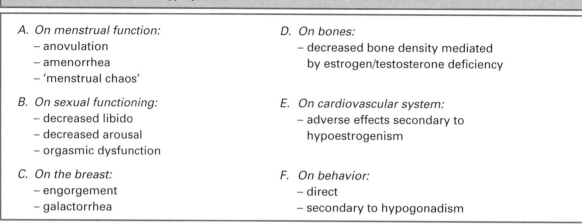

Box 17.1 Clinical effects of hyperprolactinemia

A. On menstrual function:
– anovulation
– amenorrhea
– 'menstrual chaos'

B. On sexual functioning:
– decreased libido
– decreased arousal
– orgasmic dysfunction

C. On the breast:
– engorgement
– galactorrhea

D. On bones:
– decreased bone density mediated by estrogen/testosterone deficiency

E. On cardiovascular system:
– adverse effects secondary to hypoestrogenism

F. On behavior:
– direct
– secondary to hypogonadism

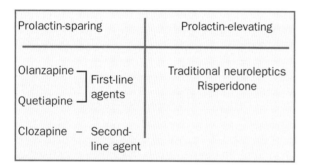

Figure 17.1 Antipsychotic drugs and prolactin

premenopausal women, risperidone increased prolactin levels to levels twice or greater than those found with typical drugs.[34,35]

Neuroleptics are thought to elevate prolactin levels mainly by interfering with the normal tonic dopaminergic inhibition of prolactin, but why some of these drugs have more profound and sustained liability to induce hyperprolactinemia is poorly understood.[36] Increases in prolactin correlate poorly with the clinical potency of the compound and are influenced by the pharmacologic and pharmacokinetic profile of the antipsychotic.[37] Females have a greater increase in prolactin following neuroleptic treatment than do

men.[37] The general belief that neuroleptics cause only modest prolactin elevations (up to six times the upper limit of the reference range) has been recently challenged with reports of much higher levels of up to 15 times normal in women taking first-generation antipsychotics.[38] Hyperprolactinemia can persist throughout chronic treatment, that is, continued neuroleptic prescription carries the risk of persistent prolactin elevations, although some individuals may develop tolerance.[39]

Hyperprolactinemia inhibits the normal pulsatile secretion of gonadotropin releasing hormone (GnRH) by the hypothalamus that is necessary for the normal pituitary secretion of luteinizing hormone (LH) and follicle stimulating hormone (FSH) and for the normal pituitary ovulatory response to the ovarian follicle's steroid signals (Figure 17.2).[29] When GnRH pulses are disrupted, there is a distortion of the menstrual cycle progressing sequentially from continued regular menses with impaired follicular growth and therefore impaired fertility, to menses that are too frequent or infrequent, and/or too heavy or too light.[15] More severe impairment of pulsatile GnRH secretion causes insufficient secretion of gonadotropins to produce an ovarian response, thus leading to an anovulatory amenorrheic

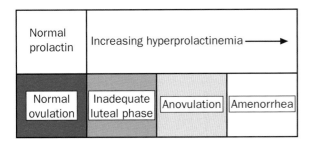

Figure 17.2 Prolactin and menstrual dysfunction. Reproduced with permission from Speroff et al (1999).[29]

state[29,40] with all the long-term sequelae of deficient estrogen secretion such as genitourinary symptoms, dyspareunia, decreased bone mineral density[41,42] and increased risk of cardiovascular disease.[43] As estrogen has a profound influence on mental functioning, psychopathology, mood state and cognition can all be affected.[9] Chronic anovulation is now considered to be a serious medical condition that requires evaluation and therapeutic management to avoid the consequences of infertility and increased risk of developing endometrial carcinoma.[29,44] These side effects have been understudied in women with schizophrenia.[16,17]

Although the etiology of hyperprolactinemia is diverse, the key point is that once the condition is diagnosed, it is amenable to therapy by treating the underlying cause, or by inhibiting pituitary secretion of prolactin with dopaminergic agonist medications.[45] With the introduction of prolactin-sparing antipsychotic drugs, there is a new treatment option should NIHP induce side effects in women with schizophrenia.[16]

Reproductive health

As women with severe mental illnesses now overwhelmingly live in community settings rather than institutions, issues affecting them are those that affect women without psychiatric illnesses. Defi-

ciencies in available contraception, unwanted/unplanned pregnancies and children, the risks of contracting sexually transmitted diseases (STDs), and abusive sex are concerns of all women.[46] There is some evidence that mentally ill women are less prepared to cope with these problems and are an especially vulnerable population.[47] Persons with schizophrenia are also at high risk of developing HIV/AIDS and have special needs for education and prevention.[48] While there are model programs that incorporate education and interventions aimed at addressing domestic and sexual violence and family planning and a full range of options in case pregnancy does occur,[12,49,50] these are the exception, not the rule in the system of care for women with schizophrenia.

Recently, treatment programs often called 'early psychosis programs' have been developed, which focus on early identification of and interventions for individuals developing psychotic illnesses. Given that the world population between 10 and 19 years of age is more than 1 billion and that the onset of schizophrenia, particularly in males, is often during mid- to late adolescence, targeting this population to research their needs in terms of sexual and reproductive health is crucial. Yet, even in the nonmentally ill population, it is not clear how to best help this group communicate their problems in an 'adolescent friendly way' so that these functions remain intact.[46] As these programs develop for persons in the early stages of illness, it is important that sexual and reproductive issues, which have historically been marginalized and of limited interest to schizophrenia researchers, are investigated.

Also, there has been little focus on 'men's reproductive health issues' for seriously mentally ill individuals. Often intimate relationships develop between patients who attend the same services and programs. Thus, ensuring that males are aware of and educated about these issues not only affects their own health, but that of women with schizophrenia. Access to counseling and services that assist individuals of both sexes to make decisions about relationships, contraception, sexuality and reproduction should be integrated into comprehensive programs for persons with schizophrenia throughout the life cycle.

Menstruation and schizophrenia

Disrupted menstrual cycles and amenorrhea associated with schizophrenia were noted before the introduction of neuroleptics. In a subsample of unmedicated institutionalized premenopausal women with schizophrenia, increased variability of menstrual cycle length, a high incidence of amenorrhea, and disruption of cycles by physical therapies used then including leucotomy, insulin coma therapy, and electroconvulsive therapy were found.[51] As antipsychotic drugs can also cause abnormal menses and amenorrhea, it is sometimes unclear in women with schizophrenia whether the disturbance is due to the disease, the drugs, or both. It is possible that women with schizophrenia, given their brain disease, will be especially vulnerable to drug-induced dysregulation of their hypothalamic–pituitary–ovarian axis.[16,17,52] See Speroff et al[29] for a current review of amenorrhea.

In people with schizophrenia it is important to acknowledge and understand psychological issues such as sexuality, and desire or lack thereof to bear children, that historically had limited clinical priority for mental health personnel. Reproductive functioning influences gender identity and feelings about fertility. Its meaning is influenced by multiple variables including education, individual experience, and cultural traditions. Psychologically, amenorrhea secondary to antipsychotic drugs may be experienced with indifference, as a loss of youth and generativity, or as a welcome development.[52] The loss of menses and/or galactorrhea may be misinterpreted as conclusive evidence of pregnancy and in women with psychosis contribute to delusional beliefs.[53,54]

Menstrual disturbances and anovulation have also been undervalued as biological side effects of antipsychotic medication, are not routinely monitored for in mental health clinics, and if they do occur may be inappropriately treated with reas-

surance. All traditional antipsychotic drugs via their prolactin-elevating properties may induce reproductive and sexual side effects. Risperidone in a small retrospective case series was reported to cause more amenorrhea and galactorrhea than traditional neuroleptic therapy,[34] a fact related to its propensity to cause hyperprolactinemia, and thus may be less well tolerated during chronic treatment of premenopausal women with schizophrenia. This has been disputed by a post hoc analysis of the risperidone clinical trial data.[33] However, it is difficult to draw conclusions about prolactin-induced reproductive and sexual side effects secondary to any of the new antipsychotics from clinical trial data, given the methodological problems encountered. These include:

1. The brief time spans of clinical trials, usually 6–8 weeks, relative to the length and variability of normal menstrual cycles.
2. The use of scales that were not designed to capture menstrual abnormalities during brief drug trials; for example, the UKU[55] requires absence of menses for 3 months to diagnose amenorrhea.
3. The lack of control for use of contraceptive pills, hormone replacement therapy, and hysterectomies.
4. Inadequate determination of menopausal status at trial initiation. Classifying menopausal status by age without evaluation of endocrinological status may either over- or underestimate the number of women capable of menstruating and hence at risk of developing abnormal menses.

Case studies have reported that switching to prolactin-sparing antipsychotics has reversed menstrual side effects,[56–58] but longitudinal, large-sample studies are needed to clarify this issue.

Obtaining an initial menstrual history before starting neuroleptics, monitoring for menstrual disturbances and for the onset of menopause, should be a routine part of clinical psychiatric practice. Prolactin-sparing drugs may be preferred initial therapy in women with histories of erratic cycles, as this eliminates one risk factor for developing amenorrhea. If menstrual abnormalities develop, concomitant with hyperprolactinemia, switching to either olanzapine, quetiapine, or clozapine may be diagnostic. However, decisions about switching antipsychotic drugs must include assessment of many variables, including efficacy of the antipsychotic, degree of response, cost of possible relapse to the patient, and other side effects. Lowering the dose of the traditional antipsychotic or risperidone may reduce the prolactin levels enough to resolve side effects. Other options are the addition of a dopamine agonist (such as bromocriptine) to lower the prolactin levels, or prescription of oral contraceptives to treat the drug-induced hormone deficiency.[16,17,59] The latter approach will not end side effects such as galactorrhea and sexual dysfunction directly related to NIHP. The clinician must keep in mind that reversal of hyperprolactinemia is a well-accepted strategy in the treatment of infertility and therefore contraceptive needs must be reviewed before lowering prolactin levels.

There is remarkably little known about menopause in women with schizophrenia given the interest of psychiatrists, gynecologists, and sociologists in psychiatric symptoms and the menopause.[60,61] The decline in estrogen levels that occurs at menopause has been suggested as a factor contributing to late-onset schizophrenia in women and higher neuroleptic doses in psychotic women in their forties than in younger women.[20] Amenorrhea secondary to NIHP in perimenopausal females with schizophrenia may be attributed incorrectly to the onset of menopause and be reversed when a switch to a prolactin-sparing antipsychotic is made. Therefore, both older and younger women should be advised of the possibility of return of menstrual cycles with a drug change.[52]

Fertility and schizophrenia

The fertility of men and women with schizophrenia has been found to be reduced compared to their unaffected siblings, with males showing greater reduction in reproductive fitness than females.[62,63] The reasons for the reduced number of children are complex and have been attributed to the illness itself, the drugs used to treat it, and societal factors such as institutionalization and stigmatization of people with serious mental illnesses. However, at least in some cultures, this may be changing. A more current American community sample of women with schizophrenia, when compared to demographically matched controls, was found to have the same average number of pregnancies but more unplanned and unwanted conceptions and more abortions.[50]

As more men and women with severe mental disorders are treated in community settings, achieve better control of their psychiatric symptoms, and receive drugs that cause fewer sexual and reproductive side effects, theoretically more pregnancies may occur.[64–66] However, there have not been any epidemiological studies describing differences in the gravidity of psychotic patients at a population level comparing women on the new versus the old antipsychotics. As clozapine, olanzapine, and quetiapine are the first prolactin-sparing antipsychotics marketed, and as these drugs may reverse menstrual dysfunction in a subgroup of neuroleptic-treated women, this may lead to fertility trends over time in the population of women with psychotic disorders.

Whether or not birth control measures are used obviously affects rates of conception. Women with schizophrenia may have more difficulty understanding available options and accessing and utilizing contraception than do other women.[47] Respecting the patient's autonomy while helping her avoid an unwanted pregnancy is challenging for clinicians.[67] The concept of 'variably impaired autonomy',[68] that is, limitations in decision-making ability that are not static over time, is helpful to clinicians in developing a non-paternalistic alliance with these women and in planning effective interventions around reproductive issues. Education during a time of mental stability may address misconceptions about contraception and more effective medications may target reality impairments, thus assisting these women to make realistic decisions. This is a complex and evolving area given technological advances such as contraceptive implants and changing value systems in a more consumer-oriented mental health services system.

Pregnancy and schizophrenia

Given the common occurrence of menstrual disturbances in women with schizophrenia on antipsychotic medications, delays may occur in diagnosis of pregnancy as the regular cycles, absence of which cues other women to possible conception, may not occur. In addition, the high rate of custody loss and/or the perception that medical personnel will react negatively to a pregnancy may encourage some women to hide their pregnancy.[69,70] Others, because of psychosis, may misinterpret and/or misunderstand signs of pregnancy, or in extreme cases exhibit delusional denial of pregnancy. Denial of pregnancy is associated with a diagnosis of chronic schizophrenia, with previous loss of custody of children, and with anticipation of separation from the baby.[71] All of these factors make it necessary for the clinician to have an understanding of the patient's feelings about having children and a high index of suspicion which regard to the possibility of pregnancy, monitoring for this on an ongoing basis.

Despite clinicians' perception that women with schizophrenia improve during pregnancy, for many of these women pregnancy is a very stressful time with worsening of mental status especially in younger women with unwanted pregnancies.[47,72,73] The diagnosis of schizophrenia predicts less adequate prenatal care and more complicated births.[74] As smoking, substance abuse, and economic deprivations are associated with fetal growth retardation, premature births, and increased perinatal morbidity and mortality, efforts should be made to work with the pregnant woman with schizophrenia to reduce these additional risk factors.[50,75] A woman with delusions or psychotic denial about her pregnancy is less likely to detect signs of labor and impending delivery and is at risk of birth complications.[49] Therefore, this psychopathology should alert the clinician that intensive psychiatric follow-up and prenatal care and planning for delivery are indicated.

The patient's psychiatrist plays a key role in coordinating comprehensive care and educating other medical specialists and community workers about schizophrenia and the benefits and limitations of drug treatments when a woman with schizophrenia becomes pregnant.[70] This area is becoming more complicated given the introduction of the second generation of antipsychotics and the limited clinical experience with these drugs in pregnant and postpartum patients.

If drug treatment of psychosis is required during pregnancy, higher-potency antipsychotic medications such as trifluoperazine and haloperidol are recommended, as more clinical experience has accumulated with these drugs than with the novel antipsychotics. Adjunctive anticholinergics and low-potency antipsychotics should be avoided. Ideally, drugs should not be given in the first trimester, but realistically, for many women with schizophrenia, the risk and consequences of relapse make this impossible.[47,59,76,77] There is controversy about tapering and/or discontinuing antipsychotics for 5–10 days prior to delivery to minimize the risk of side effects, particularly extrapyramidal symptoms.[78]

Clozapine is not known to have teratogenic effects[79] but it may pose extra risks in pregnancy given the inability to monitor fetal hematology.[80] There are no case reports of neonates who are born to clozapine-treated mothers who develop agranulocytosis, but the literature is so limited that this outcome cannot be excluded. Monitoring white blood cell counts in these babies for the first 4 weeks after birth seems reasonable, as this is the protocol when adults discontinue clozapine therapy. Whether to continue clozapine treatment during pregnancy, or to initiate it in severely ill treatment-resistant women, is a risk–benefit decision that needs to be made on a case-by-case basis. In women with treatment-resistant schizophrenia, reverting to ineffective traditional antipsychotic therapy during pregnancy risks exacerbation of psychosis that may ultimately be more dangerous to the dyad than clozapine continuation. The opinion held by some psychiatrists that women who have been treatment failures with traditional neuroleptic treatment should be discouraged from getting pregnant[77] is a debatable issue. Clozapine treatment combined with intensive psychosocial support may allow these women to remain competent, cooperate with prenatal care, manage labor and delivery, and ultimately improve the odds that they will be able to retain custody of their children, a goal of many women with serious mental illnesses.[70]

Increasing glucose intolerance following clozapine initiation has been reported.[81] There have been two case reports of clozapine-treated women developing gestational diabetes.[69,70] Whether clozapine use in pregnancy increases the risk of difficult delivery (shoulder dystocia) through increased risk of maternal hyperglycemia and resulting macrosomia is unknown, but physicians should be alert to this possibility.[70]

There are no published case reports of women being prescribed olanzapine, risperidone, or quetiapine while pregnant. A case report of a woman switched from depot antipsychotic to olanzapine and subsequently conceiving,[82] with the pregnancy terminated by therapeutic abortion, is very similar to cases reported with clozapine.[70,83] Given that many women of childbearing age are prescribed the new antipsychotic drugs and that there is a lack of data on use during pregnancy, physicians should contact the manufacturers and teratology information services such as the Motherisk Program in Canada[84] should a pregnancy occur.

The postpartum period and schizophrenia

While women with mood disorders have a higher rate of acute illness exacerbation in the postpartum period, the risk of relapse of schizophrenia during this time is also significant.[85–87] It is impor-

tant to reinstitute full doses of antipsychotic medication post-delivery if they have been reduced during pregnancy, to minimize the risk of relapse and to ensure that psychosocial supports are provided during this high-risk period.

Whether a woman with schizophrenia can care for her child at birth is a major issue with profound consequences for both the woman and her baby. Ideally, decisions about child-care should be made during the pregnancy well in advance of delivery. However, the reality is that often child protection services intervene at the birth of these children given their mandate to ensure the safety of the infants, particularly in instances when a prior child has been apprehended. Social welfare systems do vary in their attitudes about women with mental illnesses retaining custody of their children and in resource availability; clinicians caring for these women must therefore explore options in their own communities.

Evaluation of parenting capabilities in women with mental illness is a very complex topic that is beyond the scope of this chapter. There are no factors that predict a woman will permanently be unable to parent even when an extreme event such as previous neonatacide has happened.[88] Schizophrenia is not a contraindication to parenting although many of these women have difficulties with this role. Programs have been described that incorporate parenting rehabilitation and provide support for women with psychotic disorders,[12,89,90] but for the most part there has been limited integration of parenting training into psychosocial rehabilitation programs for persons with severe mental illnesses. Whether the new antipsychotic drugs will improve the custody outcomes in women with severe mental illnesses is currently unknown.

Women taking antipsychotic medication are often advised not to breastfeed,[59] but this recommendation is based on remarkably scant data given that these drugs have been prescribed for over 40 years. As with the use of drugs in pregnancy, a decision about breastfeeding requires an individualised risk–benefit assessment. The goals are to treat the woman's mental illness adequately while minimizing the exposure of the infant to the drug.[78,91] Women who choose to breastfeed while taking antipsychotic medication must have the ability to monitor the infant and to access a pediatrician who is willing to work with them to minimize risk to the infant.

With atypical drugs, there is information available only on clozapine and breastfeeding. Barnas et al[92] describe the course of a planned pregnancy in a 31-year-old patient who experienced remission of symptoms on a low dose of clozapine. This case is remarkable in that maternal plasma clozapine levels were determined monthly during pregnancy, and maternal plasma, fetal plasma, and breast milk clozapine levels were determined at delivery. High levels of clozapine were found in the breast milk. The authors recommend those mothers not to breastfeed while taking clozapine.

In women requiring antipsychotic therapy during the postpartum period, there may be advantages to prescribing a prolactin-sparing antipsychotic, as lactation is often not desired. One case reports the successful use of clozapine in treating a patient with mastitis and a postpartum psychosis.[93] However, as clozapine use is restricted because of the hematological risk, the newer prolactin-sparing agents olanzapine and quetiapine may be useful in women who require antipsychotic therapy post partum, are not treatment-resistant, and who do not wish to breastfeed.

Conclusion

While schizophrenia is not a 'woman's disease', women with schizophrenia may benefit from gender-focused management including strategies such as education and counseling about contraception and sexuality, supports for parenting, and integrated medical and psychiatric care specific to the stage of the reproductive cycle. Sex differences in response to and side effects from medication and the modifying effects of hormones are evolving areas of study that may advance care for

both men and women with schizophrenia. The role of the prolactin-sparing antipsychotics in treatment needs to be better understood.

References

1. Hafner H, Maurer K, Loffler W et al, The epidemiology of early schizophrenia. Influence of age and gender on onset and early course, *Br J Psych* (1994) **(Suppl 23):**29–38.

2. Szymanski S, Lieberman JA, Alvir JM et al, Gender differences in onset of illness, treatment response, course, and biologic indexes in first-episode schizophrenic patients, *Am J Psychiatry* (1995) **152:**698–703.

3. Fennig S, Putnam K, Bromet EJ, Galambo SN, Gender, premorbid characteristics and negative symptoms in schizophrenia, *Acta Psychiatr Scand* (1995) **92:**173–7.

4. Nopulos P, Flaum M, Andreasen NC, Sex differences in brain morphology in schizophrenia, *Am J Psychiatry* (1997) **154:**1648–54.

5. Lindamer LA, Lohr JB, Harris MJ et al, Gender related clinical differences in older patients with schizophrenia, *J Clin Psychiatry* (1999) **60:**61–7.

6. Bryant NL, Buchanan RW, Vladar K et al, Gender differences in temporal lobe structures of patients with schizophrenia: a volumetric MRI study, *Am J Psychiatry* (1999) **156:**603–9.

7. Goldstein JM, Seidman LJ, Goodman JM et al, Are there sex differences in neuropsychological functions among patients with schizophrenia? *Am J Psychiatry* (1998) **155:**1358–64.

8. Seeman MV, Gender differences in treatment response in schizophrenia. In: Seeman MV, ed, *Gender and Pathology* (American Psychiatric Press: Washington, DC, 1995) 227–51.

9. Seeman MV, Psychopathology in women and men: focus on female hormones, *Am J Psychiatry* (1997) **154:**1641–7.

10. Taminga CA, Gender and schizophrenia, *Can J Psychiatry* (1997) **(Suppl 15):**33–7.

11. Kulkarni J, Women and schizophrenia, *Aust N Z J Psychiatry* (1997) **31:**45–56.

12. Seeman MV, Cohen R, A service for women with schizophrenia, *Psychiatr Serv* (1998) **49:**674–7.

13. Jensvold MF, Halbreich U, Hamilton JE, eds, *Psychopharmacology and Women: Sex, Gender, and Hor-*

mones (American Psychiatric Press: Washington, DC, 1996).

14. IMS, National Disease Therapeutic Index. November 1996 to April 1997.

15. Romach MK, Drug development for women, *Can J Clin Pharmacol* (1999) **6:**7–8.

16. Dickson RA, Glazer WM, Neuroleptic-induced hyperprolactinemia, *Schizophr Res* (1999) **35:**75S-86S.

17. Dickson RA, Glazer WM, Women and antipsychotic drugs: focus on neuroleptic-induced hyperprolactinemia. In: Lewis-Hall F, Panetta JA, Williams TS, Herrera JM, eds, *Women's Issues in Psychiatry* (American Psychiatric Press: New York, in press).

18. Szymanski S, Lieberman J, Pollack S et al, Gender differences in neuroleptic nonresponsive clozapine-treated schizophrenics, *Biol Psychiatry* (1996) **39:**249–54.

19. Cohen LS, Goldstein J, Lee H et al, Sex and neuroendocrine differences in response to treatment with olanzapine: a preliminary analysis. Presented at the New Clinical Drug Evaluation Unit Conference, Boca Raton, FL, May 1997.

20. Seeman MV, Interaction of sex, age, and neuroleptic dose, *Compr Psychiatry* (1983) **24:**125–8.

21. Lane HY, Chang YC, Chang WH et al, Effects of gender and age on plasma of clozapine and its metabolites: analyzed by critical statistics, *J Clin Psych* (1999) **60:**36–40.

22. Haring C, Meise U, Humpel C et al, Dose related plasma levels of clozapine: influence of smoking behavior, sex and age, *Psychopharmacology (Berl)* (1989) **99(Suppl):**S38–S40.

23. Seeman MV, Lang M, The role of estrogens in schizophrenia gender differences, *Schizophr Bull* (1990) **16:**185–94.

24. Alvir JM, Leiberman JA, Agranulocytosis: incidence and risk factors, *J Clin Psychiatry* (1994) **55(Suppl B):**137–8.

25. Glazer WM, Morgenstern H, Doucette JT, Predicting the long-term risk of tardive dyskinesia in outpatients maintained on neuroleptic medications, *J Clin Psychiatry* (1993) **54:**133–9.

26. Yassa R, Jeste DV, Gender as a factor in the development of tardive dyskinesia. In: Yassa R, Nair NP, Jeste DV, eds, *Neuroleptic-Induced Movement Disorders* (Cambridge University Press, 1997) 26–40.

27. Morgenstern H, Glazer WM, Identifying risk factors for tardive dyskinesia among long term outpatients maintained with neuroleptic medications, *Arch Gen Psychiatry* (1993) **50:**723–33.

28. van Os J, Fahy T, Jones P et al, Tardive dyskinesia: who is at risk? *Acta Psychiatr Scand* (1997) **96:**206–11.

29. Speroff L, Glass RH, Kase NG, *Clinical Gynecologic Endocrinology and Infertility*, 6th edn. (Lippincott, Williams & Wilkins: Baltimore, 1999).

30. Meltzer HY, Goode DJ, Schyve PM et al, Effect of clozapine on human serum prolactin levels, *Am J Psychiatry* (1979) **136:**1550–5.

31. Crawford AM, Beasley CM Jr, Tollefson GD, The acute and long-term effect of olanzapine compared with placebo and haloperidol on serum prolactin concentrations, *Schizophr Res* (1997) **28:**224–67.

32. Arvanitis LA, Miller BG, Multiple fixed doses of 'Seroquel' (quetiapine) in patients with acute exacerbation of schizophrenia: a comparison with haloperidol and placebo. The Seroquel Trial 13 Study Group, *Biol Psychiatry* (1997) **42:**233–46.

33. Kleinberg DL, Davis JM, de Coster R et al, Prolactin levels and adverse events in patients treated with risperidone, *J Clin Psychopharmacol* (1999) **19:**57–61.

34. Dickson RA, Dalby JT, Williams R, Edwards AL, Risperidone-induced prolactin elevations in premenopausal women with schizophrenia [letter], *Am J Psychiatry* (1995) **152:**1102–3.

35. Caracci G, Ananthamoorthy R, Prolactin levels in premenopausal women treated with risperidone compared with those of women treated with typical neuroleptics [letter], *J Clin Psychopharmacol* (1999) **19:**194–6.

36. Petty RG, Prolactin and antipsychotic medications: mechanism of action, *Schizophr Res* (1999) **35:**S67–S73.

37. Grunder G, Wetzel H, Schosser R et al, Neuroendocrine response to antipsychotics: effects of drug type and gender, *Biol Psychiatry* (1999) **45:**89–97.

38. Pollock A, McLaren EH, Serum prolactin concentration in patients taking neuroleptic drugs, *Clin Endocrinol (Oxf)* (1998) **49:**513–16.

39. Zelaschi NM, Delucchi GA, Rodriguez JL, High plasma prolactin levels after long-term neuroleptic treatment, *Biol Psychiatry* (1996) **39:**900–1.

40. Corenblum B, Disorders of prolactin secretion. In:

Copeland LJ, ed, *Textbook of Gynecology* (WB Saunders: Philadelphia, 1993) 447–67.

41. Halbreich U, Palter S, Accelerated osteoporosis in psychiatric patients: possible pathophysiological processes, *Schizophr Bull* (1996) **22**:447–54.

42. Biller BM, Baum HB, Rosenthal DI et al, Progressive trabecular osteopenia in women with hyperprolactinemic amenorrhea, *J Clin Endocrinol Metab* (1992) **75**:692–7.

43. Shaarawy M, Nafei S, Abul-Nasr A et al, Circulating nitric oxide levels in galactorrheic, hyperprolactinemic, amenorrheic women, *Fertil Steril* (1997) **68**:454–9.

44. Dexeus S, Barri PN, Hyperprolactinemia: an inductor of neoplastic changes in endometrium? A report of two cases, *Gynecol Endocrinol* (1998) **12**:273–5.

45. Biller BM, Hyperprolactinemia, *Int J Fertil Womens Med* (1999) **44**:74–7.

46. Khanna J, Van Look PFA, eds, *Reproductive Health Research: The New Directions.* Biennial Report 1996–97 (World Health Organization: Geneva, 1998).

47. Miller LJ, Sexuality, reproduction, and family planning in women with schizophrenia, *Schizophr Bull* (1997) **23**:623–35.

48. Gottesman II, Groome CS, HIV/AIDS risks as a consequence of schizophrenia, *Schizophr Bull* (1997) **23**:675–84.

49. Spielvogel A, Wile J, Treatment and outcomes of psychotic patients during pregnancy and childbirth, *Birth* (1992) **19**:131–7.

50. Miller LJ, Finnerty M. Sexuality, pregnancy, and childrearing among women with schizophrenia-spectrum disorders, *Psychiatr Serv* (1996) **47**:502–6.

51. Gregory BA, The menstrual cycle and its disorders in psychiatric patients – II, *J Psychosom Res* (1957) **2**:199–224.

52. Dickson RA, Seeman MV, Corenblum B, Hormonal side-effects in women: typical vs. atypical antipsychotic treatment, *J Clin Psychiatry* (2000) **61(Suppl 3)**:10–15.

53. Michael A, Joseph A, Pallen A, Delusions of pregnancy, *Br J Psych* (1994) **164**:244–5.

54. Wesselmann U, Windgassen K, Galactorrhea: subjective response by schizophrenic patients, *Acta Psychiatr Scand* (1995) **91**:152–5.

55. Lingjaerde O, Ahlfors UG, Bech P et al, The UKU side effect rating scale: a new comprehensive rating scale for psychotropic drugs and a cross sectional study of side effects in neuroleptic-treated patients, *Acta Psychiatr Scand* (1987) **334**:1–100.

56. Bunker MT, Marken PA, Schneiderhan ME, Ruehter VL, Attenuation of antipsychotic-induced hyperprolactinemia with clozapine, *J Child Adolesc Psychopharmacol* (1997) **7**:65–9.

57. Canuso CM, Hanau M, Jhamb KK, Green AI, Olanzapine use in women with antipsychotic-induced hyperprolactinemia [letter], *Am J Psych* (1998) **155**:1458.

58. Gazzola LR, Opler LA, Return of menstruation after switching from risperidone to olanzapine, *J Clin Psychopharmacol* (1998) **18**:486–7.

59. Working Group for the Canadian Psychiatric Association and the Canadian Alliance for Research on Schizophrenia, Canadian Clinical Practice Guidelines for the Treatment of Schizophrenia, *Can J Psychiatry* (1998) **43(Suppl 2 revised)**:25S-40S.

60. Beumont PJ, Corker CS, Friesen HG et al, The effects of phenothiazines on endocrine function: II. Effects in men and post-menopausal women, *Br J Psychiatry* (1974) **124**:420–30.

61. Ballinger CB, Psychiatric aspects of the menopause, *Br J Psychiatry* (1990) **156**:773–87.

62. Bassett AS, Alison B, Hodgkinson KA, Honer WG, Reproductive fitness in familial schizophrenia, *Schizophr Res* (1996) **21**:151–60.

63. McGrath JJ, Hearle J, Jenner L et al, The fertility and fecundity of patients with psychoses, *Acta Psychiatr Scand* (1999) **99**:441–6.

64. Dickson RA, Edwards A, Clozapine and fertility [letter], *Am J Psychiatry* (1997) **154**:582–3.

65. Currier GW, Simpson GM, Antipsychotic medications and fertility, *Psychiatr Serv* (1998) **49**:175–6.

66. Dickson RA, Glazer WM, Hyperprolactinemia and male sexual dysfunction, *J Clin Psychiatry* (1999) **60**:125.

67. Haggis F, Contraception without consent? [letter] *Br J Psych* (1985) **146**:91–2.

68. Coverdale JH, Bayer TL, McCullough LB, Chervenak FA, Respecting the autonomy of chronic mentally ill women in decisions about contraception, *Hosp Community Psychiatry* (1993) **44**:671–4.

69. Waldman MD, Safferman A, Pregnancy and clozapine [letter], *Am J Psychiatry* (1993) **150**:168–9.

70. Dickson RA, Hogg L, Pregnancy of a patient

treated with clozapine, *Psychiatr Serv* (1998) **49:**1081–3.

71. Miller LJ, Psychotic denial of pregnancy: phenomenology and clinical management, *Hosp Community Psychiatry* (1990) **41:**1233–7.

72. McNeil TF, Kaij L, Malmquist-Larsson A, Women with nonorganic psychosis: pregnany's effect on mental health during pregnancy, *Acta Psychiatr Scand* (1984) **70:**140–8.

73. McNeil TF, Kaij L, Malmquist-Larsson A, Women with nonorganic psychosis: factors associated with pregnancy's effect on mental health, *Acta Psychiatr Scand* (1984) **70:**209–19.

74. Goodman SH, Emory EK. Perinatal complications in births to low socioeconomic status schizophrenic and depressed women, *J Abnorm Psychol* (1992) **101:**225–9.

75. Bennedsen BE, Adverse pregnancy outcome in schizophrenic women: occurrence and risk factors, *Schizophr Res* (1998) **33:**1–26.

76. Taylor D, Duncan D, McConnell H, Abel K, *Prescribing Guidelines* (The Bethlem and Maudsley NHS Trust: London, 1997).

77. Hertz MI, Liberman RP, Leiberman JA et al, Practice guidelines for the treatment of patients with schizophrenia, *Am J Psychiatry* (1997) **154(Suppl 4):**

78. Goldberg HL, Nissim R, Psychotropic drugs in pregnancy and lactation, *Int J Psychiatry Med* (1994) **24:**129–49.

79. Altshuler LL, Cohen L, Szuba MP et al, Pharmacologic management of psychiatric illness during pregnancy: dilemmas and guidelines, *Am J Psych* (1996) **153:**592–606.

80. Pinkofsky HB, Fitzgerald MJ, Reeves RR, Psychotropic treatment during pregnancy [letter], *Am J Psychiatry* (1997) **154:**718–19.

81. Popli AA, Konicki PE, Jurjus GJ et al, Clozapine and associated diabetes mellitus, *J Clin Psychiatry* (1997) **58:**108–11.

82. Dickson RA, Dawson DT, Olanzapine and pregnancy [letter], *Can J Psychiatry* (1998) **43:**2.

83. Kaplan B, Modai I, Stoler M et al, Clozapine treatment and risk of unplanned pregnancy, *J Am Board Fam Pract* (1995) **8:**239–41.

84. Koren G, Pastuszak A, Ito S, Drugs in pregnancy, *N Engl J Med* (1998) **338:**1128–37.

85. Verdoux H, Bourgeois M, A comparative study of obstetric history in schizophrenics, bipolar patients and normal subjects, *Schizophr Res* (1993) **9:**67–9.

86. Kumar R, Marks M, Platz C, Keiko Y, Clinical survey of psychiatric mother and baby unit: characteristics of 100 consecutive admissions, *J Affect Disord* (1994) **33:**11–22.

87. Videbech P, Gouliaev G, First admission with puerperal psychosis: 7–14 years of follow-up, *Acta Psychiatr Scand* (1995) **91:**167–73.

88. Jacobsen T, Miller LJ, Mentally ill mothers who have killed: three cases addressing the issue of future parenting capability, *Psychiatric Serv* (1998) **49:**650–7.

89. Waldo MC, Roath M, Levine W, Freedman R, A model program to teach parenting skills to schizophrenic mothers, *Hosp Community Psychiatry* (1987) **38:**1110–12.

90. Miller LJ, Comprehensive prenatal and postpartum psychiatric care for women with severe mental illness, *Psychiatr Serv* (1996) **47:**1108–11.

91. Llewellyn A, Stowe ZN, Psychotropic medications in lactation, *J Clin Psychiatry* (1998) **59:**41–52.

92. Barnas C, Bergant A, Hummer M et al, Clozapine concentrations in maternal and fetal plasma, amniotic fluid, and breast milk [letter], *Am J Psychiatry* (1994) **151:**945.

93. Kornhuber J, Weller M, Postpartum psychosis and mastitis: a new indication for clozapine, *Am J Psychiatry* (1991) **148:**1751–2.

18

Patient Compliance

Roisin A Kemp and Anthony S David

Contents • Introduction • The clinical importance of patient compliance • Can we predict poor compliance? • General issues in promoting compliance • Study of compliance therapy in psychotic patients • Conclusion

Introduction

Patient compliance is an important but somewhat neglected aspect of therapeutics. It can be defined simply as suboptimal adherence to the treatment regime. Poor compliance includes failure to engage with services, non-attendance at appointments, and refusal to participate in recommended procedures or programmes. However, in this chapter we will concern ourselves with pharmacotherapy, specifically, the total or partial omission of prescribed antipsychotic medications. Recently the term 'compliance' has been criticized as too paternalistic, and suggestive of both deviance on the part of the patient and coercion on the part of the clinician. Alternative terms have been suggested to better reflect the changing nature of the doctor–patient relationship with the ideals of increased partnership in treatment, the current favourite being 'concordance'.[1]

Whatever the terminology adopted for non-compliance, its extent and costs are formidable: Weiden and Olfson[2] estimate that non-compliance with treatment in the United States contributes 40% of a $2 billion estimated annual cost of rehospitalization for patients with multiple-episode schizophrenia. In the United Kingdom, Bebbington[3] has estimated this figure to be approximately £100 million.

The clinical importance of patient compliance

Poor compliance is associated with an increase in readmission rates, severity of episode on relapse, and length of inpatient stay. It is the most important modifiable risk factor for rehospitalization.[4] Estimates of non-compliance rates vary, but figures of up to 90% have been reported depending on the setting, the patient population and the compliance measure used.[5,6] Not surprisingly, rates rise from inpatient to outpatient settings (see Table 18.1).[7–10] Weiden et al[11] found that 48% of patients were non-compliant for at least a week over a year's follow-up, rising to 70% over 2 years. Follow-up studies of patients on depot medication showed missed injection rates or refusal of up to 43%.[12–14]

Summarizing the research literature, Cramer and Rosenheck[6] found that the mean compliance rates for patients prescribed antipsychotics were 58% (range 24–90); 65% (40–90) for antidepressants and 76% (60–92) for a variety of physical disorders. These data refute the argument that the compliance rate in populations of patients with chronic schizophrenia is not different from those in other chronic illness. Apart from unfavourable health beliefs and individual and cultural prejudices regarding medication, severe

Table 18.1 Rates of non-compliance in schizophrenia.

Study	Setting	Measure	Non-compliance rate
Forrest et al (1961)[7]	Inpatient	Urine assay	15%
Irwin et al (1971)[8]	Open ward	Urine assay	32%
Scottish Schizophrenia Research Group (1987)[9]	Inpatient	Serum assay	46%
Serban and Thomas (1974)[10]	Outpatient	Self-report	42%
Weiden et al (1991)[11]	Outpatient	Observer and self-report	48% 1st year 70% 2nd year
Carney and Sheffield (1976)[12]	Depot clinics	Missed injection	40%
Falloon et al (1978)[13]			
Quitkin et al (1978)[14]			

psychiatric illness brings with it compromised reality testing and reasoning, cognitive impairment and lack of insight, all which may potentially contribute to poor compliance.

Measures of compliance used have varied from self-report, clinician rating, pill count, and urine or serum level. The electronic lid counter has only recently been used with psychotic populations (see below). The merits and problems associated with the various methods have been discussed by Babiker,[15] the principal criticisms being the following: self-report is unreliable, clinician ratings prone to overestimate compliance, pill counts are technically difficult to organize and 'medication missing' does not necessarily mean 'medication consumed'; urine assays may overestimate compliance for medications with a long half-life, and serum assay measures give an index of recent compliance only – also currently available methods may not reliably detect medication at the lower dose ranges. Clinicians tend to overestimate compliance, especially in community treatment settings.[16] One possibility whose potential in compliance research is currently under study is hair analysis, use of which to date has been confined to the examination of comorbid substance abuse, and which has been shown to be

very acceptable to patients with schizophrenia. Because of the limitations of the currently available methods, the use of more than one method of measurement in research is recommended.

Can we predict poor compliance?

We will consider in turn the evidence from the literature regarding possible 'predictors' of non-compliance. With many of these factors it is hard to disentangle cause and effect on the basis of the available evidence, but nevertheless their presence might alert the clinician to the likelihood of poor compliance (see Box 18.1).

Predictors can be considered under the headings of factors associated with the illness, the person and the treatment. Illness-related factors are known to include psychotic symptomatology, cognitive impairment, and mood. Person-related factors are known to include detention status, treatment attitudes and capacity for insight. Treatment-related factors include the quality of the doctor–patient relationship, service provision, and the treatment itself: its complexity, the mode of administration, and adverse side-effects. Finally, there are other wider factors which also deserve to be considered, such as attitudes to

Box 18.1 Checklist of non-compliance-associated factors in schizophrenia

> Service profile
>   Poor service consistency
>   No assertive outreach
>   No follow-up on appointment defaulters
> Treatment regimen
>   Complex regimen, polypharmacy
>   Poor instructions and information
>   provided
>   Depot route not used when appropriate
> Patient profile
>   Expect higher rates if:
>   Younger patients
>   Living alone or homeless
>   Comorbid substance abuse
>   Has been involuntarily detained
> Insight
>   Denial of illness
>   Denial of need for treatment
>   Denial of vulnerability to relapse
> Treatment attitudes
>   Negative views regarding subjective
>   effects of medication
>   Negative views regarding efficacy and
>   benefits of medication
> Adverse side-effects
>   Extrapyramidal symptoms, especially
>   akathisia and akinesia
>   Sedation
>   Sexual dysfunction
> Symptoms
>   Paranoid delusions
>   Thought disorder
>   Hostility
>   Grandiosity
>   Depression
> Cognitive impairment
>   Attention and memory difficulties
>   Executive dysfunction with poor planning
>   abilities, disorganization

treatment and mental disorders prevalent in society in general, and closer to home, attitudes of relatives. We will consider these aspects in turn.

Illness-related aspects

Not surprisingly, it has been shown several times that severity of acute psychotic symptomatology, including paranoid delusions, hostility, grandiosity, perplexity and thought disorder, is associated with overt treatment refusal;[17-19] no overall association with global severity and non-compliance but a specific link with grandiosity was noted by Bartko et al[20] and van Putten et al.[21] Bartko et al[22] also found that when compared to compliant relapsers, non-compliant relapsers had more severe positive symptoms on admission to hospital and again after a month's treatment. It makes sense that those with acute psychotic symptoms of the paranoid variety will be suspicious of treatment, or that patients who are grandiose are unlikely to interpret their mental state as an illness requiring treatment. Further, it seems self-evident that those with thought disorder, if this is severe, will be unable to realize the need for treatment, and further, would require considerable supervision with respect to adherence in the follow-up phase. These psychotic symptoms are commonly associated with either treatment refusal, suspiciousness of the goals of treatment or not infrequently delusional ideation regarding the medication, such as beliefs that one is being poisoned or punished.

With respect to the influence of mood, an increased risk of depressive symptoms has been found in infrequent compared to frequent attenders at a depot clinic.[23] Similar findings were noted by Young et al,[24] but here the depressive symptoms were attributed to antipsychotic side-effects (akinesia and possibly neuroleptic dysphoria) rather than the patients' psychopathology. Motivational problems as part of the deficit syndrome have been cited by Weiden et al[25] as influencing clinical attendance rates and adherence with prescribed regimes. More generally, a chronic psychotic illness is often accompanied by demoralization, social alienation and despair, given that many patients are deprived of rewards from the work, leisure and relationship opportunities available to the majority of the population.

Finally and importantly, in many patients, compliance will be affected by the cognitive impairments accompanying schizophrenia, with attention and memory difficulties as well as executive dysfunction.[26–29] They may be forgetful or disorganized with their regime, leading to both errors of omission and commission, as a result missing doses, showing erratic adherence, or making inadvertent combinations. This has implications for the degree of supervision and monitoring or prompting required, the need for regular review and rehearsal of the medication regime, the use of behavioural strategies, and the role of regular reinforcement.

Person-related aspects
Sociodemographic

Sociodemographic factors are relatively unimportant. A few studies have found that younger patients may be less compliant[30–32] although several other groups reported no difference.[33,34] Likewise, there is no clear consensus regarding gender. Men were found to be either less compliant than women[30] or equally compliant.[33,34] Marital status has not been shown to have an effect. Low socioeconomic status has been linked with worse compliance.[24,29] Two British studies have highlighted a particular problem for compliance in African-Caribbean populations.[35,36] Ethnicity was not found to be a major factor in other studies.[30,34] High rates of non-compliance are associated with homelessness and substance abuse.[37,38] Finally, family attitudes are an important variable. Smith et al[39] attempted to study this by approaching the patient's nominated 'significant other' in order to examine his or her illness beliefs. The authors found that a third of the nominated others were unco-operative and often shared similar attitudes to the patients, including failure to note the beneficial effects of medication. Families and carers may have experienced medication failures first-hand or may have felt blamed for the patient's illness by the medical profession. They too may have experienced psychiatric disorders.

Insight and attitudes

Research has increased apace in the construct of insight, now understood to be a multidimensional phenomenon comprising the following axes: recognition of illness, reattribution of symptoms, and acceptance of treatment.[40] Several studies have underlined a relationship between compliance and insight, either simply defined as acknowledgement of illness, as a single item from the Present State Examination (PSE) or rated according to a structured scale.[20,21,32,41,42] Interestingly, McEvoy et al[41] showed that there is some dissociation between insight and compliance so that insight does not automatically predict compliance and vice versa. There are now several scales for the measurement of insight[43] which may help in further elucidation of this relationship. Nageotte et al,[44] in a large cross-sectional study ($n = 202$), found that aspects of the Health Belief Model predicted compliance, so that a majority of those who believed themselves to be mentally unwell were compliant (rated on a self-report scale). Similarly, acceptance of vulnerability to relapse in the future was associated with compliance. However, this relationship was not straightforward in that 38% of those who did not believe themselves to be unwell were also compliant. Clearly other factors also play a role in this group, possibly including therapeutic alliance, family support or personality traits.

Treatment-related aspects

Several studies have shown that belief that treatment has helped is positively associated with compliance.[34,45] Some authors have suggested that indirect treatment benefits (being able to function better) may be more appreciated by patients than symptom reduction itself.[46] Adverse side-effects of antipsychotic treatment which have notoriously been linked with poor compliance include weight gain, sedation, sexual dysfunction and particularly extrapyramidal side-effects. However, despite evidence of these issues in clinical practice, the research evidence is surprisingly uncompelling with respect to adverse side-effects.

The cause and effect nature of the compliance/side-effect relationship is problematic. For example, in an early outpatient study, Willcox et al[47] found that drug side-effects on chlorpromazine were actually slightly more common in compliant than non-compliant patients (estimated by urine assay). Interpretation of results from these early studies is also problematic for the reason that often higher medication doses were used, and it is difficult to avoid the suspicion that in a cross-sectional study more patients who were compliant would have side-effects. Conversely, Nelson[48] found a significant association between the presence of antipsychotic side-effects and reduced compliance as estimated by urine assay in newly admitted patients ($n = 120$). Extrapyramidal side-effects (EPS) and akathisia in particular were linked with treatment refusal by van Putten.[49] However Marder[50] found no difference in EPS or other side-effects between refusers and consenters to treatment. Similarly, EPS did not distinguish infrequent from frequent attenders in the study by Pan and Tantam.[23] In Buchanan's 2-year follow-up study,[34] the presence of akinesia was related to worse compliance over the follow-up period, whereas no such effect was found for akathisia, dystonia, tremor and drowsiness. It should be noted that the studies cited above have generally not used comprehensive side-effect ratings.

In terms of the relative importance of side-effects with respect to adherence behaviour as reported by patients, evidence exists that side-effects may have less influence than treatment attitudes (though obviously for some patients one will affect the other). For example, in a follow-up study of 132 patients by Renton et al,[51] 46% were poorly compliant after 12 months, and side-effects came second of the cited reasons for poor compliance, the most common reason cited by the patients being that they were feeling well, and seeing no need for continued treatment. In the self-report study by Kelly et al[52] the experience of side-effects contributed to 10% of the variance in self-reported compliance. Interestingly, when reasons for non-compliance are sought, patients usually cite side-effects more often than their treating clinicians.[19] In summary, the evidence to date for the influence of side-effects on compliance is equivocal; most agree that when severe, the impact is negative, but when milder, their influence is less easily predicted and may be swamped by other factors, such as insight or treatment alliance.

Other aspects of treatment to be considered include consistency of service receipt, service provision and mode of delivery of medication. It is hardly surprising that in the large Nageotte et al[44] study, those who had little or no outpatient service contact within the previous 3 months were more likely to be non-compliant with medication. Regarding mode of treatment delivery, Wilson and Enoch[53] reported that receipt of oral medication was more associated with non-compliance. A meta-analysis of such studies suggests improved relapse rates in the second year for patients switched to depot.[54] Clearly, then the use of depot medication may provide more assured compliance in a well-organized service, when there is early follow-up of clinic defaulters. With the increasingly widespread use of novel antipsychotic medication, the compliance issue is again a concern. For example, it has been anticipated that the use of these drugs with their improved pharmacokinetic profiles and reduced incidence of adverse side-effects, particularly EPS, would obviate the compliance problems for the majority of patients.[55] However, because of issues to do with insight and attitudes to treatment, the situation may not be so simple, and we await data which clearly demonstrate the expected compliance benefits of the novel agents. In our view, the use of these agents provides very real advantages for patients but that compliance may be further optimized by the judicious combination of effective pharmacotherapy with compliance-enhancing interventions.

General issues in promoting compliance

Studies of strategies to enhance compliance with medical treatment generally have been reviewed by Haynes et al,[56] who found only 14 studies meeting their rigorous inclusion criteria, of which 8 showed significantly improved adherence, but only 6 led to consistent improvements in treatment outcomes. These included the following, all involving considerable input: the use of telephone calls and regular prompts; combining oral with written information, self-monitoring, patient support groups, special outreach nurses, family therapy and compliance therapy (see below). General compliance-enhancing measures which will be obvious to most clinicians (see Box 18.2) include providing a consistent accessible service with responsive outreach, using treatment regimes which minimize side-effects, and enlisting significant others to supervise and prompt medication-taking. Strategies which compensate for cognitive impairments and a disorganized lifestyle include using a simplified regime, regular rehearsal of regime instructions, the use of cue cards and self-monitoring calendars, and tailoring medication with daily rituals such as teeth-brushing or meals.[57] Communication can be improved by simplifying language, checking that the patients understand, repeating important messages and reinforcing verbal instructions with written ones.[58]

Didactic psychoeducational interventions appear to be less effective in psychotic disorder than behavioural or cognitive-behavioural approaches and their input needs to be sustained for any lasting benefit.[59] A few approaches deserve special mention. The labour-intensive medication management module developed in UCLA has shown considerable promise in field studies and a small randomized controlled trial,[60] though to date compliance data have not been reported. Their module uses multimedia and role play, and covers 'skills' such as correct self-administration of medication regime, knowledge of medication

Box 18.2 Compliance-enhancing strategies

1. General
Providing an accessible and responsive service
Monitoring service consistency
Early follow-up of appointment defaulters
Regular use of telephone reminder prompts
Enrolment of significant others to supervise or prompt
Training all mental health professionals in psychoeducation and medication updates
Non-punitive attitudes (expect erratic and variable compliance)
Routine monitoring of medication side-effects (not only if patients complain)
Simplified medication regimes
Bringing medication bottles to appointments
Use of novel antipsychotics with lower side-effect propensity
Consider switch to depot route especially with chaotic patients
Regularly rehearse regimen instructions with the patient
System of feedback from pharmacy on prescription filling

2. Specific
Simple behavioural strategies:
  Self-monitoring calendars
  Dosette boxes
  Cue cards
  Pairing regimen with daily rituals
Psychosocial interventions:
  Medication management module:
    Information on benefits of medication
    Tracking side-effects
    Negotiating medication issues with clinicians
  Compliance therapy:
    Uses motivational interviewing techniques
    Explores ambivalence about treatment

benefits, tracking side-effects and negotiating treatment issues with clinicians. Lecompte and Pelc[61] employed an eclectic intervention which included educational, cognitive and behavioural strategies as well as a focus on the therapeutic alliance. Subjects were selected on the basis of a good response to medication. In a randomized trial, they showed that hospitalization and remission can both be changed for the better in tandem with compliance. Most recently, Cramer and Rosenheck[62] report preliminary results on a small ($n = 60$), mixed group of psychiatric patients using a combination of instructions on how to integrate medication-taking into their lifestyle, and also microelectronic devices attached to bottle caps which provide feedback displays of medication use. A control group was not provided with the ongoing feedback and had less structured advice about medication. The proportion of days in which the number of bottle openings corresponded to prescription was calculated for each group and was 76% in the intervention group compared to 57% for controls.

Study of compliance therapy in psychotic patients

Compliance therapy (CT) is a new pragmatic intervention aimed at improving adherence with antipsychotic medication. It is an individualized intervention that can be used in the inpatient or outpatient setting as part of a general programme. We developed this intervention on the basis of the principles of motivational interviewing, a counselling technique aimed at behaviour change that has wide application in medicine (to stop smoking, lose weight, reduce substance abuse, correct eating disorder). The basic principles of this intervention were included, using reflective listening and exploring ambivalence by weighing up the pros and cons of behaviours and alternatives. The approach was modified for use with psychotic patients by adding flexible session length, making use of repetition and having less reliance on eliciting self-motivational statements.

Also, we added cognitive techniques developed for psychotic patients, and included a psychoeducational component.

Summary of the compliance therapy intervention

There are three phases (see Box 18.3).

Phase 1

The patient's illness history is reviewed, and his or her conceptualization of the illness ascertained and stance towards treatment explored. When appropriate, any link between medication cessation and relapse is emphasized. Negative treatment experiences are acknowledged. Outright denial of illness and denial of need for treatment are not directly challenged at this stage; instead gentle inquiry is made about the social or lifestyle consequences of becoming unwell for that individual.

Phase 2

Ambivalence toward treatment is further explored. Even when such reluctance has not been forthcoming from the patient, the therapist openly predicts common misgivings about treatment.[63] These include fears of addiction to medication, fears of loss of control, fears of alteration or loss of personality. Sometimes patients confuse symptoms and side-effects, and such misconceptions can be corrected. The natural tendency to

Box 18.3 Compliance therapy intervention

Phase 1
Ascertain stance towards treatment.
Link medication cessation with relapse.

Phase 2
Anticipate misgivings about treatment.
Weigh up benefits and drawbacks.

Phase 3
Offer rationale for maintenance treatment.
Establish medication as a strategy to stay well and meet goals.

stop medication when one feels well is discussed. The meaning that the individual ascribes to taking medication is discussed (for example, 'taking those pills means you are crazy'), and an attempt is made (1) to normalize use of medication and (2) to use cognitive techniques to challenge unhelpful personalizations.

The patient is invited to weigh up the benefits and drawbacks of treatment, and then the therapist 'homes in' on the benefits, especially when these emerge spontaneously. Symptoms reported by the patient are fed back as being 'target symptoms' for treatment. Indirect medication benefits are discussed (such as getting on better with one's family). Some metaphors are used, such as the value of medication as a 'protective layer'. The therapist aims to create a degree of cognitive dissonance in the patient, that poor compliance is actually disadvantageous for that individual in achieving his or her goals.

Phase 3

The final phase of the intervention deals with stigma by reframing the use of medication as a freely chosen strategy to enhance the patient's quality of life. A number of normalizing rationales are used. We make analogies with physical illness requiring maintenance treatment and ask patients for examples from their own circle of acquaintances or family to emphasize the point. The high prevalence of psychological disorders in the general population is highlighted and examples of famous sufferers are used. Medication is described as an 'insurance policy to stay well'.[64] The therapist invites the patient to think of any reasons they have for wishing to avoid becoming unwell again in the future. In turn, the patient is asked to consider the value of staying well to reach individual goals or maintain valued sources of fulfilment (interests, work, relationships). The consequences of stopping medication are predicted, and finally characteristic prodromal symptoms identified where possible, and the value of seeking early intervention to stave off a full-blown episode is emphasized.

Case vignette: 'Larry'

Larry is a 25-year-old African-Caribbean man whose previous experience of treatment had been negative. He had been detained involuntarily and found this experience extremely unpleasant. He felt that the police and psychiatrists were working together to persecute him and make his life difficult. His attitude to his treating team was adversarial and he was generally hostile and unco-operative. His view of antipsychotic treatment was that it was a kind of punishment. Additionally, he had adverse side-effects from medication including impotence, tremor and oversedation. The sessions with Larry allowed him to enumerate his reservations about receiving antipsychotic treatment. His principal concern was not wanting to be controlled by others. He was not willing to accept the concept of an illness that required treatment indefinitely. Initially he was unable to identify a single advantage for him in having medication. However, he could later accept that being calm rather than aroused was a good thing for him, and perhaps medication could offer him some protection in staying in control of himself. Larry agreed that there were times that he had 'gone off his head' and got into trouble as a result, including losing access to his child. Also, he was encouraged to discuss precisely which unwanted side-effects he found most troublesome with his treating clinician, and after an adjustment of the medication regime the tremor improved. This enabled him to 'own' some involvement with his medication regime. Later sessions focused on maintenance treatment as a strategy to stay strong in himself and avoid the consequences of relapse. Becoming tense and irritable, poor concentration and sleep disturbance were among the warning signs heralding relapse for Larry, even though he tended to view these symptoms as due to pressure from other people. This scenario was rehearsed repeatedly with Larry, with the notion of early contact and a temporary dose increase (or resumption of regime) to deal with the 'stress symptoms' and where possible, to avoid having to come into hospital.

Case vignette: 'Suzanne'

Suzanne is a 35-year-old woman who was involuntarily detained in an intensive treatment unit following an unprovoked attempted assault on a passer-by in the street. She retained an encapsulated delusion, with paranoid beliefs concerning her neighbours. She was of moderate premorbid intelligence and not significantly cognitively impaired. She complained of weight gain, lethargy and oversedation on her medication regime. The initial therapy sessions explored her frustration at being incarcerated in a medium secure unit and mistrust of mental health professionals (though she had a good relationship with her keyworker). The side-effect issues were also addressed. The value of anxiety reduction and ensuring sleep in order to keep functioning optimally were emphasized. Later a medication change to an atypical neuroleptic with less weight gain and sedation propensity was proposed. Suzanne was initially worried about 'being a guinea-pig', and her fears about starting a novel drug were allayed with further information regarding data on the drug's safety and benefits in terms of tolerability. The value of continuing treatment when well was subsequently explored. Suzanne was homeless as a consequence of events preceding her admission, and the importance for her of being able to live independently and pursue her own interests was agreed as the goal of longer-term maintenance treatment.

The study

Compliance therapy has been tested in a randomized, controlled clinical trial.[65,66] Briefly, the study population was drawn from consecutive acute admissions with Diagnostic and Statistical Manual for Mental Disorders (DSM-111-R) diagnosed psychotic disorders aged 18–65 to an acute ward serving a deprived inner London catchment area. Seventy-four subjects entered the trial and were randomized to two groups, one receiving four to six sessions of compliance therapy and a control group receiving four to six sessions of supportive counselling. In the control condition, patients could present any concerns for discussion but were advised to approach their treating teams to discuss medication issues. The interventions were additional to routine management including informal psychoeducation and the therapists were independent of the treating teams. After discharge all patients received routine aftercare as determined by their treating teams. Booster sessions were offered at 3, 6 and 12 months.

All subjects were assessed on standardized measures of psychopathology (Expanded Brief Psychiatric Rating Scale,[67] Global Assessment of Functioning Scale-Disability,[68] Scale for the Assessment of Insight – expanded version,[59] Drug Attitudes Inventory,[69] and scales to measure extrapyramidal side-effects, premorbid IQ and use of services (The Client Service Receipt Inventory).[70] Compliance was rated blind to intervention status by the patient's primary nurse and was a composite rating based on several sources for the follow-up phase (see Box 18.4). The ratings were repeated prior to discharge and evaluations repeated at 6, 12 and 18 months.

The groups were well matched with no significant differences between them in age, gender, ethnic composition, chronicity or proportion with DSM-111-R schizophrenia. It is of note that over half the patients in each group were involuntarily

Box 18.4 Observer-rated compliance measure

> 1 = complete refusal of medication
> 2 = partial refusal (e.g. refuses depot) or accepts minimum dose only
> 3 = accepts only if compulsory, or requires constant persuasion, or questions need often, e.g. once every 2 days
> 4 = occasional reluctance requiring persuasion (e.g. questions need once per week)
> 5 = passive acceptance, accepts without questioning, but little apparent interest or knowledge
> 6 = moderate participation, some interest or knowledge and no prompting required
> 7 = active participation, readily accepts and shows responsibility for the regimen

detained. The two groups received equivalent doses of antipsychotic medication; a small minority in each were being treated with novel antipsychotics including clozapine; 12 patients in the compliance therapy group and 14 in the control group were receiving depot antipsychotics; a similar proportion in each group was also receiving lithium, carbamazepine or antidepressants, 14 in the intervention group and 11 in the control group.

The group receiving compliance therapy had significantly greater gains in compliance, insight, treatment attitudes and social functioning.[65]

Finally, a survival analysis on time to readmission between the two groups over the follow-up revealed that the CT group survived longer in the community prior to readmission. The risk of readmission at any given time for a person in the control group was 2.2 times that of a person in the CT group. An evaluation of service utilization costs and outcome has revealed the intervention to be cost-effective.[71] Thus, the study showed the applicability of a pragmatic intervention which was largely acceptable to patients and easily applicable in a busy clinical setting and which produced measurable and sustained gains.

Conclusion

Non-compliance limits the efficacy of even the most powerful drugs and prevents patients with schizophrenia reaching their full potential. The problem of non-compliance can only be understood with reference to the wide variety of influences which act on medication taking. Our view is that symptom control and relapse prevention will be optimized by combining well-tolerated antipsychotic regimes, good multidisciplinary care which involves patients in their own treatment, and interventions such as compliance therapy.

References

1. Royal Pharmaceutical Society of Great Britain, *From Compliance to Concordance: Towards Shared Goals in Medicine Taking* (Royal Pharmaceutical Society: London, 1997).

2. Weiden PJ, Olfson M, Cost of relapse in schizophrenia, *Schizophr Bull* (1995) **21**:419–29.

3. Bebbington PE, The content and context of compliance, *Int Clin Psychopharmacol* (1995) **9(Suppl 5)**: 41–50.

4. Sullivan G, Wells KB, Morgenstern H et al, Identifying modifiable risk factors for rehospitalisation: a case-control study of seriously mentally ill persons, *Am J Psychiatry* (1995) **152**:1749–56.

5. Corrigan PW, Liberman RP, Engel JD, From non-compliance to collaboration in the treatment of schizophrenia, *Hosp Community Psychiatr* (1990) **41**: 1203–11.

6. Cramer JA, Rosenheck R, Compliance with medication regimens for mental and physical disorders, *Psychiatr Serv* (1998) **49**:196–201.

7. Forrest FM, Forrest IS, Mason AS, Review of rapid urine tests for phenothiazines and related drugs, *Am J Psychiatry* (1961) **118**:300–7.

8. Irwin DS, Weitzel WD, Morgan DW, Phenothiazine intake and staff attitudes, *Am J Psychiatry* (1971) **127**:1631–5.

9. Scottish Schizophrenia Research group. The Scottish First Episode Study 11. Treatment: pimozide versus flupenthixol, *Br J Psychiatry* (1987) **150**: 334–8.

10. Serban G, Thomas A, Attitudes and behaviours of acute and chronic schizophrenic patients regarding ambulatory treatment, *Am J Psychiatry* (1974) **131**:991–5.

11. Weiden PJ, Dixon L, Frances A. Neuroleptic non-compliance in schizophrenia. In: Schulz SC, ed, *Advances in Neuropsychology and Pharmacology* (Raven Press: New York, 1991) 285–96.

12. Carney MWP, Sheffield BF, Comparison of antipsychotic depot injections in the maintenance treatment of schizophrenia, *Br J Psychiatry* (1976) **129**:476–81.

13. Falloon I, Watt DC, Shepherd M, A comparative controlled trial of pimozide and fluphenazine decanoate in the continuation therapy of schizophrenia, *Psychol Med* (1978) **8**:59–70.

14. Quitkin F, Rifkin A, Kane JM et al, Long-acting versus injectable antipsychotic drugs in schizophrenics. A one year double-blind comparison in multiple episode schizophrenics, *Arch Gen Psychiatry* (1978) **35**:889–92.

15. Babiker IE, Non-compliance in schizophrenia, *Psychiatric Developments* (1986) **4**:329–37.

16. Trauer T, Sacks T, Medication compliance: a comparison of the views of severely mentally ill clients in the community, their doctors and their case managers, *J Ment Health* (1998) **7**: 621–9.

17. Appelbaum PS, Gutheil TG, Drug refusal: a study of psychiatric inpatients, *Am J Psychiatry* (1980) **137**:340–6.

18. Marder SR, Mebane A, Chien CP, A comparison of patients who refuse and consent to neuroleptic treatment, *Am J Psychiatry* (1983) **140**:470–2.

19. Hoge SK, Appelbaum PS, Lawlor T, A prospective, multi-center study of patients' refusal of antipsychotic medication, *Arch Gen Psychiatry* (1990) **47**:949–56.

20. Bartko G, Herczeg I, Zador G, Clinical symptomatology and drug compliance in schizophrenic patients, *Acta Psychiatr Scand* (1988) **77**:74–6.

21. van Putten T, Crumpton E, Yale C, Drug refusal in schizophrenia and the wish to be crazy, *Arch Gen Psychiatry* (1976) **33**:1443–5.

22. Bartko G, Maylath E, Herczeg I, Comparative study of schizophrenic patients relapsed on and off medication, *Psychiatry Res* (1987) **22**:221–7.

23. Pan PC, Tantam D, Clinical characteristics, health beliefs and compliance with maintenance treatment. A comparison of regular and irregular atten-

ders at a depot clinic, *Acta Psychiatr Scand* (1989) **79:**564–70.

24. Young JL, Zoanana HV, Shepler L, Medication noncompliance in schizophrenia: codification and update, *Bull Am Acad Psychiatry Law* (1986) **14:**105–22.

25. Weiden P, Olfson M, Essock S, Medication non-compliance in schizophrenia: effects on mental Health Service policy. In: Blackwell B, ed, *Treatment Compliance and the Therapeutic Alliance* (Harwood Academic Press: Brunswick, NJ, 1997).

26. Geller JL, State hospital patients and their medication: do they know what they take? *Am J Psychiatry* (1982) **139:**611–15.

27. MacPherson R, Double DB, Rowlands RP, Harrison DM, Long-term patients' understanding of neuroleptic medication, *Hosp Community Psychiatry* **44:**71–3.

28. Lysaker P, Bell M, Milstein R et al, Insight and psychosocial treatment compliance in schizophrenia, *Psychiatry* (1994) **57:**307–15.

29. Weiden PJ, Shaw E, Mann J, Causes of neuroleptic non-compliance, *Psychiatric Annals* (1986) **16:** 571–5.

30. Tunnicliffe S, Harrison G, Standen PJ, Factors affecting compliance with depot injection treatment in the community, *Soc Psychiatry Psychiatr Epidemiol* (1992) **27:**230–3.

31. Zito JL, Routt WW, Mitchell JE, Roerig JL, Clinical characteristics of hospitalised psychotic patients who refuse antispychotic drug therapy, *Am J Psychiatry* (1985) **142:**822–6.

32. Agarwal MR, Sharma VM, Kishore Kumar KV, Lowe D, Non-compliance with treatment in patients suffering from schizophrenia, *Int J Soc Psychiatry* (1998) **44:**92–106.

33. Atwood N, Beck JC, Service and patient predictors of continuation in clinic-based treatment, *Hosp Community Psychiatr* (1985) **36:**865–9.

34. Buchanan A, A two-year prospective study of treatment compliance in patients with schizophrenia, *Psychol Med* (1922) **22:** 787–97.

35. Sellwood W, Tarrier N, Demographic factors associated with extreme non-compliance in schizophrenia, *Soc Psychiatry Psychiatr Epidemiol* (1994) **29:**172–7.

36. Perkins RE, Moodley P, Perception of problems in psychiatric inpatients: denial, race and service

usage, *Soc Psychiatry Psychiatr Epidemiol* (1993) **38:**189–93.

37. Pristach CA, Smith CM, Medication compliance and substance abuse among schizophrenic patients, *Hosp Community Psychiatr* (1990) **41:** 1345–8.

38. Salloum IM, Moss HB, Daley DC, Substance abuse and schizophrenia: impediments to optimal care, *Am J Drug Alcohol Abuse* (1991) **17:**321–36.

39. Smith CM, Barzman D, Pristach CA, Effect of patient and family insight on compliance of schizophrenic patients, *J Clin Pharmacol* (1997) **2:**147–54.

40. Amador XF, David AS, eds, *Insight and Psychosis* (Oxford University Press: New York, 1998).

41. McEvoy JP, Freter S, Everett G et al, Insight and the clinical outcome of schizophrenic patients, *J Nerv Ment Dis* (1989) **177:**48–51.

42. Lin IF, Spiga R, Fortsch W, Insight and adherence to medication in chronic schizophrenics, *J Clin Psychiatry* (1979) **40:**430–2.

43. Sanz M, Constable G, Lopez-Ibor I et al, A comparative study of insight scales and their relationship to psychopathological and clinical variables, *Psychol Med* (1998) **28:**437–46.

44. Nageotte C, Sullivan G, Duan N, Camp PL, Medication compliance among the seriously mentally ill in a public health system, *Soc Psychiatry Psychiatr Epidemiol* (1997) **32:**49–56.

45. Chan DW, Medication compliance in a Chinese psychiatric out-patient setting, *Br J Med Psychology* (1984) **57:**81–9.

46. Adams SG, Howe JT, Predicting medication compliance in a psychotic population, *J Nerv Ment Dis* (1993) **181:**558–60.

47. Willcox D, Gillan R, Hare EH, Do psychiatric out-patients take their drugs? *BMJ* (1965) **2:**790–2.

48. Nelson A, Drug default among schizophrenic patients, *Am J Hosp Pharmacy* (1975) **32:**1237–42.

49. van Putten T, Why do schizophrenic patients refuse to take their drugs? *Arch Gen Psychiatry* (1974) **31:**67–72.

50. Marder SR, Facilitating compliance with antipsychotic medication, *J Clin Psychiatry* (1998) **59:**21–5.

51. Renton CA, Affleck JW, Carstairs GM, Forrest AD, A follow-up of schizophrenic patients in Edinburgh, *Acta Psychiatr Scand* (1963) **39:**548–81.

52. Kelly GR, Mamon JA, Scott JE, Utility of the health belief model in examining medication compliance

among psychiatric out-patients, *Soc Sci Med* (1987) **25**:1205–11.

53. Wilson JD, Enoch MD, Estimation of drugs rejection by schizophrenic patients with analysis of clinical factors, *Br J Psychiatry* (1967) **113**:209–11.

54. Glazer W, Kane J, Depot neuroleptic therapy: an underutilized treatment option, *J Clin Psychiatry* (1985) **53**:426–33.

55. Marder SR, Facilitating compliance with antipsychotic medication, *J Clin Psychiatry* (1988) **59**:21–5.

56. Haynes RB, McKibbon KA, Kanani R et al, Interventions to assist patients to follow prescriptions for medications (Cochrane review). In: The Cochrane Library, Issue 3, (Update Software: Oxford, 1998).

57. Boczkowski JA, Zeichner A, DeSanto N, Neuroleptic compliance among chronic schizophrenic outpatients: an intervention outcome report, *J Consult Clin Psychol* (1985) **53**:666–71.

58. Ley P, Communicating with patients. Improving communication, satisfaction and compliance (Chapman & Hall: London, 1992).

59. Kemp R, David A, Insight and compliance. In: Blackwell B, ed, *Treatment Compliance and the Therapeutic Alliance* (Harwood Academic Publishers: Newark, NJ, 1997) 61–84.

60. Eckman TA, Wirshing C, Marder SR et al, Technique for training patients in illness self-management: a controlled trial, *Am J Psychiatry* (1992) **149**:1549–55.

61. Lecompte D, Pelc I, A cognitive-behavioral program to improve compliance with medication in patients with schizophrenia, *Int J Mental Health* (1996) **25**:51–6.

62. Cramer JA, Rosenheck R, Enhancing medication compliance for people with serious mental illness, *J Nerv Ment Dis* (1999) **187**:53–5.

63. Goldstein MJ, Psychosocial strategies for maximising the effects of psychotropic medications for schizophrenia and mood disorder, *Psychopharmacol Bull* (1992) **28**:237–40.

64. Falloon IRH, Developing and maintaining adherence to long-term drug-taking regimens, *Schizophr Bull* (1984) **10**:412–17.

65. Kemp R, Hayward P, Applewhaite G et al, Compliance therapy in psychotic patients: randomised controlled trial, *BMJ* (1996) **312**:345–9.

66. Kemp R, Kirov G, Everitt B et al, Randomised controlled trial of compliance therapy: 18-month follow-up, *Br J Psychiatry* (1998) **172**:413–19.

67. Lukoff D, Nuechterlein KH, Ventura J, Manual for expanded BPRS, *Schizophr Bull* (1996) **12**:594–602.

68. American Psychiatric Association, *Diagnostic and Statistical Manual of Mental Disorders*, revised 3rd edn, (American Psychiatric Association: Washington, DC, 1987).

69. Hogan TP, Awad AG, Eastwood R, A self-report scale predictive of drug compliance in schizophrenics: reliability and discriminative validity, *Psychol Med* (1983) **13**:177–83.

70. Beecham JK, Knapp MRJ, Costing psychiatric interventions. In: Thornicroft G, Brewin C, Wing JK, eds, *Measuring Mental Health Needs* (Gaskell: London, 1992) 163–83.

71. Healey A, Knapp M, Astin J et al, Cost-effectiveness evaluation of compliance therapy for people with psychosis, *Br J Psychiatry* (1998) **172**:420–4.

19

Medical Management of Persons with Schizophrenia

Lisa Dixon, Karen Wohlheiter and Donald Thompson

Contents • Introduction • Mortality in schizophrenia • Morbidity in schizophrenia • Models of comorbidity • Barriers to adequate health care • Smoking and schizophrenia • Weight and exercise • Diabetes and schizophrenia • Polydipsia and schizophrenia • Summary

Introduction

A variety of changes and improvements in the clinical care of persons with schizophrenia have led to a recent focus on the somatic health and health behaviors of this population. First, antipsychotic medications reduce or eliminate psychotic symptoms with less problematic side effects for many people with schizophrenia, and most live in the community with psychosocial supports and interventions. Attention has thus been directed 'beyond the brain' to general health and quality of life. Second, changes in the health care system and the emergence of 'managed care' have led health care payers to consider the total costs of all care to persons with schizophrenia. Decisions to 'carve in' (integrate) or 'carve out' (separate) mental health services from the rest of health care require an understanding of somatic health care needs and costs. Third, the focus on health behaviors for people with schizophrenia may be motivated by the general social phenomena of increased expectations for individual personal responsibility, and increased consumer knowledge and participation in health behaviors in society at large. People with schizophrenia, their families, and mental health professionals alike take in the widespread media messages on improving general health by adjusting diet, exercise and other positive health behaviors.

This chapter will summarize current knowledge in the medical management of somatic health among people with schizophrenia. We will initially outline some general issues and then review research and clinical findings of the health behaviors relating to obesity and smoking. A detailed discussion of a specific medical illness, type II diabetes, will follow. Lessons learned from the comorbidity of diabetes and schizophrenia have implications for the comorbidity of schizophrenia and other illnesses. We will conclude with a discussion of polydipsia, a medical complication of schizophrenia itself. This chapter will not cover the use of alcohol and other illicit drugs since that is being covered elsewhere in this volume.

Mortality in schizophrenia

Persons with schizophrenia have significantly higher mortality rates than the general population.[1-7] Elevated suicide rates account for some, but not all, of this observed excess mortality.[1,2,6] Persons with schizophrenia have been reported to die prematurely due to infectious, endocrine, circulatory, respiratory, digestive, and genitourinary disorders.[1,3,4,6,7] Although the specific causes of excess mortality vary slightly by study, gender, and age, overall elevated mortality due to 'natural causes' has been found in studies conducted in different countries (see Table 19.1).

Table 19.1 Review of mortality studies of schizophrenia (adapted from Harris and Barraclough[7]).

Cause of death	Men			Women		
	No. of studies	Population size	SMR	No. of studies	Population size	SMR
All causes	12	14 619	156[a]	10	10 356	141[a]
Unnatural	12	14 619	480[a]	10	10 356	378[a]
Natural	12	14 619	129[a]	10	10 356	129[a]
Suicide	8	13 634	979[a]	6	9424	802[a]
Other violent	8	13 634	225[a]	6	9424	229[a]
Infectious	3	3645	455[a]	3	2446	490[a]
Neoplasms	8	13 457	86[a]	7	9682	115[a]
Endocrine	1	2122	182	1	1501	250
Mental	1	2122	556[a]	1	1501	600[a]
Nervous	1	2122	100	1	1501	222
Circulatory	8	13 457	110[a]	7	9682	102
Respiratory	5	12 486	214[a]	5	9331	249[a]
Digestive	3	10 756	208[a]	3	8201	163[a]
Genitourinary	3	10 756	182[a]	3	8210	130[a]

SMR, standardized mortality ratio. [a] statistically significant

Studies have followed first-break patients and more chronic patients with relatively consistent findings, Overall, Simpson and Tsuang concluded that, on average, a diagnosis of schizophrenia shortens a person's life expectancy by about 10 years.[8]

Morbidity in schizophrenia

Mortality studies tell us about death rates and immediate causes of death, but tell us little about the medical illnesses and morbidity with which individuals may have lived. Many fewer studies have focused on medical morbidity in schizophrenia, although elevated rates of comorbid medical conditions have also been found.[2,5] Investigators from Oxford conducted a record linkage study and found a markedly increased rate of cardiovascular disease and pneumonia in schizophrenia.[9,10] Dalmau and colleagues[11] recently reported a Swedish case control study comparing persons with schizophrenia and age- and sex-matched controls on numbers of inpatient admissions for different medical illnesses. Persons with schizophrenia had greater rates of hospitalization for infectious and parasitic diseases; neoplasms; endocrine disease; diseases of the respiratory, circulatory, digestive, and nervous systems; diseases of the skin and subcutaneous tissue; and injuries, as well as a category titled, 'symptoms, signs and ill-defined conditions'. These investigators addressed the important potential role of substance abuse in mediating the observed increased morbidity in schizophrenia. They found persistently elevated rates of hospitalization for persons with schizophrenia for the majority of illness categories even when substance abusers were excluded. Research has also suggested that persons with severe mental illness who suffer from somatic conditions may have more severe forms of these disorders.[5]

The Schizophrenia Patient Outcomes Research Team (PORT) interviewed 719 persons receiving treatment for schizophrenia in two different states and a variety of treatment settings. This study offers the opportunity to determine the self-reported prevalence of medical comorbidities and the association of medical comorbidity with physical and mental health status.[12] The interview asked patients whether a doctor had told them that they had any of 12 different medical problems, and if so, whether they were receiving treatment. The majority of patients reported at least one problem (see Table 19.2). Problems with eyesight, teeth, and high blood pressure were most common. The rates of non treatment for current medical conditions ranged from 14% (diabetes) to 59% (hearing problems). The study demonstrated reasonable reliability of patients' self-report of medical problems. The rates of a number of illnesses, including diabetes, heart diseases, respiratory diseases, and sexually transmitted diseases, exceed reported rates obtained by a similar methodology in the general population for persons of similar age groups.

As expected, the study also found that greater *numbers* of current medical problems were independently associated with lower perceived physical health status. Greater numbers of current medical problems were also associated with more severe psychosis and depression and greater likelihood of a history of a suicide attempt. The linkage of medical morbidity with worse mental health status highlights the importance of somatic health assessment on the mental health care of persons with schizophrenia.[12]

Models of comorbidity

Little is known about why persons with schizophrenia have increased mortality and medical morbidity. Many explanations focus on the ways schizophrenia or its treatments may predispose people to greater incidence and severity of medical illnesses. For example, the sedentary lifestyle associated with institutionalization may be linked with development of obesity and related medical illnesses. On a neurological level, persons with schizophrenia may have decreased pain sensitivity and thus not experience an internal cue

Table 19.2 Medical illnesses reported by schizophrenia patients in PORT study ($n = 719$).

Physical condition	Ever been told by a doctor that you have a physical condition n (%)
High blood pressure	245 (34.1)
Diabetes	107 (14.9)
Sexually transmitted disease	71 (10.0)
Cancer	33 (4.6)
Breathing problems	148 (20.6)
Heart Problems	112 (15.6)
Bowel problems	172 (23.9)
Seizures	84 (11.7)
Problems with hearing	93 (13.0)
Problems with eyesight	392 (54.6)
Problems with teeth	276 (38.4)
Skin problems	107 (14.9)

that they have a health problem, and so access care at a more advanced stage of illness.[5] Antipsychotic drugs may cause weight gain, higher risk of tobacco use, and the health consequences of both. Some psychotropics also interfere with glucose metabolism and may predispose to the development of diabetes.[13] The extent to which these phenomena contribute to the observed increased morbidity and mortality is uncertain. It is necessary to learn more about the reasons for the observed morbidity and mortality in schizophrenia to remedy this problem successfully.

Barriers to adequate health care

In addition to the individually oriented possible explanations for elevated comorbidity, it is also important to consider the barriers to good health care that exist for people with schizophrenia.[14] These can be conceptualized as patient-related, health-provider-related and system-related. Patient-related barriers include issues such as an inability for some patients to clearly verbalize physical symptoms through their psychotic thought process. For example, patients may at times articulate a physical symptom in such a way as to make it difficult for the health care provider to differentiate a real symptom from a somatic delusion. Communication difficulties, dissatisfaction with treatment, fears, poverty, denial, or lack of insight can lead to nonadherence to treatment protocols, affecting both somatic and mental health.

Health providers may feel uncomfortable

engaging patients who are actively psychotic, confused, or uncommunicative and may lack skills to interact with them effectively. They also may not take the extra time necessary to adequately assess a medical concern with such a patient. Some providers still practice with operant stigmas. For example, such a clinician may view the physical complaints of a person with a psychotic disorder as 'psychosomatic' and dismiss them without proper examination. In a different vein, some psychiatrists are uncomfortable getting involved with the medical problems of their patients, but may serve as their 'principal' physician. All of these can form barriers to good physical health care and services.

System-related barriers include the dichotomy of general health care and mental health care delivery systems. Good integration in these areas is rare in most systems of care. This bifurcation fragments treatment and deters coordination and holistic care. Poverty and lack of health care coverage can be further barriers to adequate health care in this population, as can limited service availability in some places.

An additional barrier to the treatment of a comorbid medical disorder may be the very phenomenon of comorbidity, if the two comorbid disorders are unrelated. Redelmeier et al[15] studied the approximately 1.3 million residents of Ontario, Canada who are 65 or older. They found that for three different pairs of unrelated medical disorders, treatment for the second disorder was less likely in the presence of the first. Patients with diabetes were 60% less likely to receive treatment with estrogen replacement therapy, patients with pulmonary emphysema were 31% less likely to receive lipid-lowering medications, and patients with psychotic syndromes were 41% less likely to receive medical arthritis treatment. There are numerous plausible explanations for these consistent observations. However, the study powerfully suggests the potential for great undertreatment of comorbidity in the setting of chronic disease.

Understanding the most significant barriers for each individual and incorporating this knowledge into active treatment planning can result in better access to medical care and reduced morbidity of medical problems for persons with schizophrenia. The rest of this chapter will discuss these and related issues in the context of specific health and behaviors and conditions.

Smoking and schizophrenia

Prevalence

Studies have shown that persons with schizophrenia smoke cigarettes at almost double the rate of the general population.[16–18] Reported prevalence rates of smoking range from 56% to 88%. One study reported that out of the people with schizophrenia interviewed, 93% had smoked cigarettes sometime during their lifetime. Similar estimates have been found internationally in a number of different countries and cultures including Ireland, Italy and Chile.[18]

The health consequences of smoking are exacerbated by the fact that persons with schizophrenia tend to smoke high-tar cigarettes,[18] inhale more deeply, and smoke for longer periods of time. In a study by Lohr and Flynn, 80% of the schizophrenic population had smoked for 18 years or more.[17] While the number of smokers in the general population decreases each year, this does not hold true for people with schizophrenia.[17]

Possible explanations

There are a number of hypotheses that could explain why so many persons with schizophrenia smoke tobacco. In the past, cigarettes have been used in hospitals and other settings as rewards.[19] Although treatment changes and the current trend toward smoke-free hospitals may have halted or attenuated this practice, it may have contributed to current nicotine addiction. High rates of unemployment, decreased amounts of social activities, and general boredom may contribute to smoking in schizophrenia.[20]

There are biological reasons why persons with

schizophrenia may be vulnerable to increased smoking rates. Research has suggested that nicotine's interaction with dopamine may contribute to the smoking behavior of people with schizophrenia.[16] Nicotine can serve as a mood regulator and improves alertness and attention. Depressed prefrontal dopamine, which is hypothesized to be related to the negative symptoms of schizophrenia, may be elevated by nicotine.[18] Therefore, some patients may use smoking as a form of self-medication to relieve negative symptoms or even extrapyramidal side effects. The short-term subjective effects of nicotine may make it even more difficult for people with schizophrenia to stop smoking once they start.

Health consequences

There are a number of negative sequelae of smoking that directly affect people with schizophrenia. First, persons with schizophrenia who smoke experience similar negative health repercussions to nonschizophrenic smokers. They have a greater likelihood of bronchial cancer, breathing problems, and lung cancer than nonsmokers in the general population. However, interestingly, one study found that persons with schizophrenia who smoke tend to experience less cancer than nonschizophrenia smokers.[21]

Smokers are more likely to use drugs and alcohol than nonsmokers. Also, smokers tend to be more sexually active than nonsmokers, which can lead to sexually transmitted diseases including HIV.[22] Heavy smoking has also been linked to polydipsia or self-induced water intoxication.[16]

Antipsychotic dosing

People with schizophrenia who smoke tobacco require higher doses of neuroleptics than nonsmokers to achieve the same antipsychotic drug effect.[23,24] One possible reason is that cigarette-smoking may increase the plasma clearance for some antipsychotic medications.[17] It has also been demonstrated that smoking may reduce the effect of benzodiazepines.[25] If dosages are not increased to compensate for the increased antipsychotic

drug metabolism, increased attentional, cognitive and mood symptoms may result.[24] To the extent that persons with schizophrenia use tobacco to self-medicate these symptoms, they may feel the need to smoke more, which might further decrease effective antipsychotic drug levels, resulting in a vicious self-medication cycle. It is thus imperative that the role of tobacco is taken into consideration when prescribing medication to patients with schizophrenia who smoke heavily.

Treatment suggestions

Persons with psychiatric disorders have been found to derive the same benefits from stopping smoking as other smokers, Thus, researchers and clinicians have made a number of suggestions for decreasing smoking among people with schizophrenia. The most important principle is that smoking cessation programs must be tailored to meet the specific needs of people with schizophrenia – such as the short-term benefits of nicotine with respect to schizophrenic symptoms. In treatment facilities where smoking is still permitted, it should be discouraged or prohibited.

Pharmacological nicotine-replacement strategies such as the transdermal nicotine patch and nicotine gum may be effective.[26] Behavioral strategies are important as well. Ziedonis and colleagues described a ten-session behavioral program using motivational enhancement techniques.[27] Recently, the American Lung Association 'Freedom From Smoking' program was modified for use with a schizophrenic population.[23] This 7-week, eight-session program paid attention to the role of smoking in the lives of persons with schizophrenia, had greater tolerance for psychotic ideation, and considered the social and financial limitations of persons with schizophrenia when designing potential rewards and behavioral alternatives to smoking.[26]

Novel antipsychotics may play a role in smoking cessation. One study demonstrated that clozapine has been shown to contribute to a significant decrease in daily cigarette use in heavy smokers in comparison to typical neuroleptics.[28]

Although there is no current evidence to suggest that nicotine withdrawal has an impact on the symptoms of schizophrenia, it is prudent for clinicians to consider the potential impact of nicotine withdrawal in treatment.

Comment

Cigarette-smoking among persons with schizophrenia is frequently ignored by clinicians. Clinicians may view attempts at smoking cessation as depriving persons with schizophrenia of one of the few pleasures they experience. It may seem almost irrelevant to address smoking given the host of other psychiatric problems that patients, clinicians and families are attempting to manage. On the other hand, the health consequences are potentially grave. Further, families and housing providers chronically worry about unextinguished, smoldering cigarettes as a potential fire hazard. Cigarettes are becoming increasingly expensive for persons with schizophrenia whose income is typically limited to their disability benefit. The negative impacts of cigarette-smoking merit the careful consideration of clinicians. Ultimately, the most important public health challenge is to prevent adolescents and persons with schizophrenia from starting to smoke in the first place.

Weight and exercise

Prevalence and diet

People with schizophrenia often have health problems related to being overweight. A recent study compared the distributions of body mass index (BMI) of persons with schizophrenia to those of other populations.[29] Persons with schizophrenia were found to be as or more obese than others. This was especially true for women. One possible contributor to obesity is the lack of proper nutrition. Dietary habits related to poverty, unstable living situations, and frequent consumption of fast food and high-fat items can contribute to obesity.[14] Also, a lack of knowledge about nutrition and healthy diet can also lead to poor eating habits.

Medication effects

Another major factor in weight gain among people with schizophrenia is medication side effects. Almost every antipsychotic medication causes some weight gain, and several typically cause significant weight gain.[14,29] In part this has been attributed to 5-hydroxytryptamine (5-HT) or H_1 activity, which can lead to an increase in food consumption.[14] A comparison study between risperidone and clozapine showed a significantly greater weight gain in people taking clozapine (23.5 lbs vs 3.7 lbs over 12 weeks). Olanzapine has also been associated with significant weight gain.[14]

Health consequences

Regardless of cause, weight gain and obesity increase risk for heart disease, cardiovascular problems and fatigue. Additionally, when antipsychotic medications cause or contribute to weight gain, resultant depression or distress may lead to medication noncompliance.[14]

Suggestions

Since weight gain and obesity can lead to a number of physical and emotional problems, doctors and therapists should address this issue when treating persons with schizophrenia. Body mass, age, gender, and predictors of weight gain should be considered when prescribing medications to these clients. Additionally, it may be beneficial to provide nutritional assessments and weight loss intervention for persons with schizophrenia, especially those taking clozapine.[14]

Exercise

Exercise programs can also be used to address obesity and weight problems.[30] Often people with schizophrenia tend to have sedentary lifestyles.[31] Numerous studies have demonstrated the myriad of benefits of exercise in the general population.[32,33] However, physical fitness among people with mental illness is an area that is often overlooked in services. Despite the potential health benefits of exercise demonstrated in the general population, the research literature on exercise programs for people with mental illnesses is scant. The few existing studies suggest that exercise confers both psychological and physiological benefits.[32,33]

In a small interview survey of subjects with schizophrenia who participated in an aerobic or nonaerobic exercise program, the vast majority reported that participation in exercise made them feel less depressed and anxious, gave them higher energy levels, and improved participation in other rehabilitation treatment modalities.[33] Comparison of participants randomly assigned to the aerobic or nonaerobic exercise conditions revealed that aerobic exercise was superior. Subjects in the aerobic program had a significant decrease in their scores on the Beck Depression Inventory in comparison to the clients assigned to the nonaerobic program. The subjects in the aerobic condition also had significantly greater improvements in their aerobic health. Clients who participated in the aerobic program had a 20.9% increase in their oxygen capacity after 12 weeks of participating in the program. While it is possible that such a large increase was due to below-average fitness before the program, some clients also lost significant amounts of weight (30–60 lbs) during the aerobic program, returning them into the normal range for their height and gender. A third study by Pelham et al[33] interviewed 15 participants in their psychiatric rehabilitation program who did not participate in formal exercise therapies. This group exhibited a negative correlation between level of depression and aerobic fitness. The higher the level of aerobic fitness, the lower the level of depression observed.

Comment

Obesity and poor physical fitness is clearly a health problem among persons with schizophrenia. Research suggests that exercise may be a beneficial, cost-effective, and safe intervention, with physical and emotional benefits. These programs can be incorporated into the rehabilitation programs with interventions that address weight problems in people with schizophrenia. As with any other health intervention, such programs must take into account the specific deficits of persons with schizophrenia.

Diabetes and schizophrenia

Schizophrenia is likely to have unique linkages with a variety of specific medical disorders. Cancer, HIV, and autoimmune diseases, among others, have been the focus of attention. Since it is not possible to review each disease, we have chosen to focus on a single disease, type II diabetes, as an example of an important medical comorbidity that may have implications for the other medical problems in schizophrenia. Type II diabetes has been of historic interest in schizophrenia dating back to the 1980s, is relatively common and is influenced by smoking and obesity, and has both acute and chronic sequelae of poor self-care. The incidence of diabetes in schizophrenia may be on the rise due to the widespread use of novel antipsychotic drugs.

Prevalence

Research has suggested that people diagnosed with schizophrenia are at high risk for developing type II diabetes.[2,34–37] For example, in the large national database of the Schizophrenia PORT study, 15% of participants reported having diabetes at some point in their lives, and 11% reported having it currently.[13] This compares with 1.2% for persons aged 18–44 and 6.3% for persons aged 45–64 in the 1994 National Health Interview Study.[38]

Schizophrenia itself has been associated with insulin resistance and impaired glucose tolerance,[37,39–42] while antipsychotic drugs often cause weight gain – all of which are associated with diabetes. Additionally, some evidence suggests that new atypical drugs may contribute directly to hyperglycemia.[35,43,44] Furthermore, tobacco use may interfere with glucose metabolism,[40] and sedentary, isolated lifestyles and poor diet may increase diabetes risk. These are all too common in the lives of people with schizophrenia.

A number of demographic characteristics were associated with a diagnosis of diabetes in both schizophrenia samples[13] and in the general population.[45–48] These include being older, African-American or a member of another ethnic/racial minority group, having less education, and having ever been married.[13]

Health consequences

In the database generated during the Schizophrenia Patient Outcomes Research Team (PORT) study, self-reported physical health status was lowest among interviewees reporting that they had diabetes but were not receiving treatment (14% of sample), and highest among people without diabetes. Diabetes was clearly associated with greater use of health services and greater costs compared to people with schizophrenia but without diabetes. Previous work with the 1992 Medicare population found that persons with diabetes had costs of care that were 1.5 times greater than other Medicare beneficiaries in 1992.[49] Roughly the same overall ratio was observed for patients in the PORT study. However, in the schizophrenic group, the ratio increased with age, suggesting a relatively increasing cost of a comorbid diabetes diagnosis in schizophrenia in older persons.[13] In the PORT study, persons with diabetes also had greater rates of other medical comorbidities in addition to diabetes.[13]

Management and treatment

Diabetes is a chronic condition that requires active self-care for optimal management. The cognitive, memory, and social skills dysfunctions common in schizophrenia make it likely that many people with both disorders would have trouble understanding, retaining, organizing, and acting on diabetes treatment and self-care recommendations. Effective communication with health care providers may be problematic. The potential impact of the new antipsychotic drugs on diabetes rates and incidence must be carefully monitored. The implications for health screening, treatment

planning, costs, and locus of care delivery are considerable.

Polydipsia and schizophrenia

Prevalence and description

People with schizophrenia frequently experience polydipsia, the excessive intake of fluids.[50] A study conducted by deLeon et al[51] at a Pennsylvania State hospital found that 26% of patients in the sample were polydipsic.[51] A total of 80% of these were patients who had schizophrenia or schizoaffective disorder diagnoses. Polydipsic patients consume large amounts of liquids, in excess of 3 litres per day, and in some cases massive quantities such as 10–15 litres per day. The polydipsic patients had a specific gravity of urine of lower than 1.009. Polyuria, the excretion of greater than 3 litres per day of urine, and water intoxication are both commonly associated with polydipsia.[51] Polydipsia and water intoxication have been associated with long hospitalizations, high neuroleptic dosages, moderate dosage of anticholinergic drugs, and heavy smoking.[51] Caucasians and males may also have a greater likelihood of being polydipsic than members of other demographic groups.[50]

It is often difficult to identify polydipsic behavior in clients. Common methods include staff reports based on observation and biological determinants such as specific gravity of urine, urine creatinine concentration, normalized diurnal weight gain.[51] Weight gain due to excessive water intake is temporary. Nonetheless, studies suggest that polydipsia among people with schizophrenia is underestimated.[51] Patients may consume excess fluids secretly if limits are imposed, making accurate behavioral observation difficult. Biological markers may only show if the behavior occurred within 24 hours of testing.[51] Polydipsia may also be overlooked in cases where water intoxication is not present.

Health consequences

Polydipsia and water intoxication can lead to other health complications, such as kidney problems and osteoporosis.[50–52] Physical complications commonly occur in clients who suffer from extended periods of water intoxication or polydipsia. Osteoporosis, secondary to increased calcium excretion in urine, can occur.[52] Chronic dilation of the urinary and gastrointestinal tracts is also associated with excessive consumption of fluids. A total of 52% of the patients in deLeon's study exhibited water retention linked with water intoxication. About 5% had a history of previous water intoxication.[51] Water intoxication occurs when low serum sodium levels lead to brain edema, causing neurological and psychiatric symptoms such as nausea, vomiting, ataxia, seizures, coma, psychosis, agitation and irritability.

Causal hypotheses

A number of hypotheses have attempted to explain the high prevalence of polydipsia among people with schizophrenia. Goldman and Blake[53] suggested that hippocampal dysfunction may be important given its regulation of vasopressin and thirst. Research has also speculated that psychotropic medications may be linked to polydipsia; however, the phenomenon was noted before certain medications were developed.[52] Suggestions have also been made that polydipsia may be related to dopamine supersensitivity, perhaps explaining why people with tardive dyskinesia have a greater likelihood of developing problems with fluid regulation.[54] While the question of cause remains unsolved, the various findings can help service providers identify clients at risk for polydipsia and its consequences.

Treatment suggestions

Both behavioral and pharmacological treatments have been tried to decrease fluid intake among people with schizophrenia, although often without success.[55] Adapting substance abuse treatment models, Millson and Smith assigned polydipsic patients to a control group (no intervention) or a treatment group (group psychoeducation twice a week for 45 minutes for 4

months). Although intervention group members became more aware of problems associated with increased fluid consumption and could monitor their weight gain, the two groups had the same mean weight increases. Also, after the study ended intervention group members quickly resumed their previous levels of fluid consumption.[55]

Clozapine has also been tried as a treatment for polydipsia.[57] Of patients receiving clozapine for treatment-resistant psychosis, 64% had significant increases in sodium serum measures taken at 6 a.m. and 4 p.m. (signaling decreased fluid intake) within the first 2 weeks. This is possibly explained by research findings that the moderate D_1 blockade clozapine has been linked to a decrease in water consumption in animals.[56]

Summary

Persons with schizophrenia have the misfortune of suffering from medical problems at a greater rate and with greater severity than the rest of the population. This morbidity is not benign, and leads to markedly elevated mortality rates for a number of different disorders. Medical risk appears in part due to the symptoms and biology of schizophrenia, its treatments, and to systems of care that are not equipped to address comorbidity effectively. Smoking and obesity are important mediators of medical illness in schizophrenia. Antipsychotic drug treatment increases the risks of obesity and may also play a role in increasing smoking risk, although more research is necessary in this area. The linkage between mental health and physical health as well as concern for the overall quality of life of persons with schizophrenia make it imperative that medical concerns of persons with schizophrenia are not ignored.

References

1. Allebeck P, Schizophrenia: a life-threatening disease, *Schizophr Bull* (1989) **15:**81–9.
2. Felker B, Yazel JJ, Short D, Mortality and medical

comorbidity among psychiatric patients: a review, *Psychiatr Serv* (1996) **47:**1356–63.

3. Baxter DN, The mortality experience of individuals on the Salford psychiatric case register I. All-cause mortality, *Br J Psychiatry* (1996) **168:**772–9.

4. Mortensen PB, Juel K, Mortality and causes of death in first admitted schizophrenic patients, *Br J Psychiatry* (1993) **163:**183–9.

5. Jeste DV, Glasjo JA, Lindamer LA, Lacro JP, Medical comorbidity in schizophrenia, *Schizophr Bull* (1996) **22:**413–30.

6. Saku M, Tokudome S, Ikeda M et al, Mortality in psychiatric patients, with a specific focus on cancer mortality associated with schizophrenia, *Int J Epidemiol* (1995) **24:**366–72.

7. Harris EC, Barraclough B, Excess mortality of mental disorder, *Br J Psychiatry* (1998) **173:**11–53.

8. Simpson JC, Tsuang MT, Mortality among patients with schizophrenia, *Schizophr Bull* (1996) **22:** 485–99.

9. Herman HE, Baldwin JA, Christie D, A record-linkage study of mortality and general hospital discharge in patients diagnosed as schizophrenic, *Psychol Med* (1983) **13:**581–93.

10. Baldwin JA, Schizophrenia and physical disease: a preliminary analysis of the data from the Oxford Record Linkage Study. In: Hennings G, ed, *Biochemistry of Schizophrenia and Addiction* (MTP Press: Lancaster, 1980) 297–318.

11. Dalmau A, Bergman B, Brismar B, Somatic morbidity in schizophrenia – a case control study, *Public Health* (1997) **111:**393–7.

12. Dixon LB, Postrado L, Delahanty J et al, The association of medical comorbidity in schizophrenia with poor physical and mental health, *J Nerv Ment Dis* (1999) **187:**496–502.

13. Dixon LB, Weiden PJ, Delhanty J et al, Diabetes in schizophrenia, *Schizophr Bull*, in press.

14. Masand P (Editor), Weight gain and Antipsychotic Medications, Journal of Clinical Psychiatry Visuals, 1999, Physicians Postgraduate Press, Memphis Tennessee.

15. Redelmeier DA, Tan SH, Booth GL, The treatment of unrelated disorders in patients with chronic medical diseases, *N Engl J Med* (1998) **338:**1516–20.

16. deLeon J, Smoking and vulnerability for schizophrenia, *Schizophr Bull* (1996) **22:**405–9.

17. Lohr JB, Flynn K, Smoking and schizophrenia, *Schizophr Res* (1992) **8:**93–102.

18. Chiles JA, Cohen S, Maiuro R et al, Smoking and schizophrenic psychopathology, *Am J Addict* (1993) **2:**315–19.

18. O'Farrell TJ, Connors GJ, Upper D, Addictive behaviors among hospitalized schizophrenic patients, *Addict Behav* (1983) 329–33.

19. Maiuro RD, Michael MC, Vitaliano PP et al, Patient reactions to a no smoking policy in a community mental health center, *Community Ment Health J* (1989) **25:**71–7.

20. Hughes JR, Possible effects of smoke free inpatient units on psychiatric diagnosis and treatment, *J Clin Psychiatry* (1993) **54:**109–14.

21. Masterson E, O'Shea B, Smoking and malignancy in schizophrenia, *Br J Psychiatry* (1984) **145:**429–32.

22. Hymowitz N, Jaffe FE, Gupta A et al, Cigarette smoking among patients with mental retardation and mental illness, *Psychiatr Serv* (1997) **48:** 100–102.

23. Ziedonis DM, Koster TR, Glazer WM et al, Nicotine dependence and schizophrenia, *Hosp Community Psychiatry* (1994) **45:**204–206.

24. Vinarova E, Vinar O, Kabvach Z, Smokers need higher doses of neuroleptic drugs, *Biol Psychiatry* (1984) **19:**1265–8.

25. Swett C, Drowsiness due to chlorpromazine in relation to cigarette smoking, *Arch Gen Psychiatry* (1974) **31:**211–13.

26. Addington J, Group treatment for smoking cessation among persons with schizophrenia, *Psychiatr Serv* (1998) **49:**925–8.

27. Ziedonis DM, Gorge TP, Schizophrenia and nicotine use: report of a pilot smoking cessation program and review of neurobiological and clinical issues, *Schizophr Bull* (1997) **23:**247–54.

28. George TP, Sernyak MJ, Ziedonis DM, Effects of clozapine on smoking in chronic schizophrenic outpatients, *J Clin Psychiatry* (1995) **56:**344–6.

29. Allison DB, Fontaine KR, Moonseong H et al, The distribution of body mass index among individuals with and without schizophrenia, *J Clin Psychiatry* (1999) **60:**215–20.

30. Skrinar GS, Unger KV, Hutchinson DS et al, Effects of exercise training in young adults with psychiatric disabilities, *Can J Rehab* (1992) **5:**151–7.

31. Layman E, Psychological effect of physical activity.

In: *Exercise and Sport Sciences Reviews*, American College of Sports Medicine Series. (Academic Press: New York, 1974) 33–70.

32. Pelham TW, Campagna PD, Benefits of exercise in psychiatric rehabilitation of persons with schizophrenia, *Can J Rehab* (1991) **4:**159–68.

33. Pelham TW, Capagna PD, Ritvo PG et al, The effects of exercise therapy on clients in a psychiatric rehabilitation program, *Psychosocial Rehab J* (1993) **16:**75–84.

34. Mukherjee S, Decina P, Bocola V et al, Diabetes mellitus in schizophrenic patients, *Compr Psychiatry* (1996) **37:**68–73.

35. McKee HA, D'Arcy PF, Wilson PJ, Diabetes and schizophrenia – a preliminary study, *Journal of Clinical Hospital Pharmacology* (1986) **11:**297–9.

36. Dynes JB, Diabetes in schizophrenia and diabetes in nonpsychotic medical patients, *Diseases of the Nervous System* (1969) **30:**341–4.

37. Richter D, Biochemical aspects of schizophrenia. In: Richter D, ed, *Schizophrenia: Somatic Aspects* (Pergamon Press: London, 1957).

38. Adams PF, Marano MA, Current estimates from the National Health Interview Survey, 1994, National Center for Health Statistics, *Vital Health Stat* (1995) **10:**193.

39. Brambilla F, Guastalla A, Guerrini A et al, Glucose–insulin metabolism in chronic schizophrenia, *Diseases of the Nervous System* (1976) **37:**98–103.

40. Holden RJ, The estrogen connection: the etiological relationship between diabetes, cancer, rheumatoid arthritis and psychiatric disorders, *Med Hypotheses* (1995) **45:** 169–89.

41. Holden RJ, Schizophrenia, suicide and the serotonin story, *Med Hypotheses* (1995) **44:**379–91.

42. Holden RJ, Mooney PA, Schizophrenia is a diabetic brain state: an elucidation of impaired neurometabolism, *Med Hypotheses* (1994) **43:**420–35.

43. deBoer C, Gaete HP, Neuroleptic malignant syndrome and diabetic keto-acidosis, *Br J Psychiatry* (1992) **161:**856–8.

44. Kamran A, Doraiswamy PM, Jane JL et al, Severe hyperglycemia associated with high doses of clozapine, *Am J Psychiatry* (1994) **151:**1395.

45. Cantor AB, Krischer JP, Antor AB et al, Diabetes-mellitus (IDDM) in relatives of patients with IDDM, *J Clin Endocrinol Metab* (1995) **80:**3739–43.

46. Casparie A, Epidemiology of type II diabetes mellitus and aging of the population: health policy implications and recommendations for epidemiological research, *Int J Epidemiol* (1991) **20(Suppl 1):**S25–S29.

47. MMWR (Morbidity and Mortality Weekly Report of the Centers for Disease Control and Prevention), Self-reported prevalence of diabetes among Hispanics – United States, 1994–1997, *Morbidity and Mortality Weekly Report* (1999) **48:**8–12.

48. Harris MI, Diabetes in America: epidemiology and scope of the problem, *Diabetes Care* (1998) **21(Suppl 3):**C11–C14.

49. Krop JS, Powe NR, Weller WE et al, Patterns of expenditures and use of services among older adults with diabetes – implications for the transition to capitated managed care, *Diabetes Care* (1998) **21:**747–52.

50. Shutty MS, Song Y, Behavioral analysis of drinking behaviors in polydipsic patients with chronic schizophrenia, *J Abnorm Psychol* **106:**483–5.

51. deLeon J, Verghese C, Tracy JI et al, Polydipsia and water intoxication in psychiatric patients: a review of the epidemiological literature, *Biol Psychiatry* (1994) **35:**408–19.

52. Blum A, Tempey FW, Lynch WJ, Somatic findings in patients with psychogenic polydipsia, *J Clin Psychiatry* (1983) **44:**55–6.

53. Goldman MB, Blake L, Association of nonsuppression of cortisol on the DST with primary polydipsia, *Am J Psychiatry* (1993) **150:**653–6.

54. Umbricht DSG, Saltz B, Polydipsia and tardive dyskinesia in chronic psychiatric patients – related disorders? *Am J Psychiatry* (1993) **150:**1536–9.

55. Millson RC, Smith AP, Self-induced water intoxication treated with group psychotherapy, *Am J Psychiatry* (1993) **150:**825–7.

56. Spears NM, Leadbetter RA, Shutty MS, Clozapine treatment in polydipsia and intermittent hyponatremia, *J Clin Psychiatry* (1996) **57:**123–8.

20(i)

Ethnic Influences in Schizophrenia: Pharmacogenetics

Katherine J Aitchison

Contents • CYP2D6 • CYP3A4 • CYP1A2 • CYP2C19 • Drug–drug interactions • Conclusions

The term 'pharmacogenetics' was coined when adverse drug reactions were first attributed to genetic factors.[1] Genetic factors affect both drug metabolism (pharmacokinetics) and drug response at the level of the target organ (pharmacodynamics). With respect to interethnic variation affecting the treatment of psychosis, pharmacokinetic genetic factors, encoding the drug metabolizing enzymes (or DMEs), have been far more extensively investigated than pharmacodynamic genetic factors.

An important subset of the DMEs is the cytochrome P450 enzyme family, or hemethiolate proteins. These enzymes metabolize not only drugs, but also endogenous compounds (for example, steroids), plant products and man-made environmental toxins. Three members of this family of enzymes are involved in the metabolism of antipsychotics; these enzymes are: CYP2D6, CYP3A4 and CYP1A2 ('CYP' stands for cytochrome P450). Other enzymes in this family, including members of the CYP2C subfamily, should also be considered, with regard to drug–drug interactions.

CYP2D6

Three different levels of activity of CYP2D6 have been identified through the use of probe drugs which are metabolized by the enzyme; an individual may be termed an ultrarapid metabolizer (UM), extensive metabolizer (EM) or poor metabolizer (PM). This variation in enzymatic activity is due to multiple allelic variants of *CYP2D6* (the gene encoding the protein), the frequencies of which differ in different ethnic groups.[2]

One might expect that individuals with relatively low enzyme activity should show a tendency towards higher serum levels of drugs metabolized by CYP2D6 for a given dose, and might therefore be more susceptible to adverse effects (be treatment-intolerant), whereas UMs might show particularly low serum levels at standard doses and might therefore appear to be treatment-refractory. In accordance with this, in studies on normal volunteers, PMs were shown to have significantly higher serum levels of perphenazine[3] and zuclopenthixol,[4] while the oral clearance of perphenazine and zuclopenthixol in patients on continuous treatment was shown to be significantly predicted by CYP2D6 genotype.[5]

CYP2D6 is also involved in the metabolism of haloperidol, fluphenazine and trifluperidol.[6] Case reports support an association between PM status and a higher susceptibility to adverse effects.[7,8] A trend towards an excess of mutant CYP2D6 alleles has been seen in schizophrenics with movement disorders.[9] However, another study has not found an excess of PMs amongst schizophrenics intolerant of typical antipsychotics (Aitchison et al, unpublished data).

In Caucasian populations, the frequency of PMs is 5–10%, while in Black Africans the frequency is 0–8%, in African-Americans the frequency is 3.7% and in Orientals it is approximately 1%. In addition, a lower population mean enzyme activity has been observed in Chinese, Zimbabweans and Ghanaians as compared to Caucasians. The low PM frequency in Orientals is caused mainly by the very low frequency of the *CYP2D6*4*† mutant allele, an allele which is associated with absent enzyme activity and accounts for about 66% of PM alleles in Caucasians.[10] The lower population mean enzyme activity has been attributed to the relatively high frequency of *CYP2D6*10* in the Chinese, and of *CYP2D6*17* in the Ghanaians and Zimbabweans, both of which alleles being associated with diminished CYP2D6 activity.[11] The *CYP2D6*17* allele also occurs at a greater frequency in African-Americans.[12]

At the other end of the spectrum of enzyme activity, the frequency of UMs also differs markedly between different ethnic groups, being 0.8–2% in Danes or Swedes, 3.6% in Germans, less than 5% in Black Zimbabweans, 7% in Spaniards, 20% in Saudi Arabians and 29% in Ethiopians.[13]

Haloperidol concentrations have been found to be elevated in Chinese patients suffering from schizophrenia.[14] Although this could also be due to interethnic variations in CYP3A4 activity (see below), it would be consistent with the lower mean CYP2D6 activity seen in Chinese. Nyberg et al[15] showed that a PM of CYP2D6 had higher concentrations of plasma haloperidol throughout a 4-week treatment period with haloperidol decanoate compared with 7 EMs of CYP2D6. Suzuki et al[16] studied 50 Japanese schizophrenic patients, and found a higher mean steady state

plasma haloperidol concentration in patients with one mutant allele (mainly *CYP2D6*10*) than in patients with no mutant alleles, and a higher mean steady state plasma reduced haloperidol concentration in patients with 1 or 2 mutant alleles as compared with patients with no mutant alleles. However, Lin et al[17] found that on a fixed-dose weight-adjusted regimen, Oriental patients had only a slightly increased mean haloperidol plasma level. Nonetheless, they had a significantly higher rating for extra pyramidal symptoms (EPS), and also higher concentrations of prolactin in response to haloperidol.[18] This could be due to a pharmacodynamic interethnic difference, due for example to variability in the dopamine D_2 receptor, or to interethnic differences in CYP3A4 (see below).

With regard to UM status, two patients have been described for whom particularly high doses of tricyclic antidepressants metabolized by CYP2D6 were required in order to achieve a therapeutic response.[19] However, in a study comparing 73 patients who were successfully treated with typical antipsychotics with 235 treatment-refractory patients, an excess of UMs was not found in the refractory group.[20] On the contrary, a trend towards an excess of UMs was found in the non-refractory group, although the numbers of UMs were very low in both groups (2 and 3 in the refractory and non-refractory groups, respectively). This argues against ultrarapid hydroxylation by CYP2D6 of typical antipsychotics being a major cause of failure to respond to treatment with these agents.

CYP3A4

CYP3A4 is present in the liver and small intestine, and plays a role in the metabolism of many typical antipsychotics, and clozapine.[21] This enzyme can be induced, inhibited or inactivated by drugs as well as environmental factors including foods. Interpopulation variation in activity may there-

†The genes, or allelic variants, of the cytochrome P450 enzymes are italicized.

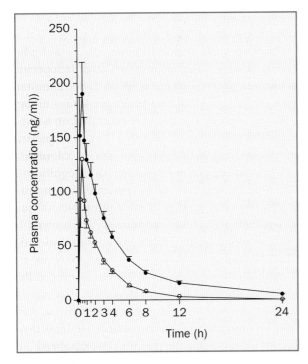

Figure 20(i).1 Plasma concentration–time curves for nifedipine after 20 mg capsules given to Caucasian subjects (open circles; $n = 27$) and South Asians (solid circles; $n = 30$). Data are mean values with standard errors shown as vertical bars. (From: Ahsan et al, 1993,[23] with permission.)

fore arise not only secondary to intrinsic variation in enzyme activity, but also secondary to the effect of environmental agents.

Nifedipine is a cardiovascular drug that is metabolized by CYP3A4 and has been used as a probe drug to investigate CYP3A4 activity in different populations. South Asians (from the Indian subcontinent) oxidize nifedipine at a significantly slower rate than Caucasians,[22,23] resulting in sustained haemodynamic changes. In the first study by Ahsan and colleagues, the South Asians had retained their original dietary practices, whereas the Caucasians consumed a typical Western diet. The effect of diet was studied in 6 of these Caucasians by giving them an Indian diet

for 3 days prior to the administration of nifedipine; no significant difference in any of the pharmacokinetic parameters was detected. This means that despite the ability of foods to affect CYP3A4 activity, the difference in nifedipine oxidation rate between Caucasians and South Asians is not due to cultural factors such as dietary practices, but is genetic in origin.

Similarly, the N-demethylation of codeine, which is catalysed by an enzyme of the CYP3A subfamily, occurs at a significantly slower rate in Chinese as compared to Caucasians.[24] Interestingly, Chinese have also been shown to have significantly lower mean codeine N-demethylation activity as compared to Japanese.[25]

Recently an A to G point mutation has been found in the nifedipine responsive region at position -289 in the $5'$ flanking region of the *CYP3A4* gene.[26] This mutation has been further analysed in 59 Taiwanese, 59 Finnish and 75 African-American subjects, and found to show an allelic frequency of 0%, 4.2% and 66.7% in these populations respectively (Sata, personal communication). Functional studies have not yet been performed, but it could be the case that this mutation is the primary mutation responsible for interethnic variations in CYP3A4 activity.

CYP3A4 is responsible for the back oxidation of reduced haloperidol to haloperidol and also for the N-dealkylation of haloperidol.[27,28] A negative correlation between clinical response and reduced haloperidol levels or reduced haloperidol/haloperidol ratios has been observed;[29] hence individuals with higher CYP3A4 activity could respond better to haloperidol than those with lower CYP3A4 activity. In a study on newly hospitalized Chinese patients with schizophrenia, Lane and colleagues[30] found that those who experienced EPS had significantly higher reduced haloperidol concentrations and reduced haloperidol/haloperidol ratios than the other patients. A trend towards higher haloperidol concentrations was also found in the EPS group. This would be consistent with individuals with lower CYP3A4 activity being more vulnerable to EPS.

CYP3A4 is readily induced by carbamazepine; for most typical antipsychotics twice as much antipsychotic is required to achieve the same plasma concentration in the presence of carbamazepine as in its absence.[21] This interaction is obviously very relevant for the treatment of schizoaffective psychoses. Other substances (such as ketoconazole and itraconazole) inhibit metabolism by the CYP3A enzymes, and valproate and cimetidine are potent CYP inhibitors. Clozapine toxicity has been reported after the coadministration of erythromycin,[31] due to the inhibition of CYP3A4 by erythromycin. Individuals who have relatively low CYPD6 activity or who are in receipt of drugs that inhibit CYP2D6 metabolism would be expected to be at increased risk of effects secondary to drug interactions at CYP3A4, and vice versa.

CYP1A2

CYP1A2 is involved in the metabolism of many typical antipsychotics, as well as clozapine and olanzapine. A preliminary study showed evidence of interethnic variation, with Japanese showing an increased maximum plasma concentration of olanzapine after a given dose, and a mean half-life of 34 hours as compared with 24 hours in Caucasians.[21] Le Marchand et al[32] also showed significantly lower CYP1A2 activity in Japanese as compared with Caucasians. Nakajima et al[33] showed that CYP1A2 activity as measured by caffeine 3-demethylation was bimodally distributed in a group of Japanese, with 14% being poor metabolizers. Relling et al[34] showed that the CYP1A2 activity was significantly lower in a group of Black subjects as compared with a group of White subjects ($p = 0.036$).

This enzyme is also involved in the metabolism of aromatic and heterocyclic amines, and in most populations is induced by smoking.[32] Oral contraceptives, postmenopausal replacement oestrogens and pregnancy appear to reduce CYP1A2 activity, and the lower CYP1A2 activity in women as com-

pared to men appears to be explained by the effect of oestrogens.[32]

Le Marchand and colleagues also found that lutein (which is found in green leafy vegetables) inhibits CYP1A2 activity. Caffeine and paracetamol (or acetaminophen) intake increase CYP1A2 activity, as does the consumption of cruciferous vegetables (cabbage, broccoli, Brussels sprouts and watercress). However the amount of cruciferous vegetable (for example, 500 g broccoli daily for 10 days) required to increase CYP1A2 activity is considerably higher than that present in a normal diet. Intake of meat cooked rapidly at a high temperature has also been shown to increase CYP1A2 activity.[35]

Although environmental factors such as the above contribute towards variability in CYP1A2 activity, Le Marchand and colleagues[32] found that 73% of the variability remained unexplained after taking into account the major environmental contributors to the variance in 90 subjects of various ethnic backgrounds in Hawaii. A mutation in the promotor region of *CYP1A2* has recently been found (Aitchison et al, unpublished data). This mutation shows significant interethnic variation: the frequencies of individuals heterozygous and homozygous for the mutation were found to be 3.4% and 0% respectively in 87 Caucasians and 19.2% and 3.2% respectively in 125 Taiwanese.

The metabolism of clozapine in vivo appears to correlate with CYP1A2 activity, although CYP3A4, CYP2C19 and CYP2D6 are also involved.[36] Levels of clozapine of at least 350–420 ng/ml are associated with therapeutic response,[37] while the incidence of seizures and EEG abnormalities also appears to increase with dose. Elevated plasma clozapine concentrations in Chinese patients have been described (steady state plasma clozapine concentration 30–50% higher than those reported in Caucasians).[38] At the opposite end of the spectrum, very low plasma clozapine levels despite high doses and compliance have been described, in association with very high CYP1A2 activity.[39] It is therefore possible that, analogous to the situation with

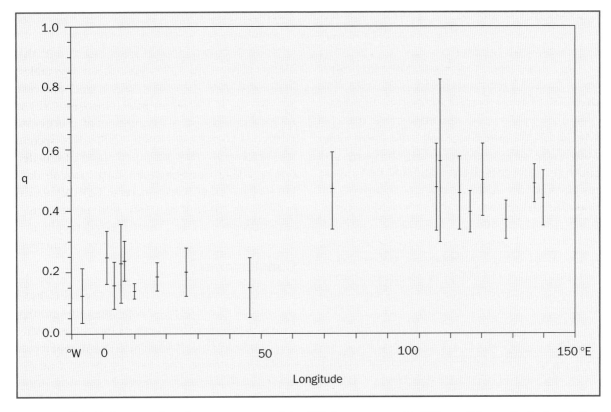

Figure 20(i).2 Estimates of q, the square root of the PM frequency, with 95% confidence limits in relation to longitude. (From: Price Evans et al, 1995,[40] with permission.)

CYP2D6, there exist individuals with ultrarapid CYP1A2 metabolizer status.

CYP2C19

There is substantial interethnic variation in frequency of CYP2C19 poor metabolizers (PMs), being 2–5% in Caucasians, 2% in Saudi Arabians, 4% in Black Zimbabweans, 5% in Ethiopians, 13% in Koreans, 15–17% in Chinese, 21% in Indians and 18–23% in Japanese.[2] Indeed, when the square root of the PM frequency was plotted versus longitude, an increase in this value was seen, with a step in the value occurring between Saudi Arabia and Bombay (Figure 20(i).2).

There are two wild-type *CYP2C19* alleles

(*CYP2C19*1A* and *CYP2C19*1B*), and seven defective alleles which are responsible for the PM phenotype.[41]

Omeprazole has been used as a probe drug in studies of CYP2C19 activity; in single-dose studies the clearance of omeprazole has been found to be higher in CYP2C19 EMs than PMs in Caucasians, Chinese and Koreans, with the clearance in Caucasian EMs being significantly higher than that in both Chinese and Korean EMs.[42] After multiple doses of omeprazole, the mean areas under the plasma concentration–time curve for the parent drug indicated that heterozygous individuals had a reduced rate of metabolism as compared to homozygous EMs. Therefore the difference in clearance between Caucasians and

Orientals may be due to the relatively high proportion of heterozygous EMs among Orientals as compared with Caucasians.

The clearance of diazepam is significantly lower in Caucasian and Korean CYP2C19 PMs than EMs.[42] However, in Chinese, no significant difference between the elimination half-life of 8 EMs and 8 PMs was found, and the mean clearance in the whole group was relatively low as compared to Caucasians. It was suggested that among the 8 Chinese EMs, 7 with a relatively low diazepam clearance might be heterozygous, which would explain the low overall clearance and the lack of significant difference between the EM and PM groups. Alternatively, differences in the contribution of CYP3A4 to diazepam pharmacokinetics in the different ethnic groups could explain the different findings. Like CYP2D6, CYP2C19 often functions as a high-affinity, low-capacity enzyme, which is more important at low drug doses. With higher doses, multiple dosing, or in the case of CYP2C19 deficiency, CYP3A4, which has a relatively high capacity and often shows relatively low substrate affinity, increases in its contribution to overall drug clearance. Schmider et al[43] have calculated that even with single doses, approximately 60% of diazepam clearance is CYP3A4-dependent. The relatively high incidence of low CYP3A4 activity in Chinese may therefore contribute to the low mean diazepam clearance and, if polymorphisms in *CYP3A4* and *CYP2C19* do not cosegregate, could contribute towards the lack of a significant difference between diazepam clearance in *S*-mephenytoin PMs and EMs. It has been noted that 'many Hong Kong physicians routinely prescribe smaller diazepam doses for Chinese than for White Caucasians';[44] this tradition is consistent with the lower clearance found experimentally.

Drug–drug interactions

When prescribing psychotropic drugs that are subject to interethnic variations in metabolism, it is important to remember that interactions with non-psychotropic drugs at these sites may occur. A summary of substrates metabolized by the enzymes discussed above is listed in Table 20(i).1. Many enzymes show overlapping substrate specificity, and only the major routes of metabolism are shown. It should also be remembered that substances may exert considerable inhibitory effect at a given route, without being metabolized by that enzyme (for example, quinidine in the case of CYP2D6). An individual who is a PM of a particular CYP enzyme will tend to be more susceptible to drug–drug interactions at the other cytochromes.

Conclusions

There is considerable interethnic variability in the activity of the DMEs. Although some studies aiming to show correlations between the activity of a single DME and clinical effects have yielded conflicting results, this may be because of the existence of alternative metabolic pathways using other DMEs. For example, in the case of CYP2D6 or CYP2C19 deficiency, CYP3A4 will often be able to play a substitutive role. Individuals who have a realtively low CYP2D6 or CYP2C19 activity will therefore be more susceptible to the effects of CYP3A4 inhibitors. Furthermore, it would be logical to hypothesize that while the clinical effects of single enzyme deficiency might not be consistent, the effects of deficiency of more than one enzyme might well be significant. This hypothesis is supported by the finding of Rojas and colleagues[45] that smokers with combined CYP1A1 and glutathione *S*-transferase M1 (GSTM1) deficiency showed significantly higher levels of activated DNA-bound potentially carcinogenic metabolites than individuals with CYP1A1 or GSTM1 deficiency alone.

I have noted the lower population mean CYP2D6 activity, lower CYP1A2 activity and higher incidence of CYP2C19 poor metabolizers in Japanese as compared to Caucasians. Similarly, a lower population mean CYP2D6 activity and a much higher incidence of a mutation in the

Table 20(i).1 Some substrates of polymorphic CYP enzymes. Taken from Aitchison et al.[2]

CYP2D6	CYP3A4	CYP1A2	CYP2C19
Haloperidol	Codeine	Valproate	Cortisol	Chlorpromazine	Clozapine
Perphenazine	Dextromethorphan	Codeine	Prednisolone	Trifluoperazine	Olanzapine
Zuclopenthixol	Methadone	Dextromethorphan	Amiodarone	Clozapine	Amitriptyline
Thioridazine	Methamphetamine	Dextropropoxyphene	Diltiazem	Olanzapine	Imipramine
Risperidone	Methylenedioxymethamphetamine[a]	Clomipramine	Nifedipine	Amitriptyline	Clomipramine
Amitriptyline	Propranolol	Orphenadrine	Nimodipine	Imipramine	Moclobemide
Clomipramine	Metoprolol	Fluoxetine	Erythromycin	Nicardipine	Clomipramine	Citalopram
Imipramine	Pindolol	Fluvoxamine	Clarithromycin	Digitoxin	Zopiclone	Diazepam
Desipramine	Timolol	Sertraline	Doxycycline	Proguanil	Tacrine	Propranolol
Nortriptyline	Flecainide	Nefazodone	Isoniazid	Quinidine	Caffeine	Phenytoin
Fluvoxamine	Mexiletine	Trazodone	Rifampicin	Cisapride	Theophylline	Ibuprofen
Paroxetine	Perhexiline	Venlaflaxine	Trimethoprim	Lidocaine	Aminophylline	Diclofenac
Mianserin	Propafenone	Diazepam	Testosterone	Terfenadine	Paracetamol/acetaminophen	Naproxen
Desmethylcitalopram	Metoclopramide	Midazolam	Androsterone	Cyclosporin		Omeprazole
Maprotiline	Orphenadrine	Clonazepam	Dapsone	Ondansetron		Pantoprazole
Venlaflaxine	Ondansetron	Alprazolam	Dehydroepiandrostendione	Vinblastine		Proguanil
		Zolpidem	Oestradiol			Piroxicam
		Caffeine	Tamoxifen			
		Theophylline	Progesterone			
		Carbamazepine	Oral contraceptives			

[a]Also known as 'ecstasy'.

promotor of CYP3A4 has been found in Black subjects, while impaired CYP3A4 activity and a high frequency of CYP2C19 poor metabolizers have been found in individuals from the Indian subcontinent. Therefore, when treating patients with schizophrenia who are from these ethnic groups, lower doses of the drugs metabolized by these enzymes may be required, and susceptibility to drug–drug interactions at other sites or the effects of environmental agents such as food substances may be increased. A summary of the main clinical implications of interethnic variation in DME activity is given in Box 20(i).1.

Box 20(i).1 Clinical implications of interethnic variation in drug-metabolizing enzymes (DMEs).

- Dual or multiple DME deficiency exists in certain ethnic groups.
- Individuals with dual or multiple DME deficiency would be expected to be significantly more susceptible to the adverse effects of drugs metabolized by these DMEs.
- Similarly, it is possible that dual DME hyperactivity (e.g. CYP2D6 and CYP1A2) also exists, and that individuals with dual DME hyperactivity would be refractory to drugs metabolized by both of these enzymes.
- Dietary constituents may affect the activity of DMEs, and contribute to interethnic variation in DME activity.
- Many DMEs show overlapping substrate specificity, complex drug–drug interactions may occur and individuals who are poor metabolizers of particular DMEs will be more susceptible to drug–drug interactions or the effects of dietary constituents at other DMEs.

References

1. Vogel F, Moderne Probleme der Humangenetik, *Ergebn Inn Med Kinderheilk* (1959) **12**:52–125.
2. Aitchison KJ, Jordan BD, Sharma T, The relevance of ethnic influences on pharmacogenetics to the treatment of psychosis, *Drug Metabol Drug Interact* (2000) **16**:15–38.
3. Dahl-Puustinen M-L, Liden A, Nordin AC, Bertilsson L, Disposition of perphenazine is related to polymorphic debrisoquin hydroxylation in human beings, *Clin Pharmacol Ther* (1989) **46**:78–81.
4. Dahl M-L, Ekqvist B, Widén J, Bertilsson L. Disposition of the neuroleptic zuclopenthixol cosegrates with the polymorphic hydroxylation of debrisoquine in humans. *Acta Psychiatr Scan* (1991) **84**:99–100.
5. Jerling M, Dahl M-L, Åberg-Wistedt A et al, The CYP2D6 genotype predicts the oral clearance of the neuroleptic agents perphenzaine and zuclopenthixol, *Clin Pharmacol Ther* (1996) **56**:423–8.
6. Lin KM, Polan RE, Ethnicity, culture, and psychopharmacology. In: Bloom FE, Kupfer DJ, eds, *Psychopharmacology: The Fourth Generation of Progress* (Raven: New York, 1995) 1907–17.
7. Aitchison KJ, Patel M, Taylor M et al, Neuroleptic sensitivity and enzyme deficiency in two schizophrenic brothers: a case report [abstract], *Schizophr Res* (1995) **18**:140.
8. Gill M, Hawi A, Webb M, Homozygous mutation at cytochrome P4502D6 in an individual with schizophrenia: implications for antipsychotic drugs, side effects and compliance, *Ir J Psych Med* (1997) **14**:38–9.
9. Armstrong M, Daly AK, Blennerhassett R et al, Antipsychotic drug-induced movement disorders in schizophrenics in relation to CYP2D6 genotype, *Br J Psychiatry* (1997) **170**:23–6.
10. Marez D, Legrand M, Sabbagh N et al, Polymorphism of the cytochrome P450 *CYP2D6* gene in a European population: characterization of 48 mutations and 53 alleles, their frequencies and evolution, *Pharmacogenetics* (1997) **7**:193–202.
11. Droll K, Bruce-Mensah, Otton SV et al, Comparison of three CYP2D6 probe substrates and genotype in Ghanaians, Chinese and Caucasians, *Pharmacogenetics* (1998) **8**:325–33.

12. Leathart JBS, London SJ, Steward A, CYP2D6 phenotype–genotype relationships in African-Americans and Caucasians in Los Angeles, *Pharmacogenetics* (1998) **8:**529–41.

13. Bathum L, Johansson I, Ingelman-Sundberg M et al, Ultrarapid metabolism of sparteine: frequency of alleles with duplicated CYP2D6 genes in a Danish population as determined by restriction fragment length polymorphism and long polymerase chain reaction, *Pharmacogenetics* (1998) **8:**119–23.

14. Potkin SG, Shen T, Pardes H et al, Haloperidol concentrations elevated in Chinese patients, *Psychiatry Res* (1984) **12:**167–72.

15. Nyberg S, Farde L, Halldin C et al, D_2 dopamine receptor occupancy during low-dose treatment with haloperidol decanoate, *Am J Psychiatry* (1995) **152:**173–8.

16. Suzuki A, Otani K, Mihara K et al, Effects of the CYP2D6 genotype on the steady-state plasma concentrations of haloperidol and reduced haloperidol in Japanese schizophrenic patients, *Pharmacogenetics* (1997) **7:**415–18.

17. Lin KM, Polan RE, Nuccio I et al, A longitudinal assessment of haloperidol dosage and serum concentration in Asian and Caucasian schizophrenic patients, *Am J Psychiatry* (1989) **146:**1307–11.

18. Lin KM, Poland RE, Lau JK, Rubin RT, Haloperidol and prolactin concentrations in Asians and Caucasians, *J Clin Psychopharmacol* (1988) **8:**195–201.

19. Bertilsson L, Dahl M-L, Sjöqvist F et al, Molecular basis for rational megaprescribing in ultrarapid hydroxylators of debrisoquine [letter], *Lancet* (1993) **341:**63.

20. Aitchison KJ, Munro J, Wright P et al, Failure to respond to treatment with typical antipsychotics is not associated with CYP2D6 ultrarapid hydroxylation, *Br J Clin Pharmacol* (1999) **48:**388–94.

21. Ereshefsky L, Pharmacokinetics and drug interactions: update for new antipsychotics, *J Clin Psychiatry* (1996) **57(suppl 11):**12–25.

22. Ahsan CH, Renwick AG, Macklin B et al, Ethnic differences in the pharmacokinetics of oral nifedipine, *Br J Clin Pharmacol* (1991) **31:**399–403.

23. Ahsan CH, Renwick AG, Waller DG et al, The influences of dose and ethnic origins on the pharmacokinetics of nifedipine, *Clin Pharmacol Ther* (1993) **54:**329–38.

24. Yue QY, Svensson JO, Alm C, Sjöqvist F, Säwe J, Interindividual and interethnic differences in the demethylation and glucuronidation of codeine, *Br J Clin Pharmacol* (1989) **28:**629–37.

25. Yue QY, Svensson JO, Alm C, Sjöqvist F, Säwe J. Interindividual and interethnic differences in the demethylation and glucuronidation of codeine. *Br J Clin Pharmacol* (1989) **28:**629–37.

26. Rebbeck TR, Jaffe JM, Walker AH et al, Modification of clinical presentation of prostate tumors by a novel genetic variant in CYP3A4, *J Natl Cancer Inst* (1998) **90:**1225–9.

27. Pan LP, De Vriendt C, Belpaire FM, In-vitro characterization of the cytochrome P450 isoenzymes involved in the back oxidation and *N*-dealkylation of reduced haloperidol, *Pharmacogenetics* (1998) **8:**383–9.

28. Fang J, Baker GB, Silverstone PH, Coutts RT, Involvement of CYP3A4 and CYP2D6 in the metabolism of haloperidol, *Cell Mol Neurobiol* (1997) **17:**227–33.

29. Bareggi SR, Mauri M, Cavallaro R et al, Factors affecting the clinical response to haloperidol therapy in schizophrenia, *Clin Neuropharmacol* (1990) **13(Suppl 1):**S29–S34.

30. Lane H-Y, Hu O Y-P, Jann MW et al, Dextromethorphan phenotyping and haloperidol disposition in schizophrenic patients, *Psychiatry Res* (1997) **69:**105–11.

31. Funderburg LG, Vertrees JE, True JE et al, Seizure after the addition of erythromycin to clozapine treatment, *Am J Psychiatry* (1994) **151:**1840–1.

32. Le Marchand L, Franke AA, Custer L et al, Lifestyle and nutritional correlates of cytochrome CYP1A2 activity: inverse associations with plasma lutein and alpha-tocopherol, *Pharmacogenetics* (1997) **7:**11–19.

33. Nakajima M, Yokoi T, Mizutani M et al, Phenotyping of CYP1A2 in Japanese population by analysis of caffeine urinary metabolites: absence of mutation prescribing the phenotype in the CYP1A2 gene, *Cancer Epidemiol Biomarkers Prev* (1994) **3:**415–21.

34. Relling MV, Lin J-S, Ayers GD, Evans WE, Racial and gender differences in *N*-acetyltransferase, xanthine oxidase, and CYP1A2 activities, *Clin Pharmacol Ther* (1992) **52:**643–58.

35. Sinha R, Rothman N, Brown ED et al, Panfried meat containing high levels of heterocyclic aromatic amines but low levels of polycyclic aromatic hydrocarbons induces cytochrome P4501A2 activity in humans, *Cancer Res* (1994) **54:**6154–9.

36. Shader RI, Greenblatt DJ, Clozapine and fluvoxamine, a curious complexity, *J Clin Psychopharmacol* (1998) **18:**101–2.

37. Byerly MJ, DeVane CL, Pharmacokinetics of clozapine and risperidone: a review of recent literature, *J Clin Psychopharmacol* (1996) **16:**177–87.

38. Chang WH, Lin SK, Lane HY et al, Clozapine dosages and plasma drug concentrations, *J Formos Med Assoc* (1997) **96:**599–605.

39. Bender S, Eap CB, Very high cytochrome P4501A2 activity and nonresponse to clozapine, *Arch Gen Psychiatry* (1998) **55:**1048–9.

40. Price Evans DAP, Krahn P, Narayanan N, The mephenytoin (cytochrome P450 2C19) and dextromethorphan (cytochrome P450 2D6) polymorphisms in Saudi Arabians and Filipinos, *Pharmacogenetics* (1995) **5:**70.

41. Goldstein JA, Polymorphisms in human *CYP2C19*.

Proceedings of the Twelfth International Symposium on Microsomes and Drug Oxidations, Montpellier, France, July 1998.

42. Bertilsson L, Geographical/interracial differences in polymorphic drug oxidation. Current state of knowledge of cytochromes P450 (CYP) 2D6 and 2C19, *Clin Pharmacokinet* (1995) **29:**192–209.

43. Schmider J, Greenblatt DJ, von Moltke LL, Shader RI, Relationship of in vitro data on drug metabolism to in vivo pharmacokinetics and drug interactions: implications for diazepam disposition in humans, *J Clin Psychopharmacol* (1996) **16:**267–72.

44. Kumana CR, Lauder IJ, Chan M et al, Differences in diazepam pharmacokinetics in Chinese and white Caucasians – relation to body lipid stores, *Eur J Clin Pharmacol* (1987) **32:**211–5.

45. Rojas M, Alexandrov K, Cascorbi I et al, High benzo[a]pyrene diol-epoxide DNA adduct levels in lung and blood cells from individuals with combined CYP1A1 *MspI/MspI-GSTM1*0/*0* genotypes, *Pharmacogenetics* (1998) **8:**109–18.

20(ii)

Cultural Influences on Schizophrenia

Julian Leff

Contents • Can schizophrenia be recognized across cultures? • Does the incidence of schizophrenia vary across cultures? • Does the outcome of schizophrenia vary across cultures? • Does the treatment of schizophrenia vary across cultures?

In this chapter I will consider the influence that culture may exert on the recognition of schizophrenia, on its incidence, its outcome and its treatment. It is necessary to start with a definition of culture in order to avoid misunderstandings. More than a hundred definitions have been proposed,[1] but I will not attempt to review these. Instead I will work with a simple definition: culture encompasses everything that has been constructed or devised by humankind as opposed to those things that stem directly from the fact that human beings are biological systems. Of course this definition raises the complex problem of sorting out those characteristics that are biologically determined from those that are cultural in origin. For example, there are convincing arguments that the deep structure of language is built into the human brain, whereas the form of individual languages is clearly determined by the culture of upbringing. The intricate problem of deciding the relative contributions of culture and biology will surface again and again in this chapter.

Can schizophrenia be recognized across cultures?

Folk categories of mental disturbance

This is an essential question to be answered before we can study the frequency of the condition in different cultures. Objections have been raised to using Western trained psychiatric professionals to study this question, on the grounds that the training will have blinkered them to states of mind that are not recognized in the Western diagnostic system.[2] To avoid this trap it is necessary to discover what local people recognize as mental disturbance, an endeavour which needs to draw upon anthropological techniques of enquiry. In addition to interviewing ordinary members of the public, it is desirable to question community leaders and traditional healers. All cultures that have been investigated in this way have a word for madness, although the categories used to subdivide this overall term vary considerably. The Serer of Senegal recognize seven varieties of 'illnesses of the spirit', among which is O Dof – people who become mad as a result of spirit attack, and who show hostile, excited and destructive behaviour.[3] The Yoruba of Nigeria have a term *were*, which refers to people who laugh for no reason, tear off their clothes, set fires and hit people without warning.[4] The word *nuthkavihak* in the Yupik language of the Inuit is used for people who talk to themselves, run away, drink urine and threaten others.[4] Another source of such information is classical texts written well before the emergence of Western psychiatry. The Ayurvedic texts from India date back at least 3000 years and contain recognizable descriptions of psychosis.[5] The New Testament is also a source of descriptions of mental disturbances. Both Mark and Luke depict a mentally ill man, who was cured by Jesus casting out the devils that were supposedly causing his condition. The composite picture that emerges from their accounts is of a man who wandered about naked and homeless, but who usually returned to a cemetery, where presumably he found some shelter from the elements. He had been violent, causing him to be put in chains, but he had broken out of this restraint. His illness is described as chronic and he is recorded as shouting, possibly in response to voices, and cutting himself with stones. This may have been either attempted suicide or self-mutilation. This portrait from the Middle East two millenia ago is recognizable as a person suffering from a chronic psychosis, almost certainly schizophrenia.

It is apparent that these folk categories of madness are defined largely by observed behaviour rather than by psychological symptoms, but this is hardly surprising since it is only by careful enquiry that the latter are elicited. The image of the mentally ill person held by the contemporary public in Europe and North America is also characterized mainly by behavioural qualities such as difficulty in communication, bizarre behaviour, poor self-care, aggression and unpredictability.[6,7] The form of severe mental disturbance recognized by lay people across the world and over the centuries corresponds quite closely to the nineteenth-century professional category of madness, before Kraepelin separated schizophrenia from manic-depressive psychosis. However, a Kenyan traditional healer interviewed by Onyango[8] clearly recognized manic-depression as a distinct category. He ascribed the symptoms to worms in the head and stated:

> The worms have hairy bodies and these interfere with brain function. When the worms are awake in the head the patient becomes very excited, talkative, his voice changes and the eyes become red. But when the worms are sleeping the patient becomes too sad, never talks, refuses food and he may become very violent.

The diagnosis of schizophrenia across cultures

In the continuing absence of laboratory tests for the diagnosis of schizophrenia, diagnosis remains a matter of consensus between psychiatric professionals. As such it is subject to the vagaries of fashion and the prevailing climate of opinion about the nature of schizophrenia. In this sense the diagnosis of schizophrenia reflects the psychiatric culture of the time, which may vary considerably from place to place. This phenomenon was brought into prominence by two international studies in the 1970s, the US:UK Project and the International Pilot Study of Schizophrenia (IPSS). The US:UK Project was designed to explore the observation that there were dramatic differences between the first admission rates for schizophrenia and manic-depressive psychosis between American and British hospitals.[9] There was a strong suspicion that this reflected differences in diagnostic practices rather than a true difference in incidence rates. The strategy employed was to establish a project team of research psychiatrists who were trained to use a standardized assessment of symptoms and signs, the Present State Examination (PSE),[10] and to apply, as far as possible, the same diagnostic rules to the psychopathology. The use of this team on both sides of the Atlantic demonstrated that when a standardized assessment of symptoms and diagnosis was applied, the apparent differences in admission rates disappeared.[11] It emerged that American psychiatrists held a much broader concept of schizophrenia than British psychiatrists and included under this rubric many patients that the British would have diagnosed as suffering from mania, depression or personality disorder. How did this gulf between psychiatrists speaking the same language develop? The main influence seems to have been the dominance of psychoanalysis in American psychiatry at the time, as opposed to its negligible influence on British psychiatry. Psychoanalysis focuses on dynamic mechanisms underlying the surface appearance of behaviour. There is only a small range of postulated mechanisms, such as projection and denial, and these mechanisms are seen to be common to patients exhibiting psychotic and neurotic symptoms, as well as to apparently asymptomatic members of the public. Hence a focus on underlying psychodynamics broadens the view of pathology and largely explains the all-inclusive American diagnosis of schizophrenia prevalent at the time. The British concept was largely shaped by the phenomenological approach of German psychiatry.

The International Pilot Study of Schizophrenia (IPSS) was initiated at about the same time as the US:UK Project, but was much more ambitious and included a refinement of methodology. This was a computerized algorithm, Catego, which processed data from the PSE to provide standardized diagnostic classes. The IPSS included centres in nine countries, five of which were in America and Europe, including Moscow, while four were in developing countries: Agra in India, Cali in Colombia, Ibadan in Nigeria, and Taipei in Taiwan. The aim was to collect 100 consecutive cases of schizophrenia in each centre and to compare the diagnoses made by local psychiatrists with the standardized PSE-Catego system. What emerged was a close consensus on the diagnosis of schizophrenia between psychiatrists from seven of the centres.[12] The two outliers were Washington and Moscow. The reasons for the divergent views of American psychiatrists have already been explored, but the situation in Moscow has a completely different explanation. Moscow psychiatry was dominated by one man, Snezhnevsky, who headed the psychiatric institute. A school of psychiatry developed under his leadership in which the course taken by the illness and the level of social functioning between episodes were given greater diagnostic importance than the symptoms themselves. Any psychiatric illness that was recur-

rent or was associated with decline in social adjustment between episodes was labelled schizophrenia. Social adjustment was judged largely by the ability of individuals to conform to the Soviet system. This criterion was readily exploited by the authorities, who were able to have political dissidents diagnosed as schizophrenic. Interestingly, psychiatrists from St Petersburg recognized the idiosyncratic nature of the Moscow diagnostic system and asserted that their concepts were much closer to mainstream European views.

These two international studies reveal that culture not only exerts an influence on patients, but that psychiatric professionals are also embedded in a culture of ideas and beliefs, which can be intensely local, as it was in Moscow, and profoundly affects psychiatric diagnosis, including that of schizophrenia. The diagnostic culture has changed in Moscow as a result of successive political upheavals, and even more dramatically in America, where there has been a widespread rejection of psychoanalytic theory and practice. But we should be under no illusion that the current diagnosis of schizophrenia is culture-free. The prevailing ethos in Western medicine is biological and reductionist. The expectation is that molecular genetics will provide the answer to most diseases, including schizophrenia. Diagnostic systems are reshaped to concur with this ethos. We need to be very cautious about accepting the current diagnosis of schizophrenia as being permanent and conclusive. The culture of ideas in psychiatry can change radically, as we have seen, and views about the diagnostic limits of schizophrenia which are heretical today may become tomorrow's orthodoxy.

Does the incidence of schizophrenia vary across cultures?

Early epidemiological studies

Before structured interviews and standardized diagnostic techniques were introduced, a few epidemiological studies of psychosis were carried out on specific cultural groups. Two studies in particular became famous because they recorded a very high and a very low incidence of schizophrenia respectively. Böök[13] surveyed a Swedish community north of the Arctic Circle and found an exceptionally high incidence of schizophrenia. This was explained on the grounds that only people with a schizoid personality could tolerate the harsh physical conditions and the social isolation of this region.[14] investigated the Hutterite community in America and recorded a very low incidence. Alternative explanations were that the cohesive and supportive nature of the community protected vulnerable people against developing schizophrenia, or that people predisposed to schizophrenia migrated out of the community because they found the enforced intimacy intolerable. Unfortunately the lack of standardized methodology at the time makes it difficult to compare these intriguing studies with later research. Valid international comparisons of incidence rates had to wait until the IPSS established a viable and rigorous set of procedures.

International studies of incidence and outcome

The success of the IPSS led to the initiation of an ambitious cross-national project, the Determinants of Outcome of Severe Mental Disorders (DOSMD). The aim was to collect all psychotic patients in the catchment areas of the centres who made contact with the psychiatric services during the study period. Thus the samples were intended to be truly epidemiological allowing a comparison of first contact rates for schizophrenia across centres. One of the main points of interest was to compare rates between developed and developing countries in view of major social and cultural differences between them which might be implicated in aetiology.[15] Two of the participating centres were in developing countries, Ibadan in Nigeria and Chandigarh in north India. Chandigarh itself is a modern city, designed by the French architect Le Corbusier, with a relatively literate and urbanized popu-

lation. It is surrounded by rural areas in which villagers still carry on a traditional way of life.

The problems of establishing a comprehensive case-finding network in a developing country are enormous, considering the paucity of psychiatric facilities and personnel, and the need to gain the co-operation of traditional healers. In the event, it was decided that too great a leakage of cases occurred in Ibadan for the data to be included. The rates from the other centres are shown in Table 20(ii).1.

The left-hand column displays the rates for narrowly defined schizophrenia: S+ in the Catego system, which indicates the presence of at least one of Schneider's first-rank symptoms. The right-hand column shows the rates for non-Schneiderian schizophrenia, mostly patients with paranoid delusions in the absence of first rank symptoms. It can be seen that the incidence rates for narrowly defined schizophrenia do not vary significantly across centres.[16] This striking finding has attracted much interest since no other disease has an invariant incidence across the world. If correct, it suggests that the causal factors for Schneiderian schizophrenia are likely to be independent of the social and cultural environment. By contrast, the rates for non-Schneiderian schizophrenia show a fourfold difference between the lowest, in Aarhus, Denmark, and the highest, in rural Chandigarh, which is highly significant. Variation in incidence of this magnitude across centres is highly likely to be due to environmental factors, although what they may be remains open to speculation.

Within the category of schizophrenia there is one subtype which has shown remarkable changes in frequency over time and across cultures, namely catatonia. Over the past century catatonia has progressively disappeared from the wards of psychiatric hospitals in the West and from psychiatric practice in general hospitals. For example, the records of the Bethlem Royal Hospital in London (the original Bedlam) show a decline of catatonia from 6% of all admissions in the 1850s to 0.5% in the 1950s. A similar picture emerges from the records of Iowa State Psychopathic Hos-

Table 20(ii).1 First contact rates of schizophrenia according to different diagnostic definitions (adapted from Jablensky et al 1992)[16]

Centre	First contact rate per 100 000 population	
	S+	non-S+
Aarhus	7	8
Chandigarh rural	11	31
Chandigarh urban	9	26
Dublin	9	13
Honolulu	9	7
Moscow	12	16
Nagasaki	10	10
Nottingham	14	8
X^2	7.7	61.8
d.f. = 7	$p > 0.1$	$p < 0.000001$

pital in the US.[17] Study of the first admission rates shows that catatonia as a proportion of all schizophrenia dropped from 14.2% during the years 1920–44 to 8.5% between 1945 and 1966, a highly significant decrease. These figures are particularly telling because the first admission rate would not be affected by the introduction of innovative pharmacological or social treatments, one of the explanations proposed for the disappearance of catatonia.

The picture in developing countries is quite different. The proportion of catatonia out of all patients with schizophrenia attending Ain Shams University Clinic in Cairo during 1966 was found to be 14.4%,[18] while the figure for a psychiatric unit in Kandy, Sri Lanka during the 1970s was 21%.[19] The DOSMD study provides the most reliable cross-cultural data available on the incidence of catatonia. This diagnosis was made in 10% of cases of schizophrenia from centres in developing countries, but in only a handful of cases in the developed countries. It is difficult to think of a plausible biological explanation for the virtual extinction of catatonia in the West while it continues to flourish in developing countries. One

possible explanation rests on the fact that catatonia is the non-verbal form of schizophrenia. Some if not all of the characteristic signs of catatonia can be seen as non-verbal equivalents of delusions and hallucinations. Waxy flexibility, echopraxia and echolalia represent behaviours of the patient which are imposed by the actions of another person. These could be viewed as the bodily equivalents of delusions of control. Posturing and mannerisms are stances and gestures adopted by the patients which appear to have some symbolic meaning for them and can be interpreted as the bodily expression of delusions. The correspondence between these somatic signs of catatonia and the psychological symptoms of other subtypes of schizophrenia is close enough to support the speculation that the disappearance of catatonia in the West is a consequence of the shift in the general population from bodily to psychological modes of expression. If this explanation is correct, then the incidence of catatonia in developing countries should decline over the next few decades as they become increasingly westernized in outlook.

The incidence of schizophrenia in ethnic minority groups

One of the earliest epidemiological studies of schizophrenia, the survey by Faris and Dunham[20] of psychiatric admissions from different districts of Chicago, found a high rate of admissions for schizophrenia for Black citizens. The rate was particularly elevated for Blacks living in predominantly White areas, leading the researchers to postulate social isolation as an aetiological factor. Considerable controversy has subsequently surrounded this hypothesis, with the competing explanation of social drift gaining ascendancy over the years, although the issue has recently been revived by studies showing that urban births are associated with a higher risk for schizophrenia.[21,22] Research into possible social and cultural factors augmenting the risk for schizophrenia has been advanced by studies of ethnic minority communities.

A number of early studies showed a high incidence of schizophrenia in the African-Caribbean population in the UK[23-25] but were weakened by the use of hospital admission diagnoses or unstructured interviews. In recent years a series of studies has been published which have employed standardized interviewing and diagnostic techniques and have been rigorously conducted.[26-28] Each has found an incidence of schizophrenia for African–Caribbeans which is significantly higher than that for the White population. Harrison's study in Nottingham found rates that were 12–13 times higher, but the population denominator used may not have been very accurate. The two later studies, both conducted in London, used data from the 1991 census which collected information on self-ascribed ethnicity for the first time. King's study found a fourfold increase in the incidence of schizophrenia for African–Caribbeans, while the excess from the study by Bhugra and colleagues was twofold. Both the later studies also collected data on Asian groups, but differed in their findings. King and colleagues found the rate for Asians to be higher than that for Whites, while in the study by Bhugra

and colleagues these two ethnic groups had similar rates. Bhugra's group collected three times as many Asian patients as King's so that their result bears more weight.

The work in the UK has been supported by one study in the Netherlands.[29] The researchers used data from the Dutch national register to determine first admission rates for schizophrenia for four immigrant groups, from Surinam, the Netherlands Antilles, Turkey and Morocco. The age stratified rates for people from Surinam and the Antilles ranged from twice to five times the rate for the native-born. Young males from Morocco also had very high rates, but those for people from Turkey did not exceed the rates for the native-born. This body of work indicates an exceptionally high incidence of schizophrenia in African–Caribbeans who have migrated to Europe or who are born of migrant parents. While other migrant groups have elevated rates, they do not appear to have the same level of susceptibility as African–Caribbeans. The fact that these high rates persist, and are even augmented, in the second generation excludes the stress of the migratory experience as an explanation. Three epidemiological studies in the West Indian islands have failed to show high incidence rates of schizophrenia in these populations.[30-32] Therefore the most likely explanation for the high rate in African–Caribbeans in Europe is that factors in the physical or social environment are responsible. It has recently been found that siblings, but not parents, of UK African-Caribbean patients have a higher risk of schizophrenia than their White counterparts,[33] and this has been independently confirmed.[34] This finding focuses attention on the socio-cultural environment and a number of candidate factors have been proposed. These include the gap between expectations and achievement, which is likely to be much higher in African–Caribbeans than in Whites because of their greater socio-economic deprivation. Some evidence for this gap in the area of housing has been found[35]. Another possible factor is cultural marginalization, affecting those African–

Caribbeans who aspire to become assimilated into the dominant White culture, but who find themselves rejected.[36] Ongoing research into these socio-cultural issues is likely to provide some resolution in the next few years.

Does the outcome of schizophrenia vary across cultures?

From the early 1970s onwards a series of studies was conducted on the outcome of schizophrenia in developing countries, some of which suggested that it might be better than in the West. These studies were carried out on the island of Mauritius,[37] and in Hong Kong,[38] Chandigarh[39] and Sri Lanka.[40] Further suggestive evidence was provided by the IPSS, in which follow-ups after both 2 years and 5 years showed a higher proportion of patients with the best outcome in the developing countries than in the developed countries.[41,42] However the IPSS did not collect an epidemiological sample, rendering interpretation of the results problematic. This problem was avoided by the DOSMD study, which was based on catchment area populations. The 2-year follow-up of the schizophrenic patients collected in this study confirmed the findings of the IPSS.[16] Patients with the best outcome, recovering completely from the episode of inclusion and remaining well during the follow-up period, formed 37% of the samples in developing countries compared with 15.5% of those in developed countries. In the samples from the developing countries there was a higher proportion of patients with an acute onset, which is associated with a good prognosis. Susser and Wanderling[43] reanalysed the DOSMD data, applying a definition of non-affective acute remitting psychosis as characterizing patients who developed a psychosis within 1 week without any prodrome and who then recovered completely. They found that the age of onset and sex distribution of these cases were significantly different from those of other types of schizophrenia, and argued that this may represent a different diagnostic entity with a particularly good prognosis. However, when patients with an onset within 1 month of contact were excluded from the original analysis, the better outcome for patients in developing countries remained significant,[16] indicating that an explanation other than that of a separate diagnostic entity must be considered.

The finding of a better outcome has met with some scepticism given that biomedical facilities are scarce in developing countries and that very few patients with schizophrenia receive maintenance antipsychotic medication in these countries. Nevertheless, the consistency of this finding over increasingly more rigorous studies is convincing evidence of its validity. There are likely to be a number of social and cultural factors accounting for this phenomenon, but to date only one has been investigated, namely the emotional climate in the home. Since the 1950s research has been conducted on the relationship between relatives' Expressed Emotion (EE) and the course of schizophrenia. EE is measured by applying the Camberwell Family Interview (CFI).[44,45] The interview is given to a family member at a time of onset or exacerbation of the patient's illness, is audiotaped, and ratings of EE are made later from the tape. The key elements of EE are criticism, hostility and overinvolvement. Numerous studies in the US and Europe have replicated the original finding that patients living with high EE relatives have more than twice the risk of relapse over a 9-month period than those in low EE homes. Bebbington and Kuipers[46] have conducted an aggregate analysis of 25 of these studies, with a total of more than 1300 patients. Until recently, however, no study had been conducted in a developing country. The DOSMD programme provided the opportunity to conduct such research, and a study of EE was incorporated in the protocol for the centre in Chandigarh, north India. Back-translation was used to check the accuracy of the translation, and ratings by an independent psychiatrist, bilingual in English and Hindi, were employed to assess the validity of the transfer of the techniques between languages.[47] Relatives of 70 first-onset patients were successfully rated and their data compared with first onset patients in London. It was found that the Chandigarh relatives had much lower levels of criticism and over-involvement than the London relatives, although the proportion showing hostility was almost the same in London and in the city of Chandigarh. The rural relatives were even lower than the city dwellers on all measures of EE.[48] When the 1-year follow-up data were examined, it was found that only the element of hostility was significantly related to relapse. The outcome for the Indian patients was significantly better than that for the London patients, as expected, with a relapse rate of 14% compared with 29%. This better outcome was largely explicable in terms of the lower proportion of Indian relatives who were rated as high EE, 23% compared with 47%.[49]

These findings indicate that the high level of tolerance shown by the relatives of the Chandigarh patients goes a long way to explaining their better outcome. Since more than 90% of people with schizophrenia in developing countries live with their family, it is likely that the same factor is influential throughout these cultures. There are a number of important implications of these results. Firstly, the higher levels of EE in urban relatives than in rural relatives in Chandigarh constitute a warning that as urbanization and industrialization advance in developing countries, tolerance for the symptoms and behaviour of people with schizophrenia is certain to be reduced, following which their outcome will approach that of patients in the West. Secondly, it means that the work with families which has been proved to be efficacious in reducing the relapse rate of schizophrenia[50] is currently of less importance in developing countries, although it may gain in relevance with time. Thirdly, the question arises of whether families migrating from a developing country to the West retain their traditional tolerance for people with schizophrenia, or whether it attenuates with increasing acculturation. This question remains to be answered.

Does the treatment of schizophrenia vary across cultures?

The role of the traditional healer

We have seen that all cultures investigated recognize madness, although the local term may cover a varied collection of conditions as defined by Western diagnostic systems. The majority of patients exhibiting the positive symptoms of schizophrenia will be included, although those with only negative symptoms might not be. In traditional cultures, people designated as mad are taken to the traditional healer as the first resource. This is partly because of the scarcity of Western psychiatric facilities, often accessible only by a long journey, but mostly on account of a general classification of diseases found in many traditional cultures.

A common response of a traditional culture to the impact of Western biomedicine, with its conspicuous success against infectious diseases such as smallpox, has been to divide illnesses into an indigenous variety and those that belong to the West. Indigenous illnesses are characterized as strong, being sent from outside the sufferer, and responding to traditional practices, whereas Western illnesses are seen as weak, originating from inside the person, and responsive to Western medicine.[51]

Conditions which biomedicine is relatively ineffective in treating remain within the domain of the indigenous. This applies to the whole range of psychiatric conditions. Consequently the traditional healer is the first to be consulted about madness and some healers specialize in mental illness.[52,53] Have traditional healers anything to offer patients with schizophrenia other than mumbo jumbo? The answer is a resounding yes. Healers use an extensive variety of techniques to manage madness. Restraint with chains now strikes Westerners as abhorrent, but in conjunction with this, healers in India and Africa are known to use the herb *Rauwolfia serpentina* (snakeroot) from which rauwolfia was extracted by Western chemists. This was found to be an effective antipsychotic drug and was introduced into Western psychiatry in the early 1950s, but was soon displaced by chlorpromazine. It is a sobering thought that this specific antipsychotic agent was used by Indian Ayurvedic practitioners for thousands of years before biomedicine developed an equivalent. Although no written records exist in Africa, there is evidence for the use of rauwolfia by traditional healers for at least 100 years.[52]

Apart from using drugs, some healers are aware of the importance of rehabilitation. Once the patient's disturbed behaviour is controlled, the chains are removed and he or she is progressively involved in increasing amounts of work in and around the healer's compound.[54] The combination of an effective antipsychotic and a graded return to activities parallels the best practice of Western psychiatry. By contrast, exorcism is regularly practised by traditional healers, while very few religious functionaries in the West would offer it to patients with schizophrenia. In many traditional cultures madness is believed to result from evil spirits entering the affected person and the cure is achieved by expelling the offending spirit(s). A variety of techniques is employed, but they share in common the involvement of the family and other members of the patient's social circle in a public ceremony which is dramatic in form. The effectiveness of such procedures for schizophrenia has never been studied, but their value in integrating the patient into their social support network should not be dismissed.

Ethnic minority groups in the West

Traditional healers are not confined to developing countries. Some travel with their countryfolk migrating to Western countries, while others make the journey after the ethnic minority group is well established in the host country. Additionally, many Westerners utilize alternative practitioners alongside or in preference to biomedical services. Hence traditional practitioners are plentiful in Western countries. The Western psychiatrist needs to be aware of and to respect the cultural traditions of patients from ethnic minor-

ity groups, who may well have consulted a traditional healer before arriving at the clinic. There are three major issues that need to be kept in mind. The patient is rarely an isolated social unit: as already mentioned, over 90% of people with schizophrenia in developing countries live with their family. Family members will expect as a matter of course to attend with the patient and to be involved in the consultation with the psychiatrist. The concepts of privacy and confidentiality are peculiar to Western culture and are likely to baffle and offend unacculturated members of ethnic minorities. As argued above, part of the explanation for the better outcome for schizophrenia in developing countries is the supportive attitude of the family. Consequently the involvement of the family with the patient's consultation and care should be seen as a positive asset.

Traditional medicine recognizes the principle of prevention: remedies can be prescribed for a client to ward off evil magic that may be worked by others. However, the concept of maintenance treatment does not exist in the canon of traditional practice. A remedy that does not work over a short period of time is considered to be a failure. Hence great care must be taken in explaining the value of maintenance antipsychotic medication to patients and their families from ethnic minority groups. Compliance can be improved by exploring the family's concepts of mental illness and negotiating the differences between those and the biomedical model of schizophrenia. The god-like status of the doctor is a thing of the past in the West; the hierarchy of power has flattened, and many doctors now practise defensive medicine through fear of being sued by their patients. The authority of the traditional healer remains unquestioned, backed as it often is by the power of the spirit world. The healer is expected to be omniscient. A traditional healer I interviewed in South Africa told me, for example, that three men will come to his house and stand silently in the doorway. He informed me that he is expected to be able to announce to them that they have come to him to find the lost cattle they are seeking. The Western medical approach of close questioning about events and behaviour will appear alien to many clients from traditional cultures, who will see this as a lack of skill on the part of the doctor.

In conclusion, there can now be few places in the Western world from which ethnic minorities are absent. It behoves the psychiatrist to become as familiar as possible with the traditions and beliefs of the cultures in his or her locality, in order to diagnose, treat and manage people with schizophrenia effectively. It should also be borne in mind that the psychiatrist is part of a professional culture, the beliefs of which are subject to social influences and can change drastically over time.

References

1. Kroeber AL, Kluckhohn C, *Culture: A Critical Review of Concepts and Definitions* (Papers of the Peabody Museum, Cambridge: Massachusetts, 1952).
2. Kleinman A, Depression, somatisation and the new 'cross-cultural psychiatry', *Soc Sci Med* (1977) **11**:3–10.
3. Beiser M, Ravel J-L, Collomb H, Engelhoff C, Assessing psychiatric disorder among the Serer of Senegal, *J Nerv Ment Dis* (1972) **154**:141–51.
4. Murphy JM, Psychiatric labelling in cross-cultural perspective, *Science* (1976) **191**:1019–28.
5. Bhugra D, Psychiatry in ancient Indian texts: a review, *History of Psychiatry* (1992) **3**:167–86.
6. Reda S, Public perceptions of former psychiatric patients in England, *Psychiat Serv* (1996) **47**:1253–5.
7. Wolff G, Pathare S, Craig T, Leff J, Public education for community care. A new approach, *Br J Psychiatry* (1996) **168**:441–7.
8. Onyango PP, The views of African mental patients towards mental illness and its treatment. MA Thesis, University of Nairobi, Kenya, 1976.
9. Kramer M, Cross-national study of diagnosis of the mental disorders: origin of the problem, *Am J Psychiatry* (1969) **125**:1–11.
10. Wing JK, Cooper JE, Sartorius N, *The Measurement and Classification of Psychiatric Symptoms* (Cambridge University Press: London, 1974).
11. Cooper JE, Kendell RE, Gurland BJ et al, *Psychiatric Diagnosis in New York and London*, Maudsley Monograph No. 20 (Oxford University Press: London, 1972).
12. World Health Organization, *The International Pilot Study of Schizophrenia*, vol 1 (WHO: Geneva, 1973).
13. Böök J, A genetic and neuropsychiatric investigation of a North-Swedish population with special regard to schizophrenia and mental deficiency, *Acta Genet et Stat Med* (1953) **4**:1–139.
14. Eaton JW, Weil RJ, *Culture and Mental Disorders* (Free Press of Glencoe: New York, 1955).
15. Sartorius N, Jablensky A, Korten G et al, Early manifestations and first-contact incidence of schizophrenia in different cultures, *Psychol Med* (1986) **16**:909–28.
16. Jablensky A, Sartorius N, Ernberg G, Anker M, Schizophrenia manifestations, incidence and course in different cultures. A World Health Organization Ten Country Study, *Psychol Med* (1992) **20**:1–97.
17. Morrison JR, Changes in subtype diagnosis of schizophrenia: 1920–1966, *Am J Psychiatry* (1974) **131**:674–7.
18. Okasha A, Kamel M, Hassan AH, Preliminary psychiatric observations in Egypt, *Br J Psychiatry* (1968) **114**:949–55.
19. Chandrasena R, Rodrigo A, Schneider's first rank symptoms: their prevalence and diagnostic implications in an Asian population, *Br J Psychiatry* (1979) **135**:348–51.
20. Faris REL, Dunham HW, *Mental Disorders in Urban Areas* (Chicago University Press: Chicago, 1939).
21. Marcelis M, Navarro-Mateu F, Murray RM et al, Urbanisation and psychosis: a study of 1942–1978 birth cohort in the Netherlands, *Psychol Med* (1998) **28**:871–9.
22. Mortenson PB, Pedersen CB, Westergaard T et al, Effects of family history and place and season of birth on the reisk of schizophrenia, *New Engl J Med* (1999) **340**:603–8.
23. Cochrane R, Mental illness in immigrants to England and Wales, *Soc Psychiatry* (1977) **12**:25–35.
24. Rwegellera GGC, Psychiatric morbidity among West Africans and West Indians living in London, *Psychol Med* (1977) **7**:317–29.
25. Dean G, Walsh D, Downing H, Shelley E, First adminissions of native-born and immigrants to psy-

chiatric hospitals in South-East England 1976, *Br J Psychiatry* (1981) **39**:506–12.

26. Harrison G, Owens D, Holton A et al, A prospective study of severe mental disorder in Afro-Caribbean patients, *Psychol Med* (1988) **18**:643–57.

27. King M, Coker E, Leavey G et al, Incidence of psychotic illness in London: comparison of ethnic groups, *BMJ* (1944) **39**:1115–19.

28. Bhugra D, Leff J, Mallett R et al, Incidence and outcome of schizophrenia in whites, African Caribbeans and Asians in London, *Psychol Med* (1997) **27**:791–8.

29. Selten JP, Sijben N, First admission rates for schizophrenia in immigrants to the Netherlands, *Soc Psychiatry Psychiatr Epidemiol* (1994) **29**:71–7.

30. Bhugra D, Hilwig M, Hossein B et al, First contact incidence rates of schizophrenia in Trinidad and one-year follow-up, *Br J Psychiatry* (1996) **169**:587–92.

31. Hickling F, Rodgers-Johnson P, The incidence of first contact schizophrenia in Jamaica, *Br J Psychiatry* (1995) **167**:193–6

32. Mahy GE, Mallett MR, Leff J, First-contact incidence rate of schizophrenia on the island of Barbados, *Br J Psychiatry* (1999) **175**:28–33.

33. Sugarman PA, Craufurd D, Schizophrenia and the Afro-Caribbean community, *Br J Psychiatry* (1994) **164**:474–80.

34. Hutchinson G, Takei N, Fahy T et al, Morbid risk of schizophrenia in first-degree relatives of White and African-Caribbean patients with psychosis, *Br J Psychiatry* (1996) **169**:776–80.

35. Mallett R, Leff J, Bhugra D et al, Ethnicity, goal striving and schizophrenia: a case-control study of three ethnic groups in the United Kingdom, *Soc Sci Med* submitted.

36. Leff J, The culture and identity schedule: a measure of cultural affiliation. In preparation.

37. Murphy HBM, Raman AC, The chronicity of schizophrenia in indigenous tropical peoples, *Br J Psychiatry* (1971) **118**:489–97.

38. Lo WH, Lo T, A ten-year follow-up study of Chinese schizophrenics in Hong Kong, *Br J Psychiatry* (1977) **131**:63–6.

39. Kulhara P, Wig NN, The chronicity of schizophrenia in North West India: results of a follow-up study, *Br J Psychiatry* (1978) **132**:186–90.

40. Waxler NE, Is outcome for schizophrenia better in nonindustrial societies? The case of Sri Lanka, *J Nerv Ment Dis* (1979) **167**:144–58.

41. World Health Organization, *Schizophrenia. An International Follow-up Study* (John Wiley & Sons: Chichester, 1979).

42. Leff J, Sartorius N, Jablensky A et al, The International Pilot Study of Schizophrenia: five-year follow-up findings, *Psychol Med* (1992) **22**:131–45.

43. Susser E, Wanderling J, Epidemiology of nonaffective acute remitting psychosis vs. schizophrenia, *Arch Gen Psychiatry* (1994) **51**:294–301.

44. Brown GW, Rutter M, The measurement of family activities and relationships: a methodological study, *Hum Relat* (1966) **19**:241–63.

45. Vaughn C, Leff J, The influence of family and social factors on the course of psychiatric illness: a comparison of schizophrenic and depressed neurotic patients, *Br J Psychiatry* (1976) **129**:125–37.

46. Bebbington P, Kuipers L, The predictive utility of Expressed Emotion in schizophrenia: an aggregate analysis, *Psychol Med* (1994) **24**:707–18.

47. Wig NN, Menon DK, Bedi H et al, Expressed Emotion and schizophrenia in North India. I. Cross-cultural transfer of rating of relatives' expressed emotion, *Br J Psychiatry* (1987) **151**:156–60.

48. Wig NN, Menon DK, Bedi H et al, Expressed emotion and schizophrenia in North India. II. Distribution of expressed emotion components among relatives of schizophrenic patients in Aarhus and Chandigarh, *Br J Psychiatry* (1987) **151**:160–5.

49. Leff J, Wig NN, Ghosh A et al, Expressed emotion and schizophrenia in North India. III. Influence of relatives' expressed emotion on the course of schizophrenia in Chandigarh, *Br J Psychiatry* (1987) **151**:166–73.

50. Anderson J, Adams C, Family interventions in schizophrenia, *BMJ* (1996) **313**:505–6.

51. Orley JH, Leff JP, The effect of psychiatric education on attitudes to illness among the Ganda, *Br J Psychiatry* (1972) **12**:137–41.

52. Prince R, Indigenous Yoruba psychiatry. In: Kiev A, ed, *Magic, Faith and Healing* (Free Press of Glencoe: New York, 1964) 84–120.

53. Gatere S, Patterns of psychiatric morbidity in rural Kenya. MPhil Thesis, University of London, 1980.

54. Harding T, Psychosis in a rural West African community, *Soc Psychiatry* (1973) **8**:198–203.

21

Systems of Care for Persons with Schizophrenia in Different Countries

T Scott Stroup and Joseph P Morrissey

Contents • Introduction • Developing countries • Developed countries • Summary observations

Introduction

The current understanding of schizophrenia internationally is greatly informed by cross-cultural research conducted by the World Health Organization (WHO), including the International Pilot Study of Schizophrenia (IPSS),[1] the Determinants of Outcome of Severe Mental Disorder study (DOSMeD),[2,3] and the International Study of Schizophrenia (ISoS).[4] Although these studies have been widely criticized on methodological grounds and the researchers' interpretations of the findings have been questioned,[5,6] the studies consistently support the view that something that can reliably be called schizophrenia exists across many cultures, and that the prognosis of schizophrenia is better in developing countries than in industrialized nations.

Several hypotheses have been advanced to account for the ways social and cultural influences might contribute to a less severe course of mental illness in developing countries.[7] These hypotheses call attention to commonly held stereotypes that emphasize disabling rather than enabling conceptions of the cause and course of schizophrenia, the influence of extended families and their levels of expressed emotion, opportunities for people who suffer mental illness to engage in meaningful paid employment, and the

characteristics of treatment settings and specific treatments. Evidence concerning the first three of these hypotheses is considered elsewhere in this text (see Chapter 20(ii)). Here, we will focus on differences and similarities of formal service systems in developing and developed countries as potential contributing factors in the observed variations in the outcomes of schizophrenia.

One difficulty in doing this needs to be acknowledged from the outset. Namely, there are no up-to-date, comprehensive, and consistent descriptions of the systems of care for people with schizophrenia in various countries around the world. Available reports in the English language literature tend to be based on case studies of individual programs, local research projects, first-person observations, or dated materials. Consequently, it is difficult to assemble current and accurate profiles of national systems of care for persons with schizophrenia based on common categories and descriptors. Here, we try to capture some of the global characteristics of care systems in the developing and developed worlds in an effort to discern the likelihood that these systems might offer an explanation for the variations in the international epidemiological data about schizophrenia. We will include several countries that participated in the WHO studies both in the developing (Nigeria, India) and developed worlds (United Kingdom and United States). In addition, we include China and Italy as complementary cases of interest.

Almost all countries in the world recognize an officially sanctioned Western medical and mental health system.[8] Beginning in the nineteenth century, the spread of Western models of psychiatric treatment to the developing world was a byproduct of European colonization. As in the West, the asylum or mental hospital model became the focal point of mental health care. During the 1970s and 1980s, again following Western trends, most developing countries began to adopt deinstitutionalization and community care policies that called for a shift away from exclusive reliance on large, centralized mental hospitals towards a balanced service system that encouraged the growth of community-based treatment programs as alternatives to hospital care.[9] The World Health Organization (WHO) has been a major proponent for the development of biomedical psychiatry and psychosocial community mental health in countries throughout the developing world.[10]

The goal of replicating Western mental health care programs to developing countries has not gone unchallenged, however. Higginbotham,[11] for example, has argued that the Western model of biomedical psychiatry, suitable for industrialized settings that can afford an intensive investment of resources, cannot be championed as even remotely feasible as a standard for nationwide service delivery in the developing world. Based on case studies in Taiwan, the Philippines, and Thailand, he notes a variety of formidable barriers preventing diffusion of that model. These include weak governmental support and leadership for mental health relative to other development priorities; a 'brain drain' of qualified professionals to Western industrial countries; extreme maldistribution of mental health resources which are concentrated mostly in a few urban centers in each country; and the failure of institutional psychiatry to gain community acceptability, integration, and continuity with prevailing health beliefs and customs.

In countries with few resources, mental health systems inevitably are geared toward the most needy population – those with overt symptomatology who suffer from schizophrenia and other major psychiatric disorders. Most of the developing world is still dependent on a few large, isolated mental hospitals, with short-term clinical care limited to major cities and few community-based resources such as halfway houses or psychosocial rehabilitation programs.[8] Rather than developing community-based psychiatric programs, most developing countries have utilized the primary health care system as a way of extending basic mental health services to the broader population.[10] 'These nations simply cannot allocate sufficient political, economic, educational, and manpower resources to generate a fully functioning (mental health) delivery system beyond one or two metropolitan enclaves).[11] Consequently, it is primarily the richer countries that have been able to afford training and services oriented toward mental health as well as mental illness.

Developing countries

Nigeria

In 1998 Nigeria had a population of 106.4 million people and an annual growth rate of 2.7% over the prior 20-year period.[12] Three main ethnic groups populate the country: the Hausas, who mainly reside in northern districts, and the Yorubas and the Igbos in the south. Islam is the predominant religion overall, and especially in the north, whereas Christianity predominates in the south. Most of the people live in rural settings and cultivate the land. Since the early 1960s, oil production has been the mainstay of the nation's economy. This has led to rapid industrialization and urbanization over the past 30 years. For the past decade, however, declines in international oil prices and persistent political upheavals in Nigeria have curtailed government spending on community mental health services.

Most psychiatrists in Nigeria today practice in tertiary institutions in urban centers.[13] Provision of mental health services is largely hospital based; very few psychiatric services are available in general hospital units and in primary health care centers. In 1990, there were a total of 27 hospitals providing psychiatric services and a workforce of approximately 2000 mental health professionals.[14] The array of hospitals included 10 state psychiatric institutions, 9 university teaching hospitals, 4 general hospital psychiatric units, and 4 specialty hospitals. More than 90% of the professionals were psychiatric nurses, 6% psychiatrists or medical doctors, and 4% social workers or psychologists. Community-based mental health centers, as seen in Europe and America, do not exist in Nigeria. Health workers with very basic medical and psychiatric training staff most of the primary health care centers.

Traditional and religious healers remain popular with many segments of the population for the treatment of mental illness. Studies of pathways to care have shown that many persons with schizophrenia and other mental illnesses come to psychiatric facilities only after first receiving care (often for extended periods of time) from traditional or religious healers.[13,15,16] Efforts have been made to engage traditional healers into psychiatric care and to improve their referral skills.

Lack of organized social welfare services of the type seen in developed countries makes the extended family the only consistent source of social support for the mentally ill.[17] In the 1950s, the Aro village system was created as an innovative and highly acclaimed effort to involve families in the care of members who were hospitalized with a severe mental illness.[18,19] This Gheel-like model was based upon two considerations: (1) the existence of a closely knit kinship system which prescribes definite roles and mutual obligations; and (2) the need to have the simplest treatment method which takes local customs into consideration. The village system started as a day hospital program and then evolved into a comprehensive village-based service system. Initially four villages surrounding Aro Hospital, a newly opened 200-

bed psychiatric hospital in Abeokuta, participated. Each patient was admitted to the villages on the condition that a well relative came to live with him there to look after his basic needs (cooking, washing of clothes, etc.), taking him to the hospital in the morning, and bringing him back to the village in the afternoon. Each village could accommodate 200–300 patients and patients were kept until both staff and relatives were satisfied that the patient was well enough to go home. Soon clinics were established in the villages and the emphasis was on treating the patient in the village community without the patient going to the hospital at all. Traditional healers were engaged in developing social and group activities for the patients. Health councils, involving village elders and hospital staff, were formed to plan and administer the clinics and public health projects.

Although never subjected to a rigorous comparative evaluation, the advantages claimed for the village system were the increased social integration and acceptance of the patient, relatively quick recovery and reduction of the risk of social disability, and low cost.[19] These gains have helped to spread the village system to other African countries.

Although nationwide expansion of this program in Nigeria was planned, it had not occurred by the mid-1980s, when only one of the original villages was still operational.[17,19] Reasons for the demise of the village system at Aro are many, including personnel turnover and lack of funding. However, Jegede[19] points to a number of societal changes that have combined to erode the agrarian underpinnings of the village system. Chief among these are urbanization, the growth of a wage economy, and the concomitant difficulty of finding relatives able and willing to travel to rural areas and stay with patients indefinitely.

As in the West, homelessness among seriously mentally ill persons cut off from family ties and other social supports has been a growing problem since the early 1980s.[17] Odejide et al[20] describe this situation in the following way:

[T]heir frequent relapses put them out of favor not only with their relatives but also with the society at large. They are therefore left to wander aimlessly on the streets, sleeping anywhere and eating discarded food. When they are not seen as vagrant psychotics, they are dumped in long-stay hospitals, a process that provides a sort of release to their relatives. This category of patients is also subjected to social disgrace, such as loss of jobs, divorce, and jail sentences, with no reference to the nature of their illness (p. 102).

Asuni[21] has also offered a recent report on the care, treatment, and rehabilitation of people with severe mental illness in Nigeria which suggests that, although improvements have occurred in the management of persons with serious mental illnesses in recent years, major advances have yet to be achieved. Belief in and acceptance of traditional and religious healing methods are still widespread, persons with schizophrenia receive treatment primarily from state mental hospitals often on an involuntary basis, and organized psychosocial rehabilitation programs are available only on a limited basis in urban centers. Costs of antipsychotic drugs have been reported to be 53% of mean total costs of illness for persons with schizophrenia seen on an outpatient basis in Nigeria, whereas the corresponding figure in Euro-American reports is 2–5%.[22] The lack of social welfare programs and nursing homes in Nigeria considerably reduces the cost of schizophrenia to the state budget, but the costs of care are a burden on many relatives who live under financial difficulties.

India

In 1998, India had a population of 982.2 million people and an annual growth rate of 2% over the period 1978–98.[12] It has been described as a 'vast multi-ethnic, agrarian, secular, developing democracy with a population … [living predominantly] in rural areas'.[23] In 1990, the country's mental health manpower resource consisted of

approximately 3000 professionals including 1500 psychiatrists and an equal number of clinical psychologists and psychiatric social workers. There are 42 state mental hospitals with a combined capacity of about 25 000 beds. This works out to about 1 mental health professional per 266 000 persons and one mental hospital bed per 32 500 population. General hospital psychiatric units do exist in the major urban areas, providing mostly acute psychopharmacological treatment. No nationwide epidemiological data are available on the prevalence of severe mental illness, but one estimate based on a variety of regional and local surveys indicates that about 5 per 1000 (4 000 000 persons) are severely mentally ill and in urgent need of services.[23]

In 1987, a National Mental Health Programme (NMHP) was enacted. This owed much to several years of work stimulated by the WHO collaborative study for extending mental health care in developing countries.[10] The NMHP sought to ensure availability of basic mental health care for all by decentralizing and integrating mental health services in primary care settings, training primary care personnel for the role of first level management of mental health problems, and promoting community participation in the development of mental health services. The initial appropriations for this plan, however, have been extremely modest given the magnitude of unmet need.[23]

Persons with severe mental illness have very few organized, community-based services for their rehabilitation. Most of the mental hospitals have campus-based occupational and vocational rehabilitation programs.[24] Several of the teaching centers (for example, the National Institute of Mental Health and Neurosciences in Bangalore, the Central Institute of Psychiatry in Ranchi, and the Institute of Mental Health in Madras) operate occupational and psychosocial rehabilitation programs each with a capacity for about 100–150 persons. A small number of voluntary agencies, mostly urban-based and poorly funded, also provide assistance to persons with severe mental illness.

Public policies toward the severely mentally ill are complexly interwoven with the matrix of Indian society's internal conflicts.[23] As in other developing countries no suitable, cost-effective, easily replicable model of rehabilitation for people who are severely mentally ill has emerged. Western models cannot be transplanted in their entirety due to the wide disparity in manpower and funding resources in India relative to the developed world.[11] This situation is reinforced by national problems of poverty, inadequate housing, unemployment, negative social attitudes towards mental illness, widespread belief in traditional healers, illiteracy, extreme geographic disparities in the distribution of manpower and facilities, and professional apathy towards working with this population on a long-term basis.[23]

Despite these seemingly staggering obstacles and barriers, a number of innovative community-based treatment and rehabilitation programs have been developed in various locales throughout the country.[23,24] These projects attempt to use existing personnel, already in place at the village and neighborhood level, rather than create an additional mental health infrastructure. These include health workers, village leaders, employers, clergy, indigenous healers, and family members.

China

In 1998, China had a population of 1.255 billion people and an annual growth rate of 1.3% over the period 1978–98.[12] As the world's most populous country, China is presumably home to more persons with schizophrenia than any other country. Although many parts of China are rapidly developing and there are several major metropolitan areas, the majority of its citizens continue to live in rural areas. The availability of mental health treatment is severely limited throughout the country, although service systems are relatively well developed in Shanghai and a few other large cities.[25] Psychiatric services are generally provided in psychiatric hospitals located in urban locations.[25]

Pearson[26] references Chinese documents that assert that over 80% of persons with mental illness get no treatment, and that hospitalization is unavailable to 95%. The intense stigma of mental illness in China means that people with less severe mental disorders do not seek treatment.[27] Mental illness is so severely stigmatizing in China that families rarely disclose that one of their members has schizophrenia.[26]

Because mental health services are provided through several national ministries with no central authority, there are no reliable data on system capacity or on the number of providers.[25] The best available estimate is that there are about 1.1 psychiatric hospital beds per 10 000 population.[25] Most patients seen by Chinese psychiatrists are diagnosed with schizophrenia.[26,27] Doctors and nurses provide formal mental health services almost exclusively. There are virtually no psychologists, social workers, or occupational therapists due to political policies outlawing social sciences beginning in the 1950s.[26] Psychiatry and mental health nursing are low-status jobs.[28] Professionals adhere to a biological model of care that developed largely in the post-1949 era while social sciences were banned.[26]

Mental health care in China continues to emphasize collective over individual interests. Thus the priority is to control dangerous behaviours, to limit social problems, and to prevent relapse rather than to provide rehabilitation. The official attitude, however, is that community treatment and rehabilitation has replaced institutionalization and control of social disruption as the preferred site and goal of the mental health system.[25]

The economic reforms that began in China in 1978 in the aftermath of the Cultural Revolution have accelerated long-standing trends in China and have intensified economic rationing of health services. Although medical treatment was never free or universal in China, price controls and state subsidies prior to 1978 meant that treatment was far more affordable than now, when hospitals must operate like other businesses in order to achieve economic self-sufficiency.[27] Phillips and colleagues[27] documented that the costs of hospitalization and psychiatric treatment increased dramatically between 1984 and 1993.

Further, requirements that hospitals become self-sufficient have led to competition for paying patients and have created incentives for hospitals and doctors to provide treatments for which they can collect fees, for example medications and electroconvulsive therapy.[25] There are incentives to prolong hospitalizations, and Phillips and colleagues[27] have documented longer lengths of stay for insured patients than for patients who are self-pay. Because community treatment has less revenue-producing potential, there is little incentive for a hospital to provide these services, especially because they may reduce the need for more lucrative inpatient services.[25]

Health insurance in China is linked to employment. Only 10–15% of people have comprehensive health insurance that covers psychiatric hospitalization.[25] Pearson[26] finds it ironic that China, still officially a socialist nation, finds itself in the situation – although this is a familiar theme across nations – that persons with chronic illness and disability often have the most limited access to treatment.

Psychiatric hospitals are virtually always free-standing – general hospitals in China do not have psychiatric wards.[27] Most resources are allocated for inpatient treatment, but the supply of hospital beds is commonly reported to be too low.[26] The previously quoted figure of 11 psychiatric beds per 100 000 population means that large-scale institutionalization of persons with schizophrenia has not occurred in China, but this is the result of resource limitations rather than conscious policy.[25]

The availability of community-based treatment is extremely limited – some of the largest urban centers have model programs, but these are rare.[29] Such services are 'virtually non-existent' in rural areas.[25] Over 90% of persons with chronic schizophrenia in China live with family.[27] The dramatically rising cost of treatment and the decline in insurance coverage since 1978 has placed a great burden on families, who are the central players in the long-term care of patients with schizophrenia.[25]

Rehabilitation services are extremely rare beyond a few model programs. An emphasis on rehabilitation is official policy, but a lack of funding has meant that changes have not been implemented. Pearson and Phillips[25] report that rehabilitation is occupational rather than psychosocial – in China, the goal of reintegration into society requires a job. The Chinese constitution states that work is the right and duty of all Chinese citizens. Because living with family is socially valued, the Western goal of helping patients with schizophrenia to live independently is irrelevant.

Developed countries

United Kingdom

In 1998, the United Kingdom had a population of 58 649 million people and an annual growth rate of 0.2% over the period 1978–98.[12] Persons with schizophrenia receive care from a diverse network of formal and informal providers in a vast array of settings.[30] Hospital services are funded through the National Health Service (NHS) and include inpatient, day patient and outpatient services in addition to depot injection clinics. Community care is provided through general practitioners, community psychiatric nurses, and day care. Other sources of care include social workers, sheltered accommodations, informal caregivers (usually family members), private sector agencies (providing care through contracts with public agencies or to private-pay patients), and volunteer organizations.

Since 1949, psychiatric services in the United Kingdom have been provided through the NHS, which provides services to each member of the population free of charge. In England and Wales, the direct costs of schizophrenia accounted for

2.8% of NHS and adult social services expenditures in 1992–93.[30] This figure is comparable to the proportion of expenditures for schizophrenia in other industrialized nations.[30,31]

The National Health Service and Community Care Act of 1990 was implemented in 1993.[32,33] Since then, responsibility for community care of persons with mental illness rests jointly with health and social services departments, which are accountable for needs assessment and case management. Outpatient treatment is available at Community Mental Health Centres (CMHCs) and day centers run by the NHS and social services departments. Community treatment is promoted but is poorly funded. Enhancement of community treatment programs will require additional money allocations because it is not feasible to shift money away from the already underfunded hospitals.

In a pattern strikingly similar to that observed in the United States, the peak population in large psychiatric hospitals was in 1955, when there were approximately 150 000 hospital residents. By the mid-1990s, this figure was down to about 50 000.[32] The large NHS hospitals are now largely out of date and inadequately funded.[32] Many closed in the late 1980s and 1990s, leaving mainly patients who require many services. Rogers and Pilgrim[32] maintain that psychiatry in the UK is still hospital-oriented, but with a shift from the 'Victorian asylums' to the district general hospitals. They point out that 90% of the NHS budget for mental health is allocated to hospitals.

Knapp[30] reports that although 44% of schizophrenia patients received services from specialty psychiatric clinics at hospitals, general practitioners were the most commonly used service provider (55%). Community psychiatric nurses (CPNs) were seen by only 21% of people with schizophrenia.

Thirteen percent of schizophrenia patients are in hospital at any given point in time,[34] two-thirds of whom are on long-stay wards. The same authors reported that 55% of schizophrenia patients who are receiving treatment live at home, with an additional 16% living in supported accommodations. Housing for persons with schizophrenia in the United Kingdom is in a variety of settings. Sixty percent of patients live with family.[35] Other options include residential care, hostels, and group homes.

United States

In 1998, the United States had a population of 274 million people and an annual growth rate of 1.0% over the period 1978–98.[12] The United States mental health system is remarkable for its relatively high expenditures, for its fragmented services, and for its isolation from other medical fields. Contrary to the care in any developing countries, schizophrenia is not the most common diagnosis leading to contact with the formal service system. However, schizophrenia accounts for a disproportionate share of direct medical expenditures. Rice[31] reports that schizophrenia accounts for about 3% of all personal health care spending for illnesses in the United States, a proportion that is similar to that in other industrialized nations.[30]

Private health insurance is linked to employment in the United States but there are two important government-sponsored programs – a social insurance progam (Medicare) and a public assistance program (Medicaid) that provide coverage for health care services for large numbers of disabled persons with schizophrenia. The Veterans Administration also provides psychiatric services for a large number of veterans disabled by schizophrenia. In 1999, in spite of this multitude of payers, 43 million persons in the United States had no health benefit. For these uninsured persons, systematic psychiatric treatment is available only through state and locally financed facilities or inconsistently through other means of charity.

Community Mental Health Centers (CMHCs) and state hospitals are the primary sites of publicly supported services for persons with schizophrenia. Privatization of public assistance programs like Medicaid and social insurance programs like Medicare have exacerbated the fragmentation of services. Vendors who contract to provide medical services have little incentive to provide the social services that many persons with schizophrenia are likely to need.

In the second half of the twentieth century there was a dramatic decrease in the number of persons hospitalized in state psychiatric hospitals. This deinstitutionalization saw state hospital censuses drop from over 500 000 in 1955 to less than 100 000 in 1990s. Hospitalization shifted to a more acute model of care provided in the psychiatric wards of general hospitals and nonpublic specialty hospitals.

Outpatient treatment is provided in diverse settings, including teaching hospital clinics, CMHCs, private offices, and clinics associated with Veterans Administration (VA) and state hospitals. Case management is generally provided at CMHCs and VA medical centers. Assertive Community Treatment teams are relatively rare but are mandated by some states. The availability of rehabilitation services varies widely across locations.

According to Torrey,[36] 40% of schizophrenia patients in the United States live with family members. There is tremendous variation by geographic area in the availability of residential services – some states provide an extensive range of options through their state mental health agency, while others rely on nursing and board and care homes that have less oversight and fewer trained personnel.

Italy

In 1978, Italy enacted national mental health legislation that has been hailed by many as the most radical shift in Western mental health policy in modern times.[37,38] The Mental Health Act (Law 180) mandated the development of a public mental health system without asylums. The law prohibited new admissions to public mental hospitals (state asylums) after January 1981, called for the eventual closing of these hospitals, made involuntary commitment more difficult, and required that community-based services (15-bed psychiatric units in general hospitals and

community mental health centers) be developed to replace the functions previously served by the old asylums. The goal was to shift the Italian mental health system from institutional segregation and control to rehabilitation and the reintegration of persons with a mental illness into the community and all aspects of social life. The legislation was part of a broad-based social reform movement in Italy during the 1970s which led to the passage of national health insurance that same year, factory safety reform, dramatic changes in divorce and abortion laws, and the introduction of an Italian National Health Service.[37]

Psychiatric reform had its origins within the old asylum system during the 1960s. A group of radical psychiatrists, led by Franco Basaglia[39] who served as medical director for public mental hospitals in Gorizia and later in Trieste, began to introduce open door policies, therapeutic communities, and patient work cooperatives. As the movement spread it became increasingly politicized in an effort to overcome resistance and inertia within the government bureaucracy. In 1972, the reformers created *Psichiatria Democratica* (Society for Democratic Psychiatry) to gain public support and to further nationwide psychiatric reform. Alliances were formed with the mostly leftist and Communist political parties in the industrialized regions of northern Italy to gain political clout for fundamental legal and policy changes in the way the Italian mental health system operated.

Today, 20 years after passage of Law 180, what can be said about its success? No controlled studies with random assignment, standardization of treatment, and follow-up by independent raters have been performed.[40] Most of the evidence comes from analyses of national trends in the delivery of mental health care and from two case registers in northern Italy where concerted efforts have been made to implement a comprehensive network of mental health services.[41] These sources clearly indicate that dramatic changes have occurred in the Italian mental health service system, but the results fall short of the 1978 reform goals.

Responsibility for implementing the legislation was assigned to the 20 regional governments that have considerable administrative autonomy but vary widely in their geographic, socioeconomic, and political characteristics. As a result, implementation of the legislation is more advanced in the central and northern (industrial) regions than in the southern (agrarian) regions of Italy. (Prior to 1978, the northern and central areas had many more patients in public hospitals than the southern areas.) Services are also more widely available in the smaller cities than in the large urban areas. The political instabilities and economic downturn of the 1980s and early 1990s had a dampening effect on government funding which slowed the development and expansion of community services.[37,38,42]

In the inpatient service sector, the pattern of utilization changed markedly after 1978.[38,41] There was an overall decline in the use of psychiatric beds from about 478 per 100 000 in 1975 to about 278 per 100 000 in 1987 (−42%). Moreover, the locus of these beds shifted from the public mental hospitals to general hospital psychiatric units. In 1979, there were about 62 000 psychiatric admissions to general hospitals; by 1987, there were about 92 000 (48% increase). The use of private mental hospitals (funded primarily by public dollars and similar in role to public mental hospitals) peaked in 1977 at about 50 000 admissions and remained relatively constant while the number of residents slowly declined over the following decade. Although new admissions to the public mental hospitals were shut off following enactment of Law 180, the hospitals did not disappear altogether. In 1987, about 25 400 inpatients (representing about 42% of those hospitalized in 1977) were still being cared for in public mental hospitals and, although prohibited by law, there were 14 000 readmissions to these facilities in that year.[41] According to some reports the patients left behind are mostly elderly, long-stay patients with high proportions of organic brain disorders and substantial social disabilities.

In the outpatient service sector, there was a rapid growth in the number of community mental health centers (CMHCs) from 249 to 674 (171% increase) between 1978 and 1984.[41] National data are not collected on the CMHCs and most available commentaries rely upon data from a special 1984 survey. As of that time, most of the patients seen had severe and/or chronic mental disorders. In some areas, particularly in the North, CMHCs provided a fully integrated system of community mental health services, including clinic and home care, rehabilitative services, and assisted housing.[38] In these areas, the use of public mental hospitals had all but been eliminated. In other areas, more so in the south, few CMHCs existed, and those that did provided a much less comprehensive array of services. In these areas, mental hospitals and other inpatient facilities continued to be used heavily.[38]

In the community residential area, there were a total of 248 (mostly public) residential care facilities operating in Italy at the end of 1984.[38] On average these facilities accommodated 12 residents each with a total capacity of about 3000 beds nationwide. Over half of these facilities were located in the north. Level of care was almost equally divided among programs providing high (24 hours/day), medium (9–18 hours/day), and low (4–8 hours/day) levels of supervision. Mostly nurses, many of whom were formerly employed in the public mental hospitals, provided staffing. Treatment in these facilities included social and daily living skills, and other rehabilitative tasks. Some studies have raised concern about the number of long-term residents in these facilities and the prospects that they are taking on institutional-like environments.

Worker cooperatives were another innovation spawned by the Democratic Psychiatry movement as a way to end the exploitative use of patient labor in the prereform public mental hospitals.[38] By 1985, a total of 1400 members were employed by 50 worker cooperatives: 19 in the North, 23 in central Italy, and 8 in the south. By 1989, the number of cooperatives had doubled, as had the number of mentally ill members employed by them. Cooperatives are involved in manufacturing and service enterprises of various types such as restaurants, mail delivery services, cleaning services, and beauty shops.

The shift from large institutions to community care in Italy was greater than in other Western countries.[41] Yet, the rate of patients still in mental hospitals in Italy today (44 per 100 000) is approximately the same as in the United States, where mental hospitals still play an important role, and marginally lower than in most Western European countries. The available data suggest that neither the private inpatient sector nor the criminal justice system has replaced the mental hospital as a source of institutional care for psychiatric patients. Economic downturns in the late 1980s and early 1990s limited the expansion of community-based services as envisioned by the early reformers. The decentralization of government in Italy and the wide differences in regional resources have led to a lot of unevenness in the availability and accessibility of community mental health services.

Summary observations

As noted in other chapters of this volume, recent decades have brought significant advances in the treatment of schizophrenia. Strong evidence supports the effectiveness of antipsychotic medications, family psychoeducation, and assertive community treatment (ACT) models in industrialized nations.[43] Antipsychotic medications are available worldwide in formal treatment settings. However, the applicability of psychosocial interventions in developing nations is uncertain. In industrial nations ACT and similar interventions can provide comprehensive support for persons without families or who otherwise need an intensive network of caregivers. In the developing world, where extended families are common and resources are scarce, ACT probably has little relevance. For schizophrenia patients with family contact, a variety of family psychoeducation interventions have been developed and shown to be effective. Because of the cross-cultural relevance of expressed emotion, family interventions aimed at reducing hostility and emotional overinvolvement may lead to improved outcomes in any setting.[44]

There is nothing in our review of systems of care to explain the differences in outcomes between developing and industrialized nations that have consistently been found in the WHO studies. Ostensibly, evidence-based treatments are far more accessible (and accessed) in developed than in developing nations. Yet these are the countries where outcomes for persons with schizophrenia are consistently worse than in less developed ones. Estroff's[45] warning that well-intended interventions may have unexpectedly adverse consequences may be relevant for understanding this seeming anomaly.

In the absence of a service system explanation for better outcomes of persons with schizophrenia in developing nations that in developed ones, can 'culture' explain the difference? Ongoing, intensive anthropologic investigations of this may lead to better answers.[46] We are left to believe that the formal service sectors are not the component of culture of sociocultural settings that leads to better outcomes in developing countries. We wonder if the studied populations in WHO reports, in spite of the use of psychometrically sound diagnostic instruments, are not fundamentally different either etiologically or diagnostically.[5,47]

The ongoing global trends towards market-based medical care and a shrinking social welfare system do not bode well for persons with schizophrenia. Indeed, schizophrenia is as much a social welfare problem as it is a medical-psychiatric one. If care systems are to be truly community-based and generally available to those in need, then provisions must be made for housing, income, and social supports in addition to formal treatment. The Western European countries, with their national health care and social welfare systems, have been better positioned in this regard relative to the United States and most developing countries. Phillips and colleagues[27] have demonstrated that market-based reforms in combination with economic rationing have led to greater financial burdens for Chinese families. Cost-saving efforts in medical care systems, including managed care in the United States, the creation of quasi-markets within the NHS in the United Kingdom, and similar efforts elsewhere, result in a narrow focus on 'medical' interventions and ignore important social aspects of illness and recovery.

The most striking commonality among the nations we examined is that while many have proposed national plans for the care of people with severe mental illness, none have yet demonstrated the political will (measured in currency units) to implement these plans fully. Resource limitations in all settings are leading to a situation in which only medical interventions thought to be cost-effective will be available, and they will be targeted only at the most disruptive or deviant individuals. In settings where there are adequate resources and there is legitimate concern about the welfare of persons with schizophrenia, social interventions will play a secondary role unless they can be proven cost-effective. In any case, resource-poor developing nations are not likely to make schizophrenia a budgetary priority.

Services for persons with schizophrenia are suboptimal worldwide except for a few model programs. There is little indication that even the model programs will garner sufficient political and financial supports so that they can be replicated on a larger scale to serve broad populations. Existing trends, including better outcomes for persons with schizophrenia in less-developed nations, are likely to continue. As nations develop economically and as market-based incentives expand to health sectors worldwide, the developed/developing world distinction will have less meaning for persons with schizophrenia, and it is most likely that they will not fare well in wage-based economies that use market forces to allocate health care resources.

References

1. World Health Organization, *Schizophrenia: An International Follow-up Study* (John Wiley and Sons: New York, 1979).
2. Jablensky A, Sartorius N, Ernberg G et al, Schizophrenia: manifestations, incidence and course in different cultures: a World Health Organization ten-country study, *Psychol Med Monogr* (1992) **20 (Suppl)**:1–97.
3. Jablensky A, Sartorius N, Cooper JE et al, Culture and schizophrenia, *Br J Psychiatry* (1994) **165**: 434–6.
4. Sartorius N, Gulbinat W, Harrison G et al, Long-term follow-up of schizophrenia in 16 countries. A description of the International Study of Schizophrenia conducted by the World Health Organization, *Soc Psychiatry Psychiatr Epidemiol* (1996) **31**: 249–58.
5. Cohen A, Prognosis for schizophrenia in the third world: a reevaluation of cross-cultural research, *Cult Med Psychiatry* (1992) **16**:53–75.
6. Hopper K, Some old questions for the new cross-cultural psychiatry, *Med Anthropol Q* (1991) **5**:299–330.
7. Desjarlais R, Eisenberg L, Good B, Kleinman A, *World Mental Health: Problems and Priorities in Low-Income Countries* (Oxford University Press: New York, 1995).
8. Lefley HP, Mental health systems in cross-cultural context. In: Scheid T, Horwitz A, eds, *A Handbook for the Study of Mental Health: Social Contexts, Theories, and Systems* (Oxford University Press: New York, 1999).
9. Goldman H, Morrissey J, Bachrach L, Deinstitutionalization in international perspective: variations on a theme, *Int J Ment Health* (1983) **11**: 153–65.
10. Sartorius N, Harding T, The WHO collaborative study on strategies for extending mental health care, *Am J Psychiatry* (1983) **140**:1470–3.
11. Higginbotham HN, *Third World Challenge to Psychiatry: Culture Accommodation and Mental Health Care* (East-West Center, University of Hawaii: Honolulu, HI, 1984).
12. World Health Organization, *Statistical Annex. The World Health Report 1999 – Making a Difference* (WHO: Geneva, 1999).
13. Abiodun O, Pathways to mental health care in Nigeria, *Psychiatr Serv* (1995) **46**:823–6.
14. Ohaeri J, Odejide O, Admissions for drug and alcohol-related problems in Nigerian psychiatric care facilities in one year, *Drug Alcohol Depend* (1993) **31**:101–9.

15. Erinosho OA, Pathways to mental health delivery systems in Nigeria, *Int J Social Psychiatry* (1977) **23**:54–9.

16. Guerje O, Acha R, Odejide O, Pathways to psychiatric care in Ibadan, Nigeria, *Tropical and Geographical Medicine* (1995) **47**:125–9.

17. Jegede R, Williams A, Sijuwola A, Recent developments in the care, treatment, and rehabilitation of the chronically mentally ill in Nigeria, *Hosp Community Psychiatry* (1985) **36**:658–61.

18. Lambo T, The village at Aro, *Lancet* (1964) **ii**: 513–14.

19. Jegede R, Aro village system of community psychiatry in perspective, *Can J Psychiatry* (1981) **26**:173–7.

20. Odejide A, Jegede R, Sijuwola A, Deinstitutionalization: a perspective from Nigeria, *Int J Ment Health* (1983) **11**:98–107.

21. Asuni T, Nigeria: report on the care, treatment, and rehabilitation of people with mental illness, *Psychosocial Rehabilitation Journal* (1990) **14**:35–44.

22. Suleiman T, Ohaeri J, Lawal R et al, Financial cost of treating outpatients with schizophrenia in Nigeria, *Br J Psychiatry* (1997) **171**:364–8.

23. Nagaswami V, Integration of psychosocial rehabilitation in national health care programmes, *Psychosocial Rehabilitation Journal* **14**:53–65.

24. Dunlap D, Rural psychiatric rehabilitation and the interface of community development and rehabilitation services, *Psychosocial Rehabilitation Journal* (1990) **14**:68–90.

25. Pearson V, Phillips MR, The social context of psychiatric rehabilitation in China, *Br J Psychiatry* (1994) **164(Suppl 24)**:11–18.

26. Pearson V, *Mental Health in China: State Policies, Professional Services and Family Responsibilities* (Gaskell: London, 1995).

27. Phillips MR, Lu SH, Wang RW, Economic reforms and the acute inpatient care of patients with schizophrenia: the Chinese experience, *Am J Psychiatry* (1997) **154**:1228–34.

28. Bueber M, Letter from China (no. 3), *Arch Psychiatr Nurs* (1993) **7**:249–53.

29. Yucan S, Changhui C, Esixi Z et al, An example of a community-based health/home care programme, *Psychosocial Rehabilitation Journal* (1999) **14**:29–34.

30. Knapp M, Costs of schizophrenia, *Br J Psychiatry* (1997) **171**:509–18.

31. Rice DP, The economic impact of schizophrenia, *J Clin Psychiatry* (1999) **(Suppl 1)**:4–6.

32. Rogers A, Pilgrim D, *Mental Health Policy in Britain* (St Martin's Press: New York, 1996).

33. Hollingsworth EJ, Mental health services in England: the 1990s, *Int J Law Psychiatry* (1996) **19**: 309–25.

34. Kavanaugh S, Opit L, Knapp MRJ et al, Schizophrenia: shifting the balance, *Soc Psychiatry Psychiatr Epidemiol* (1995) **30**:206–12.

35. Perring C, Twigg J, Aitken K, *Families Caring for People Diagnosed as Mentally Ill: The Literature Re-examined* (HMSO: London, 1990).

36. Torrey EF, *Surviving Schizophrenia: A Family Manual*, 3rd edn (Harper and Row: New York, 1988).

37. Mosher L, Radical deinstitutionalization: the Italian experience, *Int J Ment Health* (1983) **11**:129–36.

38. Burti L, Benson P, Psychiatric reform in Italy: developments since 1978, *Int J Law Psychiatry* (1996) **19**:373–90.

39. Basaglia F, Breaking the circuit of control. In: Engleby D, ed, *Critical Psychiatry* (Pantheon: New York, 1980).

40. Glick I, Improving treatment for the severely mentally ill: implications of the decade-long Italian psychiatric reform, *Psychiatry* (1990) **53**:316–23.

41. De Salvia D, Barbato A, Recent trends in mental health services in Italy: an analysis of national and local data, *Can J Psychiatry* (1993) **38**:195–202.

42. Bollini P, Mollica R, Surviving without the asylum: an overview of the studies on the Italian reform movement, *J Nerv Ment Dis* (1989) **177**:607–15.

43. Lehman AF, Steinwachs DM et al, At issue: translating research into practice: the Schizophrenia Patient Outcomes Research Team (PORT) Treatment Recommendations, *Schizophr Bull* (1998) **24**: 1–10.

44. Lefley H, Expressed emotion: conceptual, clinical, and social policy issues, *Hosp Community Psychiatry* (1992) **43**:591–8.

45. Estroff SE, *Making It Crazy* (University of California Press: Berkeley, CA, 1981).

46. Hopper K, Wanderling J, The role of culture in explaining the developed vs. developing center outcome differential in the WHO studies of schizophrenia. Presented at the Annual Meeting of the International Federation of Psychiatric Epidemiology, Taipei, Taiwan, Republic of China, 7–10 March 1999.

47. Warner R, *Recovery from Schizophrenia*, 2nd edn (Routledge: New York, 1994).

22

Economic Perspectives on the Treatment of Schizophrenia

Robert Rosenheck and Douglas Leslie

Contents • Background • A dismal discipline? • Three questions for the economic analysis of treatment for people with schizophrenia • The market and perfect competition • Conclusion

Background

Economic analysis is a tool that can be used to maximize the benefits of treatment of schizophrenia at the societal level by:

1. Identifying treatments that both maximize clinical benefit and minimize cost.
2. Determining when additional resources should be devoted to pay for treatments that cost more, but are also more effective.
3. Evaluating the benefits of treatment using measurement methods that allow comparison with other medical treatments.

This chapter reviews the current methods and recent research and highlights three central points.

First, cost-effectiveness analysis is the primary tool for determining the optimal use of current resources. Such analyses compare both costs and clinical outcomes of alternative treatments. For example, while conventional antipsychotic medications can be shown to be vastly more cost-effective than nonpharmacologic treatments provided alone, new atypical antipsychotic medications and intensive community treatments appear only modestly more cost-effective than the combination of conventional medications and outpatient care.

Secondly, since most savings from innovative treatments are based on reduced inpatient use, as hospital utilization declines in the United States, studies will increasingly find that new treatments with increased benefits will also incur increased costs. Determining whether the health benefits equal the increased costs is a major methodologic challenge for future cost-effectiveness analysis.

Thirdly, the concept of the Quality Adjusted Life Year (QALY), the equivalent of a year of healthy life, provides a potentially useful measurement tool for comparing the benefit and cost of diverse health care interventions and for placing a monetary value on health gains for purposes of comparison with other valuable goals.

Economic analysis thus seeks to assure that advances in biomedical science are used to achieve the maximum benefit for the greatest number of people. Although economic considerations typically do not, and probably should not, directly influence treatment decisions for individual patients, cost considerations are having a growing effect on the management of psychiatric care, sometimes resulting in restricted access to effective treatments. As clinicians become increasingly concerned about changes in care due to such management, they may want to become more active participants in policy-making at the institutions in which they work, and/or through their participation in professional societies and the public debate over the future of our health care system. Familiarity with economic perspectives on clinical practice is an essential foundation for such activity. The absence of knowledgeable professional input into such discussions may leave patients unrepresented by their most powerful advocates and thus increasingly vulnerable to public neglect and ignorance.

A dismal discipline?

There has been considerable concern, in recent years, that the quest for cost savings and the drive for profitability have diminished the quality and effectiveness of mental health services, especially for those with the most severe illnesses and the greatest service needs. Resource reductions of 30–40% have been observed in both private and public health care settings[1-4] and have been shown to affect severely mentally ill people no less than those with milder disorders.[5] In a world of increasing commercialization and diminishing physician authority,[6] economics and economic thinking is often viewed as the antagonist of patient-centered medicine. A recent presidential address to the American Psychiatric Association decried

> a group of economists ... slopping over the vague boundaries of their dismal discipline, [who] routinely make absolutistic pronouncements about the motivations of humans who are ill, or fear they are ill, and about the motivations of the physicians who care for those who are sick.[7]

Economics, of course, is neither a hero nor a goat in the current situation. It favors neither profits, nor healing health care services. Rather, it is an academic discipline that provides tools for studying the rational use of scarce resources, and an analytic framework for describing how our health care system operates; how it evolved; what choices we have for changing it; and what the

consequences of those choices may be for different members of society. According to Samuelson's basic college text, economics is

> the study of (a) how people and society choose to employ scarce resources (b) that could have alternative uses (c) in order to produce various commodities and (d) to distribute them for consumption ... among various persons and groups in society.[8]

Some take offense at considering health care as a commodity. A commodity is simply a scarce resource that is traded. When applied to health care this means that people who provide health care services are compensated for their efforts, and are unlikely to deliver such services in the absence of such compensation – a reality that is hard to disown. There can be no doubt that most health professionals are motivated by sincere concern and compassion for their patients. But professional training and practice are costly and time-consuming, and as a result the efforts of doctors and other health care professionals are scarce resources. Their allocation is naturally and unavoidably influenced by systems of compensation, and always has been.

By identifying health care services as scarce resources, economics provides a framework for systematic thinking about alternative ways of allocating those resources to maximize human well-being. The treatment of schizophrenia consumes substantial resources in our society and is, for that reason alone, likely to benefit from thoughtful economic analysis. It is estimated that, in 1990, the cost of schizophrenia to American society was $32.5 billion, $16 billion (49%) of which was spent on treatment and other health care services.[9] Adjusting for inflation and the impact of managed care we estimate that, in 1998, approximately $20 billion was spent on treatment and direct support of mental health organizations and providers caring for people with schizophrenia.

Three questions for the economic analysis of treatment for people with schizophrenia

The first question for the economic study of schizophrenia therefore is: 'How can we best spend this $20 billion to maximize the well-being of patients with schizophrenia, their families, and the communities in which they live? Are there treatments that are both more effective and less costly but are underutilized?' This is hardly a cold-hearted, profit-driven, selfish query. It is no more and no less caring than the question of what medication to give a patient or whether emergency hospitalization is required. It is undoubtedly more remote from direct patient care – but it is no less crucial to ultimate clinical outcomes, and it is unapproachable by the methods of conventional biomedical science. If, given a stable budget, we use a less cost-effective array of services than we might, we deprive some patients of health benefits as surely as if we refused to give them the correct prescription. In fact use of non-cost-effective treatments may be more destructive than prescribing the wrong medication because in the latter case the adverse effects become quickly apparent and can be corrected, while in the former they are invisible and thus hard to correct. We need economics, along with many other kinds of knowledge, to help us help our patients.

This first question, concerning how to spend current resources, however, is incomplete because it assumes that $20 billion is the 'right' amount to spend on care of people with schizophrenia, and that our only set of choices concerns how we should best spend that $20 billion. There is a second, far more difficult question. How much *should* we spend on treatment of schizophrenia? Perhaps we should be spending more for services for people with schizophrenia, perhaps less. Some new treatments may be more effective, but also more costly. Should we spend additional funds to make those treatments available even if it means taking money away from some other worthy program?

To think systematically about comparing the value gained by spending resources on the treatment of schizophrenia as compared to other social goods like education or cleaning up the environment, we must address yet a third question: 'How would one go about measuring the benefits associated with very different types of expenditures?' It is one thing to compare two treatments for the same group of patients. It is something quite different to compare the value of treatments for different groups of patients because one needs measures that address heath status in diverse conditions. If our task is to provide scientific underpinnings for broad societal decisions, we must be able to evaluate diverse interventions using common measures.

Economic analysis of treatment for schizophrenia thus begins by posing three very hard, but very important questions – questions that are important to patients, to their families, and to society as a whole.

1. How should we spend our current $20 billion budget for schizophrenia to maximize the well-being of our patients?
2. When should we take money from other worthy purposes and reallocate it to the treatment of schizophrenia?
3. How do we conceptualize and quantify the benefit of allocating scarce resources to diverse worthy uses?

The market and perfect competition

Before taking on the challenge of addressing these three questions, let us consider how such decisions are made in the production of other goods – let us take shirts, for example. No one holds conferences or publishes studies on how best to spend this year's 'shirt' budget. No one argues in learned journals that we should spend more on shirts than on overcoats, for example. And no one worries about developing questionnaires to determine the monetary value of the improvement in quality of life that comes from having a closet packed with fine shirts. When it comes to shirts, we do not ask 'shirt economists' or 'shirt services researchers' to provide data to inform the allocation of resources to shirt manufacturers. Rather we rely on the 'invisible hand' of the marketplace to assure that the right number of shirts are made to meet the desires of consumers with diverse tastes and different-sized budgets for clothing. In the free market, buyers and sellers meet, negotiate prices of exchange, and trade their goods. High demand for decorative designer T-shirts raises their price – signalling to manufacturers as to the tastes and preferences of consumers, and stimulating the production of similar products. Unpopular styles lie on the shelf unbought and are eventually sold at 'fire sale' or 'close out' prices, also vividly telegraphing negative public evaluation of those products to their producers. Price clearly, forcefully, and accurately communicates public preference to producers.

Why not leave the production of health care services to the free market and trust in its 'invisible hand'? Free markets can only perform their magic of maximizing the benefit from production and distribution of goods under well-specified conditions. In one formulation,[10] these conditions are described under four headings.

1. The market must be composed of numerous small firms and customers, none of which can determine prices on their own.
2. All products are the same.
3. Producers can enter and leave the market freely, i.e., without facing artificial barriers to entry or exit.
4. Producers and consumers all have perfect and identical information about the quality of the goods produced.

While these conditions are roughly approximated in the market for shirts, none of them are met in the delivery of health care services.

1. Even in the era dominated by private practice

medicine, hospitals and professional associations had a powerful influence on how health care services were priced, far beyond the influence of individual providers or patients.
2. Health care services are immensely diverse, as demonstrated definitively, years ago, by Wennberg[11] with limited homogeneity of service.
3. Providers cannot enter the market without extensive training and meticulous certification and licensure, and they cannot simply go out of business without assuring that their patients have alternative sources of care, a reality that is coming closer as some large managed care operations begin to experience major financial adversity.
4. Finally, and most importantly:
   (a) scientific information on the value of health services is, in many cases, very imprecise or unknown; and
   (b) even more crucially, there are vast differences between providers and patients in their understanding of these services – even in the era of patient education and rapid Internet access to medical information.

This last point, referred to technically as 'asymmetry of information', is especially important. The efficiency of competitive markets is based on the assumption that buyers and sellers have the same information about product quality. In medicine, expert knowledge is exactly what patients seek from their physicians and in most cases they are ready to follow their doctor's advice with few questions. Contrast this with the market for shirts. When we go to buy T-shirts, we do not pay the salespeople for their expert opinion about what designs we would like. Nor do the salespeople look at us ponderously and say: 'This is a serious situation. I'm afraid you will need to have a dress shirt. A T-shirt will only make things worse for you.'

Because of the failure of health care practice to meet the conditions under which competitive markets work, a condition called 'market failure', markets cannot be used to arrive at appropriate allocation decisions for health care. We need health economics and health services research to provide information to guide decision-making instead. What does this body of information tell us?

Optimizing current resource allocation: identifying treatments that are more effective and less costly

The tool most appropriate to the evaluation of the first of our three questions, 'How should we best spend the money we have available for the treatment of schizophrenia?', is cost-effectiveness analysis. In its simplest form, cost-effectiveness analysis compares the value of alternative treatments for the same patients. When the treatment being tested is both more effective than standard treatment *and* less expensive, the interpretation and implications are clear. In such circumstances the experimental treatment is the preferred or 'dominant' choice, and if implemented appropriately, the general welfare of society will be greater for their use. Prime examples of this kind of analysis in the treatment of schizophrenia are studies that have compared the cost-effectiveness of atypical and conventional antipsychotic medications and studies of the cost-effectiveness of intensive community care programs as compared to standard outpatient care.

In some ways research on cost-effectiveness is like other kinds of treatment effectiveness research in schizophrenia, with cost added as a systematically measured outcome. In other ways cost-effectiveness analysis is particularly sensitive to specific features of study design, analysis and interpretation. In this brief review we begin by presenting an example of an unambiguously cost-effective treatment from a period before cost-effectiveness analysis was commonly applied to health care: the use of antipsychotic medication as compared to psychosocial treatments alone. We then highlight two methodological issues that affect the design and interpretation of cost-effectiveness studies in schizophrenia and that

have substantially influenced the results of widely cited studies: (a) the use of experimental vs non-experimental designs, and (b) the variability of the cost-effectiveness of treatments across different clinical subpopulations.

Conventional antipsychotics vs placebo: a dominant choice

The use of *conventional* antipsychotic medications in the treatment of schizophrenia provides a simple and dramatic example of a cost-effective treatment that clearly dominates the alternative of no medication. Thirty-five years ago Philip May led a courageous randomized experiment in which five approaches to the inpatient treatment of schizophrenia were compared: (a) antipsychotic medications alone; (b) electroconvulsive therapy (ECT); (c) psychotherapy plus medications; (d) milieu therapy; and (e) psychotherapy alone.[12] To update that study we adjusted the cost figures for 35 years of inflation to generate costs in 1998 dollars, and added estimates of outpatient costs, since May's report only addresses inpatient service use and cost. With these adjustments, medications alone are found to be $28 888 (51%) less costly than milieu therapy alone ($33 650 vs $62 538), and $38 597 (129%) less costly than psychotherapy alone ($33 650 vs $72 247). If one considers that a year of conventional antipsychotic medications costs about $300, this amounts to a 96 to 129-fold return on the initial investment in medications, and adds 20% clinical benefit as well.[13]

Of course, conditions have changed vastly since 1964, and we can update this example to the present using a simulation with a range of explicit cost and utilization assumptions. We assume, first, that the cost of antipsychotic medications is approximately $300/year, and that the cost of a single day of hospital care is $600. Although there have been no recent long-term clinical trials of antipsychotic medication compared to placebo, a recent review suggested that conventional antipsychotic medications reduce the risk of rehospitalization among chronically ill patients by 20%, from 70% per year without medications to 50% per year on medications in typical practice.[15] Using a very conservative set of assumptions, including that each relapsing patient has only one hospitalization per year with an average length of stay of 15–30 days, regardless of their medication status, a $300 investment in antipsychotic medications results in savings of $1500–$2700 per patient, a five- to nine-fold return on the pharmacologic investment, and substantial clinical gains.

Using more realistic assumptions, one would expect patients on no medications to have far longer lengths of stay and an increased risk of relapse. If we assume that without any medications the hospitalization would last 60 days and that half of those discharged would have a second hospitalization of 60 days, still a fairly optimistic set of assumptions, savings increase to $33 300, a 111-fold return on investment, a result similar to that found with May's data. The use of conventional antipsychotic medications is clearly cost-effective in virtually all situations and such medications are appropriately available to all who need them, with great benefit to society. Even in the absence of controlled cost-effectiveness trials, society can sometimes tell a winner when it sees one.

Clinical trials vs nonexperimental outcome studies

As in any type of outcome research, randomized clinical trials are, on theoretical grounds alone, more valid than uncontrolled outcome studies. Cost-effectiveness studies have been especially important in the evaluation of atypical antipsychotic medications because, at $5000 per year, they are over ten times more expensive than conventional medications, which can cost as little as $300 per patient per year. Studies of the cost-effectiveness of atypical antipsychotics vary substantially in their results. Nonexperimental studies are especially likely to find large cost-savings in hospital care with clozapine, resulting in total savings ranging from $10 000 to over $50 000 per patient per year.

In the first of these studies to be published[16] clozapine responders (52% of those who started on the drug) were compared with dropouts and found to cost $9011 less in the second year of treatment (but not in the first year). With this study design, however, one cannot distinguish whether the observed cost reduction is attributable to the medication or the exclusion of dropouts. A second study[17] reported two sets of analyses: first that among 59 patients started on clozapine, costs dropped by $8702 from the pre-treatment phase to the treatment phase; and second, that a comparison of costs and outcomes of 37 patients who remained on clozapine treatment and 10 dropouts revealed $22 936 greater cost reductions among completers. In these analyses, too, one cannot distinguish the effect of the drug from the effects of the passage of time, or selection biases.

A third study[18] also used a pre–post design and found savings estimated at $30 000–$50 000 per year among State Hospital patients treated with clozapine. An updated study from the same group[19] extended the follow-up to 4.5 years and added a control group which included clozapine dropouts and found estimated savings of $25 000 per year.

The effect of clozapine on inpatient care and related costs in two randomized clinical trials,[20,21] however, appears to be substantially more modest than in these nonexperimental studies. A 15-site, 12 month Veterans Affairs (VA) trial of patients with 30–364 days of hospital use in the year prior to study entry is the only complete experimental cost-effectiveness study published thus far.[20] This study reported significant reduction in inpatient days resulting in $8684 lower annual psychiatric hospital costs for patients treated with clozapine ($p = 0.01$). However, after adding in the cost of clozapine treatment, total health care costs for the clozapine group were only $2441 lower than for the controls and total societal costs were only $2733 (5%) lower. Neither difference was statistically significant.

The experimental study of very long stay State Hospital patients in Connecticut found that although clozapine-treated patients were not more likely to be discharged than controls, they were less likely to be readmitted. The precise reduction in days hospitalized and costs in this study[21] have not yet been published but the authors concluded that 'at least with this patient population, clozapine did not produce the dramatic improvements ... in hospital utilization ... suggested by mirror image trials' (p. 683).

The differences in findings across these studies are primarily attributable to the greater internal validity of the experimental studies. Over the 12-month course of the VA study, for example, clozapine patients showed a 72% reduction in hospital utilization from 29 days per month early in the trial to only 7 days per month at the end. However, the controls also showed a substantial decline in hospital use over the same time period of 64%. In the absence of a randomly assigned control group the effects of clozapine would have been substantially overestimated. The bias introduced by nonexperimental studies is especially great when the target population involves inpatients, and especially those with long hospital stays.

Variability of cost-effectiveness by the level of pre-entry hospital use

While careful studies have failed to identify robust clinical predictors of the specific effectiveness of clozapine,[22] several recent reports have suggested that the results of cost-effectiveness studies can be quite specific to patients with high or low levels of service use, and thus may have limited generalizability. The studies of atypical antipsychotic medications summarized above all included patients with substantial hospital use in the previous year, ranging from 150 days[18] to 260 days[17] in the uncontrolled studies and from 110 days in the VA study[20] to 2.9 years in the Connecticut State Hospital Study.[21]

A recent reanalysis of data from the VA trial compared the cost-effectiveness of clozapine in high hospital users (mean = 215 psychiatric hospital days in the year prior to study entry) and low hospital users (mean = 58 hospital days) and found that, after including the costs of both medications and other health services, clozapine patients had $7134 lower costs than controls among high users but only $759 less than controls among low users.[23]

Furthermore, a recent pre–post design study of the use of clozapine in outpatients (with an average of only 23.5 hospital days during the year prior to treatment) showed that total treatment costs were $2363 *greater* for the clozapine group than for controls (increasing from $17 385 to $19 748).[24] In view of our previous discussion of experimental vs uncontrolled trials it could be assumed that this pre–post design overestimates savings. If we apply the 15% reduction in hospital use observed in the VA trial, we would project that costs actually increased by as much as $6700 over what they would have been with conventional medications.

A similar study of risperidone in patients with only 13.9 days in hospitals or other residential institutions found that total costs increased by $2566 (26%) in the year after the drug was initiated (from $9711 per year to $12 277).[25]

The net cost impact of atypical antipsychotic medication is thus quite sensitive to baseline inpatient utilization rates (see Figure 22.1). This observation is not hard to understand intuitively because, while the cost of clozapine is relatively constant, previous hospital use is the best predictor of subsequent use and savings from reduced inpatient utilization vary substantially by the volume of services available for reduction.[26]

Studies of intensive case management[27] and Assertive Community Treatment[28] have also found substantial cost savings among high hospital users but equal, or even greater, costs among patients with lower levels of use. A multisite VA trial of Intensive Psychiatric Community Care (IPCC) found that this high-cost intervention saved $34 000 per patient over 2 years at long-stay, high-cost hospitals (with patients averaging 452 hospital days in the 2 years before study entry), but increased costs by $5100 at short-stay, acute care hospitals (with patients averaging 123

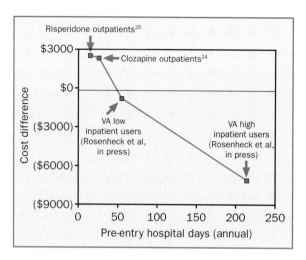

Figure 22.1 Effect of pre-entry inpatient use on difference in health care costs between atypical antipsychotic medications and conventional medications.

hospital days in the 2 years before study entry).[27] Even within each of these hospital types, IPCC-related inpatient savings were substantially greater with high-cost patients than with comparatively low-cost patients.[28]

Similar findings have been reported on the use of Assertive Community Treatment (ACT) in a State Mental Health system.[29] In that study, among patients who were outpatients at the time of program entry, ACT cost $4152 (18%) more than standard treatment ($26 635 vs $22 483). In contrast, among patients who were hospitalized at the time of program entry, ACT cost $24 894 (32%) less than standard treatment ($52 814 vs $77 708), and the cost figures are remarkably similar to those of the VA study.

These differences in cost impact are especially important because researchers have typically evaluated the cost-effectiveness of new treatments in very high cost patient populations – for the very reason that the potential for cost savings is high in such populations. Once treatments are identified

as 'cost-effective', however, they are often used in populations with much lower costs. When used with these populations, however, they are likely to incur additional costs beyond those experienced with conventional treatments. Thus, although novel treatments may be more effective than standard treatments across clinical subgroups, they are likely to be more costly in some subgroups.

When does the effectiveness of treatment merit increased expenditure?

The interpretation of cost-effectiveness studies and assessment of their implications for policy can be quite challenging. We have seen that some kinds of treatment, for example conventional antipsychotic medications in comparison with psychosocial treatments alone, are more effective and less costly under almost all circumstances. They are therefore dominant choices which are widely adopted in clinical practice, with much benefit to society. Other treatments, such as atypical antipsychotic or assertive community treatment, may result in clinical benefits for many patients but while they save money with high-cost patients they may not with others. When a new treatment is more effective than the next best alternative, but is also more costly, a decision must be made whether to allocate additional resources to pay for these treatments. From the perspective of the mental health professional this decision may seem simple. If a new treatment provides additional benefit for their patients funds should be provided to pay for it.

From the economic perspective of society, however, spending limited resources on treatment of schizophrenia would invariably take resources away from other socially valued activities like the treatment of heart disease; the education of our children; or cleaning up the environment. One of the central concepts of economics is the concept of 'opportunity cost'. This concept, one of the many brainchildren of nineteenth century economist David Ricardo, states that the cost of any activity is the difference between the value of that activity and the value of the *next best* alternative use of the resources that support it. Thus to address the question of how much more or less to spend on treatment of schizophrenia we must determine more than whether the treatment is of benefit. We must decide whether the additional well-being generated by spending an additional dollar on treatment of schizophrenia is greater than the well-being generated by spending that dollar on the next best use. This is not an easy task, but its conceptual importance cannot be overestimated.

We have many good measures of health status and quality of life among patients with schizophrenia, but for this purpose we need measures that are not specific to schizophrenia and that allow comparison of gains associated with the treatment of schizophrenia, depression, cardiac surgery, and, perhaps, even with enhanced third-grade social studies curricula, or with cleaning up toxic waste dumps.

To compare treatment of schizophrenia with other medical illness we need a universal measure of health status. However, to compare the benefits of new treatments for schizophrenia with other social goods we need an even more general measure. The standard way of comparing the value of disparate things in our world is to estimate and compare their monetary value. In other words, we need to determine the dollar value of the added health obtained by spending another dollar on treatment of schizophrenia, heart surgery, education, or the environment.

Putting a monetary value on health or happiness is clearly one of the most challenging measurement problems imaginable. Many people are put off by the very thought of putting a dollar value on such intangibles. But in fact, we make such decisions with our behavior every day. When we spend $500 000 on a heart–lung transplant that decision indicates either that the expenditure is worth the benefit, or that a powerful interest group is diverting funds from more desirable public purposes. Shrinking from the empirical task of estimating the monetary value of health gains means leaving crucial decisions to hunch,

conjecture and the societal or medical power hierarchy rather than to rational scientific argument.

As noted above, a recent study of the use of clozapine in outpatients found that treatment with clozapine was more expensive than with conventional medications, because the reduction in hospital days (even when estimated liberally using a pre–post comparison) was not sufficient to offset the cost of clozapine.[24] The authors of this study emphasized the significant reduction in hospital days as evidence of the value of clozapine treatment, but did not fully articulate the difficult but central question their study raised: whether benefits of clozapine were equal in value to their additional cost.

Similarly, in both the Connecticut ACT study and the VA study of Intensive Case Management, intensive treatment was $4000–$6000 more expensive in lower-cost patients. This type of finding will become increasingly frequent as hospital use declines and there are fewer inpatient dollars to be saved, and poses an important dilemma for both policy-setting and program-planning. For a health care system with a truly fixed budget, providing atypical antipsychotic medications to outpatients may improve the outcomes of a small number of patients, or at least reduce their exposure to uncomfortable side effects. However, as a consequence of their increased costs, some other patients may be deprived of receiving any treatment at all. Program planners must thus decide whether the additional benefit of using costly treatments with current patients equals the benefit that could be obtained from treating additional patients with standard treatment. One of the clear imperatives of economic analysis, one that is derived from the concept of opportunity cost described above, is that allocation of scarce resources always involves choices between alternatives. It is never simply a matter of identifying valuable treatments, but always of identifying treatments which are preferable to the alternative use of the same resources. Defining the nature of the problem or choice is an important step forward, and sometimes allows clear decision-making on the basis of imperfect but available data. For patients who are intolerant of conventional antipsychotic medications because of side effects, atypical antipsychotics may be the only possible medication, and such medications become a dominant choice as compared to no medication. Sometimes, however, those choices are extremely hard to make, as in a clinic with a fixed budget which must choose between providing ten patients with an atypical antipsychotic medication (at a cost of about $50 000) or adding a social worker to help homeless people find housing.

How do we quantify the benefit of allocating scarce resources to diverse worthy uses?

Almost 30 years ago health services researchers proposed a cardinal measure of health outcomes: the Quality Adjusted Life Year.[29] The ideal health index, in this conceptualization, would be an interval scale with a range from 0 (equivalent to death or no healthy life) to 1 (equivalent to perfect health) and which also admits scores representing states that are worse than death (that is, less than 0), but not scores representing states greater than perfect health (that is, greater than 1). Quality Adjusted Life Years (QALY) represent the amount of healthy life a person obtains from a treatment, taking into consideration both the duration of life (quantity) and the value of life (quality).[30,31] Consider first, for example, the situation in which a medication allows someone who was formerly living in a hospital, plagued by hallucinations and delusions, unable to participate in social or productive activities, to assume a fully productive happy life. The benefit here would be considered equivalent to a full QALY if the original state was the equivalent of death and the final state was perfect health.

Improvement more often extends from a state somewhat better than death to a state that is less than perfect health. For example, a treatment that generates 5 years of life at a QALY level increased by 0.2 over baseline (5 × 0.2 = 1) has the same effectiveness as a treatment that yields 2 years at a health status level of 0.5 (2 × 0.5 = 1): 1 year of healthy life or one QALY in both cases. A measure based on the value of years of healthy life is appealing because it can be applied, in principle, to the evaluation of benefit of treatment for any illness. It furthermore allows comparison of the cost-effectiveness of diverse treatments by comparison of their cost-effectiveness ratios – that is, the number of additional QALYs yielded per dollar expended. As we shall see below, it also suggests a method for estimating the equivalent monetary value of health gains.

To take the simplest case first, if treatment of schizophrenia, for example, prolongs life by preventing suicide, as some have suggested,[32,33] that benefit can be directly compared to the life-saving benefits of heart surgery, immunization, or preventive screening for colon cancer. For example, if a year of clozapine treatment costs $5000 and reduces the risk of suicide by 5% per year, the cost-effectiveness ratio would be $5000/0.05 = $100 000/year of life saved during the first year of treatment. On the other hand, if a coronary artery bypass graft (CABG) costing $25 000 extends life by 0.5 years, on average, it is twice as cost-effective ($25 000/0.5 = $50 000/ year of life), and is the preferred treatment at only $50 000 per year of life saved.

These examples, however, only address the number of years saved, not their quality. If, in addition, diverse health states can be converted into QALYs, that is, if we can compare the value of health states attributable to different conditions on the same 0–1 death–perfect health scale, it becomes possible to weight the increased years of life by their healthfulness. Thus, if in the example given above the health gains measured in QALYs were twice as large for clozapine as for CABG (for example 0.2 QALYs for clozapine vs 0.1 QALY for CABG), then the two treatments would be of equal value, yielding 0.2 QALYs for $100 000 (clozapine) or 0.1 QALY for $50 000 (CABG), or one full QALY for $500 000. The major measurement challenge in this example is to accurately locate diverse health states on the common death–perfect health scale.

Measuring health states in QALYs

The theoretically appropriate approach to evaluating health states is called 'the standard gamble'.[30] In this procedure a subject is asked whether they would accept a gamble in which one choice was to remain in their current health state, and the other would be to have perfect health but with an identifiable probability of dying. Through iterative questioning it is theoretically possible to use this procedure to determine, for any health state less than perfect health, what risk of death a person would accept for the chance to have perfect health. That risk, it can be shown, is equivalent to the subject's health state on a scale from death to perfect health.

As a concrete example, consider a patient confined to the hospital with severely disabling schizophrenia. Perhaps they would accept a 50% chance of death to obtain perfect health. If they maintained that state for a year, their health status would be equivalent to 0.5 QALYs. If after treatment this patient was so healthy as to be unwilling to take any gamble to improve their health, they would be scored at 1.0 on the death–perfect health scale and the improvement would be 0.5 QALY. In theory this procedure can be applied to people in various health states and with diverse medical conditions. In each case the current health state is measured against a standard and universal measure of preference, the willingness to accept a specific risk of death, and yields a standardized evaluation of their current state of health.

In fact, the standard gamble has proven to be very difficult to administer. It is either poorly tolerated or gives inconsistent results. Schizophrenic patients, in particular, but others as well, do not like to contemplate even a fictional treatment that is associated with dying. As a result several alternatives have been developed to address difficulties in administering the standard

gamble. In the time trade-off method the informant is asked how many years of life they would give up to live their remaining years in perfect health. People in poorer health states are willing to give up more years of life to attain perfect health and the proportion of years sacrificed is roughly equivalent to their health state in QALYs. An even simpler but less valid approach is to ask subjects to rate their current health by putting a mark on a simple 0–1 linear scale with extreme values labeled poor health and perfect health.

There is only one published study in which the standard gamble has been successfully applied to the assessment of health states in schizophrenia.[34] In this study psychiatrists reviewed brief clinical vignettes and evaluated them using standard gamble procedures. Efforts were made by patients and their caregivers to complete the procedure but were not successful. The psychiatrist's ratings ranged from 0.56 for an inpatient with acute positive symptoms, to 0.60 for an outpatient with severe negative symptoms, 0.70 for an outpatient with moderate functional abilities, 0.73 for an outpatient with good function and 0.83 for an outpatient with mild symptoms and excellent function.

A more recent study[35] used common psychometric instruments to develop a proxy measure of QALYs for a comparison of clozapine and haloperidol in the treatment of refractory schizophrenia. By these measures, hospitalized refractory patients with schizophrenia rated 0.47 on the death to perfect health scale, a finding that is roughly consistent with the rating of 0.56 for acute inpatients in the study by Revicki et al.[34] In this study clozapine was found to be associated with gains of 0.021–0.027 QALYs in comparison with haloperidol over a full year of treatment.

If we accept the estimate of Luchins et al[24] for the net cost of clozapine in outpatients, and the above estimates of QALYs gain during a year of treatment, we would estimate the cost-effectiveness of clozapine in such patients to range from $2636/0.021–0.027 QALYs = $8700–$112 000 per QALY. The question of whether such gains are 'worth' the cost, however, depends on the value of one QALY, and it is to this question that we now turn.

Monetizing QALYs

Another advantage of the QALY approach is that, if one can determine the monetary value of a QALY, it offers the possibility of placing a monetary value on the gains from specific treatments. Thus, if a treatment generates 0.25 QALYs over a year of treatment, and the value of a year of healthy life is estimated to be worth $100 000, one can estimate the monetary value of the treatment in question to be 0.25 × 100 000 = $25 000. If the treatment costs less that $25 000, its benefits outweigh its costs. If the treatment costs more that $25 000, its benefits are not equal to their cost. This kind of calculus, if based on precise, reliable measurements, could be an invaluable aid to evaluating the situation in which new treatments are more effective but cost more than the alternatives.

One approach to the assessment of the monetary value of a QALY is the analysis of revealed preferences.[31,36] In one example of this approach an analysis is undertaken of the increased wages that go with hazardous, life-threatening employment. If employees in a particular higher-risk profession have a 10% increased risk of death on the job, and are paid an average of $10 000 more per year, with all else held equal, the imputed value of a full year of life could be estimated to be $100 000 ($10 000/0.010). Another approach to assessing the value of a QALY using revealed preferences involves an assessment of the QALY gains from medical treatments that are widely provided and are generally regarded as worth their costs.[37] If the most expensive treatment generally provided in our health care system costs $50 000, and generates 0.5 QALYs, we may conclude that in this society a full QALY is valued at $100 000. Estimates of the value of a QALY using these methods range widely from $20 000 to $100 000 in the case of health care treatments,[31] and up to $600 000 in the case of life-threatening employment.[36] In both of these examples the value of a year of life is revealed by current conduct in markets or in clinics. The observations used in these approaches allow an estimate of apparent societal willingness to pay for additional years of life in perfect health, and thus approach a market process in which price reflects our collective willingness to pay for various commodities

Applying these estimates of society's valuation of a QALY to the treatment of outpatients with clozapine, and using the outcome and cost figures presented above, we would conclude that at $87 000–$112 000 per QALY, such treatment is at the upper limit of conventionally accepted medical technologies.

In spite of the logical appeal of the approaches outlined here, there are many methodologic problems to their implementation. We present the basic concepts because they illustrate the conceptual possibility of generating standard assessments of health states and monetizing health status improvement. Although far from applicable in conventional mental health cost-effectiveness studies, they illustrate how economic analysis holds the possibility of rationally prioritizing available health care technologies to maximize their beneficial effect on the health of the public.

Conclusion

We have considered three health economic questions that have a direct bearing on the development of a welfare-maximizing system of treatment for patients with schizophrenia. The difficulty we encounter in finding sound, convincing answers to these questions should not detract from our appreciation of their importance. Instead of disdaining the 'dismal discipline' of our colleagues we should be grateful to them for laboring since the days of Adam Smith to find useful ways of thinking about such questions. In the absence of scientific answers to these questions they will be answered through political processes – processes in which power and greed are sure to have a more determining role than compassion, fairness or justice, and in which people with mental illness are most likely to be the losers, once again. Economic analysis is thus a vital tool for psychiatric advocacy. We must learn to use it, to nurture it and to strengthen it – the old fashioned way – with research, with social experimentation, and with public dialogue.

References

1. Ma C, McGuire TG, Costs and incentives in a behavioral health care carve-out, *Health Aff* (1998) **17**:53–69.

2. Goldman W, McCulloch J, Sturm R, Costs and use of mental health services before and after managed care, *Health Aff* (1998) **17**:40–52.

3. Rosenheck RA, Druss B, Stolar M et al, Effect of declining mental health service use on employees of a large self-insured private corporation, *Health Aff* (1999) **18**:193–203.

4. Rosenheck R, Horvath T, Impact of VA reorganization on patterns of mental health care, *Psychiatr Serv* (1998) **49**:56.

5. Leslie DL, Rosenheck RA, Shifting from inpatient to outpatient care? Mental health utilization and costs in a privately insured population, *Am J Psychiatry* (1999) **156**:1250–7.

6. Krause E, Death of the Guilds: professions, states and the advance of capitalism, 1930 to the present. (Yale University Press: New Haven, 1996).

7. Eist HI, Presidential address: Strengthening psychiatry's dedication and commitment to compassionate care, educational excellence, and creative research, *Am J Psychiatry* (1997) **154**:1343–9.

8. Samuelson PA, Nordhaus WD, *Economics*, 12th edn (McGraw Hill: New York, 1987).

9. Rice DP, Miller LS, The economic burden of schizophrenia: conceptual and methodological issues, and cost estimates. In: Moscarelli M, Rupp A, Sartorius N, eds, *Handbook of Mental Health Economics and Health Policy*, vol 1. Schizophrenia (Wiley: New York, 1996).

10. Baumol WJ, Blinder AS, *Microeconomics: Principles and Policy* (Dryden Press: Forth Worth, TX, 1986).

11. Wennberg JE, Gittlesohn D, Small area variation in health care delivery, *Science* (1973) **182**:1102–8.

12. May PRA, Cost efficiency of treatment for the schizophrenic patient, *Am J Psychiatry* (1971) **127**:118–21.

13. May PRA, *Treatment of Schizophrenia* (Science House: New York, 1968).

14. Dixon LB, Lehman AF, Levine J, Conventional antipsychotic medications for schizophrenia, *Schizophr Bull* (1995) **21**:567–77.

15. Revicki DA, Luce BR, Wechsler JM et al, Cost-effectiveness of clozapine for treatment resistant schizophrenic patients, *Hosp Community Psychiatry* (1990) **41**:850–4.

16. Meltzer HY, Cola P, Way L et al, Cost-effectiveness of clozapine in neuroleptic resistant schizophrenia, *Am J Psychiatry* (1993) **150**:1630–8.

17. Reid WH, Mason M, Toprac M, Savings in hospital bed-days related to treatment with clozapine, *Hosp Community Psychiatry* (1994) **45**:261–8.

18. Reid WH, Mason M, Psychiatric hospital utilization in patients treated with clozapine for up to 4.5 years in a state mental health care system, *J Clin Psychiatry* (1998) **59**: 189–94.

19. Rosenheck RA, Cramer J, Xu W et al, for the Department of Veterans Affairs Cooperative Study Group on Clozapine in Refractory Schizophrenia, A comparison of clozapine and haloperidol in the treatment of hospitalized patients with refractory schizophrenia, *N Engl J Med* (1997) **337**:809–15.

20. Essock SM, Hargreaves WA, Covell NH, Goethe J, Clozapine's effectiveness for patients in state hospitals: results from a randomized trial, *Psychopharmacol Bull* (1996) **32**:683–97.

21. Rosenheck R, Lawson W, Crayton J et al, Predictors of differential response to clozapine and haloperidol, *Biol Psychiatry* (1998) **44**:475–82.

22. Rosenheck R, Cramer J, Allan E et al, Cost-effectiveness of clozapine in patients with high and low levels of hospital use, *Arch Gen Psych* (1999) **56**:565–72.

23. Luchins DJ, Hanrahan P, Schinderman M et al, Initiating clozapine treatment in the outpatient clinic: service utilization and cost trends, *Psychiatr Serv* (1998) **49**:1034–8.

24. Viale G, Mechling L, Maislin G et al, Impact of risperidone on the use of mental health care resources, *Psychiatr Serv* (1997) **48**:1153–9.

25. Rosenheck RA, Massari L, Frisman L, Who should receive high cost mental health treatment and for how long? Issues in the rationing of mental health care, *Schizophr Bull* (1993) **19**:843–52.

26. Rosenheck RA, Neale MS, Cost-effectiveness of

intensive psychiatric community care for high users of inpatient services, *Arch Gen Psychiatry* (1998) **55:**459–66.

27. Rosenheck RA, Neale M, Leaf P et al, Multisite experimental cost study of intensive psychiatric community care. *Schizophr Bull* (1995) **21:**129–40.

28. Essock SM, Frisman LK, Kontos NJ, Cost-effectiveness of assertive community treatment teams, *Am J Orthopsychiatry* (1998) **68:**179–90.

29. Torrance GW, Feeny D, Utilities and quality adjusted life years, *International Journal of Technology Assessment in Health Care* (1989) **5:**559–75.

30. Gold MR, Siegel JE, Russell LB, Weinstein MC, *Cost Effectiveness in Health and Medicine* (Oxford University Press: New York, 1996).

31. Weinstein MC, From cost-effectiveness ratios to resource allocation: where to draw the line. In: Sloan FA, ed, *Valuing Health Care* (Cambridge University Press: New York, 1996).

32. Meltzer HY, Okayli G, Reduction of suicideality during clozapine treatment of neuroleptic-resistant schizophrenia: impact of risk benefit assessment, *Am J Psychiatry* (1995) **152:**183–90.

33. Reid WH, Mason M, Hogan T, Suicide prevention effects associated with clozapine therapy in schizophrenia and schizoaffective disorder, *Psychiatr Serv* (1998) **49:**1029–33.

34. Revicki DA, Shakespeare A, Kind P, Preferences for schizophrenia-related health states: a comparison of patients, caregivers and psychiatrists, *Int Clin Psychopharmacol* (1996) **11:**101–8.

35. Rosenheck RA, Cramer J, Xu W et al, Multiple outcome assessment in a study of the cost-effectiveness of clozapine in the treatment of refractory schizophrenia, *Health Serv Res* (1998) **33:**1235–59.

36. Johanneson M, *Theory and Methods of Economic Evaluation of Health Care* (Kluwer Academic: Dordrecht, 1996).

37. Luapacis A, Feeny D, Detsky AS, Tugwell PX, How attractive does a new technology have to be to warrant adoption and utilization? Tentative guidelines for using clinical and economic evaluations, *Can Med Assoc J* (1992) **146:**473–81.

23

First Person Accounts

John K Hsiao

Contents • Introduction • First person account: Finding myself and loving it • First person account: A personal experience • First person account: Becoming seaworthy • First person account: Living with schizophrenia • First person account: Three generations of schizophrenia

Introduction

If there is one scientific truth that we know about schizophrenia, it is that it is a disease of the brain. The two facts most often cited to support this are: 1) schizophrenia is a genetic illness since risk is increased in biological but not adoptive relatives, and 2) brain development is abnormal since the cerebral ventricular system is enlarged. However, the majority of people with schizophrenia do not have relatives with the illness, and magnetic resonance imaging (MRI) scans of their brains are usually read as normal. This is not to suggest that schizophrenia is not a brain disease, but it is only when patients are taken as a whole and compared to nonpatients that the roles played by genetics and neuroanatomy become evident.

Similarly, clinical research is carried out and reported on groups of patients, and treatment guidelines are for the aggregate of patients with schizophrenia. Treatments, however, are applied to individuals, and schizophrenia is an illness of individual patients and families. Of necessity, mental health caregivers treat and prognosticate for each patient as if he or she were the 'average' patient, but in fact, there is no such 'average' person with schizophrenia. Each individual person with schizophrenia and each family has a unique history, personality, and circumstance. It

is difficult if not impossible to convey this individuality in a scientific paper, and while professional journals and the medical literature tell us much about the illness, its natural history, and its optimal treatment, we can find little insight into the experience of individual persons with schizophrenia or their families.

The *Schizophrenia Bulletin* has been published by the National Institute of Mental Health (NIMH) since 1969. It began as an occasional publication but since 1974 has appeared quarterly. Its primary audience is mental health professionals and researchers, but it is also read by nonprofessionals interested in schizophrenia. The *Bulletin* plays a central role in NIMH's program of schizophrenia research, providing a means for communication with an international scientific community, and helping to tie that community together. Since 1979, the *Bulletin* has included an ongoing series of First Person Accounts written by patients, ex-patients, and family members.

The five articles that follow appeared originally as First Person Accounts in the *Schizophrenia Bulletin*, and describe the individual experiences of patients and family members as they dealt with schizophrenia. 'Finding myself and loving it' appeared in 1984 and describes the experiences of a college student who had a sudden onset of psychosis but who returned to premorbid functioning with treatment. By contrast, 'A personal experience', which appeared in 1995, is the tale of a woman in her thirties who had a much more gradual onset, that took years to diagnose, and who has continued to 'struggle' despite treatment. 'Becoming seaworthy' appeared in 1985, and is written by a man who has been ill with schizophrenia for many years, expressing the regret of dreams lost due to illness as well as the importance of families in helping people with schizophrenia. The final two accounts are by family members of people with schizophrenia. The first, 'Living with schizophrenia', appeared in 1991 and is a mother's account of her daughter's illness and how devastating it has been for both of them. 'Three generations of schizophrenia' appeared in 1986, and tells of a woman's experience with multiple family members who fell ill with schizophrenia.

The same introduction has accompanied each First Person account in the *Schizophrenia Bulletin*, including these five articles. The hope is that 'mental health professionals ... will take this opportunity to learn about the issues and difficulties confronted by consumers of mental health care. In addition, ... these accounts will give patients and families a better sense of not being alone in confronting the problems that can be anticipated by persons with serious emotional difficulties.'

First person account: Finding myself and loving it

Jeanine M O'Neal

When my first episode of schizophrenia occurred, I was 21, a senior in college in Atlanta, Georgia. I was making good grades, assistant vice president of my chapter in my sorority, president of the Spanish club, and very popular. Everything in my life was just perfect. I had a boyfriend whom I liked a lot, a part-time job tutoring Spanish, and was about to run for the Ms. Senior pageant.

All of a sudden things weren't going so well. I began to lose control of my life and, most of all,

myself. I couldn't concentrate on my schoolwork, I couldn't sleep, and when I did sleep, I had dreams about dying. I was afraid to go to class, imagined that people were talking about me, and on top of that I heard voices. I called my mother in Pittsburgh and asked for her advice. She told me to move off campus into an apartment with my sister.

After I moved in with my sister, things got worse. I was afraid to go outside and when I looked out of the window, it seemed that everyone outside was yelling 'kill her, kill her.' My sister forced me to go to school. I would go out of the house until I knew she had gone to work: then I would return home. Things continued to get worse. I imagined that I had a foul body odor and I sometimes took up to six showers a day. I recall going to the grocery store one day, and I imagined that the people in the store were saying 'Get saved, Jesus is the answer.' Things worsened – I couldn't remember a thing. I had a notebook full of reminders telling me what to do on that particular day. I couldn't remember my schoolwork, and I would study from 6:00 p.m. until 4:00 a.m., but never had the courage to go to class on the following day. I tried to tell my sister about it, but she didn't understand. She suggested that I see a psychiatrist, but I was afraid to go out of the house to see him.

One day I decided that I couldn't take this trauma anymore, so I took an overdose of 35 Darvon pills. At the same moment, a voice inside me said, 'What did you do that for? Now you won't go to heaven.' At that instant I realized that I really didn't want to die, I wanted to live, and I was afraid. I got on the phone and called the psychiatrist whom my sister had recommended. I told him that I had taken an overdose of Darvon and that I was afraid. He told me to take a taxi to the hospital. When I arrived at the hospital, I began vomiting, but I didn't pass out. Somehow I couldn't accept the fact that I was really going to see a psychiatrist. I thought that psychiatrists were only for crazy people, and I definitely didn't think I was crazy yet. As a result, I did not admit myself right away. As a matter of fact I left the hospital and ended up meeting my sister on the way home. She told me to turn right back around, because I was definitely going to be admitted. We then called my mother, and she said she would fly down on the following day.

I stayed in that particular hospital for 1 week. It wasn't too bad. First I was interviewed, then given medication (Trilafon). There I met a number of people whose problems ranged from depression to having illusions of grandeur. It was quite interesting. I had a nice doctor, but he didn't tell me that I had schizophrenia – only that I had an 'identity crisis.' I was then transferred to a hospital in Pittsburgh. I did not care for my doctor. He told me that I was imagining things and constantly changed my medication. For instance, if I had a stomach ache, he would say I imagined it. At this stage of my recovery I was no longer imagining things, but I was afraid. I feared large crowds of people and therefore avoided going shopping, dancing, or riding buses (anywhere large crowds existed). It took me from September until March to recover. By the way, this particular doctor diagnosed my case as an 'anxiety-depression reaction.' In the meantime my family was very supportive of me.

In April, I decided that I was well and didn't need medication anymore (not knowing that I had schizophrenia and that it was incurable), and I also stopped going to the doctor's office. I got a job, from which I was terminated after a week. I became hypertensive and nervous without realizing it. My friends and family said I was behaving strangely, but I took no notice. I went out dancing practically every night to make up for lost time while being afraid. I felt as if I were on top of the world – as if I were free.

The summer passed quickly. I had decided to return to Atlanta in the fall and complete my senior year. After all, I only had 1 measly year toward my Bachelor of Arts degree in Spanish, and I wanted to complete my education at the college where my education began. My parents, however, suggested that I finish in Pittsburgh, in

case anything else might occur. I didn't listen, and somehow thought they were plotting against me. Next, I found myself in Atlanta and sick once again. I was taken to another psychiatric hospital. This time things were twice as bad as the first. I no longer heard voices, but the things I saw and dreamed about were far more traumatic. I recall at one point thinking I was Jesus Christ and that I was placed on this earth to bear everyone's sins.

My stay in that particular hospital was absolutely terrible. Each time I saw things I was placed in seclusion. They constantly used me as a guinea pig to discover which medicine would best suit my needs. However, I met many people (patients), some of whom became very close friends. I remained in the hospital 1 month and 2 days and was finally prescribed Loxitane, which I am presently taking.

After I was released, I returned to Pittsburgh and became an outpatient at Western Psychiatric Institute and Clinic. My doctor is very good and I respect her a lot. She's really a great person. It took me 6 months to recover. Again I was afraid of crowds of people, and I avoided them whenever I could.

Now I have been taking Loxitane for almost 2 years with considerable results. All of the symptoms seem to have vanished. I have my own apartment, I am back in college in Pittsburgh, president of my chapter of my sorority, and, above all, more confident and happier than I have ever been in my life. I reflect back on the pains of the past and consider them a learning experience. I foresee the future as a bright challenge. My doctor once asked me what do I think taking medicine means and I replied, 'not being sick.' Today I take my medicine daily, just as a person with high blood pressure or a diabetic does. It doesn't bother me. Today I am really free!

This article first appeared in the *Schizophrenia Bulletin* (1984) **10**:109–10. Reprinted with permission.

First person account: A personal experience

Elizabeth Herrig

When I was (age 12), I asked my parents if I could see a psychiatrist and they agreed. I asked him if he thought I might have schizophrenia. He told me that he would not make that diagnosis; he said that schizophrenia caused a person to have hallucinations and delusions and that I appeared to him to be rational. At the time I had not experienced anything that I would call a hallucination. I had intense fears and I was often depressed. I hated going to school and made up any excuses to stay home.

At 15 I began seeing another psychiatrist at the recommendation of a school counselor, who had noticed my strange and reclusive behavior. The problems I remember talking about with her were mostly feelings I had when I was at school. I felt different and alone. Seeing so many people in the school halls made me wonder how my life could be significant. I wanted to blend in in the classroom as though I were a desk. I never spoke. I didn't participate in any extracurricular activities or have any close friends. I loved to read. I especially enjoyed books that were not on the curriculum. I liked to read JRR Tolkien's books about Middle Earth. I enjoyed writing papers for my English classes, but I was not thought of as an exceptional student.

The high school graduation ceremony was a painful event for me. I stood alone and only one girl came to say goodbye to me. After graduation I enrolled at a college near home. I stayed only 2 years. It was difficult for me to deal with ordinary situations, such as a problem with a teacher.

My major was to be in English with an emphasis on writing. I remember thinking that I would make it through all the courses but when it came time to have my writing portfolio evaluated (a graduation requirement) I would be found lacking in writing ability and refused a diploma.

I remember those years at college as a time in which I was very angry. I couldn't understand where the anger was coming from or where it should be directed. Strong feelings of fear, anger, and depression battled for dominance within me. I decided to quit school and find a job.

During the summer after my sophomore year at college my psychiatrist decided that the drug haloperidol might help me. I remember her explaining to me that if I read about the drug I would find out that it was used to treat severely ill people. She said that she did not regard me as severely ill, but that the drug would reduce my fears. However, I remember that after taking the drug my fears intensified. I became fearful of children I saw walking down the street. I also suffered from uncontrollable jaw movements until I was also given another drug to correct it. The haloperidol had the effect of making me restless. I couldn't tolerate the effects it had on me and I was taken off it. I stopped going to see the psychiatrist because I began to doubt that seeing her would bring me any relief from the problem of being myself.

I found a job through an ad in the *Chicago Tribune*. I settled into the work. I was regarded as strange by my supervisors and co-workers, but I was soon given more difficult duties because of my ability and willingness to work.

I became obsessed with my diet and wanting to be thin, even though I had never been overweight. I began to eat only fruits and vegetables. I wanted to be weightless and to float on air, more like a spirit than a human being. Because of too much fiber in my diet, I developed an intestinal blockage and had to be rushed to hospital in excruciating pain. The doctors in the emergency room were surprised to see my skin had turned a deep orange. It was later concluded that this was the result of too much carotene from carrots in my diet.

The resident doctor called a psychiatrist to see me. He happened to be the same man who years earlier had told me I didn't have the symptoms of schizophrenia. This time he was called in to determine whether or not I had anorexia nervosa. I weighed 84 pounds at this point. He didn't diagnose me as having anorexia nervosa. He diagnosed me as having 'avoidant personality disorder' and as suffering from 'anxiety.' The blockage in my intestines cleared up and I returned to work.

That summer was a horrible time. Life took on a hellish quality that is incomprehensible to the average normal person. A book I read at about this time had a profound effect on me. The book was *Native Son* by Richard Wright. I came to identify strongly with the main character because I believed that he and I were both good people who were just misunderstood by everyone. His crime, killing a young woman, seemed logical to me under his circumstances. I also enjoyed reading classical literature such as *The Iliad* and *The Odyssey* by Homer.

It is difficult to remember the progression of my illness chronologically. The world became a more chaotic, frightening, and inexplicable place. I think it must have been in February 1984 that I began to have the perception that my thinking was beginning to change. It seemed that my mind had two parts. One part was the part that had always been there, but the other part was filled with voices that talked in the background of my thoughts. I became distracted listening to the voices and found it difficult to concentrate. As my illness progressed I couldn't understand what was happening to me. I would sit at my desk and listen to the voices. My life with my family seemed different. I remember a strange conversation while sitting in a restaurant with my parents. My father said, 'Your mother is getting old.' I looked at her and saw that she was crying. I can only suppose that she was sad about the changes in me and didn't know what she could do.

Going to work was pure hell. I continued to hear voices. One day while sitting at my desk I saw a fly land on my arm. It was the biggest fly I had ever seen. It could not have been real, not in February. One of my duties was to read information intended for military personnel. I remember reading about Hellfire missiles. I imagined the manmade hellfire killing people. I became convinced that I was reading top secret information and that someone would try to have me killed so that I couldn't talk.

Many of the thoughts I had at this time would seem embarrassing to me now if I looked at them in a judgmental way. Some thoughts seem evil or just petty and childish. I accept them all the way most people accept their dreams. I couldn't control them so I don't blame myself for any of them. Only by thinking of them in this way can I tell the story as I am doing. I hope that the average person's understanding of mental illness will become such that such episodes will be regarded as altered states of consciousness and won't be used to judge mentally ill persons as bad people.

The morning of the day I had to be hospitalized I told my mother that I didn't want to go to work because someone there would shoot me. She asked me a question and I answered in a rhyming phrase that made no sense. I left the house without letting her know and decided that I would go to work after all. I believed that I would pass every person in the world that day and that each of them would share a secret with me. I believed that the gestures of people had a special significance. This was how they told me their secrets. When I heard people talk I thought they were talking about me. At work I punched in at the timeclock, oblivious to the time. It was the middle of the morning. I sat at my desk. I don't know if I tried to work.

Someone came and handed me a note that said, 'Call the doctor.' I saw this note as coming from a mysterious force that was giving me directions. I left work and took the train to see our family doctor. It was a miracle that I came to no harm walking around in the state of mind I was in. I thought that traffic would automatically stop for me. Everything that had cost money I believed was now free. When I got to the doctor's office I asked the nurse why I had been called. She said that she hadn't called me. I asked her if she knew who I was. I wanted her to take control of the situation and guide me because I didn't know what was happening. It seemed that the force had led me to this point and was abandoning me.

Fortunately the doctor entered the room. My mother had called him earlier that morning and described my condition. He asked me to have a seat and left the room to call my mother to tell her where I was. It turned out that she had called my father and he had come home from work and they were searching for me. She had called the place where I worked to see if I was there and she had pretended that she was calling from the doctor's office. Even though I had developed a fear of them I went with them willingly. They put me in the car and drove me to a hospital. I remember the nurse in the emergency room asking me what the problem was. I started to talk about something I had read about Moses and the Ten Commandments. She asked that I just be quiet because she didn't understand. I signed myself in without realizing I was in a hospital. I trusted everyone as though I were a small child. I didn't think of asking anything, such as how long I was going to have to stay or what was going to be done for me.

My hospital stay lasted 3 weeks. I was started on medication right away. I was given haloperidol. I don't know when the medicine started having any effect. I wandered up and down the hall watching people. I told the nurse that there was a force leading me to hell. I had many bizarre delusions. I believed I was Eva Peron, the wife of the Argentinian dictator and the subject of the musical *Evita*, which was popular at that time. I believed that my mother had died of lung disease from smoking cigarettes. My heartbeat became so rapid that I thought I was in the hospital awaiting a heart transplant. I thought that a heart that was pounding so intensely could surely not last much longer. I listened to the radio in my room and interpreted each one of the lyrics as a message intended for me.

I believed that it was possible for a person to leave his or her body and inhabit the body of another person. I heard people I knew speaking through the mouths of the strangers around me.

As the weeks passed and the medication began to take effect, the world became saner. The voices stopped. Things started to seem ordinary. Before releasing me from the hospital, my parents were called in for a session with me, my psychiatrist, and a social worker. The social worker stressed the importance of my learning how to live independently. I decided that seeing the psychiatrist was necessary but that seeing the social worker was an unnecessary interference in my life. I now regret that I didn't get the help of a social worker at that time.

One pleasant aspect of being in the hospital was that it gave me a chance to think about what I really wanted to do with my life. I no longer wanted to continue working at a dull job where I was unhappy. It seemed that there should be more to life. I had a catalog from the University of Illinois at Chicago. I learned that the university had a classics department. I wanted to study about ancient Greece and Rome. I considered earning an advanced degree and teaching. My interest in the classics has been replaced over the years by stronger interests in other subjects, but I am glad I had the interest then to motivate me.

When I got out of the hospital I returned to work, or I should say I made the attempt to return. The medication had the effect of making me restless and my job required that I sit in one place all day. I would come to work and have to leave 20 minutes later. My frustrated attempts to do an ordinary thing, to stay at work, were very difficult for me. What made it harder was that no one understood my problem. I was called to personnel where I had to explain why I couldn't work a full day. The woman wouldn't believe me and insisted on calling my psychiatrist to see if it was true.

Nine years have passed since I was hospitalized. I went on to earn a bachelor's degree in political science. I tried to earn a master's but I found the course work in library science too difficult. These 9 years have been filled with many disappointments. I've gone through long periods of unemployment. At 31 I am single and unable to support myself. I live with my parents. I am searching for a job that I will really enjoy.

Even though I am struggling, I feel the worst is behind me and that the illness will not return. I regret that I went so long being ill. The time I lost would have been better spent having friends and developing my skills and talents. I hope that in the future it will be much easier for a child or young adult to get help for emotional problems so that they do not have to have an experience similar to mine. As mental health care is now, people can go without receiving the treatment they need until their lives are devastated.

This article first appeared in the *Schizophrenia Bulletin* (1995) **21**:339–42. Reprinted with permission.

First person account: Becoming seaworthy

Mark Stakes

A heavy fog hovered over a warm morning ocean. Not many of us were awake this early – only a handful of dedicated teens whose life's ambition was to be king of the surf.

Jimbo, a freckled-faced 14-year-old with red hair, was somewhere out in the distant surf bobbing unseen in the turbulent water. I was also bobbing in 6-foot swells, looking for Jimbo, to share a swell with him and ride the wave in heated competition.

We were veterans of 6 and 10 years, respectively, with wave-riding experience that made us brave in the rough seas of a prehurricane swell. Our motivation and lust for life was as strong as the tides. But that is now a bygone day; although my motivation is now not as misdirected as it was when I was a teen, I continue to feel at sea.

I no longer enter the ocean with the zeal I had then. I've changed, not by choice but by fate. I'm more cautious, more reluctant to enter an activity without reassurance of its safety and my own well-being.

When I turned 20, reality escaped me. Even though I had been brave before in prehurricane waves, my fear would now rise over simple things, accompanied by what I perceived to be special messages. These messages were a trick of the mind. They caused me to sweat in fear, though there was no attendant harm. For example, one day after flying home from Florida, I sat in my basement with a fear that I could not control. I was totally afraid – just from watching my cat look out the window.

This was not the brave teen of a year ago. I realize now that an illness had hit at its most expected time. Schizophrenia is said to strike most often between the ages of 17 and 25, and I was 20. The doctors diagnosed me as schizophrenic. I now live a better life than I did at 20, but I would do better if I had no illness. Don't get me wrong, I live a good life, but I often wonder what kind of life I would lead without a disease of the mind. I have not given up hope of a successful life, but my lifestyle will always be attended by some dependency, primarily on medication.

Now my lifestyle includes frequent visits to a doctor and monthly injections of Prolixin. In contrast to the treatment of about 30 years ago, I am not confined to a large state hospital. I function well for my condition and am as free as any citizen. With that freedom, however, comes an equal amount of responsibility.

To keep my freedom, I must work to control my life in a manner that is not upsetting to my family. Families either struggle with us or choose to let us struggle alone. I am fortunate because my family is by my side instead of letting me face the difficulties of mental illness alone. My parents tolerate shortcomings, but they do not tolerate giving up. They have expectations, but patience in forgiving my not completely adhering to these expectations. I have a supportive family, a congenial family, but one that has not enjoyed all the benefits of good health. I come from a family that weathers problems rather than solving them in divorce court.

At 20 I stopped trying to be a professional surfer. I was tested by a group of psychologists to see where my aptitude lay; I had a high score in drafting (I had earned B's in drafting in high school). The State Department of Rehabilitative Services began paying for my courses at a community college for training as a draftsman. I did well at first, and then went through a quarter where poor motivation kept me from getting good grades, and I dropped out. With the help of parental discipline and an understanding but firm boss, my motivation has improved, and I have reentered college.

Between my first try at school and now, I worked mostly as a laborer, but also as a rodman on a survey party. Surveying brought my interest back to drafting, and I soon began working in engineering offices as a civil draftsman. Now that I have returned to college, I hope to finish my associate degree as an architectural draftsman. I work part-time doing architectural delineation and also work as a graphics consultant. This spring I hope to complete my education and get an apartment. I have found the most beneficial form of rehabilitation is setting small goals that lead to accomplishing larger goals. I must confess that my old surfing competitiveness still sparks up and makes me vie with those I encounter, although most of this competition is directed at accomplishing rewarding goals.

In addition to work, there is another area of activity that promotes my well-being and keeps me out of hospitals. This area is in forming friendships. I'm a member of a clubhouse for ex-mental patients that has a psychosocial rehabilitation program for the mentally ill. Here I meet friends with problems similar to mine. Our motto, work and friendship, is stressed as the key to a healthy life as a functional schizophrenic.

I date some of the girls here, and one of the members and I have shared an apartment. In the clubhouse we struggle together, instead of alone, against the obstacles of life and low income. Finances are a problem, and the clubhouse staff help many of us in this area. Before the program existed, it was up to me to earn, budget, and spend my money. In Florida, when I was alone, I believe the stress brought on by financial difficulties helped precipitate my illness.

Here at the clubhouse those of us who can't work are assisted in obtaining Social Security benefits and Supplemental Security Income. For those who can work, the clubhouse staff help us obtain part-time jobs in the community. I am fortunate because I have a skill by which to earn money. Now that the vocational rehabilitation counselor is based here at the clubhouse, the disabled can easily be served. By being on site the counselor is better equipped to ascertain who is able mentally and motivationally to attend college, vocational training, on-the-job training, etc.

In the last 15 years since I was first afflicted by this illness, there has been progress on my part as well as on the part of Federal and State agencies. There are more rehabilitation programs that act as a network of support to keep me from falling into long-term hospitalization.

I have learned to like these programs just as I learned to like water. Just as I overcame my youthful fear of the water, I have overcome my initial fear of psychiatrists' offices. I now keep my medication appointments and cooperate with social workers and psychiatrists rather than fight them. They are now counted as friends and supporters of good mental health.

This article first appeared in the *Schizophrenia Bulletin* (1985) **11**:629–30. Reprinted with permission.

First person account: Living with schizophrenia

Evelyn Smith

My daughter, Cindy, and I get together every 2 weeks for lunch – something we can now both enjoy. Sometimes we eat in a local restaurant, sometimes in a snack bar on the grounds near her dorm.

She is in her mid-thirties and I notice with sadness that she has a few gray hairs. The sadness is because she hasn't really enjoyed or participated in life yet, but nature continues its march.

Now she and I both have gray hair. Our conversation is rather disjointed, as Cindy has difficulty understanding my words, most of the time. She struggles valiantly to answer my questions, and occasionally an appropriate response comes forth. Now, after 17 years, we sometimes exchange two or three sentences which actually have the give and take of real conversation.

Cindy has been living under the shadow of schizophrenia these past 17 years. She has a severely debilitating form of this devastating and demoralizing brain disease. Schizophrenia is caused by a chemical imbalance in the brain that produces a break with reality – *not* a split personality – and the distorted dialogue going on in her head controls her thought processes with often bizarre results. She has been a patient at a State hospital for 11 years and was in and out of hospital for 5 years before that. This 'fog,' as she calls it, descended on her at age 20 when she was starting her third year of college. During the first 5 years she got progressively worse, a course that has led to a long-term stay in a mental hospital. The best we can hope for is that someday she will be able to live in a group home; at this point we're a long way from that goal.

During lulls in our conversation, as we sit in the snack bar, I observe other patients as they come and go. One is having an imaginary conversation in her head; she smiles at something humorous only she understands. I see the pleasure on a young man's face as he's asked to share a table. I watch the expressive eyes of a lady, whose own grasp of reality seems all too tenuous, as she tries to understand the conversation of another person who is not making much sense. This is the 'normal' life of those suffering from mental illness.

The saddest thing of all is to realize that the stories of family life and previous achievements that were a part of the past lives of each of these people are no longer important to them. It's as though their past lives never existed. They are basically alone in the world because sustaining or contributing to a relationship of any kind is

beyond the realm of possibility. To see a life stopped in its tracks by this ogre, schizophrenia, is a heart-rending thing to witness. The highlights of Cindy's week now are the Monday evening dances and the Friday morning bowling trips. There are many other activities at the hospital; some she participates in and some she doesn't, depending on her mood.

As we enjoy our lunch, memories of Cindy's very normal childhood and adolescence flood my mind. Memories of a girl who loved to read and who devoured many books; of a young girl practicing the piano and being able to play tunes and advertising jingles she'd heard on the radio and television; of a teenager on the swimming and diving team at the local YMCA. Memories of a good student in school; of a cheerleader in junior high school and of a member of the field hockey team in high school; and of a waitress during the summers earning money for college.

Nothing in her growing-up years could have prepared us for the shock and devastation of seeing this normal, happy child become totally incapacitated by schizophrenia. What we knew about schizophrenia in the beginning we could have written on the head of a pin. What we learned over the next few years was confusing and frightening. Theories were archaic and pertinent information hard to come by and not easy to understand. Following Cindy around and trying to convince her of the inappropriateness of something was a time-consuming and futile activity. Every ounce of my physical strength and mental stamina was directed to helping Cindy. In the beginning I had no idea how enormous a task that would be – or how impossible. I found myself neglecting my other three children, and though they said otherwise, I felt I had almost abandoned them.

Cindy has a delightful sense of humor, which still appears from time to time. She can hit the nail on the head quite often and her language sometimes is a bit salty! She will occasionally sit down and play a few tunes on the piano – all from memory – and she frequently quotes unusual passages of scripture from a Biblical translation only she has knowledge of.

Family members learn to live with schizophrenia encumbered by a great sense of loss and frustration. Friends have fallen by the wayside because 'staying in touch' with their friend is pretty much an impossibility. Cindy's relationships with her sisters and brother are as close as she can allow. She has a twin sister whom she loves dearly, which is always evident when they are together. The break in their relationship has left a void in both of their lives.

I know from Cindy's many references to her 'husband' and 'children,' neither of which she has, that family life is very important to her. I sense her feelings of loss because this aspect of life will never be a reality for her. A Raggedy Ann doll I had gotten her a few years ago became her little girl for a year or so. She would place the doll in a chair and feed it lunch or prop it beside her on the couch.

'Mom, you don't know the hell in my head,' was the way Cindy described what was happening to her during the early stages of the disease. Many times she would burn herself with cigarettes or cut herself with razor blades. In her mind there were good reasons for these actions; the fact that there was no pain associated with them made her oblivious to the danger. On one occasion she missed her jugular vein by one quarter of an inch. Yet, as we drove her to the emergency room, she sat and talked as though nothing had happened, completely ignoring the blood-soaked towels around her neck.

When you think of the utter helplessness these victims of schizophrenia must feel and all the wasted years their lives represent, your heart cries in despair. According to statistics, 1 in 100 suffer from schizophrenia in varying degrees of severity. In this day of modern medicine, we have become so conditioned to taking a few pills to alleviate or cure an illness that faith in this process turns to disbelief when symptoms are not alleviated and no cure takes place. Some people with schizophrenia do not respond well to medication, and

Cindy is one of them. However, their reactions to life are like ours – 'they call 'em as they see 'em,' – and their actions are perfectly logical responses to what is going on in their heads. The anguish is that this demon, schizophrenia, having completely deranged a brain and ravaged a life, has now released an empty shell of a person, as though shaking it like a rag doll and throwing it to the ground. Coping with the world and understanding it is still too great a task for Cindy and most of her conversation is irrelevant or incomprehensible.

Cindy's habits of daily living and personal grooming are very poor, though she sees a rhyme and a reason for the things she does. Taking a shower means just standing under the water, usually cold, and two pats with a towel and she's dry. She enjoys using fingernail polish and lipstick but can do so only under supervision, as she likes to apply it to her nose and cheeks. There are certain shoes that keep her legs thin and are worn for this purpose occasionally, and keeping track of her glasses is really beyond her capabilities.

Coming to grips with the thought of your child living in a mental hospital, possibly for many years, leaves you with a gnawing sense of helplessness that never really dissipates. You live with it the best you can. Remembering all the years of nurturing and healthy meals and dental checkups that went into the life of this daughter of mine, I am engulfed by the feeling that it was an exercise in futility. Now, as a heavy smoker, she stands a good chance of getting lung cancer. Now, she may be hit by a car, because she doesn't think to look before she crosses the street.

It's only been in the past year that Cindy can let herself glance at family snapshots. The chasm between her real life and a remembered past makes looking at them too painful. During her visits home I stay near her all the time, as it's almost like having a 3-year-old around. For Cindy, living by any kind of a routine is completely unimportant. As everyone is sitting down to dinner she finds it imperative to smoke a cigarette. Often, 20 minutes before we have planned to leave the house she has fallen sound asleep.

At the hospital the staff oversees her activities in a constructive, patient-oriented atmosphere. From observation, I can see that Cindy's relationships with the staff and patients are sometimes friendly, sometimes antagonistic, sometimes disinterested. She makes the best of the world she finds herself in.

Down through the ages the lives of the mentally ill have been a living hell, and the only salvation for those afflicted today will be the answers we find through continued research. We are fortunate that there are now several research programs that hold the promise of producing those answers. There is also a dynamic organization, the National Alliance for the Mentally Ill, with affiliates in every State, which is pursuing goals too long overlooked by many of those entrusted with the care of the mentally ill. A new drug, Clozaril, developed by the Sandoz Pharmaceutical Company, has been hailed as a major breakthrough in the treatment of schizophrenia and is working 'miracles' for some patients. An initial price tag of approximately $9,000 a year, however, put it virtually out of reach for most of those who so desperately need it. Several lawsuits have been filed against Sandoz seeking to reduce the cost of Clozaril and its very stringent monitoring system. The company has announced a price reduction, but at this time it is unclear exactly what that means. The anguished pleas of family members and the medical profession continue to bombard Sandoz.

In the past year a new Cindy has emerged. Where once there was a rather unfriendly, often unpleasant girl, there is now an amiable, more responsive person. Cindy smiles more these days, something a person with schizophrenia doesn't do very often. For years her face was a solemn mask, and she could neither give nor receive affection. She knew something terrible had happened to her and could not understand why no one would rescue her from the hell in her head. In the past few months she has become quite

loving, and the smiles that now light her face light mine as well.

I treasure the times Cindy looks at me and tells me I'm beautiful, when she tells me my dress is pretty, or when she apologizes for some verbal abuse uttered months ago. This is the 'real' Cindy speaking – my sweet, generous, funny, intelligent daughter.

How I wish she could shed this awful affliction and be that person!

This article first appeared in the *Schizophrenia Bulletin* (1991) **17**:689–91. Reprinted with permission.

First person account: Three generations of schizophrenia

Lucy Fuchs

Abstract
The author gives an account of three generations of schizophrenia from the changing perspective of childhood through adulthood, as niece, sister, and mother. She describes the impact on the family in this 50-year span and discusses changing societal attitudes to mental illness as well as changes in treatment and professional thinking.

Ibsen treated it tragically in 'Ghosts' and Gilbert and Sullivan humorously in 'Ruddigore.' I am referring to the theme of a family curse in the form of insanity passed on from one generation to another. I disliked 'Ghosts' because of its morbid outlook and enjoyed 'Ruddigore' because of its lighthearted foolishness. In neither case did I think that the idea of inherited mental illness was realistic. Years later, I recognize that during all that time my family was enacting its own tragedy affecting several generations. Although I never chose it, a small part was thrust upon me as a child and I was inexorably drawn into a larger role as the tragedy progressed. I am referring to schizophrenia.

Early in my life I became aware of the visits my father made to his brother. The trip was an exhausting 3-hour train and bus ride to a sad and mysterious place. So sad that my mother, whom I knew to be kind, was unwilling to go. She did, however, spend the previous day cooking the meal my father was to share with my uncle. Early in the morning on the day of the trip, I watched my mother and father pack additional delicacies, mended underwear, and miscellaneous items like magazines and drawing supplies chosen to entice my uncle into activity. The day after was given to a review. 'What did the doctor say?' made sense to me. 'How did Aaron behave?' was disquieting as it implied misbehavior and childishness in an adult. As I grew older, I observed my father become more exhausted from his trips and more and more disappointed in his brother's failure to improve. The saddest visits were when my father had to report that my uncle's behavior led to being moved to a 'bad ward.' At the end of the 1940s, my parents deliberated about a proposed lobotomy. They finally agreed, hoping for the best. The best never happened. My uncle died in Pilgrim State Hospital in his eighties. He had been there for 60 years.

I did not see my uncle until I was an adult, but his self-portrait hung in our living room. His handsome, brooding presence made me feel a loss, for though I had other uncles, no other was an artist or so young.

And what caused this sad illness? Without knowing the name of my uncle's disorder, we all seemed to have accepted psychoanalytic thinking. My grandmother, my uncle's mother, was a dignified but cold woman so that the belief that schizophrenia was due to maternal rejection grew on fertile ground.

My uncle's condition had a name and came on suddenly. More tragic was my brother's, which had no name and grew insidiously. A bright, handsome child, 5 years my senior, he was loved by my parents and was a delight to his teachers. He was not, however, interested in children. As he grew older, my parents became increasingly anxious about his preference for adults. I shared their anxiety and, 40 years later, I remember our enthusiasm when he spoke of two boys whom he might invite home. Although they never came, I remember their names still. So, in subtle ways, the natural order was reversed, and I was asked to understand and make allowances for my older brother.

Lacking his own friends, he bossed and teased me. Although he played with me rarely, he resented my play with other children and disrupted our games or was embarrassingly disagreeable when I brought new friends home. Hardest for me were his sudden changes of mood. I risked his anger when I did not follow his direction and my own self-respect when I bowed to pressure. These choices were all the more painful because I loved him. As he reached adolescence, he was also becoming more critical and angry toward my parents. The three of us became adept at avoiding confrontations. Things reached a climax when he was 16. He started attending a local college and began having trouble studying. Now I know one reason was the schizophrenic 'loss of thought.' My parents arranged for a psychiatrist to see him, but after one session he refused to return.

Despite these problems, my brother must have made heroic efforts. Not only was he graduated from college, but he even served in the army for a few years. He never saw active duty and was taken under the wing of his superior officers in an Intelligence Unit. They appreciated his dependability and strict and religious outlook. Despite warm and lengthy letters, he was again difficult to live with on his return. He completely disowned me because he disapproved of my engagement and did not speak to me until my mother's terminal illness 15 years later. During this time, he structured a life with which he could cope. He never married, became intensely religious, and spent much time and energy in helping our aging parents. He worked as an elementary school teacher in an inner city school and won some acclaim as a strict but fair teacher to children who needed rules and structure. He finally found friends within a strict religious community, and this was some comfort to my parents who had by then resigned themselves to his not marrying.

They derived some satisfaction in knowing that he was involved in his work and at long last had friends. I am detailing my brother's long-range adjustment because I believe attention must be paid to other 'mild schizophrenics' who are unhappy and cause pain to their loved ones but still manage a life outside treatment and without an official diagnosis. Eventually my brother diagnosed himself. His anger abated as his delusional thinking loosened its hold. He no longer sees me or my husband as evil people. He divulged his self-diagnosis when my daughter became psychotic.

My brother wanted to be helpful and told me that he noticed his own thinking became less difficult when he was taking medication for another illness. He shared with me how he talked back to his voice when it caused trouble. 'If you can't say something wise, shut-up!' Before this revelation, I had not formed a definite opinion of his problem. I considered schizophrenia as a diagnosis when he was unreasonably accusatory and punishing toward me, but leaned toward obsessive-compulsive disorder when his accusations had some basis in reality. At any rate, in the light of his own experience, he encouraged my husband and me to continue our sympathetic support of our delusional daughter, and stressed the need to be hopeful and encouraging. So, family commitment has survived years of pain, madness, and confusion and the years to come hold some promise of affording simple family contacts and pleasures.

If diagnosis eluded me for so long, so did causality. Though sympathetic toward my parents, I was also influenced by the thinking of the time and in my heart I blamed them. Now I realize that living with a mentally disturbed son had made these naturally gentle and cautious people increasingly anxious. At the time, it was easy to credit neighbors' and relatives' comments that my brother's problems were caused by my parents' insecurity and their foolish capitulation to his angry outbursts. Today, some family therapists lean dangerously close to this attitude with their theory of the 'identified patient' who acts out the pathology of the rest of the family. True in particular cases, perhaps, this theory unfeelingly ignores the inevitable changes that occur in families who live with a mentally ill member. At any rate, when I was young, I resolved that as a parent I would neither neglect one child nor indulge the other, and I was determined to live life with more joy. Good resolutions – but no proof against biological or genetic catastrophe.

Considering my early life, it is clear why I would be drawn to working with troubled people and why I would also look forward to having a happy, healthy family. Things went well, and my husband and I were confident about our children's futures in their early years. I knew, of course, that there was no perfect child and that there was a certain amount of pain and struggle in every life. For this reason, when my second child, Susan, turned out to be an unusually quiet baby and later a shy toddler, I valued these qualities as part of her unique nature. If people were less attentive to her than to her more outgoing older brother, I wondered at them and cherished her all the more. Looking back, I can see that very early I tried to fill the gap between her and the rest of the world by becoming more attentive, playful, and protective of her. So, slowly and quite naturally, I accustomed myself to her ways and to feeling responsible for her happiness. Despite her early reserve, by 7 or 8, she had become an energetic and interested child. She excelled in school, was an avid reader, and did well in many athletic activities. With all this, she still did not find making friends easy. She was shy, easily hurt, yet critical and argumentative. We thought she would eventually find a special friend or two, and we minimized her legalistic quarrels by thinking she had strong opinions and was independent. Jokingly, we said she was surely cut out to be a lawyer.

By high school Susan was more outgoing. She attracted potential friends because of her intelligence and her dynamic interest in ideas and activities. She was still easily hurt, however, and her relationships were uneven and stormy. It was a period of confusion and stress for me as well. Although I was the one she came to in tears for comfort, I was becoming aware that there was a lack of warmth and reciprocity. We no longer had the good times together that we had had earlier There was no balance, and living with my daughter became emotionally draining. Still, I accepted the common wisdom that Susan was merely going through adolescence and that I was an overly concerned mother. When Susan reached age 15, we finally sought professional help because of the appearance of a new symptom as she began to have trouble completing written assignments. Once or twice she said she thought she was going crazy, because she couldn't think. That was outside the realm of my imagination, and I assured her that most adolescents have these fears. It was apparently outside the range of possibilities for the psychiatrist as he indicated Susan had some problems in self-esteem and suggested my distancing myself more. I followed this advice as well as scrupulously keeping out of the treatment process with him and the psychiatrist who saw her in college. In college, Susan continued the same up and down life: strong commitments, painful disappointment, and trouble with written assignments. Looking back, I think that whatever good both psychiatrists did came not from their insight-oriented therapy, but as a result of their relationship and support. Susan dropped out of college in her third year and not until her first psychotic breakdown 2 years later did we realize she was schizophrenic. In looking back, I think I can see many earlier clues. Now, I question the ease with which pronouncements about 'normal adolescence' are made. I also question the theory that early identification of schizophrenia is bad and necessarily leads to self-fulfilling prophecies. What about the wrong diagnosis of neuroses? In what other field is ignorance considered an advantage? A case could just as easily be made that early identification of children-at-risk could lead to early and more appropriate help. I particularly regret that I followed professional advice and distanced myself in

her adolescence. Schizophrenics already feel too distant.

There are many other dynamics to explore. For example, was the bossy and argumentative nature of my brother and daughter a marker? When combined with shyness, could it be understood as first an attempt to get others to share their atypical perceptions, followed by hurt and angry withdrawal when they do not succeed?

Susan became catatonic at age 23, while living a nomadic life. She was hospitalized following the intervention of a policeman but released against the advice of the hospital and as a result of being informed of her rights by a patient advocate. We breathed a sigh of relief for the 3 days she was in the hospital, where we thought she would get help. We were informed of the diagnosis of schizophrenia at the same time she was released and were naturally shocked at the precipitate release. Susan wandered around various cities for another year and a half, living on the street and in shelters or crashing with friends. She was in touch every few weeks, sometimes phoning with fantastic accusations and threats. When she periodically came home, we tried to be caring and helpful and suggested she seek psychiatric help, but were afraid to push too hard. The one occasion on which we took a strong stand led to a violent outburst and flight. Her second catatonic episode mercifully came during a visit home so we were prepared. This time we arranged for her commitment to a hospital nearby and had already chosen a psychiatrist. Medication got her moving again and helped her delusional thinking. She was more warm and outgoing than I had seen her in years. Susan went to a halfway house and enjoyed the group therapy and the contacts with the staff. We began to hope again. However, although she put up with the side effects of pacing for a month, she finally stopped her medication abruptly and lost all her gains. She took up a vagabond life again. Still we hoped we were ahead and that she would voluntarily seek help because of her positive experiences. We had not yet understood the awful grip of disordered thinking. Instead, we were on the same merry-go-round with Susan: another involuntary commitment, another precipitous release with the 'help' of a patient advocate, more self-destructive behavior, cries for help, and chaotic visits home.

We do not know if she will ever accept help or have a viable life. Yet, not knowing, we must somehow get on with our own lives. We do this for ourselves, for each other, and for our son. As it is, he will carry an extra responsibility for the rest of his life and we do not want to add to it. For my healthy son, who has had only the usual amount of human pain, and for my daughter, who lives in almost constant pain, I feel I must go on living as well as I can. One must search for choices and even pleasures if only on the margins and borders of the most pervasive tragedy. As I write, I realize I have been saying this to myself as well and have done so since as a child I witnessed my father's anguish about his schizophrenic brother and son.

This article first appeared in the *Schizophrenia Bulletin* (1986) **12**:744–7. Reprinted with permission.

24

Curing Schizophrenia, Treating Schizophrenia: Translating Research to Practice

John K Hsiao

Contents • A brief history of antipsychotic drugs • Curing schizophrenia • Treating schizophrenia • Translating research into practice • Conclusion

As we enter the new millennium, looking back on 50 years that have transformed medicine, including psychiatric medicine, this is an opportune moment to ask how close we are to curing schizophrenia, the most serious of all the mental illnesses. We are on the verge of decoding the entire human genome, we have elucidated the molecular basis of many diseases, opening new avenues for prevention and treatment, and we are even able to image the workings of a living human brain. In psychiatry, however, while we have learned much about schizophrenia, our ability to treat this devastating illness has advanced only incrementally since the first antipsychotic drugs were discovered 50 years ago.

The 1990s were heralded as the 'decade of the brain', and it is no exaggeration to say that neuroscience has burgeoned and continues to do so at an exponential rate. Just as computers and information technologies transformed society over the past two decades, it is likely that mankind's next great revolution will come from advances in neurobiology. Unfortunately, knowledge accumulates most rapidly when we know the least, and one of the most important insights to come from what we have discovered about the brain so far is that we have much more to learn. Thus every neurobiological discovery makes schizophrenia seem more complicated rather than

less. Like travelers in a tunnel, the deeper we go, the darker it becomes before we are able to see a light at the end. Our understanding of schizophrenia and ability to treat it have come a great distance, but our journey is far from over.

Nevertheless, although we do not yet have a cure for schizophrenia, the path ahead has grown increasingly clear. We do not know if the breakthrough will come in a year or in a decade, but we have some idea of what must be learned and how this might lead to a cure. One guide to the future is the past. The history of the development of antipsychotic drugs, both achievements and shortcomings, since the first one, chlorpromazine, was introduced, sheds light on where we are now in treating schizophrenia, but also illuminates the way ahead, showing us what is left to accomplish.

A brief history of antipsychotic drugs

Few advances have had as significant an impact on people with mental disorders and our understanding of mental illness as did development of the neuroleptic antipsychotic drugs in the 1950s. As with most medical advances of that era, however, it was entirely serendipitous. Chlorpromazine was originally developed and utilized as an antihistamine and a preanesthetic agent.[1] The fortuitous observation that this new drug had a calming effect led eventually to trials of chlorpromazine in patients with schizophrenia, with dramatic results.[2] The number of patients institutionalized in state hospitals decreased markedly after chlorpromazine was introduced in the 1950s[3] transforming psychiatric practice and ushering in modern psychopharmacology.

The unique properties of chlorpromazine were evident not only in humans, but also in its effects on animal behavior: producing catalepsy, reducing spontaneous movement, and interfering with classical conditioning, among others.[4] These effects in animals proved to be a useful way of screening for other chlorpromazine-like drugs, and a whole series of chemically related and unrelated antipsychotics were identified in the 1950s and 1960s. As well as ameliorating psychosis, these drugs also shared a propensity for producing extrapyramidal side effects (parkinsonism, dystonia, akathisia), and the term 'neuroleptic' was coined to reflect this dual effect.[1] Carlsson and Lindquist[5] observed that the various neuroleptics altered turnover of the neurotransmitter dopamine, and suggested that they worked by blocking dopamine receptors. This was confirmed by Creese and coworkers,[6] leading to the 'dopamine' hypothesis, which guided neurobiological research on schizophrenia for the next 30 years.

Unfortunately, while the neuroleptics were effective antipsychotics, no one of them proved to be more effective than the others.[7] Moreover, none of them were particularly useful against the negative symptoms of schizophrenia, while, in addition to a propensity for acute extrapyramidal side effects, they all had a risk for tardive dyskinesia.[8] The shortcomings of neuroleptic antipsychotics impacted not only clinical care, but also mental health research. The fact that all neuroleptics had the same mechanism of action and were more or less equally effective served as a disincentive to development of new agents, while the lack of alternate, non-dopamine hypotheses greatly hindered the search for novel drugs. As a result, there was a close to 15-year interregnum when there was little interest in drug discovery and during which no new drugs for schizophrenia were approved.

What eventually revitalized both treatment and research was clozapine, the prototype 'atypical' neuroleptic. Clozapine had been used in Europe since the early 1970s, and differed from other antipsychotics in not being selective for the D_2 receptor.[9] It produced a host of side effects, the most serious of which was agranulocytosis, but there was little if any evidence of extrapyramidal reactions.[9,10] More important, however, early experience suggested that clozapine was more effective than other antipsychotics.[11] This was demonstrated conclusively in the United States in the 1980s by a multicenter randomized clinical trial,[12] and clozapine received United States Food and Drug Administration (FDA) approval in 1990 for use in patients with treatment-resistant schizophrenia.

Subsequent to clozapine's approval in the United States, several other atypical antipsychotics have been introduced. Risperidone was released in 1994, olanzapine in 1996, and quetiapine in 1997. Sertindole received FDA approval (but was withdrawn by the sponsor), and ziprasidone is awaiting approval. The atypicals are not selective D_2 antagonists. Like clozapine, they block one or more of the 5-hydroxytryptamine$_2$ (5HT2) family of serotonin receptors as well as the D_2 dopamine receptor.[13] Other than this, however, the pharmacological profiles of the different atypicals vary widely. As with clozapine, the newer atypical neuroleptics have shown little propensity to produce extrapyramidal side effects,[14] probably including tardive dyskinesia. Whether the new atypicals are more effective antipsychotics than the typical neuroleptics, however, remains an open question.

Curing schizophrenia

There are a number of lessons to draw from this history. First is the importance of serendipity: neither chlorpromazine nor clozapine were the products of a rational drug development process. However, their discovery involved more than just good fortune; careful observation and intellectual preparedness were also necessary. As we learn more about schizophrenia, we should not let knowledge or theory blind us to the unexpected. At the same time, we obviously cannot rely on serendipity alone. For over a decade no new antipsychotics were identified – in large part because nothing new was being learned about schizophrenia. Rational drug discovery requires animal models, which in turn require an understanding of the neurobiological processes that cause schizophrenia. While that level of detail is not yet within our ken, there are several promising lines of investigation. We have learned enough to anticipate that in the not too distant future, we will understand the brain and the disorder sufficiently to develop model systems for identifying new treatments.

We have known for many years that schizophrenia can be inherited. This represents only a minority of patients. Most cases of schizophrenia are 'sporadic', with only a single family member involved,[15] and even within pedigrees with multiple affected members, genotype accounts for, at best, half the diagnostic variance (if one monozygotic twin has schizophrenia, the co-twin has only a 50% likelihood of developing the illness).[16] Moreover, the disorder is polygenic, with multiple genes involved, each of which increases the risk for developing schizophrenia, but does not itself cause the illness.[16] Schizophrenia is not a Mendelian disorder like Huntington's disease or hemophilia, and it is unlikely that gene therapy will ever produce a cure. However, genetic studies provide one of our best hopes for understanding the pathophysiology of schizophrenia. Once linkage analyses or association studies identify a susceptibility gene, the protein encoded by this gene can be isolated, the role this protein plays in neural function can be elucidated, and an appropriate target for drug therapy can be selected. Studies of neuroanatomy have demonstrated that schizophrenia is associated with subtle changes in regional morphometry and cytoarchitectonics.[17] The brains of patients with schizophrenia appear either to have developed abnormally, or been altered by the disease process. Of themselves, neuroanatomic abnormalities do not point to new treatments. However, in recent years, as in vivo neuroimaging methods have improved, studies of neuroanatomy have advanced beyond structure to begin to examine regional neural function.[18] Whereas in the past, scientists tended to conceptualize brain processes in terms of the neurochemicals involved (e.g., the 'dopamine' hypothesis), the paradigm is shifting, so that now we seek to explain behavior by studying the neural circuits used to process cognitive and affective information.[19] The hope is someday to identify the aberrant 'wiring' that underlies the signs and symptoms of schizophrenia and to use this knowledge to create an animal model that can be utilized to screen new treatments.

It has long been clear that drugs that block the dopamine D_2 receptor ameliorate the 'positive' symptoms of schizophrenia. However, the illness involves much more than just hallucinations and delusions, and drugs that affect neurotransmitter systems in addition to or instead of dopamine will be important in the future. As noted earlier, all the currently available atypical antipsychotics affect the serotonin 5HT2 family of receptors,[13] an action that may be related to their decreased propensity to produce extrapyramidal reactions.[20] There is also considerable recent interest in a phencyclidine (PCP) model of schizophrenia and the role of the excitatory neurotransmitter glutamate in the illness.[21] In particular, there is evidence to suggest that drugs that act at glutamatergic receptors may affect 'negative' symptomatology.[22] How many, if any, of these preliminary results will lead to new treatments remains to be seen, but the direction being taken – away from dopamine and towards management of specific symptoms, rather than the illness as a whole – appears promising.

Treating schizophrenia

While the ultimate goal of treatment research is a cure, there are very few illnesses for which we have a 'magic bullet', a treatment that reverses all signs and symptoms, returning a patient to normalcy. Modern therapeutics, particularly of chronic illnesses with multifactorial causes, aims to improve function and minimize adverse sequellae. Similarly, in schizophrenia, research should not be limited to searching for a cure. We must also investigate methods for managing symptoms, minimizing disability, improving long-term outcome, and maximizing quality of life.

Unfortunately, long-term outcome has not been a focus of psychopharmacologic research, particularly studies supported by the pharmaceutical industry.[23] While the new atypical antipsychotics are a tremendous step forward, providing more and better (at least in terms of side effects) options for treatment, most of what is known about them has to do with safety and short-term efficacy against psychotic symptomatology. There is a paucity of data on their effectiveness in long-term treatment, or how other realms such as quality of life, disability, and psychosocial function are affected. However, these are the outcomes that have the most practical relevance for patients and caregivers. In the United States, the National Institute of Mental Health has undertaken a major initiative (Clinical Antipsychotic Trials of Intervention Effectiveness, CATIE) to investigate the public health impact of the new atypical antipsychotics, and to define better how these new drugs should be utilized to optimize outcomes in patients with schizophrenia.[24]

For many years, there was an unfortunate degree of therapeutic nihilism towards patients with schizophrenia: a sense on the part of mental health professionals and society that the diagnosis was a sentence to a lifetime of chronic psychosis, deteriorating function, and disability. Clozapine and the other new atypicals have reversed much of this pessimism by demonstrating that poor outcomes are not inevitable. This optimism (particularly after so many years without progress) has generalized to nonpharmacological interventions, as well. Even before the atypicals were introduced, psychoeducational approaches had been shown to reduce hospitalization.[25] Now, however, there is increasing interest and research into rehabilitative approaches, with evidence of benefits in interpersonal interactions, cognitive function, and even vocational outcomes.[26] How lasting and generalizable these effects will be remains to be seen, but the most important result may be the realization that interventions are possible in these important domains.

Along with a resurgence of research on rehabilitation, and increased optimisim about outcome, has come a newfound interest in prevention. A first episode of schizophrenia is typically preceded by months or years of gradual deterioration in functioning and onset of symptoms.[27] The intriguing question is whether intervention during this prodrome might prevent or delay onset of schizophrenia and/or improve the subsequent course of illness. Research in this area remains quite limited, and is fraught with difficulties. Case identification is an issue, since most of the symptoms that make up the prodrome are not specific to schizophrenia.[28] There are anecdotal data on psychosocial and pharmacological interventions in prodromal individuals,[29] but treating subjects who may never become psychotic raises a number of ethical issues. Nevertheless, since complete recovery is rare in schizophrenia, preventive intervention in the prodrome may be a critical strategy for improving course and outcome.

Translating research into practice

The therapeutic advances we anticipate in years to come will have little impact unless they are used by practitioners and accepted by patients. Applying research results in community mental health settings may not be simple or straightforward, however. We already know that one of the most important determinants of outcome in schizophrenia is compliance.[30] Second only to the intrinsic severity of illness, whether an individual adheres to treatment, particularly maintenance pharmacotherapy, is the best predictor of how he or she will do in the long term.[30] Adherence to treatment is an issue in all disorders, psychiatric and nonpsychiatric, but in schizophrenia, noncompliance seems as much the rule as the exception (it is noteworthy that long-acting depot medications are unique to the schizophrenia formulary). In part, this is attributable to the unpleasant side effects of antipsychotics, particularly the older, conventional neuroleptics. There is also evidence to suggest that impaired insight may be intrinsic to the illness.[31] Whatever the underlying causes, insofar as compliance is a limiting factor, then improved outcomes in schizophrenia will require not just better treatments, but better adherence to treatment as well.

While noncompliance is usually thought of as a patient problem, it can also be an issue for care providers. Just as treatment adherence affects outcome for individual patients with schizophrenia, adherence to treatment guidelines can determine how effectively a practitioner or a clinic manages schizophrenia as a whole. Few (if any) guidelines in psychiatry are absolute, and considerable latitude is afforded clinicians in managing individual patients, but as a whole, most patients and most providers should fall within a broad range of standard care. Unfortunately, this does not appear to be uniformly true for treatment of schizophrenia in the United States. The Schizophrenia Patient Outcomes Research Team (PORT) examined how well mental health caregivers in two different states adhered to evidence-based treatment guidelines for schizophrenia.[32] The rate of conformance to recommended treatment was modest at best, particularly for psychosocial interventions. There may be many reasons for this, but the solution will require both improved dissemination of treatment research results as well as improved efforts at self-education by practitioners.

Conclusion

As we enter the twenty-first century, schizophrenia remains the most devastating of all the mental illnesses. It is much too premature to claim that we see a light at the end of this tunnel, yet there is reason to hope. Schizophrenia is not the mystery it once was, and even though a cure is not in sight, we have some idea of how we will find one. Identifying a gene or genes that predispose to schizophrenia could lead to novel targets for drug therapy. Elucidation of the functional neuro-anatomy underlying schizophrenia could result in better animal models for drug screening. New neurochemical models of the illness and its symptomatology may provide new approaches for drug development. At the same time, the search for a cure must now overshadow the search for better treatments. The new atypical antipsychotics are a major advance, but considerably more information is needed on their long-term effectiveness. Rehabilitation of the functional deficits associated with schizophrenia is an area of increasing interest. Early identification of prodromal cases and prevention of psychosis onset is a tantalizing possibility. Finally, although future prospects may be bright, the impact of any therapeutic advance is limited by how it is accepted and whether it is used by patients and practitioners in the community. Patient compliance with treatment must improve, as must physician adherence to guidelines.

Chlorpromazine was nothing less than a miracle when it was first introduced, but it was a singular advance, a large leap forward that provided little direction for the future. In the 40 years since, treatment of schizophrenia has advanced only incrementally, but our understanding of the illness has increased dramatically. We are not on the verge of a miracle, but now at least, we can see the path ahead. We do not have to rely on hope alone, but can anticipate that someday soon, schizophrenia will no longer mean a lifetime of disability, and no longer be the scourge it is now.

References

1. Frankenburg FR, History of the development of antipsychotic medication, *Psychiatr Clin N Am* (1994) **17**:531–40.

2. Delay J, Deniker P, Harl JM, Traitment des étas d'excitation et d'agitation par une méthode médicamenteuse derivée de l'hibernothérapie, *Ann Med-psychol* (1952) **110**:267–73.

3. Brill H, Patton RE, Analysis of population reduction in New York state mental hospitals during the first four years of large-scale therapy with psychotropic drugs, *Am J Psychiatry* (1957) **116**: 495–508.

4. Lehmann HE, Ban TA, The history of the psychopharmacology of schizophrenia, *Can J Psychiatry* (1997) **42**:152–62.

5. Carlsson A, Lindquist M, Effect of chlorpromazine and haloperidol on formation of 3-methoxytyramine and normetanephrine in mouse brain, *Acta Pharmacologica Toxicologica* (1963) **20**:140–4.

6. Creese I, Burt DR, Snyder SH, Dopamine receptor binding predicts clinical and pharmacological potencies of antischizophrenic drugs, *Science* (1976) **192**:481–3.

7. Cole JO, the NIMH Psychopharmacology Service Center Collaborative Study Group, Phenothiazine treatment in acute schizophrenia, *Arch Gen Psychiatry* (1964) **10**:246–61.

8. Kane JM, Marder SR, Psychopharmacologic treatment of schizophrenia, *Schizophr Bull* (1993) **19**:287–302.

9. Coward DM, General pharmacology of clozapine, *Br J Psychiatry* (1992) **160**:5–11.

10. Alvir JMJ, Lieberman JA, Safferman AZ et al, Clozapine-induced agranulocytosis: incidence and risk factors in the United States, *N Engl J Med* (1993) **329**:162–7.

11. Tamminga CA, The promise of new drugs for schizophrenia treatment, *Can J Psychiatry* (1997) **42**:265–73.

12. Kane J, Honigfeld G, Sunger J, Meltzer H, Clozapine for the treatment-resistant schizophrenic. A double blind comparison with chlorpromazine. *Arch Gen Psychiatry* (1998) **45**:789–96.

13. Meltzer HY, Clinical studies on the mechanism of action of clozapine: the dopamine-serotonin hypothesis of schizophrenia, *Psychopharmacology (Ber)* (1989) **99**:S18–S27.

14. Dawkins K, Lieberman JA, Lebowitz BD, Hsiao JK, Antipsychotics: past and future, *Schizophrenia Bull* (1999) **25**:395–405.

15. Gottesmann II, Shields J, Hanson DR, *Schizophrenia: The Epigenetic Puzzle* (Cambridge University Press: Cambridge, 1982).

16. Moldin SO, Gottesman II, At issue: genes, experience, and chance in schizophrenia – positioning for the 21st century, *Schizophr Bull* **23**:547–61.

17. Buchanan RW, Carpenter WT, The neuroanatomies of schizophrenia, *Schizophr Bull* (1997) **23**:367–72.

18. Weinberger DR, Berman KF, Zec RF, Physiological dysfunction of dorsolateral prefrontal cortex in schizophrenia: I. Regional cerebral blood flow evidence, *Arch Gen Psychiatry* (1986) **43**:114–25.

19. Andreasen NC, Paradiso S, O'Leary DS, 'Cognitive dysmetria' as an integrative theory of schizophrenia: a dysfunction in cortical–subcortical–cerebellar circuitry? *Schizophr Bull* (1998) **24**:203–18.

20. Lieberman JA, Mailman RB, Duncan G et al, Serotonergic basis of antipsychotic drug effects in schizophrenia, *Biol Psychiatry* (1998) **44**:1099–117.

21. Olney JW, Farber NB, Glutamate receptor dysfunction and schizophrenia, *Arch Gen Psychiatry* (1995) **52**:998–1007.

22. Goff DC, Tsai G, Manoach DS, Coyle JT, Dose-finding trial for D-cycloserine added to neuroleptics for negative symptoms in schizophrenia, *Am J Psychiatry* (1995) **152**:1213–15.

23. Norquist G, Lebowitz B, Hyman S, Expanding the frontier of treatment research, *Prevention and Treatment* 2: Article 0001a, 1999. Available on the World Wide Web. http://journals apa.org/prevention/volume2/pre0020001a.html.

24. National Institute of Mental Health, New antipsychotic drug trials. NIH Guide NOT 98-155 (RFP NIMH-99-DS-001), Nov 6, 1998. Available on the World Wide Web: http://grants.nih.gov/grants/guide/notice-files/not98-155.html.

25. Falloon IRH, Boyd JL, McGill CW et al, Family management in the prevention of exacerbations of schizophrenia: a controlled study, *N Engl J Med* (1982) **306**:1437–40.

26. Bellack AS, Gold JM, Buchanan RW, Cognitive rehabilitation for schizophrenia: problems, prospects, and strategies, *Schizophr Bull* (1999) **25**:257–74.

27. Hafner H, Maurer K, Loffler W, Riecher-Rosslen A, The influence of age and sex on the onset of early course of schizophrenia, *Br J Psychiatry* (1993) **162:**80–6.

28. Yung AR, McGorry PD, McFarlane CA et al, Monitoring and care of young people at incipient risk of psychosis, *Schizophr Bull* (1996) **22:**283–303.

29. Miller TJ, McGlashan TH, Woods SW et al, Symptom assessment in schizophrenic prodromal states, *Psychiatr Q* (1999) **70:**273–87.

30. Fenton WS, Blyler CR, Heinssen RL, Determinants of medication compliance in schizophrenia:

empirical and clinical findings, *Schizophr Bull* (1997) **23:** 637–51.

31. Amador XF, Strauss DH, Yale SA, Gorman JM, Awareness of illness in schizophrenia, *Schizophr Bull* (1991) **17:**113–32.

32. Lehman AF, Steinwachs DM, the Survey Co-Investigators of the PORT Project, Patterns of usual care for schizophrenia: initial results from the Schizophrenia Patient Outcomes Research Team (PORT) client survey, *Schizophr Bull* (1998) **24:**11–20.

Index